V SPECIAL POPULATIONS, 481

DATE DUE

Sheehy's Manual of

Emergency Care

Seventh Edition

Sheehy's Manual of
Emergency Care

Emergency Nurses Association
Des Plaines, Illinois

Edited by
Belinda B. Hammond, MSN, RN, CEN, CCRN
Clinical Nurse Educator, Critical Care
Cone Health System
Greensboro, North Carolina

Polly Gerber Zimmermann, MS, MBA, RN, CEN, FAEN
Associate Professor
Harry S Truman College
Chicago, Illinois

ELSEVIER

ELSEVIER
MOSBY

3251 Riverport Lane
St. Louis, Missouri 63043

SHEEHY'S MANUAL OF EMERGENCY CARE   ISBN 978-0-323-07827-6

Copyright © 2013 by Mosby, an imprint of Elsevier Inc.

Notices

Knowledge and best practice in this field are constantly changing. As new research and experience broaden our understanding, changes in research methods, professional practices, or medical treatment may become necessary.

Practitioners and researchers must always rely on their own experience and knowledge in evaluating and using any information, methods, compounds, or experiments described herein. In using such information or methods they should be mindful of their own safety and the safety of others, including parties for whom they have a professional responsibility.

With respect to any drug or pharmaceutical products identified, readers are advised to check the most current information provided (i) on procedures featured or (ii) by the manufacturer of each product to be administered, to verify the recommended dose or formula, the method and duration of administration, and contraindications. It is the responsibility of practitioners, relying on their own experience and knowledge of their patients, to make diagnoses, to determine dosages and the best treatment for each individual patient, and to take all appropriate safety precautions.

To the fullest extent of the law, neither the Publisher nor the authors, contributors, or editors, assume any liability for any injury and/or damage to persons or property as a matter of products liability, negligence or otherwise, or from any use or operation of any methods, products, instructions, or ideas contained in the material herein.

Previous editions copyrighted 2005, 1999, 1995, 1990, 1984, 1979

Library of Congress Cataloging-in-Publication Data or Control Number
Sheehy's manual of emergency care / Emergency Nurses Association.—7th ed. / edited by Belinda B. Hammond, Polly Gerber Zimmermann.
    p. ; cm.
  Manual of emergency care
  Includes bibliographical references and index.
  ISBN 978-0-323-07827-6 (pbk. : alk. paper)
  I. Hammond, Belinda Burns. II. Zimmermann, Polly Gerber.   III. Sheehy, Susan Budassi, 1948- Manual of emergency care.   IV. Emergency Nurses Association.   V. Title: Manual of emergency care.
  [DNLM: 1. Emergency Medical Services—Handbooks.   2. Emergency Medicine—Handbooks.
  3. Emergency Nursing—Handbooks.   WX 39]
  616.02′5–dc23

                                                                    2011040164

Senior Editor: Sandra E. Clark
Associate Developmental Editor: Jennifer Palada
Consulting Developmental Editor: Sophia Oh Gray
Publishing Services Manager: Jeff Patterson
Project Manager: Bill Drone
Design Manager: Teresa McBryan

Printed in the United States of America

Last digit is the print number: 9 8 7 6 5

To Gail Lenehan—
You have inspired so many emergency nurses because of your caring, mentoring, passion, advocacy, support, and friendship. Thank you for being our leader and role model.

CONTRIBUTORS

Maria E. Albright, MSN, APRN, ACNS-BC, CMSRN
Clinical Nurse Specialist for Acute Care
Ochsner Medical Center
New Orleans, Louisiana

Colleen Andreoni, MSN, ANP-BC, CEN
Assistant Professor
Loyola University Chicago, Niehoff School of Nursing
Chicago, Illinois;
Nurse Practitioner
Loyola University Health System
Maywood, Illinois;
Nurse Practitioner
Delnor Community Hospital
Geneva, Illinois

Randal Bryan Badillo, BSN, RN, CSPI
Clinical Supervisor Oklahoma Poison Control Center
University of Oklahoma College of Pharmacy
Oklahoma City, Oklahoma

Sharon L. Biby, MSN, BSN, ANP-BC, GNP-BC
Stroke Center Nurse Practitioner
Moses H. Cone Hospital
Greensboro, North Carolina

Shelley A. Calder, MSN, RN, CEN
Clinical Nurse Specialist, Emergency Department
Beth Israel Deaconess Medical Center
Boston, Massachusetts

C. J. Carringer, MSN, RN, CEN, CCRN
Policy and Procedure Coordinator
Patient Disability Officer
Piedmont Medical Center
Rock Hill, South Carolina

Sharon Saunderson Cohen, MSN, RN, CEN, CCRN
Adjunct Faculty
Broward, College
Davie, Florida;
Guest Speaker
Nova Southern University
Davie, Florida;
Interim Director and Clinical Nurse Specialist
Emergency Preparedness Department
Broward Health
Fort Lauderdale, Florida

Shelley Cohen, MSN, RN, CEN
Educator/Consultant
Health Resources Unlimited
Hohenwald, Tennessee;
PRN Staff Emergency Department Nurse
Williamson Medical Center
Franklin, Tennessee

Linda K. Cook, PhD, RN, APRN-BC, CCRN, CCNS, ACNP
Professor, Nursing
Prince George's Community College
Largo, Maryland;
Staff Nurse
Doctors Community Hospital
Lanham, Maryland

Laura M. Criddle, PhD, RN, ACNS-BS, CEN, CFRN, CCRN, CPEN, CNRN, ONC, FAEN
Affiliate Professor and Clinical Nurse
Oregon Health and Science University, School of Nursing
Portland, Oregon

Tina D. Cronin, MSN, RN, CNS, CCRN, CNRN
Director of Neurosciences
Piedmont Medical Center
Rock Hill, South Carolina

Megan DeVries, BSN, RN, NE-BC
Clinical Nurse Manager
Spectrum Health Regional Burn Center
Grand Rapids, Michigan

Jeanne Eckes-Roper, MBA, RN
Adjunct Instructor
Barry University
Miami Shores, Florida;
Adjunct Instructor
Broward College
Fort Lauderdale, Florida;
Specialty Registered Nurse
Emergency Department
Memorial Hospital Miramar
Miramar, Florida

Darcy Egging, MS, RN, C-ANP, CEN
Part-Time Faculty
Loyola University
Maywood, Illinois;
Nurse Practitioner
Delnor Hospital
Emergency Department
Geneva, Illinois

Faye P. Everson, RN
Clinical Educator for the Emergency Department
University of Massachusetts Medical Center
Worcester, Massachusetts

Nicki Gilboy, MS, RN, CEN, FAEN
Associate Chief Nurse for Emergency Medicine
University of Massachusetts Memorial Medical Center
Worcester, Massachusetts

Valerie Aarne Grossman, BSN, MA, RN
Registered Nurse, Imaging Sciences
University of Rochester Medical Center
Rochester, New York

Lynn Hadaway, MEd, RN, BC, CRNI
President
Lynn Hadaway Associates, Inc
Milner, Georgia

Judith S. Halpern, MSN, RN, FNP-BC
Instructor, School of Nursing
Ferris State University
Big Rapids, Michigan;
Nurse Practitioner, Occupational Health
Comp Care Partners
Kalamazoo, Michigan

Belinda B. Hammond, MSN, RN, CEN, CCRN
Clinical Nurse Educator, Critical Care
Cone Health System
Greensboro, North Carolina

Catherine Harris, MSN, RN, CEN, CPEN, CNE
Cape Cod Community College
Barnstable, Massachusetts;
Laboure College
Dorchester, Massachusetts;
Educator, Clinical Nurse Specialist
Massachusetts General Hospital
Boston, Massachusetts

Bernard Heilicser, DO, MS, FACFP, FACOEP
Medical Director, South Cook County EMS Systems;
Director, Medical Ethics Program
Ingallo Hospital
Harvey, Illinois

Robert D. Herr, MD, MBA, FACEP
Attending Physician
Grays Harbor Community Hospital
Aberdeen, Washington;
Medical Director
Regence Blue Shield
Seattle, Washington

Susan McDaniel Hohenhaus, MA, RN, CEN, FAEN
Executive Director
Emergency Nurses Association
Des Plaines, Illinois

Kimberly Hovseth, ND, MS, Pa-C, CSPI
Certified Specialist in Poison Information
Oklahoma Poison Control Center;
Guest Lecturer, Physician Assistant Program
University of Oklahoma Health Sciences Center
College of Pharmacy
Oklahoma City, Oklahoma

Jeane Jackson, MS, RN
Nurse Coordinator, Maternal-Fetal Medicine
Department of OB/GYN
Thomas Jefferson University Hospital
Philadelphia, Pennsylvania

Bethany Chimento Jennings, MN, APRN, FNP
Midlevel Provider Emergency Medical Services
Ochsner Medical Center
New Orleans, Louisiana

Linda Kelly, MS, RN, ANP-BC
Nurse Director Ambulatory Gynecology
Massachusetts General Hospital
Boston, Massachusetts

Mary Kemper, MSW
Medical Social Worker
Penn Presbyterian Medical Center
Philadelphia, Pennsylvania

Anne P. Manton, PhD, RN, PMHNP-BC, FAEN, FAAN
Psychiatric-Mental Health Nurse Practitioner
Cape Code Hospital
Hyannis, Massachusetts

Benjamin E. Marett, MSN, RN-BC, CEN, CCRN, NE-BC, FAEN
Director of Education
Piedmont Medical Center
Rock Hill, South Carolina

Lauren Wheatley McCauley, BSN, RN, CCRN
Staff Educator and Staff Nurse, Moderate Sedation
Piedmont Medical Center
Rock Hill, South Carolina

Jill C. McLaughlin, RN, CEN
Staff Nurse
Orange Regional Medical Center
Middletown, New York

Diana Meyer, MSN, RN, CCRN, CEN, FAEN
Clinical Nurse Specialist
Peace Health St. Joseph Medical Center
Bellingham, Washington

Rita D. Mintmier, BSN, RN, CNRN
Stroke Center Coordinator
Moses H. Cone Hospital
Greensboro, North Carolina

Julie V. O'Neal, BSN, RN, CEN
Registered Nurse IV, Clinical Educator
Moses H. Cone Hospital
Greensboro, North Carolina

Judith H. Poole, PhD, MHA/MBA, RNC-OB, C-EFM
Nurse Manager, Birthing Care
Presbyterian Hospital
Charlotte, North Carolina

Susanne Quallich, MSN, BSN, BS, ANP-BC, NP-C, CUNP
Clinical Faculty, School of Nursing;
Nurse Practitioner, Division of Sexual Reproductive
    Medicine, Department of Urology
University of Michigan
Ann Arbor, Michigan

Kathleen A. Ribbens, MSN, RN, CEN
Injury Prevention and Organ Donation Program
    Coordinator
Trauma and Burn Education, Regional Outreach
Spectrum Health
Grand Rapids, Michigan

Karen L. Rice, DNS, APRN, ACNS-BC, ANP
Adjunct Instructor, Graduate Research
School of Nursing, Health Sciences Center
Louisana State University
New Orleans, Louisiana;
Program Director, The Center for Nursing Research
Ochsner Medical Center
New Orleans, Louisiana

Diana Ropele, MSN, RN, CCRN
Pediatric Trauma Nurse Manager
Helen DeVoss Children's Hospital
Grand Rapids, Michigan

Scott Schaeffer, RPh, DABAT
Adjunct Faculty
University of Oklahoma College of Pharmacy
Oklahoma City, Oklahoma;
Managing Director
Oklahoma Poison Control Center
Oklahoma City, Oklahoma

S. Kay Sedlak, MS, RN, CEN, FAEN
Faculty, Laboratory Manager
Western Nevada College
Carson City, Nevada

William R. Short, MD, MPH
Assistant Professor of Medicine
Jefferson Medical College of Thomas Jefferson University
Philadelphia, Pennsylvania

Jeff Solheim, MSN, RN-BC, CEN, CFRN, FAEN
Adjunct Faculty
Portland Community College;
President
Project Helping Hands and Solheim Enterprises
Portland, Oregon

Leona Stout-Demps, MSN, RN, CEN
Clinical Unit Educator for Emergency Services
Orlando Regional Medical Center
Orlando, Florida

Joanne E. Thompson, MSN, RNC-OB, CNS
Perinatal Clinical Nurse Specialist
Presbyterian Hospital
Charlotte, North Carolina

Robin Walsh, BSN, RN
Clinical Nurse Supervisor
University Health Services
University of Massachusetts
Amherst, Massachusetts

Barbara Weintraub, MSN, MPH, RN, PNP-AC, CEN, CPEN, FAEN
Director, Pediatric and Adult Emergency and Trauma
    Services
Northwest Community Hospital
Arlington Heights, Illinois

Darleen A. Williams, MSN, CNS, CEN, CCNS, CNS-BC, EMT-P
Clinical Nurse Specialist for Emergency Services
Orlando Regional Medical Center
Orlando, Florida

Dawn M. Williamson, MSN, RN, PMHCNS-BC
Addictions Consultation Clinical Nurse Specialist,
    Emergency Department
Massachusetts General Hospital
Boston, Massachusetts

Fiona Winterbottom, MSN, RN, APRN, ACNS-BC, CCRN
Clinical Nurse Specialist, Critical Care
Ochsner Medical Center
New Orleans, Louisiana

Lisa Wolf, PhD, RN, CEN
Clinical Assistant Professor
University of Massachusetts
Amherst, Massachusetts;
Staff Educator
Cooley Dickinson Hospital
Northhampton, Massachusetts

Polly Gerber Zimmermann, MS, MBA, RN, CEN, FAEN
Associate Professor
Harry S Truman College
Chicago, Illinois

Colleen Andreoni, MSN, ANP-BC, CEN
Nancy M. Ballard, MSN, RN
Gwen Barnett, RN
Darcy T. Barrett, MSN, RN, CNRN
Nancy M. Bonalumi, MS, RN, CEN
Elizabeth Burke, BA
Patricia M. Campbell, MSN, RN, CCRN, ANP-CS
Patricia L. Clutter, MEd, RN, CEN
Nancy J. Denke, MSN, RN, FNP-C, CCRN
Kathy M. Dolan, MS, RN, CEN
Gretta J. Edwards, BS, RN, CEN
Faye P. Everson, RN, CEN, EMT-B
John Fazio, MS, RN
LCDR Andrew A. Galvin, MSN, APRN, BC, CEN
Tamara Gentry, BSN, RN
Nicki Gilboy, MS, RN, CEN
Chris M. Gisness, MSN, RN, CEN, CS, FNP-C
Donna S. Gloe, BSN, MSN, EdD, RN, BC
Katy Hadduck, BSN, RN, CFRN
Jeff Hamilton, BA, RN
M. Lynn Herman, MSN, RN
Robert Herr, MD, MBA, FACEP
Reneé Semonin Holleran, PhD, RN, CEN, CCRN, CFRN

Mary Jagim, BSN, RN, CEN
Anita Johnson, BSN, RN
LCDR Jeffrey S. Johnson, NC, USN, MSN, RN, CEN
Kimberly P. Johnson, BSN, RN
Mara S. Kerr, MS, RNC
Cheri Kommor, RN, CEN
Louise LeBlanc, BScN, RN, ENC(c)
Anne Marie E. Lewis, MA, BA, BSN, RN, CEN
Diana Lombardo, MSN-FNP, MHA, RN, CCRN
Dennis B. MacDougall, MS, RN, ACNPBC, CEN
Donna L. Mason, MS, RN, CEN
Kay McClain, MSN, RN, CEN, CNA
Jule Blakeley Monnens, MSN, RN
Jessie M. Moore, MSN, APRN-BC, CEN
Andrea Novak, MS, RN, CEN
Lisa Murphy Pruner, MS, RN
Terri Roberts, BSN, RN
Susan Rolniak, MSN, RN, CRNP
Anita Ruiz-Contreras, MSN, RN, CEN, MICN, SANE-A
Christopher Schmidt, MSN, APRN-BC, CEN, ENP, CDR, NC, USN
Janice R. Sisco, BSN, RN
Jeff Solheim, MSN, RN-BC, CEN, CFRN, FAEN

REVIEWERS

Jenny Bosley, MS, RN, CEN
Clinical Nurse Specialist, Emergency Department
Thomas Jefferson University Hospital
Philadelphia, Pennsylvania

Marylee Bressie, MSN, RN, CCRN, CCNS, CEN
PRN Clinical Nurse Specialist/Staff Nurse
Medical Intensive Care Unit
Providence Hospital and Samford University
Mobile, Alabama

Beth Broering, MSN, RN, CEN, CCRN, CPEN, CCNS, FAEN
Clinical Nurse Specialist
Emergency Services
St. Thomas Health
Nashville, Tennessee

Pat Clutter, MEd, RN, CEN, FAEN
Staff Nurse and Educator, Emergency Department
St. John's Hospital
Lebanon, Missouri

Vivian DeFalco, RN
Charge Nurse, Emergency Department
Doylestown Hospital
Doylestown, Pennsylvania

Laura R. Favand, MS, RN
Chief, Planning, Training, Mobilization, and Security
Ireland Army Community Hospital
Fort Knox, Kentucky

Joyce Foresman-Capuzzi, BSN, RN, CEN, CPN, CTRN, CCRN, CPEN, SANE-A, EMT-P
Clinical Nurse Educator, Emergency Department
Lankenau Hospital
Wynnewood, Pennsylvania

Douglas Havron, BSN, MS, RN, CEM
Chief Executive Office
Havron & Associates
Houston, Texas

Renee S. Holleran, PhD, APRN, CEN, CCRN, CFRN, CTRN, FAEN
Staff Nurse, Emergency Department
Intermountain Medical Center
Salt Lake City, Utah

Jill S. Johnson, DNP, APRN, FNP-BC, CCRN, CEN, CFRN
Family Nurse Practitioner, Clinic and Emergency
  Department
Take Care Health Systems and Team Health Emergency
  Services
Mount Sterling, Kentucky

Patricia N. Meza, MSN, RN, CCRN, CCNS, CEN
Lieutenant Colonel
US Air Force
San Antonio, Texas

Debra Ann Milliner, MSN, MBA-HCM, RN, APN, CEN, CFRN, NREMT-P
Registered Nurse/Paramedic
Flight Program (Care Flight)
Reno, Nevada;
Banner Churchill Community Hospital
Fallon, Nevada

Susan Moore, MSN, RN, CCRN, CEN, CFRN, FNP-C
Nurse Practitioner
Banner Churchill Community Hospital Emergency
  Department
Fallon, Nevada;
Flight Nurse
REMSA/Care Flight
Reno, Nevada

Margaret S. Surratt, MSN, MBA, RN, CFRN, CCRN, PHRN
Pediatric Intensive Care Unit (CNMC)
Children's National Medical Center
Washington, DC;
Temple Transport Team
Temple Physicians Incorporated
Philadelphia, Pennsylvania

PREFACE

No other area of health care feels the immediate impact of societal changes more than the emergency department. Today emergency nurses care for greater numbers of more acutely ill patients than ever before. The "baby-boomers" are aging and present with multiple co-morbidities. Unemployment and under-employment result in many patients with inadequate health insurance coverage and patients who can no longer afford their co-payments or medications presenting to emergency departments. Governmental budget cuts have decreased the availability of health care for some patients, particularly those with mental health issues. Recent years have seen an apparent rise in natural and man-made disasters, and as a result, patients seeking treatment following these incidents.

Advances in technology and the development of newer, improved therapies continue at a rapid pace. For example, management of patients experiencing stroke and ST elevation myocardial infarction (STEMI) has changed significantly in the past decade, and therapeutic hypothermia is now the standard of care for a select group of patients surviving sudden cardiac arrest.

As a result of these factors, emergency nurses must be life-long learners.

This seventh edition of *Sheehy's Manual of Emergency Nursing* aims to assist emergency nurses in updating their knowledge and improving the care of their patients. The intent is that this book will serve as a quick reference for the practicing emergency nurse. Much of the content is summarized in tables and charts and the bulleted format makes information easily accessible. Chapters contain boxes to emphasize important practice points.

As with the previous editions, the content is divided into five parts. Part 1, Basic Emergency Issues, now includes chapters related to disruptive behavior and violence in the workplace as well as ethical dilemmas frequently encountered in the emergency department. Part 2, Basic Clinical Issues, addresses topics critical to the care of all emergency patients, such as pain management. Part 3, Common Non-Traumatic Emergencies, includes separate chapters on stroke and sepsis in light of the frequency with which emergency nurses care for patients with these life-threatening problems. Part 4, Trauma, assumes the reader has basic trauma knowledge from the Emergency Nurses Association's (ENA) Trauma Nursing Core Course. Although this manual does not include the in-depth information needed by nurses working in a pediatric-only emergency department, Part 5, Special Populations, addresses common pediatric emergencies. This section also includes chapters on considerations for and emergencies specific to geriatric and bariatric patients, two groups seen with increasing frequency in most emergency departments.

Belinda B. Hammond

ACKNOWLEDGMENTS

I would like to thank the many authors and contributors to this edition for taking time from their busy lives to share their expertise and for their hard work and patience. I would also like to thank the ENA and Elsevier for their editorial assistance in this project.

Belinda B. Hammond

To the Emergency Nurses Association for their leadership, vision, and support:

Diane Gurney, MS, RN, CEN
ENA President 2010

AnnMarie Papa, DNP, RN, CEN, NE-BC, FAEN
ENA President 2011

Susan McDaniel Hohenhaus, MA, RN, CEN, FAEN
Executive Director

Jill S. Walsh, DNP, RN, CEN
Chief Nursing Officer

Diane Muench, MBA, RN, OCN
Editorial Consultant

Alyssa M. Kelly, MSN, RN, CNS, CEN
Nursing Education Editor

Renée Herrmann, MA
Copy Editor

To the following nurses for lending their support and expertise in the development of this manual:

Melanie Golda, MSN, RN, MICN
Nursing Editor

Janet Magnani, BS, RN, MICN
Nursing Editor

Vicki Sweet, MSN, RN, CEN CCRN, FAEN
Nursing Editor

Mary Ellen Wilson, MS, RN, CEN, COHN-S, FNP, FAEN

Dawn Herman, MBA, RN, CEN

Jeff Solheim, MSN, RN-BC, CEN, CFRN, FAEN

CONTENTS

Sheehy's Manual of

Emergency
Care

Basic Emergency Issues

Legal Issues for Emergency Nurses

Legal issues have a profound effect on the practice of nursing in today's increasingly technological and evolving health care arena. Emergency care can be a highly litigious area of practice. This chapter provides a basic overview of some of the legal issues that affect emergency nurses and their delivery of care. This chapter is not a substitute for professional advice. Nurses should discuss specific legal problems related to emergency nursing with an attorney.

NURSE PRACTICE ACTS

Licensed professional nurses are accountable to the public for their nursing judgment and the consequences of that judgment. Nurse Practice Acts (NPAs) are statutory laws created by legislative bodies that oversee the practice of nursing. State Boards of Nursing (known as Boards of Nurse Examiners in some jurisdictions) are the administrative bodies charged with enforcing the NPA of a state through rules, regulations, hearings, and investigations. NPAs were originated to do the following:

- Protect the public
- Define and limit the practice of nursing
- Provide scope of practice guidelines
- Set standards for nursing
- Allow for disciplinary action

Every state has its own NPA that determines qualifications for entry into professional nursing, defines educational responsibilities, and regulates advanced practice nurses. Each licensed practitioner should be aware of the scope of practice delineated in the NPA of the state in which he or she practices. While there is variability in the language and definitions contained in each state's NPA, some major themes have been identified, including care in the context of nursing, definition of the nursing process, supervision or delegation as well as executing the medical treatment plan and health maintenance and prevention.[1]

Some NPAs specify situations where the basic practice of nursing might overlap into either advanced nursing practice or the practice of medicine, as in the case of some nurse-driven protocols that would involve either ordering diagnostic procedures or administering medications. These protocols may be referred to as "standardized procedures" and must conform to regulations as outlined in the specific NPA. Many involve a collaboration between the medical staff and include advanced training, ongoing documentation of education and competency. It is crucial for the emergency nurse to understand the difference between nursing policies and these advanced protocols or procedures.[2,3]

UNLICENSED ASSISTIVE PERSONNEL

Supervision of unlicensed personnel is a growing responsibility of the licensed practitioner. Many hospitals use unlicensed assistive personnel (UAP); depending on the state this may include emergency medical technicians, paramedics, or certified nursing assistants. Delegation of nursing functions to these individuals can create legal problems for the licensed practitioner. A registered nurse may not delegate any task to UAPs that rightfully only a licensed practitioner should perform. These activities include tasks that involve professional clinical judgment related to the diagnosis and treatment of patients. This may include such nursing functions as assessment, planning, and evaluation, depending on the specific state NPA.[4]

CONFIDENTIALITY AND HIPAA REGULATIONS

Confidentiality is essential to the relationship between emergency nurses and their patients, and patients have an expectation of privacy regarding personal health information. In a world of computer technology, opportunities for violation of patient privacy related to easy access to medical data are increased. Federal and state laws exist to protect medical information. Emergency nurses have a legal and ethical duty to ensure patient privacy.

The Health Insurance Portability and Accountability Act of 1996 (HIPAA), enacted in part to simplify administration of health insurance, provides for protection of personal health information by directing ways it may be stored, shared, or released.[5,6] Under the regulations of the act, individuals are entitled to do the following:

- Receive information regarding how their health data will be used and disclosed
- Access their personal medical records (with an option to amend the record)
- Access a list of nonroutine disclosures of their information
- Authorize the use of their medical records
- Object to or restrict the use of their medical records
- Seek recourse through the U.S. Department of Health and Human Services if privacy protections are violated

Some states have enacted privacy legislation that might be stricter than that of the federal HIPAA laws. It is important to understand state laws as well as hospital policies regarding the release of information.

Patient confidentiality is everyone's concern. Hospitals are required to devise policies and procedures that address privacy issues, and all health care providers must be diligent in their efforts to protect personal medical data. Vigilance and sensitivity to patient privacy concerns are required whenever discussing or disclosing personal health information. Practitioners should limit conversations about patients to those persons who need to know and should discuss patient issues only in suitable areas. Severe civil and criminal penalties exist for wrongful disclosure of individually identifiable health information.

Privacy statutes do not limit authorized public health or required state regulatory reporting. In fact, federal and state laws exist that mandate reporting of certain illnesses, injuries, and suspicions, including the duty to warn third parties if a patient has made threats toward a specific individual.

EMTALA AND INTERFACILITY TRANSFERS

All personnel working in the emergency department must have a working knowledge of the Emergency Medical Treatment and Active Labor Act (EMTALA). It is also important to understand state and local regulations that might apply to medical screening examinations as well as to interfacility transfers. The law applies to all institutions with Medicare provider agreements in effect. The act defines an emergency medical condition as "any condition manifesting itself by

---

Situations That Mandate Reporting in Most States*
• Any death in the emergency department and deaths within 48 hours of hospital admission
• Child abuse
• Communicable diseases such as human immunodeficiency virus (HIV), hepatitis, and tuberculosis
• Disabled adult abuse
• Elder abuse
• Elopement of psychiatric patients
• Extensive burns
• Gunshot and stab wounds
• Homicide
• Infectious outbreaks
• Internal disasters
• Rape/sexual assault
• Serious injury, illness, or death reasonably suggested to be related to the use of a medical device
• Sexually transmitted infections
• Suicide (including attempted suicide)

*Refer to local regulations for specific state requirements.

---

acute symptoms of sufficient severity (including pain) that if medical treatment is not rendered, the individual or the unborn child would be subject to serious injury or death."[7] The act provides that a hospital with an emergency department must do the following[7]:

- Provide appropriate medical screening—to determine the nature and severity of the emergency condition—to any individual presenting to the emergency department and requesting treatment.
- Provide appropriate stabilizing treatment (within the capability of the hospital emergency department) for emergency medical conditions and active labor.
- With regard to transfers, EMTALA requires[8]:
  - Written informed consent from the patient or the patient's representative before transfer to another facility.
  - Documentation that the receiving facility has available space and qualified personnel to treat the patient.
  - Assurance that the receiving facility and an attending physician have accepted the patient.
  - Transfer of the patient with appropriate personnel, equipment, and mode of transportation.
  - Inclusion of all documents and medical records with the patient at the time of transfer.

Under the stipulations of EMTALA, stabilizing treatment must be provided for medical conditions (including active labor) that within reasonable medical certainty likely would deteriorate if not treated. Unstable patients transferred to other hospitals must have physician certification that the benefits of transfer outweigh the risk associated with the move.

Although triage is an important tool for establishing treatment priorities, it is not equivalent to a medical screening examination as defined by EMTALA. Hospital bylaws must delineate clearly which providers can perform the medical screening examination.

CONSENT

Consent is the patient's acknowledgment and acceptance of medical treatment. Treatment of a patient without consent can constitute battery, which is defined as intentional, unwanted touching. Consent may be implied or express. In health care, express consent often goes beyond a simple "yes" or "no," through a process known as informed consent. Table 1-1 summarizes types of consent.

Express consent, written or oral, is the patient's agreement to treatment. By law, consent is implied when a patient is unable or incapable of giving or denying permission for treatment, as in cases of unconsciousness, where immediate decisions must be made to prevent loss of life or limb. Additionally, emergent procedures may be performed on minors, without parental consent, to protect life or limb when a legal guardian is unavailable. In these cases the law assumes that a reasonable person, in the same or similar circumstances, would provide consent. Therefore the law implies consent on the patient's behalf.

Most health care laws concerning consent involve informed consent. Informed consent requires the capacity to consent. Sometimes the terms "capacity" and "competency" are used interchangeably; however, there is a difference. Capacity is the individual's ability to make informed decisions. Competency is a legal term and is usually only determined through the court system.[9] The age at which an individual may provide informed consent (or refusal) varies among states and according to the patient's condition. Importantly, the age of consent may differ from the age of majority. Many state regulations define situations where a minor may legally give consent, such as in the case of emancipated minors, active duty military, and married or pregnant minors. Informed consent occurs after full disclosure to the patient of the medical procedure. Essential components of informed consent include[8]:

- An explanation of the procedure
- Discussion of potential risks and benefits of the procedure
- Alternatives to the procedure
- Confirmation that the patient understands the risks, benefits, and any alternatives

Involuntary consent is a complex issue and is often invoked in the case of psychiatric, suicidal, or intoxicated patients. Patients may be involuntarily detained in order to receive psychiatric treatment. State regulations and hospital policy must be followed as, in many cases, detainees and prisoners still retain the right to consent to or refuse medical diagnostics and treatment.

Obtaining consent from patients with language or cultural barriers may be challenging. Authorized translation services must be provided to ensure that these individuals are able to ask questions and receive full disclosure related to proposed medical interventions.

Lack of consent does not remove EMTALA requirements to provide a medical screening examination. Necessary treatment should never be delayed while seeking consent to treat a minor.

REPORTABLE CONDITIONS

State laws govern situations that require a breach of patient confidentiality for the reporting of certain patient conditions. Mandatory reporting laws vary from state to state,

TABLE 1-1	**TYPES OF CONSENT**
TYPE	**DESCRIPTION**
Implied consent	Allows any appropriate treatment in an emergency situation when the patient is unable to give consent. Based on the assumption that a patient, if able, would provide consent for lifesaving treatment.
Express consent	Written or oral agreement to treatment. Examples include assessment, evaluation, medications, radiographs, and laboratory studies.
Informed consent	The patient has a full understanding of risks and benefits of the proposed treatment, is not under the influence of mind-altering substances, and has the legal capacity to consent. Examples of situations requiring informed consent include surgery, invasive procedures, and participation in research protocols.
Involuntary consent	When an individual refuses to consent to needed medical treatment a physician or police officer can ensure that the individual receives treatment. Examples include suicidal, delusional, or demented patients.

and each emergency department should have policies and procedures related to these laws, indicating which agencies require notification. Do not assume that a report has been made in cases where reporting is mandatory and there is a legal responsibility to ensure proper reporting, even if other members of the health care team, including physicians, disagree.[8] Note that some states require that patients who experienced an epileptic seizure or lapse of consciousness while driving be reported to the local health authority or Department of Motor Vehicles.

Common Reportable Events
- Errors in assessment, planning, implementation, or evaluation of patient conditions (particularly in the area of triage)
- Failure to act as a patient advocate or follow up abnormal conditions
- Failure to educate patients on their condition and the adverse consequences if patients do not follow the medical regimen
- Failure to monitor, adequately assess, and communicate patient conditions and changes in condition
- Falls
- Medication errors
- Patients likely to injure themselves or others
- Use of unsafe or malfunctioning equipment

DOCUMENTATION

Nursing documentation is an essential part of patient care and is intended to:
- Reflect the care administered to the patient
- Provide a chronology of patient progress or response to treatment
- Communicate clinically significant information to other members of the health care team
- Provide justification for charges and billing

Minimum documentation requirements vary by institution and are generally based on state and federal regulations. Hospitals accredited by The Joint Commission are required to provide certain information on the medical record.[8] The medical record should be:
- Clear and objective
- Realistic and factual
- Composed of one's own observations
- Free of opinions, generalizations, and ambiguities
- Grammatically written, without spelling errors
- Devoid of unapproved abbreviations. The Joint Commission issued a "Do Not Use" list of abbreviations (Table 1-2).

Many hospitals use electronic documentation, thereby creating an electronic health record (EHR). In February

---

The Joint Commission Required Documentation
- Initial assessment data
- Time when rapid interventions occurred
- Evidence that critically ill patients are receiving intensive care, such as frequent taking of vital signs
- Problems and procedures
- Interventions
- Patient responses to interventions (resolutions)
- Nursing observations
- Communications with other members of the health care team
- Communications with family members
- Patient teaching, including discharge instructions
- Any patient refusal of care
- Use of translators

TABLE 1-2   UNAPPROVED ABBREVIATIONS*

DO NOT USE	POTENTIAL PROBLEM	PREFERRED TERM/USE
U (unit)	Mistaken for "0" (zero), the number "4" or "cc"	Unit
IU (International Unit)	Mistaken for IV (intravenous) or the number "4" or "cc"	International Unit
Q.D., QD, q.d., qd (daily) or Q.O.D., QOD, q.o.d., qod (every other day)	Mistaken for each other Period after the Q mistaken for "I" and the "O" mistaken for "I"	Daily Every other day
Trailing zero (X.0 mg) Lack of leading zero (.X mg)	Decimal point is missed	X mg 0.X mg
MS	Can mean "morphine sulfate" or "magnesium sulfate"	Morphine sulfate
MSO₄ and MgSO₄	Confused for one another	Magnesium sulfate

*Modified from The Joint Commission. (2010, June). *Facts about the official "Do Not Use" list.* Retrieved from http://www.jointcommission.org/assets/1/18/Official_Do%20Not%20Use_List_%206_10.pdf

2009, the American Recovery and Reinvestment Act (ARRA) was signed into law and contains a section called Health Information Technology for Economic and Clinical Health Act (HITECH). This legislation provides incentives to implement an EHR. One incentive program is Meaningful Use wherein a certified technology is required to be able to show continuity of care, demonstrate allergy cross-checking, and maintain a current medication list as well as provide electronic laboratory reporting. The goal of the Meaningful Use program is to improve quality and safety as well as to promote security of medical records.[10]

UNUSUAL EVENTS

Document an unusual event in an institutional incident or occurrence report, *not* in the health care record. Incident reports function to evaluate patient care and trend risk management issues. In most states these reports are confidential. Nonetheless, use caution and complete incident reports as though they could be discoverable. Follow institutional policy regarding what types of events should be reported in this manner. The incident report should contain no language admitting liability or blaming others. State only the facts of the incident. Do not infer, assume, draw conclusions, or indicate what could have been done to prevent the incident. In the patient's chart, never refer to the existence of an incident report.

RESTRAINTS

The use of restraints can have severe legal and physical consequences. Restraining a person against his or her wishes constitutes false imprisonment when a nurse does not have a duty to restrain the patient. *False imprisonment* is defined as restraining a person or preventing a person from leaving an area and as confinement or prevention of a patient's freedom of movement, no matter how long the confinement occurs. Physical restraints have been associated with skin breakdown, impaired respiratory status, neurologic damage, and strangulation. Medical (chemical) restraints can cause respiratory distress, hemodynamic instability, decreased competency or judgment, severe neurologic damage, and death. Because of increasing concerns, concerted efforts have been made to limit or even eliminate the use of restraints in the United States. The overall standard dictates that patients have the right to be free from restraint or seclusion and that staff coercion, convenience, retaliation, or disciplinary efforts are inappropriate reasons for the use of restraints or seclusion.[11]

In addition to guidelines published by the Centers for Medicare & Medicaid Services (CMS) and The Joint Commission, state regulations may also govern the use of restraints as well as time limits, assessment, and documentation requirements. Follow institutional policies, which should be based on state and federal regulations.

ADVANCE DIRECTIVES

The Patient Self-Determination Act of 1991 is a federal law ratified to provide hospitalized patients with information about advance directives. Advance directives are written statements to health care providers regarding a patient's treatment choices in the face of terminal or irreversible illness. These documents go into effect whenever a patient is no longer able to communicate his or her wishes. Table 1-3 describes three types of advance directives.

The Patient Self-Determination Act requires institutions receiving Medicaid and Medicare to ask all patients about the existence of advance directives and to offer information about advance directives to patients. The Joint Commission has established guidelines that must be instituted in all accreditation-seeking hospitals. Review the hospital policies or procedures on this topic. Advance directives may not be transferable from one state to the next.

TABLE 1-3	TYPES OF ADVANCE DIRECTIVES
TYPE	**DESCRIPTION**
Living will	Specifies wishes regarding life-sustaining treatment to include withdrawing, forgoing, or restricting life-sustaining treatment. State statute determines the form the living will may take and how it can be revoked or changed after it has been executed. In most states, nurses and other medical professionals employed at the facility where the individual is receiving care are not allowed to be witnesses.
Durable power of attorney for health care	Appoints an agent to make decisions for the patient concerning medical treatment to include end-of-life treatment decisions.
Do Not Resuscitate (DNR) order	Instructs the physician regarding initiation of cardiopulmonary resuscitation or ventilatory support in the event of cardiac or respiratory arrest.

FORENSICS: EVIDENCE COLLECTION AND PRESERVATION

Medical forensics relates to the collection, analysis, and interpretation of medical evidence presented in legal cases. In the emergency department, forensic issues related to nursing practice include evidence collection, evidence preservation, and chain of custody. Because of the legal impact of evidence collection, it is crucial to understand processes to ensure uncontaminated evidence. Procedures for evidence collection, the role of the nurse in evidence collection, and situations in which nurses collect evidence for potential use in legal cases should be spelled out clearly in hospital policies or procedures.[12] Please refer to Chapter 6, Forensics, for more information.

Situations That Require Evidence Collection in the Emergency Department
- Criminal/legal requests for blood and urine specimens related to alcohol or illicit drug use
- Child abuse/neglect
- Deaths by fire
- Deaths related to airplane, train, and other federal transportation events
- Deaths related to military action
- Disabled adult abuse/neglect
- Domestic violence
- Elder abuse/neglect
- Employment-related requests for blood and urine specimens
- Medical examiner/coroner cases
- Persons who died without being treated by a physician
- Sexual assault
- Traumatic deaths
- Unexpected or unexplained deaths

The chain of custody involves protecting the viability of evidence (for court purposes) by establishing that no tampering has occurred. Chain of custody is a documented record of how the evidence was collected, labeled, and transferred to law enforcement representatives. Record information regarding forensic evidence collection in the medical record and clearly label each specimen. All individuals, including criminal suspects and prisoners, have rights. Medical personnel must recognize these rights, and medical professionals cannot compel individuals routinely to submit to specimen collection.[13] If principles of consent are not used in the collection of evidence, the nurse could be subject to civil liability for battery. Law enforcement officials may seek a search warrant or court order to obtain evidence from patients. However, emergency professionals should be careful not to be placed in the position of becoming agents of the law.[11]

VIOLENCE AND WORKPLACE SAFETY

Workplace violence has long been an area of risk especially for emergency nurses. Violent acts may include any act of aggression and can be physical, verbal, or emotional assaults.[14] Emergency departments, along with geriatric and psychiatric units, have higher rates of violent incidents than any other place in the hospital. When facilities do not have a violence prevention program, they have increased risk for assaultive behavior.[15] The Joint Commission requires facilities to develop written plans to provide for the safety and security not only of patients and visitors, but also of staff. Ongoing risk assessments to determine the potential for violent acts as well as strategies for mitigation of violence must be included as well as response plans in cases of violent events.[16]

REFERENCES

1. Jarrin, O. F. (2010). Core elements of U.S. nurse practice acts and incorporation of nursing diagnosis language. *International Journal of Nursing Terminologies and Classifications, 21*(4), 166–176.
2. Alabama Board of Nursing. (n.d.). *Standardized procedures.* Retrieved from http://www.abn.state.al.us/Content.aspx?id=181
3. California Board of Nursing. (2011, January). *An explanation of the scope of RN practice including standardized procedures.* Retrieved from http://www.rn.ca.gov/pdfs/regulations/npr-b-03.pdf
4. Emergency Nurses Association. (2010, September). *Delegation by the emergency registered nurse* [position statement]. Retrieved from http://www.ena.org/SiteCollectionDocuments/Position%20Statements/Delegation%20by%20the%20Emergency%20Nurse.pdf
5. Lorenzo, J. (2003, July 11). Healthcare marketing: HIPAA and healthcare communications. *HealthLeaders News.*
6. Health Insurance Portability and Accountability Act of 1996, Pub. L. No. 104–191 (1996).
7. Emergency Medical Treatment and Active Labor Act 42 U.S.C. § 1395dd (1996).
8. Jagim, M. (2007). Legal and regulatory issues. In: Emergency Nurses Association, *Emergency nursing core curriculum* (6th ed., pp. 1033–1046). St. Louis, MO: Saunders.
9. Carroll, D. W. (2010). Assessment of capacity for medical decision making. *Journal of Gerontological Nursing, 36*(5), 47–52.
10. Brusco, J. M. (2011). Electronic health records: What nurses need to know. *AORN Journal, 93*(3), 371–379.
11. Lee, G. (2001). *Legal concepts and issues in emergency care.* Philadelphia, PA: W.B. Saunders.

12. Ferrell, J. J. (2007). Forensic aspects of emergency nursing. In: Emergency Nurses Association, *Emergency nursing core curriculum* (6th ed., pp. 1025–1032). St. Louis, MO: Saunders.

13. O'Keefe, M. E. (2001). *Nursing practice and the law: Avoiding malpractice and other risks.* Philadelphia, PA: F. A. Davis.

14. Emergency Nurses Association. (2010, December). *Violence in the emergency care setting* [position statement]. Retrieved from http://www.ena.org/SiteCollectionDocuments/Position%20 Statements/Violence_in_the_Emergency_Care_Setting_-_ ENA_PS.pdf

15. Gacki-Smith, J., Juarez, A. M., Boyett, L., Homeyer, C., Robinson, L., & MacLean, S. L. (2009). Violence against nurses working in U.S. emergency departments. *Journal of Nursing Administration, 39*(7–8), 340–349.

16. The Joint Commission. (2010). Preventing violence in the health care setting. *Sentinel Event Alert, 45,* 1–3. Retrieved from http://www.jointcommission.org/assets/1/18/SEA_45.PDF

Workplace Violence and Disruptive Behavior

Polly Gerber Zimmermann

Disruptive behavior in the workplace is one of the single most important factors determining job satisfaction. Regardless of the source, the result is interference with the orderly performance of hospital business. Violence and disruptive behavior is no longer viewed as something that has to be accepted as just "part of the job." It can have an effect on patient care. Recognize its occurrence and intervene appropriately. Disruptive behaviors can include:

- Profane or disrespectful language
- Demeaning behavior, such as name-calling
- Sexual comments
- Inappropriate touching
- Racial jokes
- Outbursts of anger
- Throwing objects
- Intimidating behaviors
- Retaliation
- Aggressive physical contact or restraint by patients or visitors

DISRUPTIVE BEHAVIOR FROM PATIENTS AND FAMILIES

Disruptive behavior escalating to violence is on a continuum. Reasons listed for its increase include crowding and long waits, sense of entitlement and a lack of societal controls, impaired patients and families (because of drugs, alcohol, or psychiatric conditions), and the patients' anxiety-provoking situations. The role of the nurse is to set limits, effectively intervene early, and prevent the escalation to overt violence.

Obstacles to Addressing Disruptive Behavior

Obstacles to staff addressing disruptive behavior are as follows[1,2]:

- The "normalcy of deviancy"; that is, accepting deviancy as normal and acceptable
- Lack of communication skills
- Inconsistency among staff and providers
- Fear of reprisal and staff concerns about administrative support
- Lack of available resources

Prevention

According to the saying "an ounce of prevention is worth a pound of cure," consistent practice of good patient relations can help prevent the patient and family frustration and irritation that can escalate to violent situations. Consider the following practices to establish trust and diffuse patient and family anxiety. This approach starts with triage setting the tone that should follow throughout the emergency department visit.

Initial Contact[3–5]

- Look up and greet patients with a smile.
- Don't cross your arms over your chest.
- Repeat the complaint in the exact words so patients feel "heard." Do not discount expressed concerns.

Verbal Interactions

- Do not interrupt; speak slowly while making eye contact with the patient.
- Use the patient's name as often as possible.
- Keep patients informed. Share what is found on assessment.
- Praise what has been done correctly.
- Give generous time estimates.
- Establish nurses' availability if needed.
- Ask the patient and visitors, "Anything else?"
- "Script" with reassuring phrases such as "I'm sorry this happened to you" or "We'll take good care of your wife."

Behaviors

- Sit near the patient. (Patients will perceive the nurse was interacting with them twice as long than if standing far away and looking over.)[4]
- Do not type or write while the patient is expressing his or her main concern.
- Use touch; for example, touch the part that is hurting.

VIOLENCE

The Emergency Nurses Association's (ENA) Emergency Department Violence Surveillance Study[6] and Gacki-Smith et al.[7] found that 8% to 13% of emergency nurses are victims of physical violence every week and more than half of nurses who work in emergency departments have been physically assaulted on the job. No one indicator of potential violence or intervention is always effective, as patients or family members who become violent are a heterogeneous group.

Preventing Disruptive Behavior[1,8]

- Education in self-protective measures and de-escalating techniques
- Environmental controls such as:
  - Controlled access doors
  - Panic buttons and personal alarms
  - Breakaway glass
- Report incidents to increase awareness
- Facilities with zero-tolerance programs have reported fewer violent occurrences.[6,7]
- Identify high-risk patients and communicate this status (for instance, flagging or labeling the chart) to all involved health care professionals (e.g., "Wear goggles and gown when entering room; patient may spit.").

A key predictor for current violence is how volatile a patient was in the past.[8] Numerous scales exist to assess agitation in psychiatric patients. The Behavioral Activity Rating Scale (BARS) is a single-item, seven-point scale on agitated behavior. Schumacher et al.[9] found BARS to be effective in identifying patients likely to need behavioral management during their emergency department stay. It was also suggested that a retrospective assessment of the behavior during the two hours prior to triage may be useful in identifying the currently calm patient who is at risk for becoming agitated during the emergency department visit.[9,10] Consider the following interventions to further prevent violence in the emergency department:

- Work practices can also help prevent danger to health care providers.
  - Do not allow employees to work alone in a high-risk area.
  - Always have an exit always available.

- Promote legislation on violence prevention. At least 10 states have legislation to strengthen or increase penalties for acts of workplace violence affecting nurses. In New York it is a felony to assault nurses who are on duty.[8]

Resources for Dealing with Violence

- An adaptable model state bill is available at http://www.nursingworld.org
- The American Nurses Association's (ANA) brochure on preventing workplace violence is available at http://www.nursingworld.org
- ANA's continuing education offering "Workplace Violence: The Nurse Victim" is available at http://www.nursingworld.org
- The Center for American Nurses' policy statement on lateral violence and bullying in the workplace is available at http://www.centerforamericannurses.org
- The Emergency Nurses Association's (ENA) position statement "Violence in the Emergency Care Setting" is available at http://www.ena.org
- American Psychiatric Nurses Association's position statement is available at http://www.apna.org

---

DE-ESCALATION[11,12]

Behavior escalates along a continuum. It is important for an emergency nurse to identify behaviors that risk escalation to a violent situation and be skilled in response techniques. The goal is to intervene and diffuse the disruptive behavior early in the escalation.

Patient Behavior: Challenging the Provider

- The person challenges the health care provider's authority or competence. ("We've been waiting for an hour. You people are all incompetent here.")
- The voice changes in tone, volume, or cadence from the normal conversation.
- Body language shows muscle tenseness, anger expression, or leaning forward ("getting in your face").

Health Care Provider De-escalation Response

- Ignore the question (but not the person) and redirect to the issue at hand. Responding directly to the challenge (e.g., "Sir, we are all highly trained professionals here!") creates an unproductive power struggle.
- Let the person vent. Do not interrupt. Do not deny the complaint. Letting the person verbalize "deflates" his or her pent-up emotions.

- Respond with empathy, acknowledging the person's emotions ("I can see you are angry"). People are annoyed if their emotions are ignored. Validate the person's feelings ("I know you are upset").
- Keep body language nonthreatening. Significant communication occurs through body language. When a person is agitated, body language is of heightened importance as even less than usual is communicated verbally in these situations.
- Use the person's name often when emotions are taking over; it grabs the rational part of the brain.
- Don't quote authoritative rules or ultimatums (e.g., "You can't talk like that. This is a hospital!").
- Use "broken record" technique to repeat the same information and talk to the feelings.
  - "I've been waiting for 40 minutes."
    - "I know it is frustrating to wait."
  - "This is ridiculous."
    - "I know it is frustrating to wait."
  - "How can you be so inefficient?"
    - "I know it is frustrating to wait."
- Activate de-escalation and response resources early in an agitated situation. To improve the staff's ability to respond effectively to escalating and violent situations, emergency departments may consider:
  - Violence rapid response team (VRRT)
  - Violence response drills, including security and law enforcement activation procedures
  - Staff safety education emphasizing personal safety techniques during a violent occurrence

> Nurses should always de-escalate themselves first to remain calm in a volatile situation. Appear concerned but not frightened. The "best trained brain" stays in control.[11]

Patient Behavior: Refusal and Noncompliance

- The person increasingly challenges authority, becomes argumentative, and brings in a power struggle.

Health Care Provider De-escalation Response

- Set limits. Go beyond saying, "Stop that." Specifically identify what is unacceptable (i.e., tone, attitude, behavior, language), why it is unacceptable (e.g., disruptive, disrespectful), and the consequences. Limits are most effective when simple, reasonable, and enforceable. Anecdotally, many indicate stating "I will call security" as the consequence results in people backing down. Examples include:

- "I feel threatened by your screaming at me. I am asking you to stop that behavior because it is not appropriate."
- "If you refrain from cursing, we can discuss your concerns. If not, this conversation is ended until later."
- Give the disruptive person a responsible choice and time to decide his or her response.
- Consider a verbal contract, such as "Can you do ____ while I do ____?" (e.g., "Can you stand here and wait while I check on your wife's situation?").
- Focus on concrete needs. Ask if they want something to eat or a cup of coffee.

Patient Behavior: Emotional Release

- The person has an emotional outburst, often accompanied by screaming and swearing. The intensity is higher than earlier expressions, and there is a loss of rational thought.

Health Care Provider De-escalation Response

- Let the person vent but remove him or her from public arena. Some people enjoy the public show and de-escalate when the "audience" is removed.
- Listen to the patient and restate to clarify message.
- Listen to what is not being said.
- Give this individual your *undivided* attention: the person is at high risk to become out of control.
  - Do not answer a ringing phone.
  - Do not look away or turn your back.
- Share emotional responses. It may make the person realize (for the first time?) that he or she is losing control (e.g., "Now you are scaring me" or "This behavior is disturbing."). It is not unprofessional to be afraid; trust your gut. What determines professionalism is how the fear is handled.
- If the person cools off, then calmly state a reasonable directive.

Patient Behavior: Intimidation

- The verbal and nonverbal threats involve threats to safety of others. According to ENA's Emergency Department Violence Surveillance Study[6] and Gacki-Smith et al.[7], these threats mainly occur in the patient's room. The acting-out incidents mostly occur during triage, invasive procedures, or while restraining or subduing patients.[6,7]

Health Care Provider De-escalation Response

- Stand 2 to 3 feet away (e.g., one leg length) to be out of reach and to give personal space. Being too close physically can be perceived as a personal threat.

- Turn body at an angle with an open stance. This position is perceived as less threatening yet authoritative.
- Keep hands open and in plain view.
- Remove glasses or any other apparel that could injure or become a weapon.
- Always have an exit. Position oneself between the patient or visitor and the exit to the room or treatment area. Speak loudly so other staff members are aware that the person is escalating and can assist.
- If a gun is seen, loudly and repeatedly say, "GUN! GUN! GUN!"
- Get help early. Contact security and activate the emergency panic button or violence response team. Have a show of force.

Tension Reduction

Security secures the environment, under the direction of nursing. Once under control, establish reassuring contact with the affected individuals. It is important that when the situation is de-escalated, the patient and family understand that the incident will not affect the quality of care received by the patient.

> **De-escalation Resources**
> Crisis Prevention Institute http://www.crisisprevention.com
> Assertive Communication: De-escalation http://www.
>   thousandwaves.org/docs/VPResources/De-Escalation.pdf
> Ten Critical De-escalation Skills http://www.populararticles.com/
>   article45613.html
> De-Escalation Techniques: Addressing Problematic Behavior;
>   Wiebers and Wilson http://www.educ.drake.edu/rc/
>   downloads/PBS%20Training_Resources/PBS%20
>   ResourcesNov07/De-escalation/De-Escalation%20PPT.ppt

ADMINISTRATIVE POLICIES[13]

Informal Notice

- Informal notice is given verbally to the offender, directly at time of the incident.
- Using the techniques described above, informal notice helps avoid the "normalcy of deviancy."
- It is an active intervention that brings the issue to the forefront, rather than just ignoring it.
- It is more likely to occur if there is perceived administrative support to address irrational statements and behaviors by patients and family.

Formal Notice

- Formal notice consists of a written letter given to the offender.
- A written warning can be used for a known, repeating patient.

- Describe the unacceptable behavior, refer to the applicable policy, and explain the expectations and consequences.
- The letter should be signed by the appropriate manager or director.

Behavioral Agreements

- A behavior agreement is used for a known, repeating patient with a pattern of abusive behavior.
- It is done in connection with administration and the patient's primary provider. Sometimes a psychiatric consult or ethics consult is involved first.
- The offending behavior is specifically identified and it is explained that the behavior is greatly impeding the ability to provide necessary care. The patient is informed it must stop or the person will be asked to seek medical care elsewhere.
- The patient, physician, and administrative representative sign the agreement.

OTHER CONSIDERATIONS

Gangs[12]

- Do not disrespect gang colors or symbols or say anything to refute that the patient is "brave."

Alcohol Withdrawal[14]

- The patient's depressed neurons become hyperexcited when there is sudden withdrawal in a person who is use to chronic high intake of alcohol.
- The initial symptoms of withdrawal can start 4 to 6 hours after the last drink.
- These symptoms worsen with repeated withdrawals (kindling effect).
- For more information refer to Chapter 12, Substance Abuse, and Chapter 13, Alcohol Abuse.

Delirium

- Impaired mental status is present in 26% of emergency department patients who are older than age 70 years.[15] Yet in one study nurses failed to identify delirium in these patients 69% of the time.[15]
- Confusion Assessment Method (CAM) at least once per shift (Table 2-1).

CLINICIAN DISRUPTIVE BEHAVIOR

Clinician disruptive behavior is defined as behavior that is disrespectful or intimidating to another.[16-19] It is often recognized by how it makes the receiver feel. Some of the most common overt and passive disruptive behaviors are:

TABLE 2-1	**CONFUSION ASSESSMENT METHOD (CAM)**

Delirium is present if BOTH
- Mental status alteration from baseline
- Inattention (test by asking to spell "world" backwards)

AND at least ONE of the FOLLOWING
- Disorganized thinking (hallucinations, paranoia)
- Altered level of consciousness (anything besides alert, e.g., lethargy, agitation, etc.)

Data from Waszynski, C. (2007). How to try this: Detecting delirium. *American Journal of Nursing, 107*(12), 50–59 and Inouye, S. K., vanDyck, C. H., Slessi, C. A., Balkin, S., Siegel, A. P., & Horwitz, R. I. (1990). Clarifying confusion: The confusion assessment method. A new method for detection of delirium. *Annals of Internal Medicine, 113*(12), 941–948.

- Overt behaviors[16,17]:
  - Verbal outbursts (48%)
  - Physical threats (43%)
- Passive behaviors[16,17]:
  - Not answering questions or not returning calls (79%)
  - Condescending language or voice intonation (88%)
  - Impatience with questions (87%)

Actions are on a continuum; less aggressive actions can actually be more discouraging because it is not as obvious to everyone that the experienced behavior is out of line. As a whole, nurses tend to use passive-aggressive actions, such as cliques, inclusiveness, or gossip, to disrespect or intimidate another staff member. Examples include:
- Sighing, rolling eyes
- Gossiping, making complaints to others
- Walking away while other health care professionals are talking to them
- Disrespectful language, sarcasm, name-calling, profanity
- Criticizing a caregiver in front of patients or other staff
- Comments that undermine a patient's trust in other health care professionals
- Throwing objects, screaming

Incidence

Reports of incidence of disruptive behavior by health care professionals have varied, but The Joint Commission estimates prevalence to be between 3% and 5% of all providers.[1] A 2008 survey by Rosenstein and O'Daniel[16] found that 77% of all respondents (88% of nurses and 51% of physicians) saw disruptive behavior by a physician in their institution; 65% (73% of nurses, 48% of physicians) reported disruptive behavior by nurses. A 2009 study by Yildirim[20] revealed that 21% of the surveyed nurses had experienced

bullying by fellow nurses. It has also been reported that, when measuring a safety climate, problematic responses among health care workers are up to 12 times greater than those in the aviation industry.[21] Health care needs to promote appropriate interpersonal communication that results in the same "safety first" culture as found in the aviation industry.

Effects

Disruptive behavior leads to depression, lowered work motivation, decreased ability to concentrate, poor productivity, lack of commitment to work, and poor relationships with patients, managers, and colleagues.[20] Beyond morale and climate issues, adverse patient outcomes do result.[22] In one survey 76% of respondents reported that disruptive behaviors were linked to adverse events, such as medical errors (71%) and patient mortality (27%).[22]

Guiding Rules

The American Medical Association (AMA) indicated concerns about physician disruptive behavior as early as 2001, as seen in its policy H-140.918.[23] The Joint Commission similarly developed the 2009 Leadership Standard (LD.03.10) to address disruptive and inappropriate behaviors[1]:
- The hospital or organization has "a code of conduct that defines acceptable, disruptive and inappropriate behaviors." (EP4)
- "Leaders create and implement a process for managing disruptive and inappropriate behaviors." (EP5)

Recommended Interventions[1,13,16]

- Recognition and awareness is the first step to help change the culture.
- Provide employee assistance for substance abuse treatment. More than 6% of health care practitioners use illicit drugs; 3.9% have heavy alcohol use.[24]
- Educate staff members on and create policies for more effective communication. The following are different types of education or policies an institution can use:
  - Standardized hand-off techniques such as SBAR (**S**ituation, **B**ackground, **A**ssessment, **R**ecommendation/**R**equest)
  - Assertive communication techniques versus using aggression or avoidance: Assertive communication uses "I" statements and addresses behaviors directly. For instance: "I've noticed _____; When you _____, I feel _____; I want _____." Instead nurses tend to use avoidance.
  - DESC, a mnemonic for assertive communication:[25]
    - **D**escribe the facts—for example, "I noticed you walked away from me while I was trying to tell you about the patient's condition."

- Explain—for example, "It makes me feel devalued. I need you to hear my concerns so we have good patient care."
- State—for example, "As colleagues we need to be able to communicate."
- Consequences—for example, "If this continues, we will need to address this with the nurse manager. Safe care requires adequate report."
- Chain of command policies: Activate the chain of command, a formal line of authority and communication, when problems are not being successfully resolved. Remember, everyone has a boss.
- TeamSTEPPS' Advocacy and Assertion[26] was developed by the Department of Defense and Agency for Healthcare Research and Quality (AHRQ). It provides teachable skills for more effective, safe functioning of constantly changing teams. TeamSTEPPS teaches that any staff member should voice his or her concern when he or she is Concerned, feels Uncomfortable, or recognizes a Safety issue (CUS). The steps to take are:
  - Assert a corrective action in a firm and respectful manner
  - Make an opening
  - State the concern
  - Offer a solution
  - Obtain an agreement
  - If the provider ignores the voiced concern, the staff member is to voice it at least two times to ensure that it has been heard with the team member being challenged to acknowledge the concern. If the staff member feels the outcome is not acceptable, a stronger action such as the chain of command should be activated.
- Zero-tolerance policies and "Code of Conduct" for all staff (including physicians).
- Confidential reporting options. Reporting options include anonymous phone hotlines or web reporting as well as official written, signed reports.
- Policies regarding consistent, uniform method of addressing complaints. For example:
  - Make leveling distinctions between verbal abuse, verbal abuse directed at a specific person, and physical abuse (including sexual harassment).
  - Have progressive corrective actions similar to discipline for other unacceptable behaviors (after investigation). This includes a verbal warning, written warning, written apology to complainant, referral for behavioral disorder evaluation, and possible suspension of privileges.
- Intervention strategies. For example:
  - "Code White/Code Pink." All staff members surround a verbally attacked staff member. They stand

silent with arms crossed and stare at the disruptive individual, who usually stops this behavior.

There is no simple or universal solution. However, just as bullying is no longer accepted as part of growing up for children, the new awareness is that bullying nursing is also unacceptable. It affects not only nurses' morale, but ultimately patient care.

REFERENCES

1. The Joint Commission. (2008, July 9). Behaviors that undermine a culture of safety. *Sentinel Event Alert, 40*. Retrieved from http://www.jointcommission.org/assets/1/18/SEA_40.PDF
2. Leape, L. L., & Fromson, J. A. (2006). Problem doctors: Is there a system-level solution? *Annals of Internal Medicine, 144*(2), 107–115.
3. Boothman, N. (2000). *How to make people like you in 90 seconds or less.* New York, NY: Workman.
4. Mayer, T. A., & Zimmermann, P. G. (1999). ED customer satisfaction survival skills: One hospital's experience. *Journal of Emergency Nursing, 25*(3), 187–191.
5. Zimmermann, P. G., & Herr, R. D. (2006). *Triage nursing secrets.* St Louis, MO: Mosby.
6. Emergency Nurses Association. (n.d.). *The emergency department violence surveillance study.* Retrieved from http://www.ena.org/IENR/Pages/WorkplaceViolence.aspx
7. Gacki-Smith, J., Juarez, A., Boyett, L., Homeyer, C., Robinson, L., & MacLean, S. L. (2009). Violence against nurses working in U.S. emergency departments. *Journal of Nursing Administration, 39*(7–9), 340–349.
8. Trossman, S. (2010). Not 'part of the job.' Nurses seek an end to workplace violence. *The American Nurse, 42*(6), 1, 6.
9. Schumacher, J. A., Gleason, S. H., Holloman, G. H., & McLeod, W. T. (2010). Using a single-item rating scale as a psychiatric behavioral management triage tool in the emergency department. *Journal of Emergency Nursing, 36*(5), 434–438.
10. *Ziprasidone mesylate for intramuscular injection advisory committee briefing document appendix 1: The Behavioral Activity Rating Scale.* (2001). Retrieved from http://www.fda.gov/ohrms/dockets/AC/01/briefing/3685b2_02_pfizer_appendix.pdf
11. Russell, M. (2010, August 11). *Verbal de-escalation strategies.* Presented at Harold Washington College, Chicago, IL.
12. McNair, R. (2003–2010). *In the nature of the beast: Comprehensive triage and patient flow workshop.* Fairview, NC: Triage First.
13. Zimmermann, P. G. (2010, September 25). *Diffusing difficult situations: Handling disruptive colleagues, patients and families.* Presented at the Emergency Nurses Association Annual Scientific Assembly, San Antonio, TX.
14. Morgan, R. (in press). How to recognize and manage a patient experiencing alcohol withdrawal. *American Journal of Nursing.*
15. Waszynski, C. (2007). How to try this: Detecting delirium. *American Journal of Nursing, 107*(12), 50–59.
16. Rosenstein, A. H., & O'Daniel, M. (2008). A survey of the impact of disruptive behaviors and communication defects on

patient safety. *The Joint Commission Journal on Quality and Patient Safety, 34*(8), 464–471.

17. Rosenstein, A. H., & O'Daniel, M. (2005). Disruptive behavior and clinical outcomes: Perceptions of nurses and physicians. *American Journal of Nursing, 105*(1), 54–64.

18. Institute for Safe Medication Practices. (2003). *Results from ISMP survey on workplace intimidation.* Retrieved from http://www.ismp.org/Survey/surveyresults/Survey0311.asp

19. Porto, G., & Lauve, R. (2006). *Disruptive clinician behavior: A persistent threat to patient safety.* Retrieved from http://www.psqh.com/julaug06/disruptive.html

20. Yildirim, D. (2009). Bullying among nurses and its effects. *International Nursing Review 56,* 504–511.

21. Nance, J. J. (2008). *Why hospitals should fly: The ultimate flight plan to patient safety and quality care.* Bozeman, MT: Second River Healthcare Press.

22. Roche, M., Diers, D., Duffield, C., & Catling-Paull, C. (2010). Violence towards nurses, the work environment, and patient outcomes. *Journal of Nursing Scholarship, 42*(1), 13–22.

23. American Medical Association. (2000). *Policy H-140.918 disruptive physician.* Chicago, IL: Author.

24. Hood, J. (2010, December 9). Doctor overcomes abuse, helps others heal. *Chicago Tribune, 23,* 1.

25. Bartholomew, K. (2006). *Ending nurse-to-nurse hostility. Why nurses eat their young and each other.* Marblehead, MA: HCPro.

26. Agency for Healthcare Research and Quality. (n.d.). *TEAMSTEPPS: National implementation.* Retrieved from http://teamstepps.ahrq.gov/

Mass Casualty Incidents

Sharon Saunderson Cohen

Worldwide, disasters have killed millions of people and many more have endured all kinds of illness and injury as a result of these disasters. The risk of disasters affecting people or causing a mass casualty event is increasing mainly because the world population is increasing. Most of the world's population lives in areas prone to hurricanes, flooding, tornadoes, earthquakes, droughts, wild fires, or tsunamis. As such, the risk of human impact from natural disasters is increasing accordingly.

It does not take long for complacency to settle in following a natural or man-made disaster. In most cases only a few short months pass and the attention and emotion attached to the disaster fade and the sense of urgency to prepare wanes to a wait-and-see attitude. Vigilance eventually gives way to vagueness. This vagueness and sense of nonurgency is common, but to health care systems it can be the fatal flaw when the next disaster strikes.

For hospitals, especially emergency or casualty departments, it is no longer sufficient to develop disaster plans and dust them off if a threat appears imminent or a response is required. Rather, a system of preparedness across all areas of a health care system must be in place every day. Such systems make effective responses to emergencies possible and provide responders with a less confused and less chaotic approach to dealing with incidents of any size or kind.

DEFINING A DISASTER

Disasters are commonly categorized by their origin, such as natural, man-made, technological, or human conflict. Many definitions of disaster are found in the literature. The World Health Organization (WHO) defines a disaster as "a serious disruption of the functioning of a community or a society involving widespread human, material, economic, or environmental losses and impacts, which exceeds the ability of the affected community or society to cope using its own resources."[1]

The broad scope of the WHO definition includes disasters that cause mass casualties and those that do not involve human injury or illness. A definition of disaster often used by health care systems is "the number of patients presenting, during a given time, that exceed the capacity of an emergency department (ED)/casualty department to provide care and as such, will require additional allocation of human and durable resources from outside the ED."[1] This definition excludes disasters that do not have surviving patients presenting to the emergency department. Many incidences, such as plane crashes, leave few or no survivors. Others, such as technological disasters, often do not include human injury or illness in other settings, but within health care systems these disasters affect patients dependent on technology for survival (those on ventilators or intravenous pump machines). Though most disasters involving technology, such as large power grid failures or computer system failures, do not directly cause injury or illness, these disasters can have serious indirect effects on human lives, typically affecting those most dependent on the technology for survival.

DISASTER NURSING

Nursing during a disaster often focuses on the care of patients experiencing physical injury, illness, and emotional response to the event. To care for casualties following a disaster, nurses and health care providers must have an understanding of elements of disaster management such as mitigation, planning, response, and recovery.

Not all disaster incidents involve patients arriving at local emergency departments or casualty departments. Catastrophic incidents may affect the infrastructure of the hospital or community in which the hospital is located. These nonpatient generating disaster incidents include loss of computer system infrastructure, loss of electrical or water supply to a hospital, or loss of telephone systems within the hospital. With the goal of adopting digital medical records in the United States by 2016 and the global trend to make all hospital documentation electronic, loss of computer system function can have a stressful and often negative impact on hospitals and potentially on patient care.

Patient-generating disasters are often of a natural origin (e.g., tornadoes, hurricanes, and floods), whereas others are man-made incidents (e.g., the September 11, 2001 terrorist attacks in New York City and Washington, D.C.; the 2002 bombings at a nightclub in Bali; and the 2004 train bombings in Madrid). These man-made disasters had a direct impact on health care systems, often to the point of saturating receiving facilities closest to the incident.

Fundamentals of nursing during a disaster, mass casualty incident (MCI), special event, or even those disasters originating from error, natural causes, or man's infliction of terror, are essentially the same. Time is an important factor as lives can be saved by quick triage and decision making that allow rapid treatment for the most critically ill or injured patients. The principle of doing the most good for the most number of casualties often with limited resources is inherent to nursing during an MCI, disaster, or large-scale special event.

EMERGENCY MANAGEMENT

Emergencies can be threats to any health care organization. Since 2008 The Joint Commission has required hospitals to meet the new Emergency Management (EM) standards, which are separate and distinct from the Environment of Care standards.[2] These new EM standards are organized around the four phases of EM: mitigation, preparedness, response, and recovery (see Fig. 3-1).

Emergency Management aims to reduce or avoid potential losses, including loss of life and property, from potential or real disaster. The four phases of EM illustrate the ongoing process by which health care systems plan for and reduce the impact of a disaster, react during and immediately following a disaster, and take steps to recover after a disaster has occurred. Appropriate actions at all points in the cycle lead to:

- Greater preparedness
- Better warnings
- Reduced vulnerability
- Prevention of disasters (see Table 3-1)

The complete disaster management cycle includes shaping health care facility policies and plans that either modify the causes of disasters or mitigate their effects on people, property, and hospital and community infrastructure. The mitigation and preparedness phases occur as disaster management improvements are made in anticipation of a disaster event. Developmental considerations play

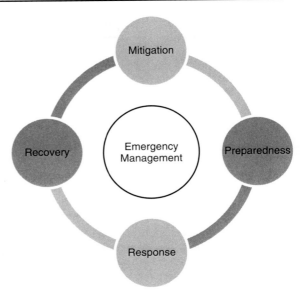

Fig. 3-1 Four phases of Emergency Management.

a key role in contributing to the mitigation and preparation of a health care system to effectively confront a disaster. The four EM phases do not occur in isolation or in this precise order. Often phases of the cycle overlap and the length of each phase greatly depends on the severity of the disaster. Because the four phases of EM are so crucial, this chapter will address each one in depth.

Mitigation

Within hospitals and health care facilities, mitigation implies the steps taken to prevent all possible hazards that may lead to a disaster. The mitigation phase of EM is unique because it focuses on long-term tasks that are effective in reducing or eliminating any risk of a disaster occurring. Obviously not all risks can be eliminated—hurricanes, tornadoes, and other disasters from natural causes are examples. However, when implemented, mitigation strategies minimize the harmful effects of these disasters on the health care facility and its operation. In hurricane-prone areas, for example, hospitals can install shutters to minimize the wind effect on the building. In flood-prone areas, a dam can be built to prevent or minimize the degree of flooding. Another mitigation strategy for hospitals in a flood-prone area is to elevate any critical infrastructure such as energy units (electrical), oxygen farms, or generators. Figure 3-2 is an example of such a mitigation plan.

The first step in mitigation is to identify risks. The Joint Commission standards EM.01.01.01 and EM.03.01.01

TABLE 3-1	**FOUR PHASES OF EMERGENCY MANAGEMENT WITH ACTIONS**
Mitigation Take places before and after an emergency occurs	Activities designed to either prevent the occurrence of an emergency or minimize potentially adverse effects of an emergency, including zoning and building code ordinances and enforcement of land use regulations. **Action:** Buying flood and fire insurance for the home, placing security cameras around the hospital, and installing hurricane shutters are examples of mitigation activities.
Preparedness Takes place before an emergency occurs	Activities, programs, and systems that exist prior to an emergency and are used to support and enhance response to an emergency or disaster. Public education, planning, training, and exercising are among the activities conducted under this phase. **Action:** Evacuation plans and stocking food and water are both examples of preparedness.
Response Takes place during an emergency	Activities and programs designed to address the immediate effects of an emergency or disaster, to help reduce casualties and damage, and to speed recovery. Coordination, warning, evacuation, and mass care are examples of response. **Action:** Seeking shelter from a tornado or turning off gas valves during an earthquake are both response activities.
Recovery Takes place after an emergency occurs	Activities involving restoring systems to normal. Recovery actions are taken to assess damage and return vital life support systems to minimum operating standards; long-term recovery may continue for many years. **Action:** Obtaining financial assistance to help pay for repairs or removing debris are recovery activities.

discuss the need for a hospital to evaluate potential emergencies that could affect demand for the hospital's services or its ability to provide those services and the effectiveness of its emergency management planning activities aimed at managing those emergencies.[2] This includes an annual review of hospital risks, hazards, and potential emergencies as defined in a hazard vulnerability analysis.

Hazard Vulnerability Analysis

A hazard vulnerability analysis (HVA) is a systematic approach to:
- Identify all hazards that may affect an organization and its community
- Assess the risk and probability of hazard occurrence
- Determine the consequence for the organization associated with each hazard
- Analyze the findings to create a prioritized comparison of hazard vulnerabilities

Table 3-2 lists potential threats for HVA consideration.

The consequence, or "vulnerability," is related to both the impact on organizational function and the likely service demands created by the hazard impact. The results of a vulnerability analysis can be used to prioritize mitigation activities and to develop disaster recovery, mitigation, and response plans. Hospital-based HVAs should be conducted with community partners such as local law enforcement, emergency medical services, and fire personnel. Community partners are vital to a true assessment and the basis

of mitigation strategies, as many of these partners will be integrated into hospital mitigation and response plans. HVAs should be conducted on an annual basis or more frequently if hospitals, health care facilities, or when populations change (hospital expansion or development of a new infrastructure in the community may affect the demographics of persons seeking health care from that facility).[3]

Preparedness

Mitigation efforts alone cannot eliminate or prevent all emergency situations. Preparedness activities ensure health care facilities that their staff, visitors, and patients are ready to react promptly and effectively during an emergency or disaster. Disasters are typically viewed as low-probability, high-impact events. Although various definitions have been used, a hospital disaster is frequently viewed as a situation in which the number of patients presenting to the facility within a given time period exceeds the ability of the hospital to provide care without external assistance or effect on the infrastructure and normal operations of the hospital. As such, the definition is facility specific, and therefore preparedness activities must likewise be specific. Health care preparedness activities often include:
- Obtaining information on threats (HVA)
- Planning an organized response to emergencies
- Providing disaster preparedness training for emergencies

Indian River County
Local Mitigation Strategy
Project Prioritization List

Project priority	Project score	Project description	Estimated project Cost and **Estimated time of completion**	Applicant	Mitigation to be accomplished	Hazards mitigated	Jurisdiction(s) involved*	Possible funding sources	Date confirmed/ added
1	93	Retrofits to the county's public schools that serve as public shelters.	$75,000 <12 months	Indian River County Emergency Management John King	Reduces vulnerability to wind and flood damage and provides for critically needed shelter (primary critical facilities) and reducing the county's safe shelter space defecit.	Wind and flood	Multiple jurisdictions	Coastal Construction Building Zone Program; CDBG; DRI; HMGP; Hurricane Program; NFMF	Confirmed 9/8/2009 (John King)
2	93	Fire escape replacement	$2 million >12 months	Indian River Medical Center Cliff Schroeder	Replacement of three fire escape towers on the patient wings of the hospital. The current towers are open-air towers that offer no protection from inclement weather. These required fire evacuation routes become unusable during a hurricane. This puts a large population of patients and healthcare workers at serious risk during a severe storm. A severe storm increases the risk of a catastrophic event that would require the evacuation of this population. The current design also increases the risk to building damage and loss of our ability to sustain operations during and post storm. Each tower serves a patient population of approximately 75 and healthcare staff of 45.	Wind	Multiple jurisdictions	HMGP	Confirmed 10/2/2009 (Cliff Schroeder)
3	93	Fellsmere paving and drainage project	$15,889,032 >12 months	City of Fellsmere Jason Nunemaker	Paving and drainage project to reduce flooding and provide for safer and more efficient evacuations for residents.	Hurricane, tropical storm, flooding	Fellsmere	CDBG, HMGP, DRI, USDA, EDA	Added 11/20/2009
4	92	Study the feasibility and appropriateness of relocating the county dune stabilization setback line (DSSL) westward.	$50,000 2011	Indian River County Community Development Roland DeBlois	Will mitigate potential impact to coastal/oceanfront structures by requiring an updated/appropriate oceanfront building setback to minimize coastal erosion damage.	Coastal erosion	Multiple jurisdictions	Florida Inland Navigation District (FIND), HMGP	Added 9/15/2009
5	92	Portable water storage system	$600,000 <12 months	Indian River Medical Center Cliff Schroeder	Install and connect a portable water tank to provide emergency water services to the hospital for patient care.	All hazards affecting water system	Multiple jurisdictions	HMGP	Confirmed 10/2/2009 (Cliff Schroeder)

Indian River County LMS
* Indicates jurisdiction interest in this project
and support wherever necessary.   December 2009   1 of 7

Fig. 3-2 Example of Indian River County mitigation strategy. (From Indian River County Florida Board of County Commissioners. [2009, December]. *Local mitigation strategy project prioritization list.* Retrieved from http://www.ircgov.com/Boards/LMS/2010_Project_List.pdf)

TABLE 3-2 POTENTIAL THREATS REQUIRING AN EMERGENCY MANAGEMENT PLAN AND RESPONSE

THREATS FROM NATURAL CAUSES	MAN-MADE THREATS	TERRORIST THREATS
Pandemic flu	Explosions	Conventional weapons
Hurricanes	Hazardous materials	Explosive or incendiary devices
Floods	Transportation accidents or incidents	Biological or chemical devices
Fire	Assaults, threats, or acts of violence	Radiological exposure devices
Tornadoes	Arson	Cyberterrorism
Ice storms	Power grid failure	Weapons of mass destruction

- Conducting emergency drills and exercises to test plans and training
- Obtaining and maintaining emergency equipment and facilities
- Establishing intergovernmental coordination arrangements
- Conducting public education related to emergencies

How does a health care facility start to prepare for any size or kind of disaster? Developing a Comprehensive Emergency Management Plan for a health care facility is the first step.

> When developing the emergency plan, gather all available relevant information, including:
> - Copies of any state and local emergency planning regulations or requirements
> - Facility personnel names and contact information
> - Contact information of local and state emergency managers
> - A facility organization chart
> - Building construction and life safety systems information

Comprehensive Emergency Management Plan

A Comprehensive Emergency Management Plan (CEMP) is the master operations document for a health care facility. The CEMP should:

- Guide the response to all emergencies and all catastrophic, major, and minor disasters
- Be broad in nature and perhaps include details and specifics as additions
- Require annual exercises to determine the ability of a health care facility, community, and, if needed, state and local governments to respond to emergencies and disasters
- Describe the basic strategies, assumptions, operational objectives, and mechanisms through which the health care facility will mobilize resources and conduct activities to guide and support a disaster response

- Be flexible, adaptable, and scalable
- Always be in effect
- Articulate the roles and responsibilities of various health care personnel
- Describe how the health care facility will interact with the surrounding community and the local government

In summary, this document focuses on the essential processes of preparing for, responding to, recovering from, and mitigating against emergencies and disasters, as well as processes for requesting and receiving assistance.

Continuity of Operations Plan

A Continuity of Operations Plan (COOP) outlines steps that a health care facility will take in the event that a disaster interrupts business. This plan must be written before the disaster occurs and should be part of the hospital's preparedness initiative. Continuity plans require the facility to designate those functions that are considered essential and nonessential. Essential functions are those job duties that must be performed regardless of circumstances. Duties can be designated as essential, intermediate, or delayed.

A COOP is designed to ensure uninterrupted performance of essential functions during a broad array of disruptions or disasters. It provides a strategic framework for health care leadership, department directors, and personnel to follow when the infrastructure of the health care system has been affected by an incident or disaster.[4]

The purpose of a COOP is to allow an organization to plan for continuation of essential functions and enable rapid response to any emergency situation. The COOP also documents:

- What will occur in a continuity situation
- How the plan will be implemented
- How quickly continuity actions must occur
- Where continuity operations will occur
- Who will participate in continuity operations

See Tables 3-3 and 3-4 for additional considerations when developing a COOP. If a disaster is protracted and working remotely is an option, the logistics of where and

TABLE 3-3	OTHER PLANS AND PROCEDURES FOR CONSIDERATION WHEN DEVELOPING A COOP

Alternate Care Sites (ATS)
Communication Failure Plan
Computer (IT) Failure or Downtime Plan
Decontamination
Emergency Credentialing Plan
Fatality Management Plan
Health Care Evacuation Plan
Hospital Surge
Infectious Disease Outbreak or Pandemic Plan
Mass Prophylaxis
Severe Weather Plan

TABLE 3-4	ELEMENTS FOR CONSIDERATION IN PLANS AND PROCEDURES

Interoperable communications
Bed and patient tracking
Resource allocation (human and durable)
Control access and lockdown
Memorandums of Agreement (MOAs), Memorandums of Understanding (MOUs), and contracts with vendors to contain "disaster language"
Work-from-home options
Disaster behavioral (mental) health and follow-up
Vulnerable populations

how to work remotely may be included in the plan. Considerations within a COOP can include how to communicate with staff, patients, visitors, and the community that "suspended services" have resumed and business is as usual.

A sample COOP template is available at FEMA's website.

Drills and Exercises

Disaster plans are of no help unless they are known to be effective. Other than during a disaster, organized drills are the only way to test a plan. Drills should not focus totally on patient treatment since, depending on the disaster, the facility may be extensively damaged and unable to provide adequate patient treatment. Disaster drills have been identified as a critical component of preparedness because they allow the health care facility to test response capabilities and plans in real time. Evaluation of these activities is essential to understand the strengths and weaknesses of an institution's disaster response.

Every disaster has its own unique characteristics. Therefore all disaster plans must be flexible and meet the needs of any disaster, regardless of size or type. A common mistake in creating disaster exercises or drills is to test only one area of the health care facility, such as the emergency department. Exercises or drills should be designed to stress the internal components of a health care system, including surgery, inpatient units, the blood bank, and specialty areas such as pediatrics and rehabilitation units. Each exercise, drill, or real incident will identify challenges, failures, or actions that need to be corrected.

Exercise and Drill Evaluation and After Action Reports and Improvement Plan. The Homeland Security Exercise and Evaluation Program (HSEEP) is a capabilities- and performance-based exercise program that provides standardized methodology and terminology for exercise design, development, conduct, evaluation, and improvement planning. This program is maintained by the Federal Emergency Management Agency's National Preparedness Directorate, Department of Homeland Security.[5]

HSEEP constitutes a national standard for all exercises. Through planned exercises, organizations can:

- Objectively assess their capabilities
- Identify strengths and areas for improvement
- Correct deficiencies
- Share information as appropriate prior to a real incident

HSEEP reflects lessons learned and best practices from existing exercise programs that can be adapted to the full spectrum of hazardous scenarios and incidents (e.g., natural disasters, terrorism, and technological disasters).[5] HSEEP is not intended to be the sole evaluation tool for disaster exercise and drill evaluation; other exercise evaluation tools are available on the Internet.

Types of Exercise Evaluations and After Action Reports and Improvement Plan

All evaluations or After Action Reports and Improvement Plans (AAR-IPs) follow the same general format. They involve the exchange of ideas and observations and focus on improving training, response to, and recovery from an incident. An AAR-IP can be formal or informal but is never meant to be punitive. It should be conducted in an open and nonthreatening manner so an accurate evaluation of the incident or exercise is obtained. Formal AAR-IPs:

- Require more resources
- Involve more detailed planning, coordination, logistical support, and supplies
- Require more time for facilitation and report preparation

The AAR-IP should follow an agenda. A facilitator guides the review discussion, using the four guiding questions to set up the "meat" of the discussion. These four guiding questions are:

- What didn't work?
- Why didn't it work?
- How can it be fixed?
- Who will be responsible to get it fixed or to implement the improvement process?

Following the AAR-IP session itself, a formal report with recommendations and actionable items is presented at a later date. The actions can be carried out and the improvements made by emergency department managers and the health care facility. Features of informal AAR-IPs include the following:

- They are usually conducted on-site immediately following an event, activity, or program and are often referred to as "hot washes."
- They require a lower level of preparation, planning, and time to complete.
- Implementation is carried out by those responsible for the activity.
- The discussion leader or facilitator can be identified beforehand or chosen by the team itself.
- As with a formal AAR, the standard format and questions guide the discussion.
- They provide instant feedback; ideas and solutions can immediately be put to use for future or similar application.[6]
- Session should begin and end with positive comments rewarding all participants for their hard work and dedication.

Training and Education

Educating health care personnel is imperative to successful planning, response, and recovery. Training provides health care first responders, leaders, and community officials with the knowledge, skills, and abilities needed to perform key tasks required by specific capabilities. Health care organizations need to include all staff in emergency management plans and processes and equipment and incident command training.

Command, Control, Communication (Incident Command): National Incident Management System

National Incident Management System (NIMS) is a comprehensive, national approach to incident management that is applicable at all jurisdictional levels and across functional disciplines. It is intended to:

- Be applicable across a full spectrum of potential incidents, hazards, and impacts, regardless of size, location, or complexity

- Improve coordination and cooperation between public and private entities in a variety of incident management activities
- Provide a common standard for overall incident management

NIMS provides an incident command system (ICS) that is a consistent nationwide framework and approach to enable government at all levels (federal, state, tribal, and local), the private sector, health care facilities, and nongovernmental organizations (NGOs) to work together to prepare for, prevent, respond to, recover from, and mitigate the effects of incidents regardless of the incident's cause, size, location, or complexity. Consistent application of NIMS lays the groundwork for efficient and effective responses, from a single agency fire response to a multiagency, multijurisdictional natural disaster or terrorism response.[7]

Hospital Incident Command System (HICS) is a methodology for using the ICS in a hospital or health care environment. It is an incident management system based on the ICS, which assists hospitals in improving their emergency management planning, response, and recovery capabilities for unplanned and planned events (see Fig. 3-3). HICS is consistent with ICS and the NIMS principles. HICS will strengthen hospital disaster preparedness activities in conjunction with community response agencies and allow hospitals to understand and implement the elements of the hospital-based NIMS guidelines. HICS is not a template hospital emergency management plan nor is it a hospital emergency operations plan.

Response

Response is the process of implementing appropriate actions *while* an emergency situation is unfolding. In short, responding means "doing what you planned to do." In contrast to most routine hospital emergencies, efficient response in disasters requires procedures for triage and casualty distribution.

The first step in responding to an incident is to recognize that an incident or something unusual is occurring. The RAIN acronym can assist in this first step of response.

RAIN
Recognize the hazard or threat
Avoid the hazard, contaminant, or injury
Isolate the hazard area
Notify the appropriate support

In any disaster the safety of all involved is the most important initial concern. Using an incident command system such as NIMS helps to maintain a safe health care

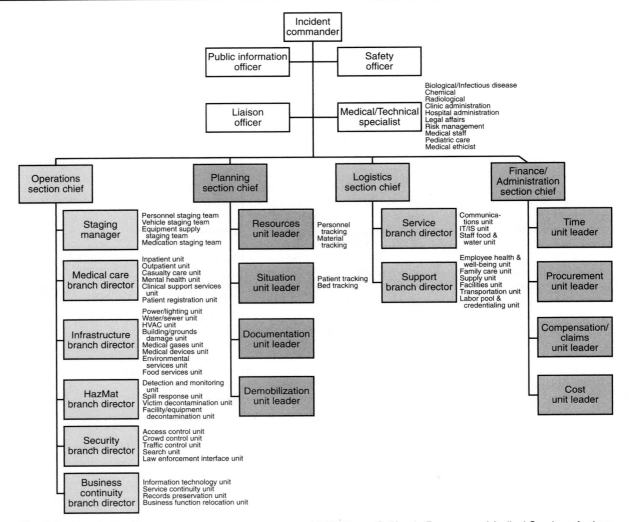

Fig. 3-3 Hospital incident management team structure: HICS. (From California Emergency Medical Services Authority. [2006, August]. *Hospital Incident Command System incident management team structure.* Retrieved from http://www.emsa.ca.gov/HICS/default.asp)

working environment during an incident. At times it may be unclear whether patients presenting to the emergency department are contaminated. A high index of suspicion will alert the health care team to potential contamination.

What Is Disaster Triage?

Traditionally, triage has been called the keystone to mass casualty management. The basic concept of disaster triage is *to do the greatest good for the greatest number of casualties,* and this involves more than just deciding who gets treated

first. It also requires maximum use of all available treatment resources. Casualties must be distributed rationally among the various hospitals and other medical treatment facilities. Generally, attention is given first to those with the most emergent conditions and those who are the most salvageable.[8] Typically, following a disaster, casualties are not distributed among the available hospitals in a rational or efficient manner. Instead, the majority of victims present to the closest hospital while other hospitals received no casualties at all. Recent world events such as Haiti's earthquake in January 2010 and Hurricane Katrina, which hit the U.S.

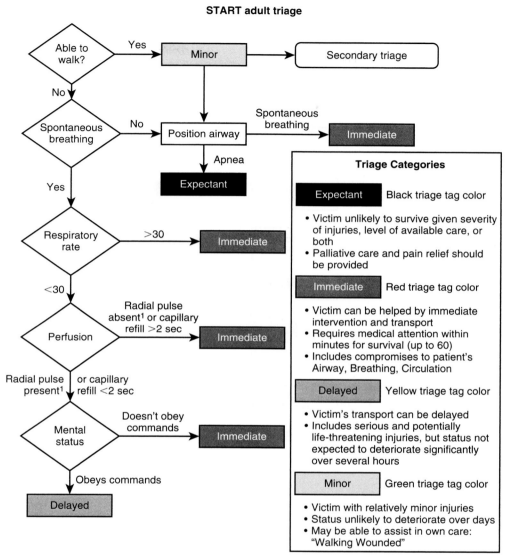

Fig. 3-4 START algorithm. (From U.S. Department of Health and Human Services. [2010, May 1]. *START algorithm.* Retrieved from http://www.remm.nlm.gov/startadult.htm)

Gulf Coast in 2005, illustrate the magnitude of the challenge of triaging casualties so as not to overwhelm one hospital or system.

Methods of Disaster Triage

START. Simple Triage and Rapid Transport (START) was developed in the 1980s in Orange County, California, as one of the first civilian triage systems.[9] This system (Fig. 3-4) was rapidly adopted across the United States and in

some international settings as well. The START triage system[10] involves:

- Making a rapid assessment (<1 minute) of every casualty
- Determining which of four categories the casualty should be assigned
- Visually identifying the categories by color coding

JumpSTART. Developed by a pediatric emergency physician in 1995, JumpSTART[11] is the first objective

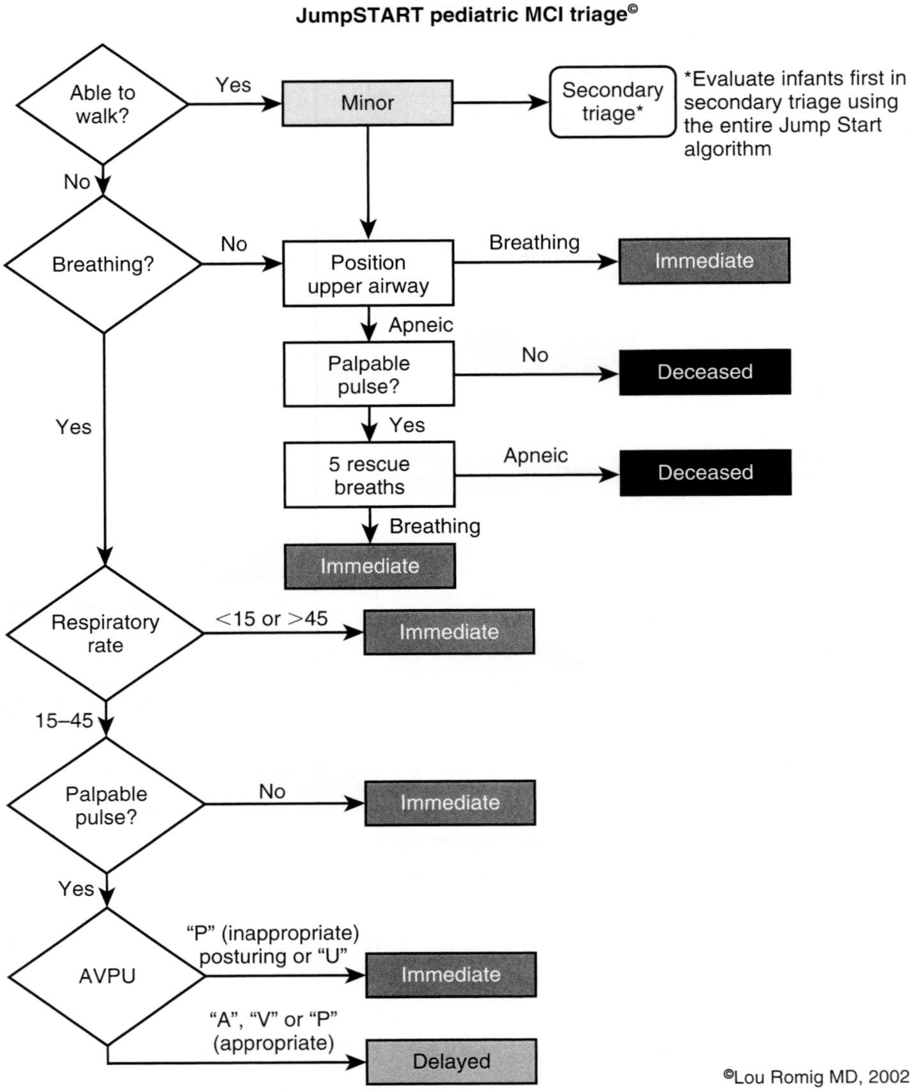

JumpSTART pediatric MCI triage©

Fig. 3-5 JumpSTART pediatric triage methodology. (Reproduced with permission from Lou Romig, MD.)

tool developed specifically for the triage of children in the multicasualty or disaster setting. Figure 3-5 shows the assessment algorithm used in JumpSTART triage.

SALT. SALT (Sort, Assess, Lifesaving Interventions, Treatment/Transport) disaster triage methodology was developed by the Centers for Disease Control and Prevention (CDC) in response to the lack of scientific data regarding the efficacy of mass casualty triage systems currently in existence. This methodology combines the best features of existing systems.[12] SALT includes a standardized naming and color-coding system to identify and prioritize patients'

medical needs, and was developed to be used to treat all types of patients (adult and pediatric) in all types of incidences (Fig. 3-6).

Multicasualty or disaster triage systems allow for lifesaving rapid assessment and interventions during the initial triage process. Mass casualty triage is a critical skill; although most hospitals use the START and JumpSTART approach, a single disaster triage methodology has yet to be adopted. Many recent studies have been conducted looking at the scientific evidence to identify one method that is most reliable and effective as well as simple to use.[13]

SALT mass casualty triage

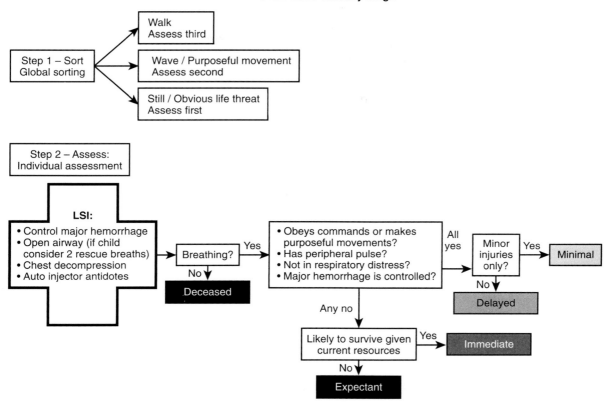

Fig. 3-6   SALT triage. (Lerner, E. B., Schwartz, R. B., Coule, P. L., & Pirrallo, R. G. [2010]. Use of SALT triage in a simulated mass-casualty incident. *Prehospital Emergency Care, 14*[1], 21–25.)

After triage, the next step in disaster response is to provide care to the injured and ill. The type of care is dependent on the agent or agents involved in the incident. A multivehicle crash may include polytrauma and possible chemical exposure to vehicle fuels or container contents (as in the case of a fuel truck carrying hazardous material). Other disasters may result from a chemical, biological, or radiological agent and include trauma from an explosive mechanism used as a dispersal device. Disasters also can result from disease outbreaks.

Disasters Resulting from Bioterrorism

Many possible agents can be the causative factor of one or many patients presenting with illness or injury. Determining whether there is malicious intent or even a terrorist nexus is the responsibility of law enforcement. However, health care workers can provide vital information to law enforcement personnel, as the patient is often an evidentiary piece of a criminal case. Recognizing and reporting something out of the norm is the health care provider's first task in identifying a potential hazard or disaster.

Many agents may be the cause of a patient's illness or injury. Tables 3-5 and 3-6 outline the most common biological and chemical agents, signs and symptoms of their use, and their medical management or treatment.

Recovery

Psychological consequences of disasters are very real and experienced by all who are involved. Physical damage and destruction are hallmarks of many but not all disasters. Disease pandemics (e.g., H1N1 pandemic in 2009), bioterrorism (e.g., anthrax-contaminated letters in 2001), cyberterrorism, and incidents involving the release of a hazardous chemical or radiation may create notable disaster events without damage to physical structures. Whether or not there is physical damage, the number of persons affected psychologically is larger than the number sustaining

Text continued on page 35.

TABLE 3-5 BIOLOGICAL AGENTS USED IN BIOTERRORISM

DISEASE OR AGENT	DIAGNOSIS	INCUBATION	VACCINE	COMMENTS	SYMPTOMS	TREATMENT
Anthrax	Possible wide mediastinum on chest radiograph Bacteria in blood, skin lesions, discharges	1–6 days (up to 45 days)	Available: 0.5 mL at 0, 2, 4 weeks and 6, 12, and 18 months Yearly booster Not available to nonmilitary persons	Spores very stable and may remain viable for >40 years	Skin lesions of depressed black eschar surrounded by erythema and edema Fever Malaise Fatigue Cough Chest discomfort Dyspnea Followed by severe respiratory distress with stridor, cyanosis, and shock Death within 6–24 hours	Ciprofloxacin Doxycycline Chloramphenicol Cephalosporins
Botulism	Clinical serology or culture	1–5 days	Pentavalent antitoxin	Very dilute concentrations will produce clinical illness	Ptosis Weakness Dizziness Dry mouth Blurred vision Diplopia Dysphonia Flaccid paralysis Respiratory failure	Ventilatory assistance IV administration of pentavalent antitoxin
Brucellosis	Blood cultures Bone marrow culture Culture of discharges Paired blood specimens for measurement of antibodies	5–60 days	None	Complications include endocarditis and encephalitis	Irregular fever, chills, sweating Headaches Fatigue and profound weakness Arthralgias Myalgias Depression	Doxycycline Rifampin Ofloxacin
Cholera	Stool culture Based on clinical presentation	4 hours to 5 days	New vaccines available outside U.S.		Little or no fever Headache Vomiting Intestinal cramps Voluminous diarrhea Dehydration Hypovolemia Shock	Tetracycline/Bactrim Doxycycline Erythromycin/ ciprofloxacin Oral or IV hydration

Agent	Diagnosis	Time	Vaccine	Notes	Symptoms	Treatment
(Glanders)	Sputum cultures Miliary lesions on chest radiograph	10–14 days	None	Necrotizing pulmonary lesions possible	Fever Sweats Rigors Myalgia Photophobia Lacrimation Diarrhea Leukocytosis Pleuritic chest pain Pneumonia Splenomegaly	Sulfadiazine/doxycycline Rifampin/ciprofloxacin Trimethoprim/sulfamethoxazole
Plague	Nasal and sputum cultures Blood cultures PCR immunoassay Culture of lymph node aspirate	1–7 days 1–4 days for primary plague	Vaccine for bubonic plague only; not available to general public	Organism lives up to 1 year in soil and 270 days in live tissue	High fever and chills Headache Hemoptysis Toxemia Rapid progression to dyspnea, stridor, and cyanosis Death due to respiratory failure if not treated in 12–24 hours	Streptomycin is drug of choice Tetracycline Chloramphenicol
Tularemia	Blood culture Serology	1–14 days 3–5 days peak	Yes	Aerosolized will cause pneumonia Tetracycline used as prophylaxis	Local ulcer Lymphadenopathy Fever Malaise Headache Substernal pain Nonproductive cough Prostration	Streptomycin Gentamicin
Ricin toxin	Clinical presentation	Latent period of 8 hours Death in 36–72 hours	None	Made from castor beans	Weakness Fever Cough Pulmonary edema Severe respiratory distress Gastrointestinal hemorrhage	No effective medications Supportive measures only
Q fever	Serology testing by indirect IFA to detect antibodies to *Coxiella burnetii* bacteria	2–3 weeks	Investigational only	Tetracycline prophylaxis	Fever Cough Pleuritic chest pain Illness may last 2 days to 2 weeks	Tetracycline Doxycycline

Continued

TABLE 3-5 BIOLOGICAL AGENTS USED IN BIOTERRORISM—cont'd

DISEASE OR AGENT	DIAGNOSIS	INCUBATION	VACCINE	COMMENTS	SYMPTOMS	TREATMENT
Smallpox	Biopsy or smear of skin lesions	7–19 days	Available from health departments Give within 2–3 days of exposure	Can be confused with varicella	Malaise Fever and rigors Vomiting Headache Backache 2–3 days later, skin lesions change from macular to pustular vesicles	No effective medications Supportive measures only
Staphylococcus enterotoxin B	Normal chest radiograph	3–12 days	None	Use a protective mask	Sudden onset of chills, fever, headache Myalgia Nonproductive cough Shortness of breath Retrosternal chest pain	No effective medications Supportive measures only
T2 mycotoxins	Blood toxicology	Death in minutes, hours, or days	None	Referred to as "Yellow Rain" in Laos	Pruitis Vesicles Necrosis of skin lesions Nasal discharge Dyspnea, hemoptysis Death due to bone marrow collapse or hypotension, tachycardia, and hypothermia	No effective medications or antidote Supportive measures only
Anthropoid-borne encephalitis	Virus isolation IgM antibody in blood CSF for specific antigen testing Collect serum 2 weeks apart for antibody test	2–15 days Varies with virus	Available through CDC for high-risk laboratory workers	Weaponized in 1960	Sudden onset Malaise Fever, rigors Severe headache Nausea, vomiting Cough Recovery 1–2 weeks	No effective medications Supportive measures
Viral hemorrhagic fevers	Viral isolation	Varies with type of virus	Only for yellow fever	Infectious by aerosol or fomites	Febrile illnesses Petechiae and bleeding Hypotension and shock Vomiting, diarrhea Headaches Microvascular damage and increased vascular permeability	Support hemodynamic, hematologic, pulmonary, and neurologic manifestations regardless of agent

CDC, Centers for Disease Control and Prevention; *CSF,* cerebrospinal fluid; *IFA,* immunofluorescence assay; *IgM,* immunoglobin M; *IV,* intravenous; *PCR,* polymerase chain reaction.

TABLE 3-6   CHEMICAL AGENTS USED IN TERRORISM

AGENT	LATENT PERIOD	DECONTAMINATION FOLLOWING REMOVAL OF CLOTHING	ANTIDOTE	SYMPTOMS	MEDICAL MANAGEMENT	COMMENTS
Pulmonary						
DP (diphosgene) PS (chloropicrin) CL (chlorine)	Seconds	Fresh air Copious soap and water irrigation	None	Eye and airway irritation Dyspnea, chest tightness Delayed pulmonary edema	Termination of exposure Enforced rest Standard treatment of airway secretions, hypoxia, bronchospasms, and pulmonary edema Positive pressure ventilation	
Cyanide						
AC (hydrogen cyanide) CK (cyanogen chloride)	Seconds	Fresh air Copious soap and water irrigation	IV sodium nitrite and sodium thiosulfate	Seizures Respiratory arrest Cardiopulmonary arrest	100% oxygen Administer antidotes	Death due to cellular anoxia
Vesicants						
HDH (mustard)	Hours Persistent agent	Copious soap and water irrigation	None	Erythema and blisters Conjunctivitis Corneal opacity Upper airway damage Bone marrow stem cell suppression Gastrointestinal symptoms	Decontaminate immediately after exposure Symptomatic management of lesions Consider antibiotics for secondary infections	Assess for secondary lesions and leukopenia
L (lewisite)	Minutes Persistent agent	Copious soap and water irrigation	British anti-Lewisite	Immediate burning Wheal skin lesions Eye damage Airway damage Pulmonary edema	Decontaminate immediately after exposure Symptomatic management of lesions	Assess for acidosis, volume depletion, pseudo-membranes
CX (phosgene)	Seconds	Fresh air Copious soap and water irrigation	None	Erythema and blisters Conjunctivitis Corneal opacity Upper airway damage Bone marrow stem cell suppression Gastrointestinal symptoms	Restore fluid volume Administer O_2 Consider early intubation Steroids	Possible inflammation and hemorrhage of GI tract

TABLE 3-6 CHEMICAL AGENTS USED IN TERRORISM—cont'd

AGENT	LATENT PERIOD	DECONTAMINATION FOLLOWING REMOVAL OF CLOTHING	ANTIDOTE	SYMPTOMS	MEDICAL MANAGEMENT	COMMENTS
Nerve Agent GA (tabun) GB (sarin) GD (soman) GF VX	Seconds VX—persistent agent	Fresh air Copious soap and water irrigation	Atropine Pralidoxime chloride Diazepam	Miosis Rhinorrhea Copious secretions Shortness of breath Loss of consciousness Sweating Nausea and vomiting Convulsions Apnea Flaccid paralysis Shock Death	Suction Ventilatory and cardiac support	Nerve agents inhibit acetyl-cholinesterase and their effects are caused by the resulting excess acetylcholine
Incapacitating BZ (United States agent) Agent 15 (Iraq agent)	30 minutes to 24 hours	Removal of agent and clothing Copious soap and water irrigation	IV physostigmine (Use with caution because of side effects)	Combination of anticholinergic symptoms: CNS—"Mad as a hatter" Peripheral nervous system—"Dry as a bone, red as a beet, blind as a bat"	General supportive measures Fluid administration Monitor core temperature for hyperthermia	
Riot Control Agent CS (tear gas) CM (mace) Cr (British)	Seconds	Fresh air Copious soap and water irrigation	Soap and water for skin Water for eyes	Burning and pain of mucous membranes and skin on exposure Tearing of eyes Respiratory discomfort	Symptoms resolve in 15–30 minutes May use bronchodilators	Less than 1% of exposed people seek medical treatment

CNS, Central nervous system; *GI,* gastrointestinal; *IV,* intravenous; *O₂,* oxygen.

TABLE 3-7   NEEDS ASSESSMENT FOLLOWING A DISASTER EXPERIENCE

BEHAVIORAL	EMOTIONAL	PHYSICAL	COGNITIVE
Extreme disorientation	Acute stress reactions	Headaches	Inability to accept/cope with death of loved one(s)
Excessive drug, alcohol, or prescription drug use	Acute grief reactions	Stomachaches	Distressing dreams or nightmares
Isolation/withdrawal	Sadness, tearful	Sleep difficulties	Intrusive thoughts or images
High risk behavior	Irritability, anger	Difficulty eating	Difficulty concentrating
Regressive behavior	Feeling anxious, fearful	Worsening of health conditions	Difficulty remembering
Separation anxiety	Despair, hopeless	Fatigue/exhaustion	Difficulty making decisions
Violent behavior	Feelings of guilt or shame	Chronic agitation	Preoccupation with death/destruction
Maladaptive coping	Feeling emotionally numb, disconnected	Other	Other
Other	Other		

Data from U.S. Department of Veterans Affairs National Center for PTSD. (n.d.). *Appendix D: Provider worksheets.* Retrieved from http://www.ptsd.va.gov/professional/manuals/manual-pdf/pfa/PFA_Appx_DWorksheets.pdf

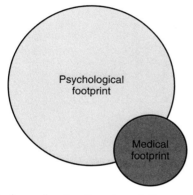

Fig. 3-7 In a disaster the size of the psychological footprint greatly exceeds the size of the medical footprint.

personal harm, damage to home, or loss of valued possessions. The psychological footprint is much larger than the medical footprint following a disaster (see Fig. 3-7).

Patients, families, and health care workers will experience psychological effects of a disaster. Table 3-7 lists signs and symptoms people may experience following a disaster and can be used as a brief assessment. Completing this assessment with disaster survivors and responders assists in establishing supportive needs and providing appropriate referral to various agencies.

REFERENCES

1. World Health Organization. (2010). *Appendix: Definition of terms.* Retrieved from http://www.wpro.who.int/NR/rdonlyres/4FAEFE0B-0194-40FC-A1F7-7BA9CC96F0CD/0/44finalDefinitions2010.pdf

2. The Joint Commission. (2010). *2011 hospital accreditation standards.* Oak Brook, IL: Joint Commission Resources.

3. Miami-Dade County Emergency Management and Homeland Security. (2008, June 30). *Ready, set, mitigated!* Retrieved from http://www.miamidade.gov/oem/library/completed_projects_manual_06-2008.pdf

4. Federal Emergency Management Agency. (2010, November 3). *IS-546.a – Continuity of operations awareness course.* Retrieved from http://training.fema.gov/EMIWeb/IS/IS546A.asp

5. Federal Emergency Management Agency. (n.d.). *Homeland security exercise and evaluation program (HSEEP).* Retrieved from http://hseep.dhs.gov/pages/1001_HSEEP7.aspx

6. United States Agency International Development. (2006, February). *After-action review technical guidance.* Retrieved from http://pdf.usaid.gov/pdf_docs/PNADF360.pdf

7. U.S. Department of Homeland Security. (n.d.). *National incident management system (NIMS) frequently asked questions.* Retrieved from http://www.fema.gov/pdf/emergency/nims/NIMSFAQs.pdf

8. Iserson, K. V., & Moskop, J. C. (2007). Triage in medicine, part 1: Concept, history, and types. *Annals of Emergency Medicine, 49*(3), 275–281.

9. Kahn, C. A., Schultz, C. H., Miller, K. T., & Anderson, C. L. (2009). Does START triage work? An outcomes assessment after a disaster. *Annals of Emergency Medicine, 54*(3), 424–430.

10. Hoag Hospital & Newport Beach Fire Department. (2001). *Simple triage and rapid treatment (START)—background.* Retrieved from http://www.citmt.org/start/background.htm

11. Romig, L. E. (2009, December 20). *The JumpSTART pediatric MCI triage tool.* Retrieved from http://www.jumpstarttriage.com/JumpSTART_and_MCI_Triage.php

12. Lerner, E. B., Schwartz, R. B., Coule, P. L., & Pirrallo, R. G. (2010). Use of SALT triage in a simulated mass-casualty incident. *Prehospital Emergency Care, 14*(1), 21–25.

13. Lerner, E. B., Schwartz, R. B., Phillip, L. C., Weinstein, E. S., Cone, D. C., Hunt, R. C., & O'Connor, R. E. (2008). Mass casualty triage: An evaluation of the data and development of a proposed national guideline. *Disaster Medicine and Public Health Preparedness, 2*(Suppl 1), S25–S34.

Patient Safety in the Emergency Department

Susan McDaniel Hohenhaus

Patient safety has become a major concern for clinicians, policy-makers, and health care consumers. This interest began to gain momentum in 1999 with the publication of the Institute of Medicine's (IOM's) report *To Err is Human: Building a Safer Health System.*[1] In its report the IOM highlighted the risks of medical care in the United States and provided information about the large numbers of medical error–related deaths per year, as well as other serious adverse events.[1] Yet 10 years later consumer groups warn that little progress has been made in the recommended areas of focus for improved safe medication practices, accountability through transparency, monitoring, coordinating and tracking of patient safety issues, and raising the standards of clinical competency.[2]

The goal of any emergency department is to provide safe, highly effective medical care that optimizes the use of information, people, and resources to achieve the best clinical outcomes. Despite these goals, in 2010, hospital emergency departments were the source of 4.4% of all reported hospital sentinel events and just over half of all reported sentinel event cases of patient death or permanent injury, especially events resulting in delays in treatment.[3] Of the 55 cases of delays in treatment, 52 resulted in patient death.[3] Commonly cited root causes include staffing, availability of physician specialists, and overcrowding.[3] However, these issues are being addressed. Emergency department teams are attacking overcrowding by focusing on social factors with community coalition-building to reduce the need for emergency department visits and to address the needs of a variety of patient populations.[4] There is an increased use of pharmacists in the emergency department for the purpose of enhancing medication safety.[5] In addition, the Emergency Nurses Association (ENA) has drawn attention to the issue of patient safety by the creation of both a white paper and a position statement regarding patient safety in the emergency department.[6,7]

WHAT IS PATIENT SAFETY?

The National Patient Safety Foundation (NPSF) defines patient safety as "the prevention of health care errors, and the elimination or mitigation of patient injury caused by health care errors."[8] NPSF defines health care error as the "unintended health care outcome caused by a defect in the delivery of care to a patient."[8] These errors may be "ones of commission (doing the wrong thing), omission (not doing the right thing), or execution (doing the right thing incorrectly)."[8]

"Quality" in health care has been defined as the "degree to which health services for individuals and populations increase the likelihood of desired health outcomes and are consistent with current professional knowledge."[9] Patient safety is a subset of quality that provides for "the *avoidance, prevention, and amelioration of adverse outcomes or injuries stemming from the processes of health care.*"[8] The Agency for Healthcare Research and Quality (AHRQ) describes *patient safety* practice as a type of process or structure whose application reduces the probability of adverse events resulting from exposure to the health care system across a range of diseases and procedures.[10]

BUILDING A CULTURE OF SAFETY

Involving the "Front Line"

In order to fully achieve a culture of safety in the emergency department, those who are working at the "front line," those providing direct care to the patients, must be involved and act as champions for improvement. It is unlikely that this will occur universally until there are major changes to the emergency nursing work environment, specifically by improving the organizational support that nurses need to provide safe care. Studies of work environments have found that nurses may experience greater professional fulfillment when strategies are implemented that promote autonomous practice environments, provide financial incentives, and recognize professional status.[11] Particular attention should be paid to safe staffing. Short staffing can increase nursing stress, increase workload, and ultimately may adversely affect patient outcomes.

Leadership Support

Nursing leaders should be involved, visible, and active in their support of patient safety. Methods that have proven successful to leadership engagement and support of safety include error reporting systems, root cause analyses of errors, culture surveys, and audits and surveillance. Feedback regarding any issues identified, including routine acknowledgment of best practices, should be provided to all employees. Once error reports are analyzed and contributing factors are identified, action that includes input from frontline staff should be discussed.

One promising intervention for emergency nursing leadership is the implementation of Patient Safety Leadership WalkRounds. WalkRounds have been shown to improve the safety culture of hospitals.[12] Leadership WalkRounds consist of a core group of senior leadership staff walking through the hospital on a weekly basis. During these rounds, members of the group ask frontline staff questions about their opinions and perceptions regarding near misses, adverse events, and system issues contributing to these events.

Unit-based patient safety rounds are a modification of these safety rounds. Implementation of safety walk-rounds led by the emergency department director, associate director, nurse director, clerical staff manager, and leaders of the Nurses' Quality Council in the pediatric emergency department at the Children's Hospital of Philadelphia resulted in an improvement in safety culture and quality of care.[13]

It is imperative that emergency nurse leaders model patient safety behaviors and skills. Good leadership is an essential ingredient in creating safe emergency departments. Emergency nurse leaders who focus attention on high-quality care and patient safety create a workplace where safety consciousness is the norm. Safe patient care practices should be promoted, encouraged, and rewarded. Those who violate safe patient care practices should be held accountable.

Technology

Technology can play an important role in the prevention of patient harm from medical error. However, in order for these strategies to be fully successful, there is a need for further standardization, universality, redundancy, and simplification of processes. There remains a significant need for the development of systems that seamlessly interact with one another, regardless of vendor origin.

Health information technology (HIT) has been suggested as a possible solution for reducing harm from medical error.[14] This may include:

- Electronic error reporting systems
- Electronic medical records
- Computerized prescriber order entry
- "Smart pump" technology
- Barcode-enabled point of care (BPOC) technology
- Standardized order sets[15]

> Further study is needed for the development and implementation of processes that decrease reliance on memory and promote the judicious use of technology.[20]

Teamwork and Communication

A key recommendation of the IOM is that health care organizations should establish "interdisciplinary team training programs for providers that incorporate proven methods of team training."[1]

Human factors research, studies of how human beings interact with their environment, has shown that even highly skilled, motivated professionals are vulnerable to error because of human limitations. However, promising research has also shown that clinicians who communicate effectively and back each other up reduce the potential for error, which results in enhanced safety and improved performance.[16]

It is important for emergency department staff to build teams using validated, evidence-based teamwork and communication programs. One such program, TeamSTEPPS, developed by the Department of Defense and supported by the AHRQ, offers techniques and tools gathered from high-reliability organizations and leveraging evidence from other high-consequence industries such as aviation and nuclear power that enhance communication and other teamwork skills. The TeamSTEPPS model includes four core "pillar" competency areas: leadership, situation monitoring, communication, and mutual support.[16] Team leadership sets the tone for a team, directs and coordinates activities, provides feedback through the assessment of team performance, and models team behaviors. Situation monitoring, the ability to scan the environment for threats and hazards, helps to coordinate the team to create a "shared mental model."[17] A mutually supportive environment is one in which it is expected that team members both offer and accept help and provide "back-up behavior" to balance workload. Communication includes standardized methods of exchanging critical and routine information regarding the patient and the health care team and environment.[16]

SYSTEM CHALLENGES

Two of the most daunting issues facing staff in the emergency department are crowding and prolonged wait times. To improve patient safety, quality, and efficiency and to reduce the effects of crowding and prolonged wait times, the emergency department *system* should be assessed, monitored, and modified. Best practices need to be further developed, shared, and replicated. Systems in the emergency department that most commonly affect the speed and efficiency of patient flow include:

* Adequate and competent staffing
* Laboratory and radiology turnaround times
* Flow of information
* Admission times from the emergency department

While there remains a need to assess and investigate the impact of hospital bed capacity on emergency department overcrowding, there is also a need to assess the system for variability in staff time and patient management.

Emergency department flow is also heavily influenced by the inability of patients to gain access to primary and other specialized care outside the hospital.[18] Streamlining patient flow through the emergency department is often hampered by the absence of broader health system reform. Public policy efforts to assist hospitals in this task would benefit from regular surveillance of hospital patient flow measures and other efficiency indicators.

Additionally, there is a need for further study of the impact on patient safety of novel approaches to emergency department patient flow. For example, the recent phenomenon of public reporting of emergency department wait times for the purpose of allowing patients to "choose" an emergency department based on shorter wait times should be carefully studied and monitored.

It is difficult to focus attention and resources on safe care when received with the mixed messages of production pressure. In the safety critical environment of the emergency department, nurses often must respond to the command to never compromise safety coupled with an admonishment to be productive while using limited resources.

PEDIATRIC SAFETY ISSUES

Most emergency departments are primarily built around the needs of adults. Many settings lack trained staff oriented to pediatric care, pediatric care protocols and safeguards, and up-to-date and easily accessible pediatric medication standards and reference materials. Emergency departments may be particularly risk-prone environments for children.[19]

> Children are at increased risk for medication errors because of:
> * Weight-based dosing
> * Medicine dilution
> * The decreased ability of the child to communicate his or her needs or responses

While there will never be a perfect process for the safe and effective emergency care of children, there is a need for the study, development, and implementation of simplified, standardized, redundant, and universal processes that decrease reliance on memory and promote the judicious use of technology.[20]

> **Pediatric Medication Safety Recommendations[23,26]**
> * Limit the number of medication concentrations and dose strengths.
> * Provide standardized instructions for home care, discussed and verified with adult caregivers before patient discharge.
> * Use only oral syringes to administer oral medications to prevent inadvertent intravenous administration of oral medications.

Emergency nurses can promote the development and use of standardized protocols and checklists. Current dosing tools need more human factors study.[20] Best practice and evidence-based dosing and administration guidelines should be evaluated and widely disseminated and used.

A "JUST CULTURE"

The phrase "just culture" was first coined by David Marx. According to Marx, the principles for achieving a culture in which frontline personnel feel empowered to report errors is critically important.[21]

For example, nursing practice and education has long focused on the "five rights" as the method for ensuring safe medication practices: the right medication, at the right dose, at the right time, by the right route, to the right patient. While no one argues that these "rights" are important to patient safety, the method's success does not rest solely with nursing. In fact, the nurse who is administering the drug often has little or no control over much of the process, reinforcing the traditional, though inappropriate, focus on individual performance rather than on system improvement.[22] Furthermore, safe medication practices are a culmination of multidisciplinary efforts where responsibility for accurate drug administration lies with multiple individuals and reliable systems to support safe medication use.[22]

DISRUPTIVE BEHAVIOR

Disruptive behavior is behavior that shows disrespect for others, or any interpersonal interaction that impedes or threatens the safe delivery of patient care. Two elements important for the creation of a safe culture, teamwork across disciplines and a just culture environment for discussing safety issues, are negatively affected by disruptive behavior. The seriousness of this issue is underscored by a Joint Commission sentinel event alert,[23] which calls attention to this problem and states that "Intimidating and disruptive behaviors can foster medical errors, contribute to poor patient satisfaction and preventable adverse outcomes, increase the cost of care, and cause qualified clinicians, administrators, and managers to seek new positions in more professional environments. Safety and quality of patient care is dependent on teamwork, communication, and a collaborative work environment. To assure quality and to promote a culture of safety, health care organizations must address the problem of behaviors that threaten the performance of the health care team."[23]

It is important to note that disruptive behaviors are not limited to physicians, although an abundance of literature documents abusive physician behavior. Disruptive behavior has also been documented to occur with regularity among nurses and other health care professionals.[24,25]

The Joint Commission recommendations for addressing disruptive behavior include the development of an organizational process for addressing intimidating and disruptive behaviors from an interprofessional team including representation of medical and nursing staff, administrators, and other employees; the provision of skills-based training and coaching in relationship-building and collaborative practice, including skills for giving feedback on unprofessional behavior and conflict resolution; and the development and implementation of a reporting and surveillance system for detecting unprofessional behavior.[23] See Chapter 2, Workplace Violence and Disruptive Behavior, for more information.

REPORTING MEDICAL ERRORS

The IOM's *To Err Is Human* has recommended the development of both mandatory and voluntary systems for reporting medical errors.[1] This recommendation was made as part of a comprehensive strategy to improve patient safety by creating an environment that encourages organizations to identify errors, evaluate causes, and take appropriate action to improve performance. Errors, whether or not they result in patient harm, should be reported, tracked, and prevented from recurring. In order to learn from past medical errors and prevent future harm to patients in the emergency department, there must be a standardized method for reporting that encourages easy access as well as freedom from fear of reprisal for reporting. Emergency nurse leaders should also ensure that feedback about what has been changed in light of the report is important. This validates the reporter's concerns and encourages other reporters to come forward when issues are identified. In one study of emergency nurses and error reporting, researchers discovered that nurses felt they had not been provided with appropriate education and training regarding error reporting, even when reporting was mandatory.[20] Fundamental questions, such as what information should be reported to improve patient safety and to whom it should be reported, should be answered and disseminated. Formal, standardized training should be developed and provided so that emergency nurses understand not only their obligation to report medical error but also the process by which to do so.

RESOURCES

Several organizations and agencies are available to emergency nurses for the purpose of recommendations and resources needed to enhance the safety of patients in the emergency department.

- *Medication Safety:* Institute for Safe Mediation Practices (ISMP) (http://www.ismp.org)
- *Just Culture:* Outcome Engineering/Just Culture Community (http://www.justculture.org)
- *Teamwork and Communication:* TeamSTEPPS (http://teamstepps.ahrq.gov)
- *Disruptive Behavior:* Joint Commission Sentinel Event Alert #40 (http://www.jointcommission.org/sentinel_event.aspx)

REFERENCES

1. Institute of Medicine. (2000). *To err is human: Building a safer health system.* Washington, D.C.: National Academies Press.
2. Consumer's Union. (2009, May). *To err is human—To delay is deadly.* Retrieved from http://www.safepatientproject.org/safepatientproject.org/pdf/safepatientproject.org-ToDelayIsDeadly.pdf
3. The Joint Commission. (n.d.). *Sentinel event.* Retrieved from http://www.jointcommission.org/assets/1/18/Stats_with_all_fields_hidden30September2010_%282%29.pdf
4. Institute for Healthcare Improvement. (n.d.). *Emergency department flow.* Retrieved from http://www.ihi.org/IHI/Topics/Flow/EmergencyDepartment/
5. Randolph, T. C. (2009). Expansion of pharmacists' responsibilities in an emergency department. *American Journal of Health-System Pharmacy, 66*(16), 1484–1487.
6. Emergency Nurses Association. (2010). *Patient safety in the emergency department* [position statement]. Retrieved from

http://www.ena.org/SiteCollectionDocuments/Position%20Statements/PatientSafety.pdf

7. Emergency Nurses Association. (2005). *Patient safety in the emergency department [white paper].* Des Plaines, IL: Author.

8. National Patient Safety Foundation. (n.d.). *About us: Our definitions.* Retrieved from http://www.npsf.org/au/

9. Committee to Design a Strategy for Quality Review and Assurance in Medicine & Institute of Medicine. (1990). *Medicare: a strategy for quality assurance* (Vol. 1). Washington, D.C.: National Academy Press.

10. Agency for Healthcare Research and Quality. (2001, July). *Making health care safer: A critical analysis of patient safety practices* (AHRQ Publication No. 01-E057). Rockville, MD: Author. Retrieved from http://archive.ahrq.gov/clinic/ptsafety/summary.htm

11. MacDavitt, K., Chou, S. S., & Stone, P. W. (2007). Organizational climate and health care outcomes. *Joint Commission Journal on Quality and Patient Safety, 22*(11 Suppl), 45–56.

12. Frankel, A., Graydon-Baker, E., Neppl, C., Simmonds, T., Gustafson, M., & Gandhi, T. K. (2003). Patient safety leadership WalkRounds. *Joint Commission Journal on Quality and Patient Safety, 29*(1), 16–26.

13. Shaw, K. N., Lavelle, J., Crescenzo, K., Noll, J., Bonalumi, N., & Baren, J. (2006). Creating unit-based patient safety walk-rounds in a pediatric emergency department. *Clinical Pediatric Emergency Medicine, 7,* 231–237.

14. Bates, D. W., Evans, S., Murff, H., Steston, P. D., Pizziferri, L., & Hripcsak, G. (2003). Detecting adverse events using information technology. *Journal of the American Medical Informatics Association, 10*(2), 115–128.

15. Institute for Safe Medication Practices. (2010, March 11). *ISMP develops guidelines.* Retrieved from http://www.ismp.org/newsletters/acutecare/articles/20100311.asp

16. Clancy, C. M., & Tornberg, D. N. (2006). *TeamSTEPPS: Integrating teamwork principles into healthcare practice.* Retrieved from http://www.psqh.com/novdec06/ahrq.html

17. Salisbury, M., & Hohenhaus, S. M. (2008). Know the plan, share the plan, review the risks: A method of structured communication for the emergency care setting. *Journal of Emergency Nursing, 34*(1), 46–48.

18. Burt, C., & McCaig, L. F. (2006). Staffing, capacity, and ambulance diversion in emergency departments: United States, 2003–04. *Advance Data,* Sept. *27*(376), 1–23.

19. Institute of Medicine. (2007). *Emergency care for children: Growing pains.* Washington, D.C.: National Academy Press.

20. Hohenhaus, S. M. (2008). Emergency nursing and medical error—a survey of two states. *Journal of Emergency Nursing, 34*(1), 20–25.

21. Marx, D. (2001, April 17). *Patient safety and the "just culture": A primer for health care executives.* Retrieved from http://www.mers-tm.org/support/Marx_Primer.pdf

22. Institute for Safe Medication Practices. (1999, April 7). *The "five rights."* Retrieved from http://www.ismp.org/Newsletters/acutecare/articles/19990407.asp

23. The Joint Commission. (2008, April 11). *Sentinel Event Alert: Preventing pediatric medication errors.* Retrieved from http://www.jointcommission.org/assets/1/18/SEA_39.PDF

24. Institute for Safe Medication Practices. (2003). *Results from ISMP survey on workplace intimidation.* Retrieved from http://www.ismp.org/Survey/surveyresults/Survey0311.asp

25. Rosenstein, A. H., & O'Daniel, M. (2005). Disruptive behavior and clinical outcomes: Perceptions of nurses and physicians. *American Journal of Nursing, 105*(1), 54–64.

26. Institute for Safe Medication Practices. (2000, April 19). *Hospital survey shows much more needs to be done to protect pediatric patients from medication errors.* Retrieved from http://www.ismp.org/newsletters/acutecare/articles/20000419.asp

Ethical Dilemmas in Emergency Nursing

Bernard Heilicser

Ethics are what a person's conduct and actions *should be* with regard to self, other human beings, and the environment. Ethics does not necessarily represent what is actually happening or what the law demands.

Ethical dilemmas arise as emergency nurses are often placed in situations where they are expected to be simultaneously agents or advocates for patients, physicians, and the organization. They may have conflicting needs, wants, and goals, as well as different personal ethical beliefs. How the emergency nurse handles these situations affects patient care and the nurse's moral satisfaction.

Emergency nurses sometimes need to choose among the available, but less than ideal, options. Using a systematic approach and available ethical tools will help nurses make better ethical decisions and feel confident about them.

> Conflicts between the medical provider and the patient or family, within the family, or between medical providers often signal an ethical dilemma.

ETHICAL FRAMEWORKS FOR DECISION MAKING[1,2]

Ethical frameworks assist in clarifying values and beliefs. Table 5-1 lists some of the most common ethical frameworks used in decision making.

PRINCIPLES[1-3]

The most fundamental ethical principle is respect for all people. Major ethical principles stem from this concept. They include the following:

- Autonomy: self-determination or freedom of choice
  - The patient may make a decision that is contrary to prudent medical treatment but, if done with full decision-making capacity, it is the patient's right.
- Beneficence: promote good
  - Nurses desire to do what is believed to be in the patient's best interest. The dilemma occurs when it conflicts with patient autonomy. Professionalism is working with the patient to achieve a compromise or balance rather than erecting a barrier. Improved patient care will result from this compromise.
  - Included in the principle of beneficence is paternalism. Paternalism exists when one individual believes that he or she knows what is best and attempts to influence decision making for another. This occurs when the health care professional does not give full regard to a patient's wishes (e.g., advanced directives).
- Nonmaleficence: do no harm
  - Hippocrates first declared it: do not interfere with normal healing processes nor impose individual beliefs on the patient. Withholding or withdrawing life support is included in this principle.
- Justice: fairness
  - The uninsured patient has as much right to the same treatment as the chief executive officer of the hospital. Adhering to this principle demonstrates humanity and professionalism. However, circumstances and triage decisions in the emergency department can certainly challenge the nurse's ability to do the same for everyone.
- Utility: good of many outweighs the wants and needs of the individual

TABLE 5-1 ETHICAL FRAMEWORKS

FRAMEWORK	BASIC PREMISE	EXAMPLE
Utilitarian	Provide the greatest good for the greatest number of people	Disaster scenario
Rights-based	Individuals share basic inherent rights that should not be interfered with	Right to refuse
Duty-based	A duty to do something or to refrain from doing something	Nurse does not scream back when a patient is yelling at the nurse
Intuitionist	Each case weighted on a case-by-case basis to determine relative goals, duties, and rights	Should a patient with severe lung disease be put on a mechanical ventilator when there is little chance of successful weaning?

- An infection-control measure that isolates a patient is one example of utility. Paternalism and utility are often related in cases when an individual's right must be restricted.
- Veracity: truth telling
  - The truth should be told, or a good reason should exist to present a deception. Hellen describes the role for a "therapeutic fib" in caring for Alzheimer's patients.[4] For instance, the nurse might tell an elderly woman with Alzheimer's who insists on "feeding her baby" that the baby has been fed since the woman is incapable of comprehending and processing the truth (e.g., that her babies are grown up).[4]
  - Truth telling also encompasses admitting a medical error. Although there is an instant fear of medical liability when an error occurs, an obligation to be honest with the patient exists. A patient or family, upon learning of a medical error that has not been disclosed, will certainly be more apt to pursue medical-legal redress than if honest disclosure of human error is revealed.[5] Additionally, a patient who is left unaware of a mistake may be in greater clinical jeopardy when future symptoms or complication occur or when significant decisions become necessary. An example is a patient who received an inappropriate dose of anticoagulant medication and then has a bleeding episode and attributes this to something else, potentially requiring unneeded, dangerous medical procedures.
- Fidelity: keeping promises, loyalty, and accountability
  - The focus of fidelity is the importance of honoring commitments. If there is conflict between multiple fidelity duties, the American Nurses Association's (ANA) Code of Ethics indicates that the primary commitment is to the patient.[6]

One study of nurse practitioners found that the most frequent ethical issue encountered was patient refusal of appropriate treatment with a conflict between patient autonomy and beneficence.[9]

CODE OF ETHICS

Professional codes of ethics do not have the power of law; however, they do provide a guide for nursing practice, providing implicit standards and values for the profession. ANA's Code of Ethics has existed since 1950. The current 2001 edition includes the following concepts[6]:

- Specifically indicating that the most fundamental accountability is to the patient
- Assuring that the workplace is safe
- Addressing duty to self

Table 5-2 lists the provision statements guiding the nursing practice in the ANA's Code of Ethics.

Other nursing associations, such as the Canadian Nurses Association and the International Council of Nurses, have also adopted ethic codes to help guide ethical decisions.

DECISION MAKING

Various processes can be used in determining an ethical decision.

The Traditional Problem-Solving Process

- Define objectives clearly.
- Gather data carefully.
- Generate many alternatives.
- Think logically.
- Choose and act decisively.

Data should be taken in context and be evidence-based. Understanding why something is appropriate and how it came into practice helps contribute to better application. A common error is not considering enough alternatives. As a

TABLE 5-2   ANA CODE OF ETHICS PROVISIONS

1. The nurse, in all professional relationships, practices with compassion and respect for the inherent dignity, worth, and uniqueness of every individual, unrestricted by consideration of social or economic status, personal attributes, or the nature of health problems.
2. The nurse's primary commitment is to the patient, whether an individual, family, group, or community.
3. The nurse promotes, advocates for, and strives to protect the health, safety, and rights of the patient.
4. The nurse is responsible and accountable for individual nursing practice and determines the appropriate delegation of tasks consistent with the nurse's obligation to provide optimum patient care.
5. The nurse owes the same duties to self as to others, including the responsibility to preserve integrity and safety, to maintain competence, and to continue personal and professional growth.
6. The nurse participates in establishing, maintaining, and improving health care environments and conditions of employment conducive to the provision of quality health care and consistent with the values of the profession through individual and collective action.
7. The nurse participates in the advancement of the profession through contributions to practice, education, administration, and knowledge development.
8. The nurse collaborates with other health professionals and the public in promoting community, national, and international efforts to meet health needs.
9. The profession of nursing, as represented by associations and their members, is responsible for articulating nursing values, for maintaining the integrity of the profession and its practice, and for shaping social policy.

Reproduced with permission of the American Nurses Association.
American Nurses Association. (2001). *Code of ethics for nurses with interpretive statements.* Washington, DC: American Nurses Publishing.

whole, the more alternatives that can be generated, the more likelihood there is that the final decision will be sound.

The Nursing Process

- Assess.
- Analyze and diagnose.
- Plan.
- Implement.
- Evaluate.

The MORAL Process[7]

- **Massage** the dilemma. Collect data about the problem and who should be involved.
- **Outline** options. Identify alternatives and analyze the causes and consequences.
- **Review** criteria and resolve. Weigh the options against the values of those involved in the decision.
- **Affirm** position and act.
- **Look** back. Evaluate the decision.

Ethics Committees

Hospitals are required to have a process to resolve medical-ethical dilemmas within their institution. The ethics committee, or an ethics consultant, should be readily available to the emergency nurse when such a dilemma exists.

Institutional Review Boards

Institutional review boards are primarily formed to protect research subjects according to the ethical principles articulated by the National Commission for the Protection of Human Subjects of Biomedical and Behavioral Research. There is a trend toward more ethical oversight of any project that collects data; use of institutional review boards has been encouraged for this purpose.[8]

SPECIFIC SITUATIONS

Advance Directives

Individuals have the right to indicate in advance what medical treatment they do or do not want in the event that they are unable to make those decisions at the time. This conversation and discussion should be encouraged.

- Power of attorney for health care: The individual approves an agent who is empowered to make all medical decisions for that person when he or she cannot (e.g., lacks decision-making capacity). The agent can be anyone of the patient's choosing.
- Living will: A popular although not as comprehensive document, it tells the medical providers what the patient wants to happen in the event that he or she has no hope for a meaningful survival. This differs from the power of attorney for health care in that the prognosis must essentially be without hope. If that prognosis is not documented, the living will does not come into play.
- Health Care Surrogate Act: When a patient does not have an advance directive, a state's Health Care Surrogate Act can be invoked. It prescribes a specific surrogacy order for medical decision making. Generally a legal guardian has primary standing, followed by spouse, children, siblings, etc.

The advance directive or designated agent for the patient overrides other family members' wishes and should be honored. If family members challenge the current decisions (e.g., believe the decisions are being made for financial gain), they can go to court to seek guardianship.

> Before any advance directive is in effect, the patient must lack decision-making capacity. Always make a careful determination regarding the patient's decision-making capacity. Patients have that autonomous right.

Do Not Resuscitate

Cardiopulmonary resuscitation (CPR) is one of the few aggressive medical treatments that is presumed, and would be performed, in the event of a cardiopulmonary arrest. To avoid this modality, an individual may refuse this in advance. Indicating a desire to avoid CPR is a right and may be requested by anyone with decision-making capacity at any time. Some issues include:

- A patient is identified as Do Not Resuscitate (DNR) but documentation is inadequate, incomplete, or absent. When this occurs, health care providers are obligated to treat the patient and CPR should not be withheld. Consequently, good communication between patients and their health care providers is essential to avoid any conflict.
- A patient with a poor prognosis still wants a full resuscitation. Although this can be very frustrating for the emergency nurse, patients have autonomous rights and this desire should be honored. Health care providers should not impose their judgment regarding quality of life on a situation.

Informed Consent or Refusal

Proper consent involves many aspects. Does the adult or emancipated patient:

- Understand the proposed course of treatment, its benefits, and its risks?
- Understand the alternative treatment, its benefits, and its risks?
- Understand the consequences of no treatment?
- Have a value system to appreciate what is happening?
- Have the ability to make a decision without coercion from family or friends?

The discussion of this information is best provided by the person who is going to perform the medical treatment. The nurse's responsibility is only *to witness* the consent process. The same criteria should be applied and well documented when a patient refuses a medical recommendation.

Leaving Against Medical Advice or Leaving Without Treatment

Regardless of the patient's behavior or appearance, it must be determined objectively whether the patient can make decisions. Competency is a judicial determination, but decision-making capacity is a medical determination. The most important aspect is not a signature on the paper but that the patient fully understands the ramifications of the action. Does the patient (who is not a minor):

- Demonstrate he or she is alert and fully aware of his or her condition?
- Understand the risks of his or her refusal, including potential complications and side effects?
- Repeat back the understanding of these consequences?
- Have a safe environment to which he or she is going?

An honest effort should be made to convince the patient to do what is in his or her best interest. To preclude abandonment, patients should be encouraged to return to the emergency department or seek medical attention if they change their minds. Appropriate follow-up information should still be provided. This entire process should be fully and specifically documented and witnessed.

Confidentiality

A primary responsibility in patient care is to respect a patient's confidentially. The trust of a patient is predicated on this. The emergency department is often a chaotic environment; although difficult, all health care providers must be cognizant of the patient's confidentiality. Conversations with patients or families and among staff should not be conducted within earshot of others. Additionally, only individuals relevant to the patient's care should be privy to this information. The patient has the right to choose with whom they want information shared and this choice should be honored.

Treating Minors

There is often controversy when a minor presents for emergency care, especially in the following instances:

- Unaccompanied minor presents to the emergency department
- A parent or guardian refuses treatment

This dilemma is easily resolved by determining what is in the child's best interest and whether it would constitute neglect or abuse to do otherwise. An unaccompanied minor should be treated if his or her medical condition necessitates emergency intervention or pain control. Assessment and stabilization is indicated. When the parent arrives, treatment can be explained with a concerned approach. If the parent would have refused treatment, this would have constituted neglect or abuse and the patient would have been treated anyway. Waiting for parental consent at the jeopardy of the child is inappropriate.

If a child presents with the parent and essential medical care is refused (e.g., lumbar puncture for suspected meningitis or refusal of insulin on religious grounds), protective custody of the child is indicated. Adults have autonomous rights, but these cannot be imposed on a child.

There are circumstances where a minor may consent to treatment. This usually relates to a presentation for treatment of a sexually transmitted infection, alcohol or drug problem, or psychiatric disorder. State-specific laws apply. An emancipated minor is also subject to state legislation. Often an individual under the age of 18 years who is a parent, married, or living independently may be emancipated.

Triage

Triage in the emergency department can be most challenging for the emergency nurse. Questions that affect triage in the emergency department include:

- Who gets seen first?
- Who gets the last intensive care bed?
- What if resources are limited?
- Is a mass casualty different?

The normal paradigm in emergency medicine calls for rendering treatment to the most critical patient. This is followed by the noncritical patient and then by the stable or nonemergent patient, essentially the red, yellow, green triage pattern. See Chapter 7, Triage, for a more detailed discussion.

An ethical challenge occurs when a more critical but less desirable patient is competing for care with, perhaps, his or her victim. Ethical medical professionals ought to treat the more critical patient first and not make individual value judgments at the bedside.

In a similar manner, priority for inpatient admission should be based on medical assessment and need. Presumed human value should not be a criterion.

When medical resources are limited, treatment decisions are complex. Again, who can be best served by the health care provider's abilities and capabilities? A mass casualty incident (MCI) demonstrates this dilemma. During an MCI, the treatment paradigm is reversed. Doing the greatest good for the greater number may be in opposition to treating the most critical patient. If supplies and staff cannot fully meet the needs of the entire patient population, profound decisions as how best to focus responses must be made. Where nurses would normally attempt a comprehensive resuscitation, the resources required for this may deprive many others, putting their survival in jeopardy. This is best exemplified in a response to a major environmental catastrophe.

Telephone calls to the emergency department present a different set of ethical issues. Many patients call the emergency department for various, and sometimes interesting, concerns. How these calls are handled certainly provides an opportunity for education, comfort, and even lifesaving advice. Responses to simple questions that do not offer medical advice (e.g., how often to take a prescribed medication or explanation of a medical term) represent good community relations. Reassurance to a frightened parent can be most beneficial. Instructing a caller to call 911 (or obtaining the information and doing it yourself) can prevent a catastrophe. However, the altruistic desire to give medical advice can be dangerous and should be avoided. The patient is not in front of the health care provider. Nurses should instruct callers to come to the emergency department if medical help is the answer. The medical-legal ramifications of inaccurate telephone information or advice can be devastating.

REFLECTION: HANDLING DIFFICULTIES WITH INTEGRITY AND ETHICS

Adhering to ethical principles, even with "difficult" patients, affirms an emergency nurse's humanity and professionalism. Overcrowding, staffing issues, and other difficulties of the emergency department that often cannot be solved by nurses can add stress that may compromise decision making. To maintain ethical decision making, nurses should keep the following in mind:

- People should be treated as patients, not as customers.
- A frequent visitor to the emergency department may eventually experience a terminal event, so he or she should be treated with the same respect and care as a first-time patient.
- Every patient is a human being looking for help.
- Decisions should be based on patients' needs.
- Ethical decisions should be made by considering:
  - Will you be able to look at yourself in the mirror in the morning?
  - How relevant will your decision be in 5 years?
  - What would your mother tell you to do?
- Remember why you decided to become a nurse.

An emergency nurse can stay engaged in this profession with his or her conscience intact by knowing that the right steps were taken for a patient when presented with an ethical dilemma.

REFERENCES

1. Marquis, B. L., & Huston, C. J. (2009). Ethical issues. In *Leadership roles and management functions in nursing: Theory and application* (6th ed., pp. 69–92). Philadelphia, PA: Lippincott, Williams & Wilkins.

2. Heilicser, B. (2006). Ethics. In P. G. Zimmermann & R. D. Herr (Eds.), *Triage nursing secrets.* St. Louis, MO: Mosby.

3. Beauchamp, T., & Childress, J. (2008). *Principles of biomedical ethics* (6th ed.). New York, NY: Oxford University Press.

4. Hellen, C. (1998). *Alzheimer's disease: Activity-focused care* (2nd ed.). Burlington, MA: Butterworth Heinemann.

5. Kachalia, A., Kaufman, S. R., Boothman, R., Anderson, S., Welch, K., Saint, S., & Rogers, M. A. (2010). Liability claims and costs before and after implementation of a medical error disclosure program. *Annals of Internal Medicine, 153*(4), 213–221.

6. American Nurses Association. (2001). *Code of ethics for nurses with interpretive statements.* Washington, DC: American Nurses Publishing.

7. Crisham, P. (1985). MORAL: How can I do what is right? *Nursing Management, 16*(3), 42A–442N.

8. Foss, G. F. (2005). Modifications of graduate public/community health nursing internships to facilitate compliance with Institutional Review Board and Health Insurance Portability and Accountability Act (HIPAA) regulations. *Public Health Nursing, 22*(2), 172–179.

9. Laabs, C. A. (2005). Moral problems and distress among nurse practitioners in primary care. *Journal of the American Academy of Nurse Practitioners, 17*(2), 76–84.

6

Forensics

Jeanne Eckes-Roper

The Chinese symbol for "truth" bears the meaning of the body of real things, events, and facts. Forensics is the use of scientific tests or techniques in the investigation of crimes to arrive at the truth. The assessments and clinical evaluations conducted by emergency and trauma practitioners' assessments and clinical evaluations play a pivotal role in seeking the truth when managing forensic evidence.

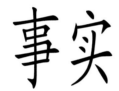

Chinese Symbol of Truth

Violence has become a public health problem because traumatic death or near-death situations affect millions of American citizens each year. Health care professionals share the responsibility, with their law enforcement partners and other legal entities, for responding to the needs of crime victims. This includes not only caring for the patient, but also understanding, preserving, and protecting any forensic evidence that may be present. Emergency and trauma personnel regularly interact with law enforcement agencies, crime scene technicians, medical examiner death investigators, and forensic pathologists. Collaboration among these professionals is essential as it relates to the collection and preservation of clinical physical evidence.

The primary responsibility for collection and preservation of forensic evidence remains with the criminalists and investigating law enforcement agency, however, emergency and trauma personnel frequently assist in this process. The emergency nurse can be the first to recognize the presence of forensic evidence on a patient, which could serve as a vital piece of evidence relevant to a criminal investigation. When a victim presents as a critically injured or ill patient, the need for emergent lifesaving treatment is a priority and the collection of forensic evidence is often lost. Understanding basic forensic principles and incorporating these guidelines as part of current practice in the emergency department is critical and can influence future medical-legal cases.

Many popular television shows dramatize crime scene investigations; however, these depictions are meant to entertain or intrigue viewers rather than portray actual forensic procedures.

BASICS OF FORENSICS

Forensics pertains to the law and more specifically to the scientific analysis of evidence. While the roots of forensics date back to ancient Greece, it has evolved into a specialized field.[1] Types of evidence include any object or asset belonging to a patient, any foreign material removed from the clothing or body of a patient, and any organ or tissue removed from a patient that is used for information before a court to prove or disprove a fact. Evidence can establish the facts, connect a person or persons to a crime or potential crime, or link a person's action to the outcome of an event. Evidence can be touched or seen and is perceptible by the senses.[2] Dr. Edmond Locard, a French scientist, developed the techniques that are considered to be the cornerstone of modern forensic sciences. During World War I, after evaluating stains on uniforms and clothing, Locard identified the location where French soldiers and prisoners died. Locard's exchange principle was thus formed by applying the scientific method and logic to criminal investigations.[3] Locard personally did not reference an exchange principle but did observe that "it is impossible for a criminal to act, especially considering the intensity of a crime, without leaving traces

TABLE 6-1 EXAMPLES OF EVIDENCE FOUND IN THE HOSPITAL SETTING

TRACE	PHYSICAL	TRANSIENT	PATTERNED
• Fingerprints • Hairs • Fibers • Glass • Paint chips • Soil samples • Botanical materials • Gunshot residue • Explosives residue • Volatile hydrocarbons (arson evidence)	• Clothing • Projectiles and missiles • Blood, bloodstains • Hairs • Fibers • Knives • Markings or injuries on the patient • Small pieces of material such as fragments of metal, glass, paint, and wood	• Odor • Temperature • Smoke • Indentations or imprints from fire or light	• Blood spatter • Glass fragments • Tire marks • Burn patterns • Projectile and missile trajectory directions

of this presence."[4] Based on these observations, the term "principle of exchange" first appeared in the publication *Police and Crime-Detection* in 1940.[4]

Emergency and trauma nurses need to understand Locard's exchange principle when evaluating patients and look for cross-transfer of evidence. Nurses who know how to recognize evidence can provide it to criminalists and technicians for processing within the parameters of the judicial system.

Evidence Classifications

There are four classifications of evidence. The most common—trace and physical evidence—are the most likely pieces of evidence to establish the facts of a crime. Emergency nurses are regularly in contact with essential physical evidence in criminal cases and often unknowingly either discard or damage vital evidence. The classifications of evidence are characterized by the following:

- *Trace evidence* is normally caused by objects or substances coming in contact with one another (no matter how slight the contact), resulting in a minute sample left on the contact surfaces.
- *Physical evidence* is any evidence that is a physical object. Facts or issues are proven based on demonstrable physical characteristics that can establish that a crime has been committed. Physical evidence can also provide a link between a crime and its victim or the perpetrator. It can conceivably include all or part of any object.
- *Transient (conditional) evidence* is any evidence that is temporary in nature.
- *Patterned evidence* occurs when there is physical contact between persons or objects.

Table 6-1 provides examples of the various types of evidence.

Uses of Forensic Evidence

The following situations (although not an all-inclusive list) demonstrate where forensic evidence is used:

- Medical-legal cases: A medical treatment situation with legal implications is defined as a medical-legal case. Medical-legal considerations are a significant part of the process of making many patient care decisions, including determining definitions and policies for the treatment of mentally incompetent people and minors, performing sterilization or therapeutic abortion, and providing care to terminally ill patients. Medical-legal considerations, decisions, definitions, and policies provide the framework for informed consent, professional liability, and many other aspects of current practice in the health care field.[5] Suspicious deaths or crime-related injuries are viewed as medical-legal cases.
  - Unintentional injuries and accidents: It is not always possible to predict whether an unintentional injury or accident will have medical-legal implications.
- Mass casualty incidents: An event where institutional resources are overwhelmed by the number or severity of victims or the resources consumed to care for these individuals. This determination will vary by facility.
- Terrorism or weapons of mass destruction: As defined by the Federal Bureau of Investigation, weapons of mass destruction would include[5]:
  - Any explosive or incendiary device, as defined in Title 18 USC Section 921: bomb, grenade, rocket, missile, mine, or other device with a charge of more than four ounces
  - Any weapon designed or intended to cause death or serious bodily injury through the release, dissemination, or impact of toxic or poisonous chemicals or their precursors

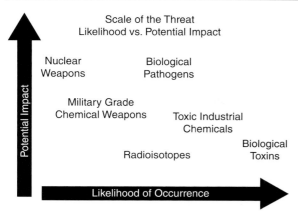

Fig. 6-1 Scale of the threat. (Modified from Federal Bureau of Investigation. [n.d.]. *What is a weapon of mass destruction?* Retrieved from http://www2.fbi.gov/hq/nsb/wmd/wmd_definition.htm)

• Any weapon involving a disease organism
• Any weapon designed to release radiation or radioactivity at a level dangerous to human life. Figure 6-1 illustrates the scale of threat in terms of likelihood of occurrence and potential impact of these weapons of mass destruction.[6]

Evidence Collection and Preservation

While the primary responsibility for forensic evidence remains with the investigating law enforcement agency, the emergency nurse may assist in the collection of forensic evidence. When a victim presents as critically injured or ill, the emergent need for lifesaving treatment is the priority, with forensic evidence collection delayed. As part of the initial team caring for injured or ill patients, emergency nurses should protect any clinical physical forensic evidence, making every effort to preserve its integrity. Evidence, regardless of type, should not be discarded and, when appropriate, evidentiary items are retrieved within an appropriate time period. Staff should document the evidence collection process in writing in the patient's medical record and, when appropriate, with photo documentation following institutional policy and procedure for these activities.

> Forensic evidence collected in a known or suspected terror incident involving chemical, biological, radiological, nuclear, or explosive materials may be processed and transported by the Federal Bureau of Investigation in addition to local law enforcement agencies.

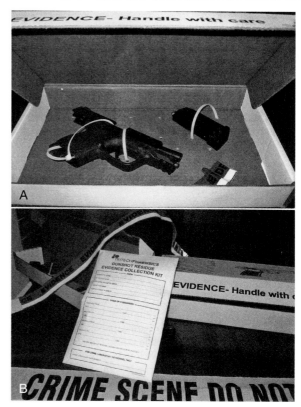

Fig. 6-2 Firearm evidence box **(A)** and Gunshot Residue Kit **(B)** used by law enforcement personnel. (Photos courtesy of J. Eckes.)

Collection and Management Principles

• *Always wear gloves during the handling of all evidence collection.* Change gloves often while the evidence is collected. Hospital personnel should wear the proper personal protective equipment (PPE).
• DO NOT cut through tears, rips, and holes, if possible.
• Check for blood, bloodstains, body fluids, gunshot residue (GSR), or trace elements. Minimize the handling of potential evidence as much as possible prior to packaging.
• Place all evidence collected in a paper bag or in a cardboard evidence box. Label the evidence box with the patient's name, medical record number, date, and signature or initials of the collector (see Fig. 6-2).

> Use paper bags instead of plastic bags to allow air to circulate. Moisture can collect within the plastic bag and alter the evidence.

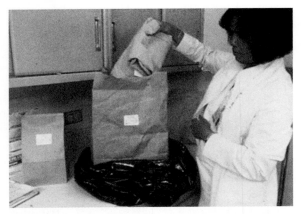

Fig. 6-3 This forensic nurse is ensuring that each evidentiary item is handled carefully and individually packaged in a paper bag. (From Lynch, V. A., & Duval, J. B. [2010]. *Forensic nursing science* [2nd ed.]. St. Louis, MO: Mosby.)

- Bag each item of clothing upon removal independently. Place each article in a separate paper bag to prevent cross-contamination (see Fig. 6-3).
- Secure all evidence retrieved and place in a designated location identified within the institution until retrieved by the appropriate investigating agency. A file cabinet with ventilation holes easily converts to a locked evidence storage locker. Access to this locker should be limited to those knowledgeable about chain of custody procedures.
- For questions concerning the collection, preservation, and documentation of evidence obtained from a deceased patient, refer to the investigating law enforcement agency, the medical examiner's or coroner's office, and institutional policy and procedure.
- Questions involving living patients should be directed to the appropriate investigating law enforcement agency.
- If the patient is pronounced dead on arrival to the emergency department (or shortly thereafter) and is *not* resuscitated:
  - Do not remove clothing.
  - Wrap the patient in a white sheet until a forensic examination is properly completed.
  - Do not dispose of or return any item to the patient's family or significant other prior to law enforcement arrival and approval.
- Notify the investigating law enforcement agency and the medical examiner's or coroner's office.
- Place paper bags over both of the patient's hands. This will preserve any potential evidence that could be under the patient's nail beds or on the hands.

- Wrap bullets in gauze to preserve trace evidence and place in a peel-pack, cup, or envelope. *Do not touch bullets with metal instruments.*

Wounds

- Observe the size, shape, and character of the wound. Create a diagram and describe all characteristics in detail.
- Avoid incising or cutting through the wound.
- Identify the presence or absence of any residue around gunshot wounds.
- Identify the number of wounds (holes) observed as well as location of the wounds. *DO NOT identify or document the wound as an entrance or exit wound.*
- Place a marker at the site of all wounds when taking radiographs to assist in the identification of location of projectiles or trajectory of projectiles. Place the marker to one side of the wound and not directly in or on the wound.
- Place paper bags over both hands, if there is consideration or knowledge of a weapon having been fired. If it is unknown at the time of admission whether a weapon has been fired, place bags over hands in preparation of crime scene investigator's evaluation.

Foreign Objects, Hairs, Fibers, and Debris[7]

- Retrieve and collect all foreign objects as potential evidence sources
- Carefully remove hairs, fibers, or other debris from the patient's body using forceps with plastic-coated tips and place each item into paper envelopes.
- Gently scrape dry debris onto a glass slide. Consult institutional protocols as they may differ.
- Place sharp objects (needles, blades, knives, glass fragments) in double peel-packs (heavy-gauge polyethylene pouch with tamper-evident adhesive closures) or in plastic (such as a urine specimen container), glass, or cardboard containers.

Overdose

- Save all pills, bottles, toxin containers, and gastric lavage fluid for evidentiary evaluation.
- Send specimen to the pathology department for evaluation.
- Use Poison Control resources as needed.
- Assure chain of custody as needed.

SPECIAL CONSIDERATIONS

Biological Evidence

Biological evidence in forensics is the study of blood, fluids, and other physiological material related to the establishment of facts surrounding a criminal or medical-legal

Scene

Victim

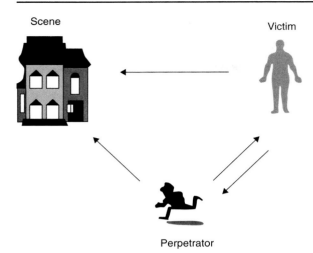

Perpetrator

Fig. 6-4 Biological evidence transfer. (Courtesy of National Center for Forensic Science, http://www.ncfs.org/bio_evd.html)

investigation.[8] Types of biological evidence the emergency nurse will encounter include but are not limited to blood, saliva, semen, vaginal secretions, urine, and bone. Biological evidence transfers in various ways, between the scene, the victim, the perpetrator, and even with the weapon if there is one. Figure 6-4 describes the most common direction of evidence transfer.[8]

Biological samples related to sexual assault are discussed in Chapter 51, Sexual Assault.

Biological Agents

With the increasing number of terrorist events in the world and focus on emergency preparedness, the emergency nurse must be aware of biological agents and the potential threat they pose. The primary responsibility of the emergency nurse is to maintain self-protection and therefore the nurse must strictly observe all guidelines as they relate to PPE.

Biological agents are bacteria, viruses, fungi, or toxins that can cause disease in humans and animals. While many biological agents occur naturally in the environment, some are altered and used for nefarious purposes, such as biological weapons, and pose a risk to national security. Agents such as smallpox, anthrax, plague, tularemia, and hemorrhagic fevers are of greatest forensic concern. Suspicion or actual identification of a biological agent automatically warrants notification of law enforcement personnel. Often specialized evidence recovery teams are responsible for evidence collection in these cases and the emergency nurse should be ready to provide support as indicated. See Chapter 3, Mass Casualty for additional information.

TABLE 6-2	**BLOODSTAIN DO'S AND DON'TS**

- Never mix dried stains together.
- Place each stain in a separate envelope.
- Do not wipe dried stains from an object with a wet cloth.
- Secure blood samples as quickly as possible.
- Preserve bloodstains from contamination.
- Protect blood specimens from decomposition.

Karagiozis, M., & Sgaglio, R. (2005). *Forensic investigation handbook: An introduction to the collection, preservation, analysis and presentation of evidence.* Springfield, IL: Charles C. Thomas.

Other biological specimens evaluated forensically and through laboratory testing are blood alcohol concentration (BAC) levels and carbon monoxide (CO) levels. When BAC is determined, the emergency nurse needs to be specific as to who drew the specimen (hospital personnel or law enforcement) and how it was obtained. This distinction has a significant impact in court based on the medical treatment provided and the timing associated with the BAC draw. Carbon monoxide levels can help to establish the source of CO inhalation.

Blood Stains and Patterns

In violent crimes, blood evidence is common. When criminalists test blood, they are able to determine if it is human or nonhuman in origin. If the blood is nonhuman, the specific animal family can be determined. Protect the blood from destruction (e.g., not cleaning the patient prior to crime scene evaluation), identify patterns, and communicate these findings to the appropriate investigating agency.

If dried blood is present, place it in a paper bag sealed and labeled with the patient's identification. Table 6-2 lists some guidelines for handling bloodstains. Patterned injuries are the result of an object leaving a distinct mark on the patient's body. This could occur because of blood spatter, dirt, or from the mechanism of action that created the injury. Identify pattern injuries and describe his or her findings in detail. Some patterned injuries or wounds are intentional and occur because of customs, rituals, or cultural beliefs as exhibited in Figure 6-5.

During the interview and assessment phase of care, the emergency nurse can determine the origin of the patterned markings and decide if there has been any harm or wrongdoing. Once determined and if necessary, the nurse must follow applicable state laws if reporting is necessary.

Deoxyribonucleic Acid

Deoxyribonucleic acid (DNA) is the blueprint of human genetic makeup. Portions of our DNA are responsible for the hereditary traits passed by parents, such as eye and hair

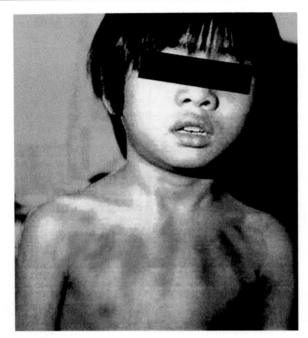

Fig. 6-5 This is an example of bruising resulting from coining. (From Price, D. L. [2004]. *Thompson's pediatric nursing: An introductory text* [9th ed.]. Philadelphia, PA: Saunders.)

color, height, and bone structure. DNA is collected from a crime scene for evidentiary purposes. DNA can be extracted from biological and blood samples from any area where saliva may have transferred to the patient, such as bite marks.

When done correctly, DNA analysis is considered the most accurate evidence available because it is as individual as a fingerprint. Crime labs do not need or want blood samples for DNA testing; rather, buccal swabs provide the best specimens. When possible, allow access to the patient or assist the criminalist in retrieval of such samples. Once the swabs have been retrieved, DNA is matched through a database operated by the FBI called CODIS (Combined DNA Index System). The database consists of four indices of DNA records: forensic index, convicted offender index, missing persons index, and a general population file of anonymous DNA profiles.

Evidence Collection of Biological Materials

Regardless of the source, collect biological specimens or evidence of any type in the following manner if law enforcement is not present:

- Don appropriate PPE, including a mask and eye protection. Change gloves frequently.
- Send biological or laboratory samples of evidence to an appropriate laboratory for analysis at direction of law enforcement.
- Use specific packaging based on the substance or agent involved. Biological specimens have special requirements. Consult the accepting laboratory for assistance.
- Consult local law enforcement, health department officials, and the local FBI office as necessary.
- Allow wet clothing to air-dry before packaging, if possible. If unable to accomplish drying, communicate to law enforcement personnel that clothing is in a damp condition.
- Take photos of blood patterns for investigating agency.
- Place dried blood flakes in an envelope or paper bag.
- Do not mix evidence samples.
- Provide assistance to investigators with other evidence collection if requested.

Penetrating Injuries
Gunshot Wounds

The handgun is the most commonly used firearm in the United States for both homicides and suicides.[9] Handguns are low-velocity, low-energy weapons with muzzle speeds below 1400 feet per second.[9] In evaluating the evidentiary value of a gunshot wound (GSW), inspect the wound for size, shape, and characteristics for determination of distance, powder stippling, and contact wounds. Although entrance and exit wounds have distinguishing features (see Table 6-3), they are not identified as such in the medical record.

> Do not document the wound as an entrance or exit wound in the medical record. Let ballistics and firearm experts identify the wound as such and provide testimony in court.

Gunshot Wound Characteristics. Firearm wounds are divided into four categories depending on the distance from the gun muzzle to the target. These classifications are contact, near contact, intermediate, and distant (see Fig. 6-6).

Contact wounds: All contact wounds exhibit a scorching of the wound edges and leave a deposit of soot in the wound area.
- The muzzle of the gun is in a hard, loose, or angled position of contact with the body.
  - Loose contact results in the deposit of a wider zone of soot (powder burning and blackening) around the entrance wound.

TABLE 6-3   DETERMINATION OF ENTRANCE AND EXIT WOUNDS

WOUNDS OVER SKIN	
ENTRANCE	**EXIT**
• Reddish zone of abraded skin results from bullet scraping against the skin as it penetrates • Tend to be small, circular or oval, and regular • Symmetrical abrasion rings indicate a head-on shot • Concentric rings suggest an angled shot	• Usually larger and more irregular than entrance because of the bullet tumble or yaw and bullet deformation • Usually no abrasion ring present • May have a stellate, crescent, circular, or completely irregular shape
WOUNDS OVER BONE	
ENTRANCE	**EXIT**
• Stellate or cruciform appearance • Hole is beveled inward	• Beveled or cratered • Hole is beveled outward

Data from Eckes-Roper, J. (2003). Forensics in trauma. In S. S. Cohen (Ed.), *Trauma nursing secrets* (pp. 25–36). Philadelphia, PA: Hanley and Belfus Medical Publishers.

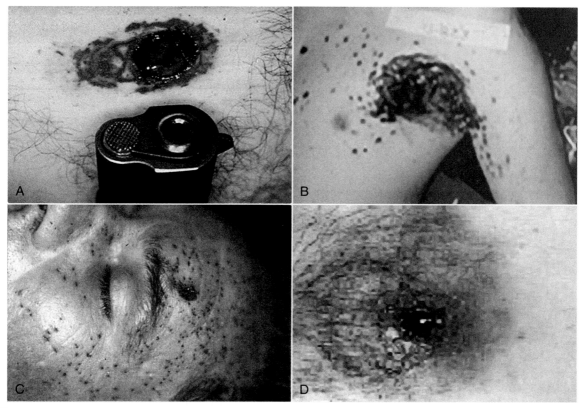

Fig. 6-6   A, Contact wound. **B,** Near contact wound. **C,** Intermediate wound. **D,** Distant wound. (Photo courtesy of J. Eckes.)

- Angled contact produces are an oval-shaped zone of soot.
- Hard contact will often leave an impression of the weapon used.
- Contact wounds over bone produce a stellate pattern wound at the entrance point because of the expansion of powder gases between the skin and the bone.
- Contact over clothing usually means that the clothing absorbs the soot and powder elements but powder grains, soot, and clothing particles may be driven into the wound track.

Near contact wounds: The muzzle of the weapon is not in contact with the skin and the entrance wound has a wide zone of soot overlying seared, blackened skin. The soot in the seared zoned cannot be wiped or washed away because it is baked into the skin.

Intermediate wounds: Since the muzzle of the weapon is not in direct contact with the skin, the powder grains produce a "tattooing" or stippling of the skin. The powder cannot be washed away, is reddish-brown to orange-brown in color, and is located around the entrance wound.

Distant wounds: These wounds exhibit no soot or tattooing so the exact range of fire cannot be determined. The bullet penetrating and bruising the skin produces the only mark on the patient. Other GSW characteristics to consider:

- Because of skin elasticity, the caliber of the bullet cannot be identified by the size of the entrance wound.
- Radiograph distortion does not allow for the identification of the caliber of the bullet in the body.
- The trajectory of the bullet through the body depends on the following factors:
    - Angle at which the weapon was held
    - The position of the victim
    - The position of the assailant
- Shotgun and automatic weapon wounds and injuries vary significantly from handgun and semiautomatic weapons.

Gunshot Residue. Emergency nurses need to recognize that GSR may be present on patients who present with gunshot wounds. Because of the immediate life- or limb-saving care needed by the patient, GSR is often overlooked or destroyed in emergency departments and trauma centers. GSR appears as minute particles of metal components (consisting of antimony, barium, and lead) that come from the primer composition and the projectile.[10] It is found on the hands, hair, skin, and clothing of any person who has fired or been in the immediate area of a discharged firearm.

To preserve GSR for law enforcement, forensic nurses or emergency personnel should follow these guidelines:

- Do not wash the patient's hands or arms.
- Place paper bags over both hands and secure with evidence tape. If evidence tape is not available, use surgical tape. If it is unknown or uncertain at the time of admission if a weapon was fired, place bags over hands in preparation of crime scene investigator's evaluation. Permit the investigator or forensic nurse access to the patient to perform a GSR test.
- Remove gunpowder residue with tape and then apply it to a glass slide in preparation for evaluation only if instructed by the criminalist or law enforcement agency.

Stab Wounds

A stab wound is an incised wound usually caused by a sharp instrument, such as a knife, that creates a deep puncture where the length on the surface is less than the depth of penetration into the body.[11] The characteristics of stab wounds are dependent on the type of instrument used and the location on the body receiving the puncture. During the assessment of the patient with a stab wound, the emergency nurse should evaluate if defensive wounds are present. Defensive wounds are injuries a victim sustains while trying to ward off an attacker and protect himself or herself. These wounds can be located on the hands or forearms of the victim.

HANDLING AND DISPOSITION OF EVIDENCE

Documentation of Evidence

- Ensure all packages used to collect evidence are sealed and labeled with the date, time, patient's name, description and source of the material (including anatomic location), name of the health care provider, and names and initials of every person that handled the material.
- Document in writing, including the use of diagrams, drawings, or photographs, the evidence collected and its disposition in the patient's medical record.
- Identify where the projectile was recovered from and by whom; document this information in the medical record.
- Document the disposition of any foreign objects, missiles, projectiles, hairs, fibers, and other debris collected as evidence.
- Document the color, type, odor, and amount of any body fluids recovered.
- If gastric fluids are collected, document the disposition of this specimen in the patient's medical record and on the chain of custody form.
- Ensure a completed chain of custody form or a property receipt in the patient's medical record before the evidentiary items are released to law enforcement.

Sketching, Drawing, and Diagramming the Injury

A written description of the assessment findings, including details about the patient's injuries, must be documented. Precision is important; measure wounds in centimeters and describe wound size, shape, appearance, and location using readily recognized anatomic landmarks. Sometimes the results of abuse or neglect can be subtle and not immediately recognized.

Body diagrams (body charts) are sometimes used to describe the exact anatomical location of a person's injuries. Diagrams are visual supplements to written assessment findings. Drawings are also important when a pattern or constellation of wounds is present. Some emergency department and trauma center documentation allows for marking a body diagram to note the specific location of the injury or wound. Diagrams, descriptions, and subsequent photographs will aid the emergency nurse if called to court to provide testimony as a witness.

Photographic Documentation

A photograph is visual proof of the victim's injury. It will maintain evidentiary value long after the trace evidence is gone and the wounds heal. Photography creates a permanent historical record and can be invaluable in later reconstruction of events. It is not, however, a substitute for written documentation. Photographs are real physical evidence that will provide graphic credibility and convincing proof in both civil and criminal cases. Photographic documentation provides consistency of the nurses' assessment findings and prevents conflicting injury interpretation.

Properly taken photographs, digital images, or video provide corroborating evidence to an investigator's reports. Digital technology has facilitated the incorporation of photographs into computer-generated reports. Photographs need to become a permanent part of the patient's medical record. When taking photos the nurse needs to use a reference scale such as a ruler in each photo (see Fig. 6-7).

Photo documentation should not delay care or written documentation. When possible, take photographs with appropriate reference scales (ruler) before injuries are treated and from different angles, including full body pictures to capture the person's face and body in one frame. Photograph close-up, both with and without a scale, to show size of the focal point.

The principal requirements for admissibility of a photograph (either digital or film) into evidence are relevance and authentication. Therefore the photograph must accurately represent the injury or wound with the

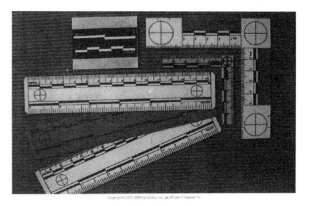

Fig. 6-7 Standards and the ABFO No. 2 scale. (From Lynch, V. A., & Duval, J. B. [2010]. *Forensic nursing science* [2nd ed.]. St. Louis, MO: Mosby.)

associated documentation. Follow institutional guidelines for evidence photography, as this is often delegated to law enforcement or specialty training forensic personnel to ensure accuracy.

Chain of Custody

Chain of custody is a legal process referring to the paper trail that assures the integrity and security of the evidence. The process identifies each person having responsibility or control over the evidentiary material or property and begins the moment the evidence is located.[12] The chain of custody process protects the integrity of the evidence. If the chain is broken or mishandled, the evidence can and will be challenged in court.

Chain of custody documentation varies by institution. To develop local protocols for evidence collection it is critical to collaborate with local stakeholders such as law enforcement, medical examiner's office or coroner, and legal counsel.

Strictly adhere to chain of custody procedures within the institution. The chain of custody routinely receives scrutiny and challenge in a court of law. If there is any suspicion that the chain of custody has been broken, the evidence is subject to allegations of mishandling or evidence tampering and has the potential for dismissal. A chain of custody form or a property receipt from the appropriate investigating agency should be completed for all transfers of evidentiary materials. Collaboration between the emergency department staff and the local law enforcement agency with jurisdiction can help design the most appropriate chain of custody form.

Legal Responsibilities when Evidence Is Collected

When participating in a potential criminal case and collecting evidence in the emergency department, the emergency nurse should follow hospital procedure defining the notification requirements of the institution's legal or risk management departments. It is important to follow documented protocol and obtain the support of these hospital resources in the event that the nurse collecting the evidence is called to testify. If subpoenaed, the emergency nurse has an obligation to appear in court. During testimony, the nurse may be asked to clarify the notes documented in the medical record, to explain what treatment was provided, or to disclose what the patient specifically told the nurse during the visit. Local laws and institutional policies should be a valuable resource.

FORENSIC NURSING OPPORTUNITIES

The opportunities for nursing practice and health care providers will continue to expand. New roles have emerged to meet the health care needs of society and deal with the violence that seems more commonplace than ever today. Forensic nursing was recognized as a specialty field in 1992.[13]

Common areas of practice for forensic nurses include but are not limited to:
- Clinical forensics—providing consulting services to nursing, medical, and law-related agencies.
- Emergency and trauma nurses—caring for ill and injured patients.
- Correctional nurses—working with criminals in prison.
- Sexual Assault Nurse Examiner (SANE)—caring for victims of domestic violence, elder, and child abuse.
- Legal nurse consulting—working with attorneys and law firms.
- Death investigators—working with the medical examiner's or coroner's office.

REFERENCES

1. Karagiozis, M., & Sgaglio, R. (2005). *Forensic investigation handbook: An introduction to the collection, preservation, analysis and presentation of evidence.* Springfield, IL: Charles C. Thomas.
2. Swanson, C., Chamelin, N., Territo, L., & Taylor, R. (2009). *Criminal investigation* (10th ed.). New York, NY: McGraw-Hill.
3. O'Connor, T. (2006, September 30). *An introduction to criminalistics.* Retrieved from http://www.drtomoconnor.com/3220/3210lect01b.htm
4. Lerner, K. L., & Lerner B. W. (Eds.). (2006). *World of forensic science: Locard's exchange principle.* Retrieved from http://www.enotes.com/forensic-science/locard-s-exchange-principle
5. *Mosby's medical dictionary* (8th ed.). (2008). St. Louis, MO: Mosby.
6. Federal Bureau of Investigation. (n.d.). *What is a weapon of mass destruction?* Retrieved from http://www2.fbi.gov/hq/nsb/wmd/wmd_definition.htm
7. Stokowski, L. (2008, March 6). *Forensic nursing: Part 1. Evidence collection for nurses.* Retrieved from http://www.medscape.org/viewarticle/571057
8. National Center for Forensic Science. (2011, February 25). *Biological evidence.* Retrieved from http://www.ncfs.org/bio_evd.html
9. DiMaio, V. J. M. (1999). *Gunshot wounds: Practical aspects of firearms, ballistics and forensic techniques* (2nd ed.). Boca Raton, FL: CRC Press.
10. Pavlik, K. A. (2005). The importance of gunshot residue. *Forensic Nurse, 4*(1), 8–9.
11. Forensic Medicine for Medical Students. (n.d.). *Characteristics of stab wounds.* Retrieved from http://www.forensicmed.co.uk/wounds/sharp-force-trauma/stab-wounds/
12. Cabelus, N. B., & Spangler, K. (2006). Evidence collection and documentation. In R. M. Hammer, B. Moynihan, & E. M. Pagliaro (Eds.), *Forensic nursing* (pp. 489–517). Sudbury, MA: Jones & Bartlett.
13. International Association of Forensic Nurses. (n.d.). *About forensic nursing.* Retrieved from http://iafn.org/displaycommon.cfm?an=1&subarticlenbr=137

Basic Clinical Issues

Triage

Nicki Gilboy

Triage is the process of rapidly sorting patients who present to the emergency department (ED) to determine who needs to be seen immediately and who is safe to wait. This process requires the skills of an experienced emergency nurse. Recently, improving the flow by streamlining the triage process has been the focus of many process improvement efforts in emergency departments.

> The National Hospital Ambulatory Medical Care Survey, Emergency Department Summary, estimated that 123.8 million visits were made to U.S. emergency departments in 2008.[1]

ENVIRONMENT

In today's busy ED, the triage function has become even more critical. The number of persons seeking medical care in EDs grew by 32% between 1996 and 2006.[2] This number is expected to continue to grow in light of the aging population, the number of uninsured patients, and issues surrounding access to primary care. In fact, in 2005, 20% of the United States population had made one or more visits to an ED within the past year.[2] In 2002 The Joint Commission[3] released a sentinel event alert that identified EDs as the location for more than half of all reported sentinel events involving patient death or permanent disability because of delays in treatment. In nearly one third of these occurrences, overcrowding was deemed to be a contributing factor. Given this environment, an effective triage process is crucial to the smooth functioning of an ED.

The word "triage" comes from the French word *trier,* which means to sort or choose. Today, hospital triage refers to the quick sorting of patients who present to the ED for care. The purpose of triage is to put the right person in the right place at the right time for the right reason. The triage concept has been used since Napoleonic times when soldiers wounded in battle were sorted according to injury severity. Those with mortal wounds were separated from combatants who potentially could be saved. The goal of rapid treatment was to maximize survival and return as many soldiers as possible to the battlefield. The triage concept is still in use in the military and has since become a standard part of civilian ED operations.

In the late 1950s and early 1960s, health care delivery models in the United States changed dramatically. Physicians moved away from independent practices and formed office-based practice groups with regular clinic hours. Instead of house calls, patients now were seen by appointment. At the same time, a nationwide move toward medical specialization began, leaving fewer doctors available for primary care. Hospitals were also evolving. As a result of advances in diagnostic technology and the introduction of intensive care units, hospitals assumed a new role, becoming 24-hour medical resources rather than just a place to stay when seriously ill. With the growth of hospital-based services, EDs began to deal with an onslaught of patients, many with nonurgent complaints. The practice of seeing patients on a first-come, first-served basis rapidly became outmoded, so severity-based triage systems were implemented.

TRIAGE SYSTEMS

Currently, most EDs in the United States use some type of triage system. These systems differ along a number of key dimensions, including who is conducting the triage, the depth of the assessment, and the amount of information obtained from the patient.

Comprehensive

Comprehensive triage is the most advanced system and is the process currently recommended by the Emergency Nurses Association's (ENA) Standards of Emergency Nursing Practice, which defines the practice as follows: "The

TABLE 7-1	**ADVANTAGES OF COMPREHENSIVE TRIAGE**

- An experienced emergency nurse greets the patient.
- Patients in need of immediate care are identified quickly.
- A knowledgeable professional performs an assessment.
- Immediate reassurance is provided to the patient and the family.
- First aid and comfort measures are initiated as needed.
- The patient, family, and visitors can be informed about emergency department processes.
- During the assessment, the emergency nurse has an opportunity for patient teaching.
- The emergency nurse decides which area of the emergency department is most suitable for the patient.
- If protocols are in place, medications for fever, pain relief, and tetanus prophylaxis may be administered.
- Emergency nurses may initiate laboratory work and order radiographs based on triage guidelines.
- Waiting patients are reassessed regularly according to departmental policy.
- A strong communication link is maintained between the triage area and the treatment area.

[emergency nurse] triages each patient and determines the priority of care based on physical, developmental, and psychosocial needs as well as factors influencing access to health care and patient flow through the emergency care system."[4] The backbone of this approach is the experienced emergency nurse who has completed a competency-based triage orientation process. Advantages of comprehensive triage are highlighted in Table 7-1.

Comprehensive triage systems have policies, procedures, and protocols (or standards) in place to serve as guidelines. The assessment process involves collecting the chief complaint and any other relevant subjective or objective information. The goal of the comprehensive triage assessment is to gather sufficient information to support a triage severity rating decision. Ratings will vary depending on whether the institution is using a two-, three-, four-, or five-level system. The triage nurse documents initial findings in the medical record and reassesses patients according to individual needs and departmental policy. The ENA recommends that the triage encounter take no more than 5 minutes and possibly as few as 2 minutes.

Two-Tiered Triage Systems

In an ideal world every patient would have a triage assessment within minutes of arrival at the ED. Because of high patient volumes, many facilities have recognized that this goal cannot be achieved and instead have adopted a two-tiered system. With this approach the triage process is broken down into steps. First, an experienced triage nurse greets the patient within minutes of arrival and determines the chief complaint while simultaneously conducting a brief assessment of airway, breathing, and circulatory status. This nurse decides whether the patient needs to be seen immediately or can wait safely for further assessment. With this type of system, patients who require immediate care are promptly taken to the treatment area and are registered at the bedside. This system quickly identifies the patient who is not safe to wait. Stable patients have a patient chart initiated by the first nurse, who documents chief complaint and then directs these patients to the assessment nurse. This second nurse completes a more detailed (but focused) evaluation and may initiate laboratory work and radiographic studies according to protocols. In many EDs, the patient is "quick" registered upon presentation. Enough information is obtained to generate a medical record and an identification band and allow diagnostic procedures to be ordered. The registration process is then completed later in the visit, usually at the bedside.

A two-tiered system has several advantages. In crowded EDs, there is legitimate concern that patients who present to the ED with a serious or life-threatening complaint will have to wait to be seen by the triage nurse. The two-tier system's advantages include the following:

- A patient with a serious complaint is immediately identified.
- The first triage nurse will know every patient in the waiting room and can keep an eye on them.
- The first triage nurse can answer any questions, address changes in patient status, and perform reassessments as appropriate.
- The detailed assessment performed by the second triage nurse builds on the rapid initial assessment. If the patient omitted vital information, the triage decision can always be changed.

Changes to the Triage Process

Recent changes have been made to the triage processes to improve ED flow. Increase in patient volume and the difficulty moving admitted patients out of the ED, are causing many EDs to focus their effort on improving the "door to doctor time"—in other words, the time of patient arrival in the ED to the time the patient is seen by a licensed independent practitioner. The traditional triage process has been identified as a bottleneck or barrier to patient flow, especially when the number of arriving patients overwhelms the triage process and patients end up waiting to be triaged and then registered. Triage bypass and team triage are two efforts to improve ED throughput.

Triage Bypass

One of the solutions to improve patient flow through the ED is the use of triage bypass. When there are open, staffed beds in an ED there is no reason to determine if the patient is safe to wait. The patient does not need to be formally triaged. Instead the patient is screened by the "greeter" nurse to determine the best location for care and then taken directly to an open, staffed bed in the treatment area. An initial assessment, including vital signs, is then completed by the primary nurse and the patient is registered at the bedside. The licensed health care provider sees the patient in a timelier manner. This movement away from the traditional, linear triage process can have a significant impact on patient flow, but it will require a culture change. Most EDs have open, staffed beds at certain times of the day, and it makes sense to bring the patient to the bed as quickly as possible. Triage bypass makes sense during these times and can reduce the queue of patients waiting to be seen.

Team Triage

In a true team triage system, the emergency physician or emergency nurse practitioner and emergency nurse triage the patient together. Based on the triage findings the physician or nurse practitioner will complete the examination and discharge the patient to home or begin the patient evaluation by ordering diagnostic procedures. For example, if the patient needed a radiograph, the test would be ordered at triage. Once the radiograph was completed the patient would be returned to an internal waiting area and never taken to an ED bed. The value of this type of system is that the patient is seen rapidly by a provider during peak hours when there are no open beds. Patients are evaluated in a timely manner. Concerns about this type of system include cost and how patient handoff will occur between the triage team and the treatment area staff.

> The goal of triage bypass and team triage is to decrease the time the patient has to wait to be seen by a licensed independent practitioner and to improve ED throughput.

TRIAGE SEVERITY RATING SYSTEMS

Several different triage severity rating systems are described in the literature and are used in various parts of the world. Each system has unique features that are described briefly later.

Triage severity rating systems are evaluated along several dimensions; two important considerations are validity and reliability. Validity refers to the accuracy of the triage severity rating system. In other words, how well does it measure what it is intended to measure? Do the different triage levels truly reflect differences in severity? For example, you would expect a high admission rate for patients identified as very ill.

Reliability is another important characteristic of a triage severity rating system. This refers to the degree of consistency (or agreement) among those using the method. Will different triage nurses assign the same patient the same severity level? Over time, will each triage nurse consistently assign similar patients the same severity level? Importantly, criteria for each triage level need to remain constant. A patient's assigned severity rating cannot vary simply because the department is busy or a particular nurse is performing triage.

> If triage data are collected accurately and consistently, an ED can use this information to analyze and trend various patient outcomes such as ED length of stay and hospitalization rates.

A triage severity rating system serves as more than just a means of scoring an individual's severity of condition; it becomes a language, a precise shorthand, for communicating patient severity to the ED as a whole. Reliable data also make it possible to compare different EDs and to look at changes within an ED over time. For example, staff may report that the pediatric population they are caring for is sicker. ED leadership can look at the case mix data for the pediatric population over time to determine if the staff's perception is correct. Another example, staff may report that fast track needs to open earlier in the day because so many low-acuity patients are waiting for a long time to be seen. ED leadership can look at arrival time and patient acuity to see if a change in hours is prudent.

Studies have demonstrated poor inter-rater (between different raters) and intra-rater (the same rater on another occasion) reliability with three-level triage severity rating systems.[5-7] This is largely because there are no universal definitions for each level. Table 7-2 defines two-, three-, and four-level triage systems and the definitions for each triage level.

Five-Level Triage

In 2003, The ENA's Board of Directors approved the following position statement developed by ENA and the American College of Emergency Physicians' (ACEP) Joint Five-Level Triage Task Force:

> ACEP and ENA believe that quality of patient care would benefit from implementing a standardized ED triage scale and acuity categorization process. Based on expert consensus of currently available evidence, ACEP and ENA support the adoption of a reliable, valid 5-level triage scale.[8]

TABLE 7-2	OVERVIEW OF TWO-, THREE-, AND FOUR-LEVEL TRIAGE ACUITY RATING SYSTEMS
SYSTEM	**LEVELS**
Two-level	Sick or not sick
Three-level	Emergent: Immediate care required. Threat to life, limb, or organ. Examples: cardiopulmonary arrest, major trauma, and respiratory failure.
	Urgent: Prompt care required but the patient may wait safely several hours if necessary. Examples: abdominal pain, fractured hip, and renal calculi.
	Nonurgent: The patient needs to be seen but time is not critical and the patient can wait safely. Examples: sore throat, rash, and conjunctivitis.
Four-level	Life threatening
	Emergent
	Urgent
	Nonurgent

In 2004 the Joint Five-Level Triage Task Force identified the Canadian Triage and Acuity Scale (CTAS) or the Emergency Severity Index (ESI) as good options based on a review of the published evidence on five-level triage systems.[9]

> The Joint Five-Level Triage Task Force statement was a large step toward the recommendation and adoption of a single five-level acuity rating system in U.S. emergency departments.

Currently, there are four research-based, five-level triage severity rating scales in use around the world. In each scale, level 1 represents the highest severity (most acute), whereas level 5 is used to designate the patients with the least acute conditions.

The Australasian Triage Scale

The Australian emergency medical community adopted the Australasian Triage Scale in 1993, and it remains in use in every ED in Australia (Table 7-3). Based on research and expert consensus, each category lists clinical descriptors or conditions that correspond to a specific severity level. Objective time frames for physician evaluation are set for each classification. This "time to treatment" is the maximum interval a patient should expect to wait for further assessment and medical intervention. The clock starts when a patient first presents to the ED. The triage nurse selects an Australasian Triage Scale category based on his or her response to the statement: "This patient should wait for medical assessment and treatment no longer than . . ."[10] Vital signs are obtained only if they will assist in making the triage severity decision. Performance thresholds are set for each level and indicate what percent of the time the ED must comply with time-to-treatment goals. Research has shown the Australasian Triage Scale to be valid and reliable.[11,12] In addition to assigning individual patient severity of condition, this scale has been used to examine case mix and to relate triage levels directly to common outcome measures such as ED length of stay, intensive care unit admission, and resource consumption. Educational materials are available online.[13]

The Canadian Triage and Acuity Scale

A group of Canadian emergency physicians developed the five-level CTAS based on the Australasian system[14] (Table 7-4). Working with the National Emergency Nurses Affiliation, the tool was adopted as the countrywide standard and has become part of the ED data regularly reported to the Canadian government. The CTAS continues to be updated based on the consensus of the National Working Group, research, and EDs' experience working with the scale.[15] In 2003 the Canadian Emergency Department Information Systems (CEDIS) published a standardized presenting complaint list.[16] The CTAS adult and pediatric guidelines have incorporated the CEDIS complaint list as well as the concept of first-order and second-order modifiers.[16] The patient's chief complaint is determined by the triage nurse. This automatically generates a complaint-specific minimum CTAS level, but this level can be altered by the use of objective first- and second-order modifiers. Based on the chief complaint the triage nurse then evaluates first-order modifiers, which are defined as modifiers that are broadly applicable to many different chief complaints. First-order modifiers include vital signs, level of consciousness, pain level, and mechanism of injury. Then second-order modifiers specific to the chief complaint are assessed. The CTAS level assigned is based on the highest level identified by any of the modifiers. Studies have indicated that the Canadian Triage and Acuity Scale is valid and reliable.[17,18] Standardized educational materials are available online.[13]

The Manchester Triage Scale

The Manchester triage scale was developed in England by a group of emergency nurses and physicians who created a detailed, flowchart-based system. Each triage level is given a name, number, and color code that identifies the target time frame for a patient to see a treating clinician[19] (Table 7-5). Based on the presenting complaint, the triage nurse chooses from 52 different flowcharts. To arrive at a triage level decision, the nurse follows the flowchart, asking about

TABLE 7-3   AUSTRALASIAN TRIAGE SCALE

LEVEL		TIME TO TREATMENT	PERFORMANCE THRESHOLD PERCENT	EXAMPLE
1	Immediately life threatening	Immediate	100	Cardiac or respiratory arrest
2	Imminently life threatening	10 minutes	80	Chest pain, stridor
3	Potentially life threatening	30 minutes	75	Severe hypertension, immunocompromised with a fever
4	Potentially serious	60 minutes	70	Abdominal pain
5	Less urgent	120 minutes	70	Minor wound

Australian Government Department of Health and Aging. (2009). *Emergency triage education kit and triage workbook.* Retrieved from http://www.health.gov.au/internet/main/publishing.nsf/Content/5E3156CFFF0A34B1CA2573D0007BB905/$File/Triage%20Workbook.pdf

TABLE 7-4   CANADIAN TRIAGE AND ACUITY SCALE

LEVEL	COLOR	NAME	TIME TO REASSESSMENT
1	Blue	Resuscitation	Continuous nursing care
2	Red	Emergent	15 minutes
3	Yellow	Urgent	30 minutes
4	Green	Less urgent	60 minutes
5	White	Nonurgent	120 minutes

Canadian Association of Emergency Physicians. (2011). *The Canadian Triage and Acuity Scale.* (n.d.). Retrieved from http://www.caep.ca/template.asp?id=B795164082374289BBD9C1C2BF4B8D32

TABLE 7-5   THE MANCHESTER TRIAGE SCALE

NUMBER	NAME	COLOR	TARGET TIME
1	Immediate	Red	0
2	Very urgent	Orange	10 minutes
3	Urgent	Yellow	60 minutes
4	Standard	Green	120 minutes
5	Nonurgent	Blue	240 minutes

Manchester Triage Group. (2006). *Emergency triage* (2nd ed.). Malden, MA: Blackwell Publishing.

signs and symptoms (or discriminators). A positive answer to a discriminator determines the severity rating. Documentation consists of simply identifying the presentational flowchart used, which discriminator defined the triage score, and the associated triage level. The Manchester triage scale is used throughout the United Kingdom and updated training materials have been published.[18]

The Emergency Severity Index

Two American emergency physicians working with a team of emergency physicians and nurses created the Emergency Severity Index (ESI).[20] This research-based, five-level scale categorizes patients by severity and expected resource needs (Fig. 7-1). *Severity* is defined as the stability of vital functions and the potential for life, limb, or organ threat. *Resource consumption*, a component unique to the ESI, is defined as the number of different resources a patient is expected to consume to reach a disposition. The experienced emergency nurse is capable of estimating resource consumption based on previous, similar patient encounters.

Like other five-level systems, research has demonstrated that the ESI is valid and reliable.[20–24] The system itself consists of an easy-to-use algorithm designed to rapidly sort patients into one of five mutually exclusive categories. Educational materials include an online course, a training DVD, and a handbook.[25,26]

THE TRIAGE PROCESS

The triage assessment should be timely and brief. The purpose of this process is to gather sufficient information about the patient to make a triage severity rating decision. The goal should be for all patients to receive an initial triage assessment within 5 minutes of arrival in the ED. Ideally, triage begins with an across-the-room assessment and then continues in the privacy of the triage booth or room. If at

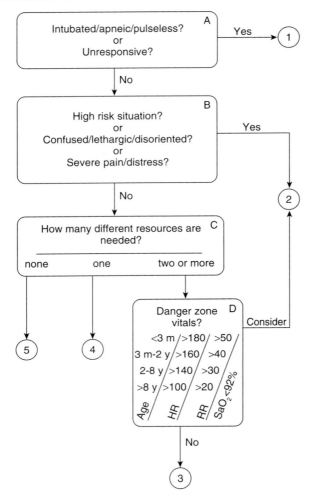

Fig. 7-1 Emergency severity index. *HR*, Heart rate; *m*, months; *y*, years; *RR*, respiratory rate; *SaO₂*, oxygen saturation in arterial blood. (ESI version 3. Copyright 1999–2001. David R. Eitel, MD, MBA, and Richard C. Wuerz, MD.)

any time the triage nurse identifies a life-threatening airway, breathing, or circulatory problem, the nurse initiates appropriate interventions immediately and the patient is transferred to a care area.

Across-the-Room Assessment

The triage assessment begins when the triage nurse first sees the patient; the nurse should observe closely, listen for abnormal sounds, and even be aware of any odors. In most cases an experienced triage nurse can take one look at a patient and, based on general appearance, decide whether

TABLE 7-6	THE PEDIATRIC ASSESSMENT TRIANGLE
Appearance	Muscle tone
	Intractability or consolability
	Look or gaze
	Speech or crying
Work of breathing	Nasal flaring
	Retractions
	Abnormal airway sounds
	Position of comfort
	Altered respiratory rate
Circulation or skin	Pallor
	Mottling
	Cyanosis

Emergency Nurses Association. (2004). *Emergency nursing pediatric course provider manual* (3rd ed.). Des Plaines, IL: Author.

immediate care is required. In such cases triage is considered complete and the patient is taken directly to a treatment room. If the patient is stable, the triage process continues. The Emergency Nursing Pediatric Course refers to this quick once-over glance as the pediatric assessment triangle[27] (Table 7-6). Table 7-7 lists information that can be obtained from an across-the-room assessment.

The Triage Interview

In a two-tier triage system the triage interview is very short. The patient or parents arrive in the ED and inform the triage nurse that they would like to see a doctor and then identify the reason.

In most triage systems the nurse introduces himself or herself and then briefly describes the triage role. The nurse determines the chief complaint and the history of the present injury or illness. Based on findings, the nurse conducts a focused assessment of the problem and measures vital signs per protocol. The nurse derives a triage severity level from this information. Next, the patient either goes immediately to a room for treatment and bedside registration or is directed first to the registration area and then to the waiting room.

> A few kind words from the triage nurse, such as "I bet that really hurts" or "You don't look like you feel very well today," can have a positive impact.

The initial greeting by a triage nurse can set the tone for the whole ED visit. Although the experienced nurse may view an illness or injury as minor, patients can be stressed and may consider the situation a crisis. Nurses need to be nonjudgmental and empathetic. Patients and their families

TABLE 7-7 ACROSS-THE-ROOM ASSESSMENT

SENSE	FINDINGS
Observe	Airway patency
	Respiratory rate, obvious distress, use of oxygen devices
	Signs of external bleeding
	Level of consciousness: interacting, unconscious, crying, moaning
	Signs of pain: grimacing, holding, guarding
	Skin color and condition
	Chronic illness: cancer, chronic obstructive pulmonary disease, neuromuscular disorders
	Deformities
	Body habitus: cachectic, morbidly obese
	Activity: ability to ambulate, balance, bear weight
	General behavior: agitated, angry, flat affect
	Presence of splints, dressings, casts, medical equipment
	Clothing: clean, appropriate
Listen	Abnormal airway sounds
	Speech pattern, tone of voice, language
	Interactions with others
Smell	Stool, urine, vomit, ketones, alcohol
	Poor hygiene, cigarettes, infection, chemicals

Emergency Nurses Association. (2004). *Emergency nursing pediatric course provider manual* (3rd ed.). Des Plaines, IL: Author.

may feel greatly relieved merely because a professional is now involved in their care. Triage nurses must possess strong interpersonal skills, respond tactfully to questions, and be able to allay anxiety with information and reassurance.

A crucial triage skill is the ability to multitask. Obtaining all necessary triage information within the 2- to 5-minute time frame recommended by ENA requires skill, and every second must be used efficiently. It is recognized that triaging geriatric and pediatric patients often takes longer.

Gathering vital information is critical for making appropriate triage decisions. However, to communicate accurately the nurse and patient need to speak a common language. In some hospitals medical interpreters are available for non–English-speaking patients. If no interpreter is immediately accessible, family members or others may be used for initial triage; however, this practice is discouraged. Several interpreter services are available via telephone. Triage documentation should make reference to the use of an interpreter.

> Open-ended questions such as "How can we help you?" or "What seems to be the problem today?" are usually effective to elicit why the patient came to the ED.

The objective of the triage interview is to establish the chief complaint, obtain a description of relevant signs and symptoms, perform a targeted history and examination, and assign a patient severity rating. The first question asked of patients usually relates to the reason the patient came to the ED. The chief complaint should be documented in the patient's own words. If the patient identifies several issues, the triage nurse needs to focus the patient to determine the proximate reason for the ED visit. When a patient is transported by ambulance, much of the triage information can be obtained from prehospital providers, but it is important to acknowledge the patient and to verify information.

> Patients who recite a whole list of medical ailments can be asked by the triage nurse: "What is different now?" or "What was it that made you decide to come in today?"

Pediatric triage can be especially challenging. The nurse needs to keep in mind the developmental level of the patient and should tailor the assessment accordingly. For the younger child, the chief complaint and subjective data must be obtained from a caregiver. Older children and adolescents may be able to supply information themselves. The Emergency Nursing Pediatric Course uses the mnemonic CIAMPEDS to describe the components of the pediatric assessment (Table 7-8).[27] Family members and caregivers also can be invaluable when triaging elderly individuals.

Multiple tools are available to assist nurses with gathering data relative to the patient's chief complaint. The PQRST (provocation/palliation, quality, radiation, severity, timing) pain mnemonic is a systematic approach to assessing pain that is frequently used by emergency nurses. If the patient arrives with a traumatic injury, obtain and document data regarding the mechanism and pattern of injury (Table 7-9). Once the nurse has obtained sufficient information about the chief complaint, the focus shifts to a brief medical history. The mnemonic AMPLE (allergies; medications; pertinent or past medical history; last meal, medications, and menstrual period; events and environment surrounding accident) can be used to guide questioning.

Triage Vital Signs

The role of obtaining vital signs at triage is controversial and is clearly an area that warrants further research. The triage policy of each ED should address when and whether vital signs need to be measured. Care of the emergent patient should never be delayed to obtain vital signs at triage. Many departments have chosen to assess vital signs on all lower-severity patients to collect data to support the assigned severity rating. Regardless of the severity rating

TABLE 7-8 CIAMPEDS

	MNEMONIC	ASSESSMENT COMPONENT
C	Chief complaint	Determine reason for the child's visit to emergency department and duration of complaint (e.g., fever for past 2 days).
I	Immunizations	Evaluate the child's current immunization status. • The completion of all scheduled immunizations for the child's age should be evaluated. • If the child has not received immunizations because of religious or cultural beliefs, document this information.
	Isolation	Evaluation of the child's exposure to communicable diseases (e.g., meningitis, chickenpox, shingles, whooping cough, and tuberculosis). • A child with active disease or who is potentially infectious must be placed in respiratory isolation on arrival to the emergency department. • Other exposures that may be evaluated include exposure to meningitis and scabies.
A	Allergies	Evaluate the child's previous allergic or hypersensitivity reactions. Document reactions to medications, foods, products (e.g., latex), and environmental allergens. The type of reaction also must be documented.
M	Medications	Evaluate the child's current medication regimen, including prescription and over-the-counter medications and herbal and dietary supplements: • Dose administered • Time of last dose • Duration of use
P	Past medical history	Review the child's health status, including prior illnesses, injuries, hospitalizations, surgeries, and chronic physical and psychiatric illnesses. Evaluate use of alcohol, tobacco, drugs, or other substances of abuse, as appropriate. The medical history of the neonate should include the prenatal and birth history: • Maternal complications during pregnancy or delivery • Infant's gestational age and birth weight • Number of days infant remained in hospital after birth The medical history of the menarche female should include the date and description of her last menstrual period. The medical history of sexually active patients should include the following: • Type of birth control used • Barrier protection • Prior treatment for sexually transmitted diseases • Gravida (pregnancies) and para (births, miscarriages, abortions, living children)
	Parents' or caregivers' impression of the child's condition	Identify the child's primary caregiver. • Consider cultural differences that may affect the caregiver's impressions. • Evaluate the caregiver's concerns and observations of the child's condition (especially significant in evaluating the special needs child).

E	Events surrounding the illness or injury	Evaluate the onset of the illness or circumstances and mechanism of injury.
		• Illness
		  • Length of illness, including date and day of onset and sequence of symptoms
		  • Treatment provided before visit to emergency department
		• Injury
		  • Time and date injury occurred
		  • *M:* Mechanism of injury, including the use of protective devices (seat belts, helmets)
		  • *I:* Injuries suspected
		  • *V:* Vital signs in prehospital environment
		  • *T:* Treatment by prehospital providers
		  • Description of circumstances leading to injury
		  • Witnessed or unwitnessed

Emergency Nurses Association. (2004). *Emergency nursing pediatric course provider manual* (3rd ed.). Des Plaines, IL: Author.

TABLE 7-8 CIAMPEDS—cont'd

MNEMONIC	ASSESSMENT COMPONENT
D Diet	Assess the child's recent oral intake and changes in eating patterns related to the illness or injury: • Changes in eating patterns or fluid intake • Time of last meal and last fluid intake • Usual diet: breast milk, type of formula, solid foods, diet for age and developmental level, cultural differences • Special diet or diet restrictions
Diapers	Assess the child's urine and stool output: • Frequency of urination over last 24 hours; changes in frequency • Time of last void • Changes in color or color of urine • Last bowel movement; color and consistency of stool • Change in frequency of bowel movements
S Symptoms associated with the illness or injury	Identify symptoms and progression of symptoms since the time of onset of the illness or injury event

TABLE 7-9 GUIDELINES FOR TRIAGING AN INJURY

MECHANISM OF INJURY	TRIAGE QUESTIONS
Motor vehicle collision	Speed of the vehicle; direction of impact; patient position within the vehicle; use of restraints; airbag deployment; ejection; rollover; fatalities; ambulatory at the scene; entrapment or prolonged extrication
Penetrating injury	Type of object (knife, bullet, impaled object); left in place, removed, broken off
Fall	From how high; landed on which body part(s); what kind of landing surface; why the patient fell
Motorcycle crash	Impact speed; helmet use; other protective clothing; thrown, skidded, pinned, or run over; position of patient relative to the motorcycle
Bicycle crash	Helmet use; collided with a vehicle or object; thrown or run over; impact speed; landed on which body parts

Emergency Nurses Association. (2004). *Emergency nursing pediatric course provider manual* (3rd ed.). Des Plaines, IL: Author.

system used, vital signs outside of age-appropriate parameters can be used to justify up-triaging a patient.

> Cooper et al.[28] studied more than 14,000 patients and concluded that vital signs were an important part of the triage decision process in certain vulnerable populations: individuals with communication problems, those less than 2 years of age, and the elderly.

Objective Data

The triage nurse performs a focused physical assessment related to the patient's chief complaint. This physical examination is limited not only in purpose but also by time, space, and privacy constraints. Inspection, palpation, and (occasionally) auscultation can be used to gather information related to the chief complaint. The triage nurse must remove dressings from wounds to assess and document the actual extent of injury. Table 7-10 addresses the focused physical assessment at triage. Assess only parameters pertinent to the chief complaint or patient presentation; this is not a system-by-system or head-to-toe examination.

Triage Severity Rating

Based on the chief complaint and on subjective and objective data, triage nurses use their knowledge, experience, and triage guidelines to assign a severity rating. This decision will be derived logically from the information obtained. The triage decision has a major impact on patient outcomes and patient safety. Undertriaged patients receive delayed care and risk deterioration. The patient who is overtriaged diverts valuable resources away from those who need them the most. (See Triage Severity Rating System above for a detailed discussion of various types.)

Limited first aid may be rendered at some point during the triage process to decrease pain and promote comfort. This treatment may include dressing a wound, splinting potential or obvious fractures, applying ice, elevating affected extremities, and controlling bleeding. Once a severity rating is determined, radiographic and laboratory studies also can be initiated (per protocol). Some triage protocols include the administration of medications for fever control, pain management, and tetanus prophylaxis.

TABLE 7-10   FOCUSED PHYSICAL ASSESSMENT AT TRIAGE

SYSTEM	ASSESSMENT PARAMETER
Respiratory/cardiac	Respiratory rate, rhythm, depth
	Work of breathing; accessory muscle use
	Skin color, temperature, moisture, turgor, mucous membrane status
	Oxygen saturation; peak expiratory flow rate
	Peripheral edema
	Breath sounds
	Position of comfort
	Chest excursion
	Level of consciousness
Gastrointestinal/genitourinary Musculoskeletal (Compare side to side)	Abdominal distention, tenderness, rigidity, scars, bruising
	Circulation, sensation
	Motor function, strength
	Deformity, wounds
	Edema, discoloration
Endocrine	Skin color, turgor; mucous membrane status
	Fingerstick blood glucose
	Level of consciousness
Neurologic	Facial symmetry, droop, ptosis, drooling
	Grip strength, pronator drift
	Speech clarity and articulation
	Level of consciousness
	Behavior
	Pupils size, shape, equality, response to light
	Motor function and sensation in all extremities
	Glasgow Coma Scale score; mental status
	Fingerstick blood glucose
	Oxygen saturation
Psychiatric	Appearance; grooming
	Speech
	Affect
	Behavior: bizarre, appropriate
	Thought content and process
	Memory; orientation
	Potential for danger to self or others
Skin	Description of wounds: size, location, depth, cause, age, bleeding
	Contamination; foreign body
	Signs of infection: general or local
	Rashes, bites, stings, other lesions
Eye	Inflammation, drainage, trauma, foreign body, tearing, photophobia
	Visual acuity: Snellen eye chart, light and dark, shapes

Be sure to reassess patients if analgesics or antipyretics are administered.

Safety and Security

The incidence of physical assault on ED nursing staff is increasing.[28] There are many factors that contribute to ED violence, including the fast-paced, stressful environment, overcrowding, long wait times, patients under the influence of drugs and alcohol, mental health issues, and gang violence.[29,30] Knowledge of what safety measures are in place in the department is essential for the triage staff. These measures may include panic buttons, restricted access doors, security cameras, and visible security guards or police officers.

The triage nurse should keep one eye on the waiting room constantly, checking for situations in which the behavior of patients, families, or visitors is escalating. While conducting a triage patient interview, the nurse also must be alert for signs of agitation and potential for violence. Objective indicators of increasing agitation include a piercing stare, pacing, fist clenching, talking rapidly, and using language that is loud or abusive. Triage nurses should not place themselves or others at risk, nor should they allow themselves to become the target of aggressive verbal or physical behavior. Often the presence of one or more security guards will deescalate the situation. Triage nurses need to be able to identify psychiatric patients who cannot remain safely in the waiting room and need to be escorted directly to a secure room in the treatment area. See Chapter 2, Workplace Violence and Disruptive Behavior.

> The triage nurse should trust his or her instincts. If a patient makes you uncomfortable, stop the interview, exit the triage booth, and seek assistance.

Triage Documentation

Triage assessment documentation should be clear, be concise, and support the assigned severity rating. Each hospital needs to have a triage policy that includes documentation requirements. See Table 7-11 for elements of a comprehensive triage documentation. Usually a specific area on the patient chart exists for the nurse to record triage findings. This section of the medical record often consists of pick lists or check boxes, or it simply may be a space for narrative notes. Many EDs now use computerized documentation systems. A description of these systems is beyond the scope of this text.

Each ED needs to decide whether mandated screening assessments (e.g., barriers to learning, nutritional needs, or domestic violence) will be completed at triage or as part of the patient's bedside assessment.

EMERGENCY MEDICAL TREATMENT AND ACTIVE LABOR ACT

The Emergency Medical Treatment and Active Labor Act (EMTALA) has profoundly affected EDs. The act is a federal law, originally passed in 1985 in an effort to stop hospitals from "dumping" nonpaying patients on another facility. The act came about in response to reports of patients being refused care at an ED or being transferred to another facility before receiving appropriate emergency treatment. Laws now mandate that all persons presenting to an ED that receives federal funding must be given a medical screening examination to determine whether an emergency exists. If an emergency does exist, stabilizing care must be provided. The act has clear implications for the triage process.

TABLE 7-11	ELEMENTS OF COMPREHENSIVE TRIAGE DOCUMENTATION

- Date and time of arrival at the emergency department
- Patient age
- Chief complaint
- Triage interview time
- Allergies (medications, food, latex)
- Current medications (prescription, over-the-counter, supplements)
- Triage severity rating
- Vital signs
- First aid measures
- Reassessments
- Assessment of pain
- History of current complaint
- Subjective and objective assessment
- Significant medical history
- Last menstrual period
- Last tetanus immunization
- Diagnostic procedures initiated
- Medications administered at triage
- Signature of registered nurse
- Consider including the following:
  - Mode of arrival
  - Use of an interpreter

The Centers for Medicare and Medicaid Services has made it clear that the triage process is not the same thing as a medical screening examination. The purpose of triage is to identify severity and to determine the order in which patients will be seen. The medical screening examination is an individual patient assessment process (which may include diagnostic procedures) designed to establish whether a medical emergency actually exists. See Chapter 1, Legal Issues for Emergency Nurses, for additional information on EMTALA.

> In 2006 more than 2.4 million persons (2% of registered visits) walked out of U.S. emergency departments without being seen by a licensed independent practitioner.[2]

LEFT WITHOUT BEING SEEN

An ED's left without being seen (LWBS) rate is an important measure of ED performance. Overcrowding has contributed to this growing number. Patients who have been triaged and registered may have to wait for hours before they receive medical care; some prefer to leave. Hospitals must have policies and procedures in place to guide triage staff in such situations because EDs are responsible for documenting patient disposition. Patients, of course, have the right to leave, but the physician on duty should be notified in situations where the nurse feels a significant illness or injury that requires emergency care exists.

Patients may or may not let the triage staff know that they are leaving. If they do, the triage nurse has an opportunity to discuss the situation. Patients with questionable capacity can be stopped from leaving. Many EDs request that patients sign a form before departure. These forms document that the patient was offered a medical screening examination but preferred to leave before being seen. If a patient walks out of the department without notifying staff, the triage nurse should document the time it was first noted that the patient was no longer in the ED. Also, the nurse should document any efforts to locate the patient (e.g., "overhead paged × 3 with no response").

THE JOINT COMMISSION

The Joint Commission has several standards applicable to the triage process and considers assessment a nursing function. Therefore triage should be performed by an emergency nurse and not by ancillary personnel. Each ED needs to have triage policies and procedures in place that include a system for assigning patient priority.

The Joint Commission standards also address the issue of staff competency. How does the hospital know that a particular nurse is competent to triage patients? Does the hospital maintain records of orientation and competency validation? The Joint Commission acknowledges that the ED has become the safety net of the health care system—the only place an individual is guaranteed access to health care—and addresses ED overcrowding as part of a greater, hospital-wide problem, mandating a hospital-wide response.

INFECTION CONTROL

The triage nurse must use standard infection control precautions in any situation where contact with blood or body fluids could occur. Hand cleansing between patients with soap and water or with a waterless alcohol-based hand sanitizer is essential to reduce the spread of infection. The ED is often the portal of entry for patients with contagious diseases. Therefore all patients should be screened with infection in mind.

Any patient identified as potentially having a communicable condition must have the appropriate precautions initiated to prevent transmission to staff, patients, and visitors. The nurse should document initiation of infection control precautions in the medical record and provide the patient with an explanation as to why precautions are necessary.

If a patient shows signs of a potential contagion, it is important to inquire about recent foreign travel and to determine whether anyone else in the household has similar signs or symptoms. Once a patient with a suspected communicable condition is triaged, the triage area needs to be cleaned before the next patient enters. Table 7-12 lists suggested infectious disease precautions.

> When a patient arrives in the triage area complaining of a cough, rash, or diarrhea, the nurse must always explore the possibility of an infectious cause.

If a patient presents to triage with signs and symptoms consistent with exposure to a biologic (bioterrorism) agent, it is essential that the nurse recognize this immediately and initiate appropriate precautions to prevent further spread of the disease. Chapter 22, Infectious Diseases, includes infection control procedures to be implemented in the event of possible exposure to a biological agent.[31]

The triage nurse also needs to identify patients who are severely immunocompromised. These individuals must be protected carefully from exposure to anyone with even a minor infectious process. Place a surgical mask on the patient and escort the patient to a positive pressure room as quickly as possible.

MANAGING THE WAITING ROOM

The goal in any ED is to have no patients waiting to be seen. Obviously this is not always possible, so it is important for an ED to have guidelines in place to monitor and reassess waiting patients. Is the timing of the reassessment based on triage acuity rating or duration of wait? What are the components of reassessment? The important concept is that the waiting patients are the responsibility of the ED staff and that a periodic determination needs to be made that their conditions have not deteriorated.

> Routine rounding in the waiting room is important for patient and family satisfaction and patient safety.

TELEPHONE TRIAGE

Telephone triage is "the practice of performing a verbal interview and making an assessment of the health status of the caller."[33] EDs frequently receive calls from the public

TABLE 7-12   INFECTIOUS DISEASE ISOLATION PRECAUTIONS

PATIENT SYMPTOMS	INITIAL PRECAUTIONS DURING TRIAGE	POSSIBLE DIAGNOSES	FINAL PRECAUTIONS FOLLOWING ASSESSMENT
Rash and fever	**Airborne and Contact** Put surgical mask on patient. Place patient in a negative pressure (Airborne Infection Isolation) room. If chickenpox is suspected, nonimmune staff should not enter the room. Gowns and gloves are required for anyone entering the room. If smallpox (variola) is possible, use an N95 mask or powered air purifying respirator (PAPR) for all staff entering the room. Contact the infection control department immediately.	1. Chickenpox (varicella) 2. Measles (rubeola) 3. German measles (rubella) 4. Smallpox (variola)	Airborne and contact precautions 1. Vesicular rash and lesions commonly occur in successive crops, with several stages of maturity evident at the same time; itching is possible; rash is more abundant on covered parts of the body (trunk); slight fever is common before rash. Only immune staff should have patient contact. Airborne precautions 2. Red, maculopapular rash; rhinorrhea; Koplik's spots on buccal mucosa. Droplet precautions 3. Maculopapular rash, sometimes resembles measles or scarlet fever; low-grade fever, malaise, lymphadenopathy; upper respiratory symptoms and conjunctivitis usually precede rash. Airborne and contact precautions 4. Generalized rash with vesicles or pustules; high fever (≥104°F [40°C]) 1–4 days before onset of rash; vesicles and pustules all in the same stage of development; rash starts on face, forearms, oral mucosa, or palate and spreads to trunk.
Headache, stiff neck, and fever	**Droplet** Put surgical mask on patient. Place patient in a private room.	Meningitis	Viral vs. bacterial? Lumbar puncture can aid in the differential. 1. Viral No special precautions required 2. Bacterial; consider meningococcal meningitis Droplet precautions
Cough and fever	**Airborne** Put surgical mask on patient. Place patient in a negative air pressure room. If tuberculosis is possible, use N95 respirator mask or PAPR for all staff entering the room.	1. Tuberculosis 2. Pertussis (whooping cough) 3. Influenza (flu)	Airborne precautions 1. Night sweats, cough >2 weeks, weight loss (≥10 lb), history of exposure to tuberculosis Droplet precautions 2. Starts with rhinorrhea, sneezing, and low-grade fever for 1–2 weeks, and then cough becomes more severe and persistent or paroxysmal. Droplet precautions 3. High fever, headache, dry cough, nasal congestion, sore throat, muscle aches. (Usually during November–April "flu season.")

Infection control manual. (n.d.). Boston, MA: Brigham & Women's Hospital.

Continued

TABLE 7-12	INFECTIOUS DISEASE PRECAUTIONS—cont'd		
PATIENT SYMPTOMS	INITIAL PRECAUTIONS DURING TRIAGE	POSSIBLE DIAGNOSES	FINAL PRECAUTIONS FOLLOWING ASSESSMENT
	Contact		
Diarrhea	Put patient in a private room. Use gown and gloves for staff entering the room.	*Clostridium difficile*– associated diarrhea	Contact precautions Associated with recent history of antibiotic usage.
	Strict		
Cough, fever, and history of possible exposure to severe acute respiratory syndrome (SARS)	Place surgical mask on patient. Put patient in a negative air pressure room. Use N95 mask or PAPR, gown, gloves, and eye protection for anyone entering the room. Contact infection control immediately.	SARS	Strict precautions (airborne, and contact precautions, eye protection). Consider this diagnosis if World Health Organization or Centers for Disease Control and Prevention report the occurrence of SARS and patient has had possible exposure to SARS. Upper respiratory symptoms with fever >100.4°F (38°C); may also have cough, shortness of breath, or difficulty breathing.

asking for general medical information, inquiring about what health care actions they should take, and seeking advice as to whether they should come to the ED. ENA's position statement on telephone advice clearly addresses this issue: nurses working in facilities with no established telephone triage program should not offer medical advice over the telephone. The nurse should inform the caller that the ED is open 24 hours a day and that services are available to anyone who wishes to be seen. Hospitals should have a written telephone advice policy.

TRIAGE QUALIFICATIONS

Rapid, accurate triage requires an emergency nurse with the right qualifications, education, and experience. The ENA recommends the following qualifications for any nurse who functions in a triage capacity[30–32,34]:

- Registered nurse
- Complete a standardized triage education course that includes a didactic component and clinical orientation with a receptor prior to being assigned triage duties.
- Certified in cardiopulmonary resuscitation and Advanced Cardiac Life Support
- Emergency Nursing Pediatric Course Verification
- Trauma Nursing Core Course verification
- Geriatric Emergency Nurse Education verification
- Certified Emergency Nurse certification or Certified Pediatric Emergency Nurse (preferred)
- Effective communication skills and ability to work collaboratively
- Ability to use the nursing process effectively
- Flexible personality and adaptable to change

- Role model and suitable hospital representative
- Excellent decision-making skills

The decision as to the competency and what qualities make an effective triage nurse lies ultimately with ED leadership, who should make sure that the triage nurse receives appropriate education and demonstrates additional qualities to be successful in this role.

THE TRIAGE ROLE

Working as a triage nurse can be mentally challenging and sometimes exhausting. The triage area frequently is noisy and overcrowded; telephones ring constantly; children cry; and patients, families, and visitors are stressed and demanding. Determining which patients need to be seen immediately and which patients can wait safely requires knowledge and experience. The front-end or triage processes are being redesigned in many EDs to ensure that the ultimate goal is met: getting the right patient in the right place at the right time for the right reason.

REFERENCES

1. Centers for Disease Control and Prevention. (n.d.). *Emergency department visits.* Retrieved from http://www.cdc.gov/nchs/fastats/ervisits.htm
2. McCaig, L. F., & Ly, N. (2002). National Hospital Ambulatory Medical Care Survey: 2000 emergency department summary. *Advance Data, 326,* 1–30.
3. The Joint Commission. (2002). Delays in treatment. *Sentinel Event Alert, 26,* 1–2.
4. Emergency Nurses Association. (1999). *Standards of emergency nursing practice* (4th ed.). Des Plaines, IL: Author.

5. Gill, J. M., Reese, C. L., & Diamond, J. J. (1996). Disagreement among health care professionals about the urgent care needs of emergency department patients. *Annals of Emergency Medicine, 28*(5), 474–479.

6. Travers, D. A., Waller, A. E., Bowling, J. M., Flowers, D., & Tintinalli, J. (2002). Five-level triage system more effective than three-level in tertiary emergency department. *Journal of Emergency Nursing, 28*(5), 395–400.

7. Wuerz, R. C., Fernandes, C. M., & Alarcon, J. (1998). Inconsistency of emergency department triage. Emergency Department Operations Research Working Group. *Annals of Emergency Medicine, 32*(4), 431–435.

8. Emergency Nurses Association; American College of Emergency Physicians. (2010). *Standardized ED triage scale and acuity categorization: Joint ENA/ACEP statement.* Retrieved from http://www.ena.org/SiteCollectionDocuments/Position%20Statements/STANDARDIZEDEDTRIAGESCALEANDACUITYCATEGORIZATION.pdf

9. Fernandes, C., Tanabe, P., Gilboy, N., Johnson, L., McNair, R., Rosenau, A., … Suter, R. E. (2005). Five-level triage: A report from the ACEP/ENA Five-Level Triage Task Force. *Journal of Emergency Nursing, 31*(1), 39–50.

10. Australasian College for Emergency Medicine. (n.d.). *Guidelines for implementation of the Australasian Triage Scale in emergency departments [policy document].* Retrieved from http://enw.org/AustralianTriageScales%20Guidelines.pdf

11. National triage scale. (1994). *Emergency Medicine Australia, 6*(2), 145–146.

12. Jelinek, G. A., & Little, M. (1996). Inter-rater reliability of the National Triage Scale over 11,500 simulated occasions of triage. *Emergency Medicine Australia, 8*(4), 226–230.

13. Australian Government Department of Health and Aging. (2009). *Emergency triage education kit and triage workbook.* Retrieved from http://www.health.gov.au/internet/main/publishing.nsf/Content/5E3156CFFF0A34B1CA2573D0007BB905/$File/Triage%20Workbook.pdf

14. Canadian Association of Emergency Physicians. (2011). *The Canadian Triage and Acuity Scale.* Retrieved from http://www.caep.ca/template.asp?id=B795164082374289BBD9C1C2BF4B8D32.

15. Warren, D., Jarvis, A., LeBlanc, L., & Gravel, J.; CTAS National Working Group; Canadian Association of Emergency Physicians; National Emergency Nurses Affiliation; Association des Médecins d'Urgence du Québec; Canadian Paediatric Society; Society of Rural Physicians of Canada. (2008). Revisions to the Canadian Triage and Acuity Scale Paediatric Guidelines (PaedCTAS). *Canadian Journal of Emergency Medical Care, 10*(3), 224–243.

16. Bullard, M., Unger, B., Spence, J., & Grafstein, E.; CTAS National Working Group. (2008). Revisions to the Canadian Emergency Department Triage and Acuity Scale (CTAS) adult guidelines. *Canadian Journal of Emergency Medical Care, 10*(2), 136–151.

17. Beveridge, R., Ducharme, J., Janes, L., Beaulieu, S., & Walter, S. (1999). Reliability of the Canadian emergency department triage and acuity scale: Interrater agreement. *Annals of Emergency Medicine, 34*(2), 155–159.

18. Manos, D., Petrie, D. A., Beveridge, R. C., Walter, S., & Ducharme, J. (2002). Inter-observer agreement using the Canadian Emergency Department Triage and Acuity Scale. *Canadian Journal of Emergency Medical Care, 4*(1), 16–22.

19. Manchester Triage Group. (2006). *Emergency triage* (2nd ed.). Malden, MA: Blackwell Publishing.

20. Wuerz, R. C., Milne, L. W., Eitel, D. R., Travers, D., & Gilboy, N. (2000). Reliability and validity of a new five-level triage instrument. *Academic Emergency Medicine, 7*(3), 236–242.

21. Tanabe, P., Gimbel, R., Yarnold, P. R., Kyriacou, D. N., & Adams, J. G. (2004). Reliability and validity of scores on the Emergency Severity Index version 3. *Academic Emergency Medicine, 11*(1), 59–64.

22. Wuerz, R. C., Travers, D., Gilboy, N., Eitel, D. R., Rosenau, A., & Yazhari, R. (2001). Implementation and refinement of the emergency severity index. *Academic Emergency Medicine, 8*(2), 183–184.

23. Tanabe, P., Travers, D., Gilboy, N., Rosenau, A., Sierzega, G., Rupp, V., … Adams, J. G. (2005). Refining Emergency Severity Index triage criteria. *Academic Emergency Medicine, 12*(6), 497–501.

24. Travers, D. A., Waller, A. E., Katznelson, J., & Agans, R. (2009). Reliability and validity of the emergency severity index for pediatric triage. *Academic Emergency Medicine, 16*(9), 843–849.

25. Gilboy, N., Tanabe, P., Travers, D. A., Rosenau, A. M., & Eitel, D. R. (2005). *Emergency Severity Index, version 4: Implementation handbook* (AHRQ Publication No 05-0046-2). Rockville, MD: Agency for Healthcare Research and Quality.

26. ESI Triage Research Team. (n.d.). *Welcome to the Emergency Severity Index.* Retrieved from http://esitriage.org

27. Emergency Nurses Association. (2004). *Emergency nursing pediatric course provider manual* (3rd ed.). Des Plaines, IL: Author.

28. Cooper, R. J., Schriger, D. L., Flaherty, H. L., Lin, E. J., & Hubbell, K. A. (2002). Effect of vital signs on triage decisions. *Annals of Emergency Medicine, 39*(3), 223–232.

29. Gacki-Smith, J., Juarez, A. M., Boyett, L., Homeyer, C., Robinson, L., & MacLean, S. L. (2009). Violence against nurses working in U.S. emergency departments. *Journal of Nursing Administration, 39*(7–8), 340–349.

30. Emergency Nurses Association. (2010). *Violence in the emergency care setting* [position statement]. Retrieved from http://www.ena.org/SiteCollectionDocuments/Position%20Statements/Violence_in_the_Emergency_Care_Setting_-_ENA_PS.pdf

31. Allen, P. (2009). *Violence in emergency departments: Tools and strategies to create a violence free ED.* New York, NY: Springer.

32. *Infection control manual.* (n.d.). Boston, MA: Brigham & Women's Hospital.

33. Emergency Nurses Association. (2010). *Telephone triage* [position statement]. Retrieved from http://www.ena.org/SiteCollectionDocuments/Position%20Statements/Telephone%20Triage.pdf

34. Emergency Nurses Association. (2011, February). *Triage qualifications* [position statement]. Retrieved from http://www.ena.org/SiteCollectionDocuments/Position%20Statements/TriageQualifications.pdf

Airway Management

Julie V. O'Neal

Management of the airway is always a first priority when caring for patients. Airway management can be as simple as positioning the patient to optimize air exchange or may entail more complex interventions such as cricothyrotomy.

> Management of the airway is always a first priority.

ASSESSMENT

Assessing airway patency and spontaneous breathing is an essential first step in the care of the patient with an airway emergency. Observe for level of consciousness and determine if apnea is present. If spontaneous breathing is noted, assessment includes the following:

- Airway patency
  - Stridor, drooling, snoring respirations
  - Possible upper airway obstruction—presence of foreign body, blood, vomitus
  - Ability to vocalize
- Respiratory rate, depth, and pattern
- Work of breathing—retractions, accessory muscle use, nasal flaring
- Breath sounds bilaterally
- Patient position
- Skin color, moisture, and temperature
- Vital signs including oxygen saturation (SpO_2)

HISTORY

The history should include:

- Onset and description of symptoms
  - In children, it is important to evaluate for foreign body aspiration
- Medical history

- History of tobacco use: type, amount, length of use
- Patient's occupation, past and present
- Recent travel history
- Recent exposure to infectious disease

AIRWAY EMERGENCIES

Soft Tissue Swelling or Edema in the Airway

Upper airway obstruction resulting from edema or soft tissue swelling can be a frightening experience for the patient. The most common causes are allergic reaction, infectious process or mass, and angioedema.

Allergic Reaction

An allergic reaction is a hypersensitive response by the immune system from exposure to a previous antigen. The initial antigen exposure causes the immune system to develop antibodies that are activated with subsequent exposures. Reactions may range from mild to severe. The most severe reaction, anaphylaxis, occurs suddenly causing complete airway obstruction. Significant airway swelling requires immediate airway management. Anaphylaxis can lead to anaphylactic shock (see Chapter 20, Shock, for more information).

Signs and Symptoms

- Skin flushing
- Hives
- Urticaria
- Coughing
- Sneezing
- Dyspnea
- Facial and upper airway edema
- Muffled voice
- Wheezing
- Stridor
- Nausea, vomiting, diarrhea

Therapeutic Interventions

- If patient is alert, allow position of comfort optimizing good air exchange.
- Administer high flow oxygen (O_2).
- Establish intravenous access.
- Continuously monitor cardiac rhythm and oxygen saturation.
- Obtain emergency airway equipment including cricothyrotomy tray.
- Prepare for early endotracheal intubation; do not delay if symptoms are severe.
- Anticipate administration of the following:
  - Bronchodilators
  - Epinephrine: subcutaneously for moderate reactions, intravenously for severe reactions
  - Antihistamines: diphenhydramine (Benadryl)
  - Histamine (H_2) blockers: famotidine (Pepcid)
  - Corticosteroids

Infectious Process or Mass

An infection such as a peritonsillar abscess or a mass from throat cancer can cause edema and lead to gradual respiratory distress and airway obstruction. These are most often seen in the upper airway. Airway edema is also seen in patients with epiglottitis or inhalation or burn injuries.

Signs and Symptoms

- Drooling
- Dyspnea
- Stridor
- Muffled voice

> With airway obstruction resulting from infectious process or mass, allow the patient to assume a position of comfort.

Therapeutic Interventions

- Allow patient to assume a position of comfort.
- Provide supplemental oxygen by any means the patient will tolerate.
- Establish intravenous access.
- Continuously monitor cardiac rhythm and oxygen saturation.
- Obtain emergency airway equipment including cricothyrotomy tray.
- Anticipate administration of corticosteroids and antibiotics.

Angioedema

Angioedema is the development of large welts causing edema below the surface of the skin. The welts are primarily around the eyes and lips but are also seen on the throat, hands, and feet. This condition may be hereditary or may be precipitated by allergen exposure or stress.

Although the symptoms are similar to those of an allergic reaction, angioedema is not a true antigen-antibody response, so treatment with antihistamines and corticosteroids is not very effective. Angioedema that does not affect breathing may be uncomfortable but generally resolves in a few days. Patients with airway compromise require aggressive airway management because angioedema can cause life-threatening airway obstruction.

Signs and Symptoms

- Facial edema (lips, nose, ears, eyelids)
- Wheals
- Urticaria
- Stridor
- Abdominal pain
- Nausea, vomiting

Therapeutic Interventions

- Provide supplemental oxygen by any means the patient will tolerate.
- Establish intravenous access.
- Continuously monitor cardiac rhythm and oxygen saturation.
- Obtain emergency airway equipment including cricothyrotomy tray.
- Prepare for early endotracheal intubation; do not delay if symptoms are severe.
- Proceed to surgical airway management if intubation is not possible.
- Consider administration of fresh frozen plasma for hereditary angioedema.

Foreign Body Aspiration

Foreign body aspiration occurs most frequently in children under the age of 9 years. Symptoms vary widely and may be delayed depending on the extent of the obstruction and the stability of the object causing the obstruction. Patients may initially be asymptomatic or may immediately exhibit acute airway compromise.

Signs and Symptoms

- Sudden onset of choking or gagging
- Stridor
- Wheezing
- Cough
- Drooling
- Dyspnea
- Diminished breath sounds (bilateral or unilateral)
- Cyanosis
- Sense of impending doom

Therapeutic Interventions

- Rapidly assess airway for patency and spontaneous breathing.
- Facilitate emergent endotracheal intubation in the unconscious, nonbreathing patient.

If the patient is not moving air:

- Perform abdominal thrusts (chest thrusts in infants) to attempt to remove the object.
- Direct visualization of the upper airway with a laryngoscope may facilitate observation and removal of the foreign object.
- If unable to remove object, attempt oral intubation. If unable to intubate, immediately proceed to surgical airway.

If the patient is moving air:

- Encourage coughing, leaning forward to facilitate expulsion of object.
- Remove any objects visible in the mouth (with fingers, suction, or Magill forceps). Do not perform a blind finger sweep.
- Provide supplemental oxygen by any means the patient will tolerate.
- Continuously monitor cardiac rhythm and oxygen saturation.
- Obtain emergency airway equipment including cricothyrotomy tray.
- Chest and soft tissue lateral neck radiographs can be used to localize objects but should never delay care.

AIRWAY MANAGEMENT

Management of the patient's airway is one of the first priorities in emergency care. Failure to anticipate potential airway decline or to successfully ventilate and oxygenate the patient can lead to hypoxic brain injury or even death.

The recommended method of establishing a patent airway in an unresponsive or minimally responsive patient who is not suspected of having cervical spine injury is the head-tilt chin-lift. If the patient is at risk for cervical spine injury, the airway is opened with a jaw thrust movement while providing in-line cervical spine immobilization.

Common Airway Adjuncts

Oxygen

Oxygen administration is a fundamental therapy used to treat many conditions. Oxygen therapy can be administered by a variety of methods delivering low to high concentrations. Potential side effects include dryness of the airways and irritation of the nose, face, or ears from the delivery device. Table 8-1 summarizes common oxygen therapy devices.

Oropharyngeal Airways

- An oropharyngeal airway (OPA) is a curved plastic device that is inserted over the tongue into the posterior pharynx.
- The OPA is used to prevent the tongue or epiglottis from falling back against the posterior pharynx and occluding the airway in an unconscious or heavily sedated patient.
- Oral airways facilitate suctioning of the pharynx and prevent patients from biting their tongues or grinding their teeth. In the intubated patient the OPA can also serve as a bite block to prevent biting on the endotracheal tube
- This device should *not* be used in patients with an intact gag reflex. It may induce gagging and possible aspiration.
- The OPA comes in a variety of sizes. To select the correct size, measure from the corner of the patient's mouth to the tip of the earlobe. Be sure the correct size is used.
- If the device is too short, it will push the tongue back and occlude the airway. If the device is too long, it may stimulate gagging and emesis.
- There are two methods used for insertion. First, insert the device upside down (curved side up) until the soft pallet is reached, then rotate the device 180° and advance over the tongue. Do not use this method in children.
- Another method is to use a tongue blade to depress the tongue and insert the device (curved side down) into the posterior pharyngeal area.
- When correctly inserted the plastic flange should rest against the outer surface of the patient's teeth.

> Improperly sized and placed oral and nasal airways can cause airway obstruction.

Nasopharyngeal Airway

- Nasopharyngeal airways (NPA, nasal trumpet) are made of soft semirigid rubber and are inserted through a nonobstructed nostril to provide air passage between the nose and nasopharynx.
- This device is preferred for conscious patients because it is better tolerated and less likely to produce a gag reflex.
- Select a size that extends from the nares to the tragus of the ear. If the device is too long, the tip can stimulate laryngospasm.
- Be sure the NPA is well lubricated with a water soluble lubricant or topical anesthetic (lidocaine jelly 2%).
- Insert it into the nostril with the bevel toward the septum and advance into the posterior pharyngeal area.

TABLE 8-1 SUMMARY OF OXYGEN THERAPY DEVICES

TYPE OF BREATHING DEVICE	OXYGEN FLOW RATE	OXYGEN CONCENTRATIONS	ADVANTAGES	DISADVANTAGES
Nasal cannula	2–6 L/min	24%–44%	No rebreathing of expired air	Can be used only on patients breathing spontaneously; actual amount of inspired oxygen varies greatly
Face mask	5–10 L/min	40%–60%	Higher oxygen concentration than nasal cannula	Not tolerated well by severely dyspneic patients; can be used only on patients breathing spontaneously
Partial rebreather mask	8–12 L/min	50%–80%	Higher oxygen concentration than nasal cannula or face mask	Must have tight seal on mask; can be used only on patients breathing spontaneously; actual amount of inspired oxygen varies greatly
Nonrebreather mask	12–15 L/min	85%–100%	Highest oxygen concentration available by mask	Must have tight seal on mask; do not allow bag to collapse; can be used only on patients breathing spontaneously
Venturi mask	2–12 L/min	24%–50%	Oxygen concentration can be adjusted	Can be used only on patients breathing spontaneously
Pocket mask	10 L/min	50%	Avoids direct contact with patient's mouth; may add oxygen source; may be used on apneic patient; may be used on children; can obtain excellent tidal volume	Rescuer fatigue
Bag-mask	Room air 12 L/min	21% 40%–90%	Quick; oxygen concentration may be increased; rescuer can sense lung compliance; may be used on both apneic and spontaneously	Air in stomach; low tidal volume; difficulty obtaining a leak-proof seal
Oxygen-powered breathing device	100 L/min	100%	High oxygen flow, positive pressure; improved lung inflation	Gastric distension; overinflation of lungs; standard device cannot be used in children without special adapter; requires an oxygen source

- The NPA can also be useful for endotracheal suctioning in the nonintubated patient and can improve ventilation when used in conjunction with bag mask ventilation.
- Complications may include epistaxis, laryngospasm, or vomiting.
- The NPA is contraindicated in patients who are anticoagulated, have confirmed or suspected facial or basilar skull fractures, or have nasal deformities.

Bag-Mask Ventilation

Manual assisted ventilation is indicated:
- If the patient becomes apneic
- If spontaneous ventilation is not effective
- To reduce work of breathing
- If patient is hypoxic
  Successful-bag mask ventilation depends on:
- Maintaining an open airway
- Establishing a seal between the patient's face and the mask
- Delivering adequate tidal volume

> Be sure the bag-mask device is attached to an oxygen source prior to use.

Points to remember when manually ventilating the patient:
- Deliver 100% oxygen by maintaining O_2 flow rate of 15 L/min to the resuscitation bag.
- Deliver ventilations 8 to 10 times per minute, observing for easy rise and fall of the chest.
- Excessive tidal volume or airway pressure can cause gastric distention or pneumothorax.
- If spontaneous breathing is present, synchronize bag ventilations with the patient's inspiratory efforts.
  When no cervical spine injury is suspected, use these procedures for providing bag-mask ventilation:
- An oropharyngeal airway or nasopharyngeal airway may be placed to help maintain a patent airway.
- Stand behind the patient's head and place the appropriate-sized mask securely on the face.
- Place the narrow part of the mask at the bridge of the nose, being careful to avoid pressure on the eyes. The base of the mask should rest at the tip of the chin.
- Stabilize the mask in the left hand with gentle downward pressure, with the thumb and first and second fingers on the mask forming a "C" and the other fingers along the mandible.
- Compress the resuscitation bag with the right hand, observing for easy rise and fall of the chest.
  If cervical spine injury is suspected or if the patient has a large face or a beard and it is difficult to maintain a good mask seal:

- Two-handed technique is preferred. Mask placement and position of the operator is the same as above.
- Hold the face mask in place with both hands. Place the mask against the face and secure each side of the mask with both hands forming a "C" on each side.
- A second operator compresses the resuscitation bag observing for easy rise and fall of the chest.

Endotracheal Intubation

Endotracheal intubation is the preferred method of airway management in the apneic patient. This procedure requires practice, preparation, and skill. Endotracheal intubation is a two-handed procedure where the provider holds the laryngoscope in the left hand and positions the head with the right hand. Once the head is tilted back in position the trachea is intubated by passing the endotracheal tube (ETT) through the right side of the mouth and advancing it to the glottic opening and through the vocal cords.[1] There are circumstances when nasotracheal intubation may be the preferred method.

Indications for endotracheal intubation include:
- Airway protection
- Relief of obstruction
- Route for mechanical ventilation and oxygen delivery
- Respiratory failure
- Shock
- Intracranial hypertension
- Reduce work of breathing
- Facilitate suctioning of the airway
  The role of the assistant during the intubation procedure:
- Pass equipment to the airway provider
- Hold the head in position
- Hold open the right corner of the mouth during intubation

> The American Heart Association no longer recommends cricoid pressure as a routine procedure in cardiac arrest.

Assessment of Endotracheal Tube Placement. Once the endotracheal tube has been placed, it is imperative to confirm correct placement in the trachea. The most common method is to attach a colorimetric capnometer to the end of the ETT to detect exhaled carbon dioxide (ECO_2). The colorimetric capnometer will quickly change color from purple (poor) to yellow (yes) when carbon dioxide is detected. The color change often occurs within the first two breaths but may be delayed for up to six breaths. If the color does not change to yellow, confirming ECO_2, the ETT is not correctly placed in the trachea. If the color turns tan, this may also indicate incorrect placement. If ETT placement is incorrect, it must be removed and reinserted. Continuous capnography monitoring may be done where waveform and numeric carbon dioxide values can be monitored.

Auscultation of bilateral breath sounds over the right and left chest and axilla and over the epigastrium, as well as observation of chest rise and fall during ventilation, should be done to confirm successful intubation. A chest radiograph will verify position of the endotracheal tube and rule out right mainstem bronchial intubation.

The ETT must be well secured after confirmation of placement and correct placement must be frequently assessed thereafter.

Rapid Sequence Intubation

Rapid sequence intubation (RSI) begins with preoxygenation and is followed by the administration of a potent sedative agent and a rapidly acting neuromuscular blocking agent to facilitate rapid endotracheal intubation. The purpose of RSI is to render the patient unconscious and paralyzed in order to intubate the trachea without the need for bag-mask ventilation, which can cause gastric distension and risk of aspiration.[2]

> Always give a sedative prior to administering a neuromuscular blocking agent.

- Successful RSI requires a detailed knowledge of the sequence of steps to be taken as well as the time required for each step to achieve success.
- RSI is the preferred method of preparation prior to intubation in the conscious patient.
- This process is not used for patients that are apneic.
- RSI begins with preoxygenation and is followed by administration of a series of medications. These include giving an induction agent followed immediately by a rapidly acting neuromuscular blocking agent.
- The sequential steps are often referred to as the "seven P's": preparation, preoxygenation, pretreatment, paralysis, placement, placement verification, and post intubation management. See Table 8-2.

TABLE 8-2   RAPID SEQUENCE INTUBATION

TIME	STEP
Zero minus 5–10 minutes	**Preparation** Establish good intravenous access. Prepare necessary equipment (bag-mask, suction, endotracheal tube, stylet, laryngoscope, tube holder or tape, ventilator).
Zero minus 5 minutes	**Preoxygenation** Preoxygenate with 100% oxygen (by nonrebreather mask or bag-mask). (High PaO_2 levels will allow up to 8 minutes of apnea before desaturation occurs.)
Zero minus 3 minutes	**Pretreatment** Administer an appropriate sedating agent (midazolam, fentanyl, etomidate, thiopental, ketamine) Give drugs to minimize the effects of intubation such as increased intracranial pressure (lidocaine), bradycardia (atropine), and muscle fasciculations (a small dose of a defasciculating paralytic such as vecuronium, pancuronium, rocuronium).
Zero	**Paralysis** Inject a short-acting neuromuscular blocking agent (succinylcholine, vecuronium, rocuronium, pancuronium). Begin (or continue) manual ventilation.
Zero plus 45 seconds	**Placement** Perform the Sellick maneuver (compression of the larynx against the esophagus) to prevent aspiration. Do not release pressure until the endotracheal tube cuff has been inflated. Intubate the patient and inflate the cuff.
	Placement Verification Confirm tube placement by auscultation, chest rise and fall, and a carbon dioxide detection device. Secure the tube.
	Postintubation Management Provide additional sedation as needed for ventilator management.

Modified from Roberts, J. R., & Hedges, J. (Eds.). (2004). *Clinical procedures in emergency medicine* (4th ed.). Philadelphia, PA: Saunders.

TABLE 8-3　RAPID SEQUENCE INDUCTION MEDICATIONS

PURPOSE	MEDICATION	DOSE	COMMENTS
Sedative	Midazolam	0.1–0.3 mg/kg IV	
Analgesic	Fentanyl	2–3 mcg/kg IV	
Protective agent	Atropine	0.01–0.02 mg/kg (children)	Prevents bradycardia
		0.5–1 mg IV (adults)	
	Lidocaine	1.5 mg/kg IV	Suppresses cough reflex
			Blunts intracranial pressure response
Anesthesia	Etomidate	0.2–0.4 mg/kg IV	May cause myotonic or myoclonic activity
			Reduces bronchospasm; contraindicated in head injury
	Ketamine	1–2 mg/kg IV	Contraindicated in asthma; may cause hypotension and laryngospasm
	Thiopental	2 mg/kg IV	Contraindicated in hyperkalemia, burns, neuromuscular disease, eye injuries
	Propofol	0.5–2 mg/kg IV	Contraindicated if patient allergic to eggs
Paralytic	Succinylcholine	1–2 mg/kg IV	Contraindicated in head and eye injuries, cardiovascular disease
	Pancuronium	0.01 mg/kg IV (defasciculating dose)	
	Rocuronium	0.6–1 mg/kg IV	Contraindicated in head and eye injuries, cardiovascular disease
	Vecuronium	0.01 mg/kg IV (defasciculating dose)	
		0.1 mg/kg IV (paralyzing dose)	

IV, Intravenous.
From Roberts, J. R., & Hedges, J. (Eds.). (2004). *Clinical procedures in emergency medicine* (4th ed.). Philadelphia, PA: Saunders.

- Administration of a sedation agent prior to neuromuscular blockade is essential. Table 8-3 lists medications commonly used in RSI.

Alternative Invasive Airways

- Endotracheal intubation is the "gold standard" for effective ventilation, oxygenation, and protection of the airway from aspiration. However, successful intubation requires skill and training.
- Failure to successfully intubate the patient and maintain ventilation and oxygenation leads to significant morbidity and mortality.

Over the past two decades several alternative rescue device airways have been developed. These devices should not be used in patients with an intact gag reflex. The most commonly used devices are described below.

Laryngeal Mask Airway

- There are several different laryngeal mask airways (LMAs) available. They come in a variety of sizes to be used for children as well as adults.
- Although training is required, these devices are easy to use.

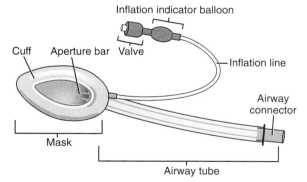

Fig. 8-1　Laryngeal mask airway. (From Fultz, J., & Sturt, P. [2005]. *Mosby's emergency nursing reference.* St. Louis, MO: Mosby.)

- LMAs do not prevent aspiration of gastric contents but do allow for effective oxygenation and ventilation of the patient until a more definitive airway can be placed.
- The LMA is inserted through the mouth and is advanced over the tongue to position over the larynx. See Figure 8-1.

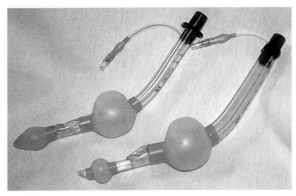

Fig. 8-2 King LT-D and LTSD airways. (Image courtesy of King Systems Corporation.)

- Once in place, the collar is inflated with air to seat it in position.
- Some LMAs are disposable and others are designed to allow for intubation with a endotracheal tube through the device after the LMA is in place.

Combitube

- The Combitube is a latex dual lumen, dual cuff airway that is designed to be inserted into the esophagus but can function short term as an ETT if placed into the trachea.
- Like the LMA, the Combitube is inserted by hand into the mouth and advanced into place while maintaining the head and neck in a neutral position.
- The Combitube has two balloon pilots that must be inflated once the tube is in place.
- Contraindications to use of Combitube:
  - Patients under 5 feet tall (Combitube) or 4 feet tall (Combitube SA)
  - Patients with esophageal disease or patients who have ingested caustic substances

King Laryngeal Tube Airway

The King airway is a disposable, latex-free single lumen tube with two cuffs. One cuff is oropharyngeal and the other is esophageal with a ventilation outlet between the two. Only one pilot balloon is used to inflate both cuffs. See Figure 8-2.

- The King LT comes in sizes that can be used in patients 4 feet (122 cm) or taller. The King LT-D can be used in patients 35 inches (90 cm) or taller.
- The King LT-D has a gastric access lumen that allows passage of a nasogastric tube to decompress the stomach.
- Patients can be mechanically ventilated, short term, using the King airway.

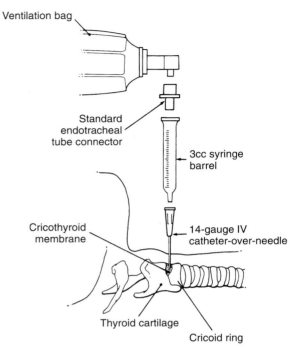

Fig. 8-3 A simple setup for transtracheal ventilation using standard equipment found in any emergency department. This setup is inadequate for adults. High-pressure (50 psi) ventilation systems are optimal. Even with the pressure relief valve on the bag valve device turned off, only a suboptimal pressure can be developed. However, this technique may be satisfactory in infants and small children. *IV*, Intravenous. (From Roberts, J. R., & Hedges, J. R. [2004]. *Clinical procedures in emergency medicine* [4th ed.]. St. Louis, MO: Saunders.)

- An endotracheal tube can be placed through the King airway with the use of a tube exchange catheter inserted through the King LTS-D ventilation channel. Once the endotracheal tube is in place the King airway is removed.

Emergency Airway Techniques

Only physicians or advanced practice nurses typically perform emergency airway techniques. They are temporary until a more definitive airway can be placed.

Percutaneous Transtracheal Ventilation

Also known as "needle cricothyrotomy" or "jet insufflation," percutaneous transtracheal ventilation is illustrated in Figure 8-3.

- Involves placing a large-bore intravenous catheter (14 gauge or larger) into the trachea through the cricothyroid membrane below the level of the vocal cords.
- When successfully placed, the connector from a 3.0 endotracheal tube is inserted into the intravenous catheter and then attached to a bag-mask device to ventilate the patient.
- If available, a high pressure oxygen source, or jet insufflator, can be used to ventilate the patient. Transtracheal jet ventilation systems consist of a high pressure oxygen source, high pressure oxygen tubing connected to a regulator to control the driving pressure, and an on–off valve to control inspiratory time.
- Assess for rise and fall of the chest with inspiration and allow adequate exhalation time to prevent carbon dioxide accumulation with this procedure.

Surgical Cricothyrotomy

- A surgical cricothyrotomy is done to establish an airway when attempts at intubation have failed or when endotracheal intubation would not be successful. Examples include but are not limited to massive facial trauma, airway obstruction resulting from edema, and masses or foreign objects occluding the airway.
- An opening is made to the trachea through the cricothyroid membrane. This can be accomplished with a commercial device or a scalpel incision. Several different cricothyrotomy techniques can be performed to secure the airway. Once the opening is made, either a endotracheal tube or a tracheostomy tube can be inserted to secure the airway and ventilate the patient.

Suctioning

To maintain a patent airway, suctioning of the oropharynx, nasopharynx, and trachea is often required.

- Patients with artificial airways, especially endotracheal tubes, have ineffective coughing and secretion removal, which requires periodic suctioning of pulmonary secretions.
- The thickness or amount of secretions in the oropharynx often requires the use of a tonsillar tip device (Yankauer).
- Suctioning should not be done routinely but only when clinically indicated.
- Refer to Table 8-4 for indications for and complications of endotracheal suctioning.
- Hyperoxygenation with 100% oxygen should always be provided prior to each suction attempt.
- Endotracheal or tracheostomy tube suctioning is a sterile procedure to prevent nosocomial infections and ventilator-associated pneumonia (VAP).

TABLE 8-4	INDICATIONS FOR AND COMPLICATIONS OF ENDOTRACHEAL SUCTIONING
INDICATIONS	**COMPLICATIONS**
Clearance of secretions, foreign matter, vomitus, or blood in the airway	Hypoxemia
Suspected aspiration of gastric contents or secretions	Laryngospasm
Auscultation of coarse or gurgling breath sounds	Damage to mucosa, leading to risk of bleeding
Increased work of breathing, or respiratory distress	Bronchospasm
To clear secretions via the endotracheal tube or tracheostomy tube	Hypertension or hypotension
Increasing respiratory rate, frequent coughing, or both	Increased intracranial pressure
A gradual or sudden decrease in oxygen saturation	Vagal stimulation leading to bradycardia and hypotension, especially in infants and young children

- Suctioning should not exceed 10 seconds per attempt, to prevent hypoxia.

Suctioning can be performed by one of two methods.

1. Open suctioning is performed using a single-use sterile suction catheter. This technique can be used for oropharyngeal, nasopharyngeal, or endotracheal suctioning.
2. The closed suction techniques, also known as in-line suctioning, is used in mechanically ventilated patients. A multiple-use suction catheter covered by a sterile sleeve is attached to the end of the endotracheal or tracheostomy tube.
   - Use of the closed suction technique allows for maintenance of oxygenation and ventilatory support while suctioning. This is beneficial to patients who require high levels of pressure support or positive end expiratory pressure (PEEP).
   - Use of the closed system is also beneficial to the health care provider as it reduces the risk of aerosolization of secretions.
   - The closed system is preferred for patients who develop instability or rapid oxygen desaturation with the open suctioning technique.

VENTILATION OF THE EMERGENCY PATIENT

Noninvasive Positive Pressure Ventilation

The advantages of noninvasive positive pressure ventilation (NPPV) include:

- Preservation of speech, swallowing, and physiological airway defense mechanisms
- Reduced risk of airway injury
- Reduced risk of nosocomial infections
- Reduced length of stay in the intensive care unit.[1]

NPPV offers short-term (typically 1–4 days) ventilatory support. It has two modes of ventilation: CPAP and BiPAP.

- Continuous positive airway pressure (CPAP) provides constant airway pressure throughout the airway cycle.
- Bilevel, or biphasic, positive airway pressure (BiPAP) provides airway pressure that cycles between inspiratory airway pressure (IPAP) and an end expiratory airway pressure (EPAP).

NPPV is administered to the patient through a variety of devices: a mask that covers only the nose, one that covers the nose and mouth, or one that covers the entire face (a helmet). These devices should be comfortable and provide a good seal to minimize air leak. Patients that would benefit from NPPV are spontaneously breathing, conscious, and alert but have a poor ventilatory drive. Patients with exacerbation of chronic obstructive pulmonary disease (COPD), decompensated heart failure, severe pneumonia, or status asthmaticus are all good candidates for NPPV.[3] BiPAP and CPAP have been shown to be effective in treating patients with sleep apnea. NPPV is contraindicated in patients who are apneic, uncooperative, or at risk of losing their airway.

Mechanical Ventilation

The basic purpose of mechanical ventilation is to provide positive pressure ventilation, maintain alveolar gas exchange, decrease work of breathing, and deliver a specific concentration of oxygen. Several modes of ventilation can be used to accomplish these goals. Mechanical ventilation can be administered through a correctly placed endotracheal, tracheostomy, or cricothyrotomy tube.

Common terms used in mechanical ventilation are defined in Table 8-5.

Precautions with Mechanical Ventilation

- Ensure proper placement of the endotracheal tube prior to initiating ventilation.
- Can cause further damage to an already injured lung or damage a previously healthy lung.
- May cause pneumothorax or tension pneumothorax.

TABLE 8-5 COMMON TERMS USED IN MECHANICAL VENTILATION

- Tidal volume (Vt): The volume of each breath measured in milliliters. Tidal volumes are usually in the range of 6 to 8 mL/kg of ideal body weight.
- Respiratory rate or frequency (f): Usual setting 12 to 20 breaths per minute.
- Fractional concentration of inspired oxygen (FiO_2): Concentration of oxygen that ranges from room air (21%) to pure oxygen (100%). When initiating mechanical ventilation, 100% FiO_2 is usually used.
- Positive end expiratory pressure (PEEP): Constant pressure that is typically set at 5 to 10 cm H_2O to keep the alveoli open.
- Common ventilation modes:
  - Assist control (AC): The preferred mode for patients in respiratory distress or failure. The patient or the ventilator can initiate the breath. If the patient initiates the breath, it will trigger the ventilator to administer the preset tidal volume.
  - Synchronized intermittent mandatory ventilation (SIMV) or intermittent mandatory ventilation (IMV): The ventilator initiates each breath at the set tidal volume. The ventilator synchronizes with the patient's respiratory efforts, delivering the set tidal volume. If the patient intiates the breath, he or she will receive only the tidal volume he or she is able to take in. This mode can lead to increased work of breathing.
  - Control mode of ventilation (CMV): Used in the operating room or in sedated and paralyzed patients.
  - Pressure support ventilation (PSV): Usually set at 5 to 10 cm H_2O. This mode augments inflation volumes during spontaneous breathing or is used to overcome the resistance of breathing through the ventilator circuit. This limits work of breathing for the patient, especially during the weaning process.

- May cause ventilator-associated pneumonia.
- An understanding of the different ventilator alarms and troubleshooting tips is important.

Caring for Mechanically Ventilated Patients

- Assess patients requiring mechanical ventilation frequently for adequacy of ventilation and the possible development of complications such as pneumothorax or tension pneumothorax.
- Ventilated patients often become anxious, which can interfere with the mechanical ventilation. Administration of sedatives or narcotics can help the patient relax,

which will decrease work of breathing and decrease oxygen consumption.

- Some patients may require neuromuscular blockade agents (NMBAs). *Always* administer adequate sedation and analgesia prior to administering an NMBA.
- Monitor continuous pulse oximetry. In some settings, continuous capnography (ECO_2) monitoring may also be done.
- If the patient has high airway pressures as noted on the ventilator, assess the patient for the need for suctioning. If after suctioning the patient continues to have high airway pressures, assess for signs of a pneumothorax.

REFERENCES

1. Walls, R. M., & Luten, R. C. (Eds.). (2008). *Manual of emergency airway management* (3rd ed.). Philadelphia, PA: Lippincott Williams & Wilkins.
2. Nestor, N. B., & Burton, J. H. (2008). ED use of etomidate for rapid sequence induction. *American Journal of Emergency Medicine, 26*(8), 946–950.
3. Rose, L., & Gerdtz, M. F. (2009). Review of non-invasive ventilation in the emergency department: Clinical considerations and management priorities. *Journal of Clinical Nursing, 18*(23), 3216–3224.

Cardiopulmonary Arrest

Belinda B. Hammond

Cardiopulmonary arrest is not an unusual occurrence in the emergency department. Causes can range from the expected terminal event of chronic or acute illnesses to sudden cardiac death. Hypoxemia secondary to severe respiratory insufficiency, intentional or accidental drug overdose, or neurologic insult can also result in unexpected cardiopulmonary arrest. Traumatic cardiopulmonary arrest is a less common and more difficult to manage cause of arrest.

The goal of basic life support (BLS) is to restore effective circulation and oxygenation and to maintain intact neurologic function. Emphasis is placed on the immediate initiation of the following steps:
- Recognize sudden cardiac death by establishing unresponsiveness and absence of normal respiration
- Activate emergency response team ("calling a code" in the hospital setting)
- Perform high-quality chest compressions
- Begin rescue breathing
- Perform rapid defibrillation if appropriate

> Emphasize to all patients with a history of heart disease the importance of calling 911 rather than having family members drive them to the emergency department.

The ABCs of BLS have been replaced by CAB—compressions, airway, breathing—to reflect the growing evidence that chest compressions are the most important aspect of early resuscitation efforts. In addition, airway management takes time and can delay the initiation of effective chest compressions.[1]

Most victims of cardiopulmonary arrest initially experience ventricular fibrillation. Chest compressions can maintain some level of cardiac output but will not convert this life-threatening rhythm; defibrillation is the only definitive treatment. The interval from collapse to defibrillation is one of the most important determinants of survival from cardiopulmonary arrest.[1] The automatic external defibrillator (AED) is useful for early defibrillation in that no specific rhythm interpretation is required by the operator. The AED will determine whether the rhythm is "shockable" or not.

It is assumed that the reader is familiar with the principles of BLS and techniques of high-quality chest compressions. Specific BLS guidelines and advanced cardiac life support (ACLS) treatment algorithms can be found on the American Heart Association's website. All emergency nurses should obtain and maintain certification in ACLS.

> - Open-access, multilingual websites that provide straightforward explanations and demonstrations of cardiopulmonary resuscitation (CPR) are available; see http://www.learncpr.org.
> - The American Heart Association has an application for smart phones called "Pocket First Aid and CPR."

MANAGEMENT OF CARDIOPULMONARY ARREST

Chest Compressions

One of four rhythms can cause cardiopulmonary arrest:
- Ventricular fibrillation (VF)
- Pulseless ventricular tachycardia (VT)
- Pulseless electrical activity (PEA)
- Ventricular asystole

The *2010 American Heart Association Guidelines for Cardiopulmonary Resuscitation and Emergency Cardiovascular Care Science*[1] emphasizes the need for quality chest compressions as fundamental in managing cardiopulmonary arrest resulting from these four rhythms.

The importance of high-quality chest compression cannot be overemphasized.
- Push hard, push fast—to the tune of "Stayin' Alive"!
- Allow complete release of chest pressure between compressions.

- Assess for femoral pulse during compressions to determine the effectiveness of compressions.
- Minimize interruptions of chest compressions.
- In the absence of an advanced airway, synchronize compressions to ventilations with a ratio of 30:2. Once an advanced airway has been placed, give continuous chest compressions at a rate of at least 100 per minute; do not pause for ventilations.
- High-quality chest compressions can quickly lead to provider fatigue. Rotate the chest compressor every 2 minutes.

Airway Control

During cardiopulmonary arrest, oxygen delivery to the vital organs is diminished because of low blood flow (perfusion) rather than arterial oxygen content (ventilation), emphasizing again the need for immediate initiation of high-quality chest compressions. Still, 100% supplemental oxygen should be initiated as soon as possible, without delaying or interrupting compressions, during resuscitation from cardiopulmonary arrest.[1]

- Open and maintain a patent airway using:
  - Head-tilt chin-lift
  - Jaw lift without head extension if suspected head or neck injury
- Do not delay chest compressions or defibrillation to establish an invasive airway.
- Refer to Chapter 8, Airway Management, for more information concerning airway management.

Breathing and Ventilation

- Assess rise and fall of chest for adequacy of ventilation.
- If bag-mask ventilation is sufficient, invasive airway management may be deferred until return of spontaneous circulation (ROSC).
- Monitor rate and depth of manual ventilation to prevent hyperventilation. Excessive ventilation can increase intrathoracic pressure, decreasing venous return to the heart.
- In the patient without an advanced airway, the rate of ventilation is two ventilations after each cycle of 30 chest compressions. Once an advanced airway is placed, ventilations should be given at a rate of 8 to 10 per minute (one ventilation every 5–6 seconds) without a pause in chest compressions.

Obtaining Circulatory Access

- Establish intravenous (IV) access.
- Use a large-gauge catheter to access a large vein, preferably in the antecubital space. Do not interrupt chest compressions while obtaining IV access.
- Consider intraosseous (IO) insertion if no venous access is available.
- Avoid central venous access via the subclavian approach during resuscitation efforts because of the need to stop compressions and the potential for complications such as pneumothorax.

Defibrillation

- Other than high-quality CPR, the only rhythm-specific treatment shown to increase survival to hospital discharge is defibrillation of VF or pulseless VT.[1]
- The main goal is to electrically terminate a shockable rhythm as quickly as possible; the earlier the defibrillation occurs, the better the chance of patient survival.
- Do not interrupt chest compressions while the defibrillator is charging if charging takes more than 10 seconds.
- Follow each shock immediately with 2 minutes of high-quality chest compressions to enhance coronary perfusion. Even if VF is terminated by the shock, almost all patients will experience a period of nonperfusing rhythm. CPR is needed to maintain circulation during this time.[2]
- Do not stop to check for a pulse after delivering the shock. Pulse checks may be performed if an organized rhythm is evident on the monitor, but chest compressions should not be interrupted for longer than 10 seconds.[2]

> Resume chest compressions immediately after a shock is delivered *without* checking for a pulse or rhythm.

- Shocks can be delivered through paddles or self-adhesive disposable pads applied to anterior-posterior or anterior-anterior position.
  - Use of self-adhesive, hands-free monitor or defibrillator pads is recommended over paddles.
  - To maximize current flow through the myocardium, the recommended pad placement is sternal-apical.
    - Place the sternal pad to the right of the upper sternum below the clavicle.
    - Place the center of the apical pad in the left midaxillary line.
    - Place the apical pad beneath the female breast.
    - Do not allow pads to touch one another.
    - Do not place pads on top of a transdermal medication patch (nitroglycerine, nicotine, hormone replacement). Remove the patch and wipe the skin clean before applying the pad.
- American Heart Association guidelines note if there is any evidence of an implantable cardioverter defibrillator

(ICD) or permanent pacemaker, defibrillation should not be delayed by pad or paddle placement. It is recommended to avoid placing the pads or paddles over the implanted device.[1]

- These devices do not need to be deactivated during resuscitation efforts.
- Anterior-posterior placement of the pads is recommended to minimize damage to the device[2] but pad placement should not delay defibrillation.
- The energy level for the initial shock with a biphasic defibrillator is 120 to 200 joules; if using a monophasic defibrillator, use 360 joules. If unsure as to whether the defibrillator is biphasic or monophasic, deliver the shock at 200 joules. Deliver subsequent shocks at the energy level that was previously successful.
- Ensure that all personnel are "clear" of the patient, bed, and equipment before delivering shocks.

Drugs

- The drugs most commonly used during resuscitation from cardiopulmonary arrest are epinephrine, vasopressin, and amiodarone.
- Epinephrine, 1 mg, either IV or IO, is given every 3 to 5 minutes during cardiopulmonary arrest in the adult.
  - Because of its vasoconstrictor effects, epinephrine increases cerebral and coronary blood flow during CPR.
  - Studies have demonstrated no benefit to higher doses or increasing doses of epinephrine during cardiopulmonary arrest.[2]
  - Epinephrine may be administered via the endotracheal tube if IV or IO access cannot be obtained. However, drug absorption is unpredictable and this route is not recommended.[2]
- Vasopressin (Pitressin), 40 units, either IV or IO, can replace either the first or the second dose of epinephrine.
  - The effects and survival rates of vasopressin use have not been shown to differ from those of epinephrine.[2]
- The recommended initial dose of amiodarone is 300 mg, either intravenously or intraosseously; this may be followed by a single 150-mg dose.
  - Amiodarone (Cordarone) can be administered in either of the following ways:
    - Direct injection of undiluted drug followed by a minimum 10 mL flush
    - Minimally diluting two 150-mg doses in two 10 mL 0.9% sodium chloride–filled ("flush") syringes[3]
  - If amiodarone is unavailable, lidocaine can be given. However, there is no evidence demonstrating improved survival with lidocaine use.[2]

TABLE 9-1	THE H'S AND T'S: COMMON CAUSES OF CARDIOPULMONARY ARREST
H'S	**T'S**
Hypoxia	Toxins (including drug overdose)
Hypovolemia	Tamponade (cardiac)
Hydrogen ion (acidosis)	Tension pneumothorax
Hypothermia	Thrombosis (coronary and pulmonary)
Hypokalemia, hyperkalemia	

- Follow bolus injections of drugs with a 20-mL bolus of IV fluid; elevate the extremity for 10 to 20 seconds following administration to facilitate delivery to the central circulation.[2]

Treat Reversible Causes

Although high-quality CPR and early defibrillation, when appropriate, are the cornerstones of successful resuscitation from cardiopulmonary arrest, possible causes of the arrest must be considered early on. Reversible causes of arrest or factors that may impede resuscitative efforts are known as the "H's and T's" and are listed in Table 9-1. A high index of suspicion and specific diagnostic measures are needed to identify and treat these conditions.

THE TEAM APPROACH

- One person, certified in ACLS, should assume the role of team leader and direct the resuscitation efforts.
- Closed-loop communication is essential. Team members should repeat orders for medications (including the dosage) and other interventions and announce the completion of these orders.
- One team member is designated to document all aspects of the resuscitation and to frequently review for the team what interventions have been used and the time frame of the resuscitation.
- Table 9-2 lists the various roles of the resuscitation team and their responsibilities.

FAMILY PRESENCE DURING RESUSCITATION

The Emergency Nurses Association (ENA) has long advocated offering family members the option of being present at the patient's bedside during resuscitative efforts[4]; some feel that nurses have a moral obligation to offer this

TABLE 9-2 ROLES AND RESPONSIBILITIES OF THE RESUSCITATION TEAM

Team Leader
- Directs assessment and interventions
- Observes team members for ability to fulfill assigned roles
- Ensures closed-loop communications
- Requests input from team members
- Teaches and reinforces efforts of team members

Airway Manager
- Maintains patent airway
- Continually monitors respiratory and ventilator status of patient
- Provides adequate ventilation via bag-mask or advanced airway
- Requests arterial blood gas studies when appropriate
- Monitors efficiency of chest compressions; reminds compressors to change to prevent fatigue
- Participates in closed-loop communications

Chest Compressors
- Perform high-quality, uninterrupted CPR
- Remain aware of fatigue and are willing to rotate with other team members
- Participate in closed-loop communications

Treatment Nurse
- Establishes and maintains IV access
- Operates defibrillator, including ensuring all are "clear" before discharge
- Monitors for femoral pulse during chest compressions
- Administers IV or IO medications
- Assesses vital signs as appropriate
- Participates in closed-loop communications

Recorder
- Documents all steps of the resuscitation effort, including accurate times using the same clock
- Frequently reviews with the team what medications and interventions have been completed
- Helps monitor compressor fatigue and calls for a change
- Advises team of patient's medical history as it becomes known
- May communicate orders to others not directly involved in the resuscitation effort
  - Calls for portable chest radiograph, other interventions, etc.
- Participates in closed-loop communication

Traffic Controller
- Clears the resuscitation room of unneeded observers.
- Provides for patient privacy by keeping doors and curtains closed and limiting noise, extraneous conversations, and other distractions

Family Advocate or Liaison
- If family chooses to be present during resuscitation efforts:
  - Stays with family to offer support and information
  - Removes disruptive family members if necessary
- If family chooses not to be present:
  - Provides family with private waiting area with telephone, tissues, and beverages
  - Maintains contact with resuscitation team and provides frequent updates to family
  - Stays with family members as needed
  - Offers to contact hospital chaplain or family's preferred spiritual adviser
  - Accompanies family to bedside when resuscitation efforts have been completed
  - Informs family of "what happens next" depending on outcome of resuscitation

CPR, Cardiopulmonary resuscitation; *IO,* intraosseous; *IV,* intravenous.
Adapted from Neumar, R. W., Otto, C. W., Link, M. S., Kronick, S. L., Shuster, M., Callaway, C. W., ... Morrison, L. J. (2010). Part 8: Adult advanced cardiovascular life support: 2010 American Heart Association guidelines for cardiopulmonary resuscitation and emergency cardiovascular care. *Circulation, 122*(18 suppl 3), S729–S767; Zimmerman, J. L. (2007). *Fundamental critical care support* (4th ed.). Mount Prospect, IL: Society of Critical Care Medicine.

opportunity.[5] In order for family presence at the bedside to be successful, one health care team member (a nurse or knowledgeable chaplain or social worker) should be assigned to care solely for the family members.
- Remain physically at the family member's side.
- Explain in simple terms what is happening and why.
- Inform team members involved in the resuscitation that a family member is present.
- If at all possible, allow the family member to hold the patient's hand and speak to the patient during the resuscitation efforts.[5]

Table 9-3 summarizes some of the concerns and benefits of family presence during resuscitation.

SPECIFIC CAUSES OF CARDIAC ARREST

Pulseless Ventricular Tachycardia/Ventricular Fibrillation
- Defibrillation is the treatment of choice for pulseless VT or VF.
- Epinephrine, 1 mg IV or IO, is repeated every 3 to 5 minutes and makes VF more responsive to defibrillation.

TABLE 9-3	**BENEFITS AND CONCERNS RELATED TO FAMILY PRESENCE DURING RESUSCITATION EFFORTS**

POTENTIAL BENEFITS	POSSIBLE CONCERNS
Families understand the seriousness of the patient's illness or injury and see that all possible interventions were performed to save their loved one's life.	Family members may interfere with the resuscitation efforts.
Families are able to begin the grieving process; closure and healing may be facilitated.	Family members may misinterpret resuscitation activities in a way that increases the potential for litigation.
Family members can provide additional information concerning the patient's medical history and possible events leading to the cardiopulmonary arrest.	Events and procedures may be too traumatic for the family members.
Family members are given a chance to say "good-bye."	Safety of family members may be compromised; members may faint or be accidentally exposed to blood or body fluids.
Family fear and anxiety may be reduced and their feelings of isolation minimized.	Family's response to grief may be anger or violence.

Adapted from Fell, O. P. (2009). Family presence during resuscitation efforts. *Nursing Forum, 44*(2), 144–150; Laskowski-Jones, L. (2007). Should families be present during resuscitation? *Nursing, 37*(5), 44–47; and Tomlinson, K. R., Golden, I. J., Mallory, J. L., & Comer, L. (2010). Family presence during adult resuscitation: A survey of emergency department registered nurses and staff attitudes. *Advanced Emergency Nursing Journal, 32*(1), 45–58.

- Vasopressin, 40 units IV or IO, can be substituted for the first or second dose of epinephrine.
- Amiodarone is the preferred treatment for shock-refractory VF.

Asystole or Pulseless Electrical Activity

- Ventricular asystole is often an end-stage rhythm in which there is a total absence of ventricular contraction. PEA refers to a heterogeneous group of organized electrical rhythms that fail to produce effective contraction and a palpable pulse.[2]

- Support circulation with high quality CPR while considering the cause. Treating possible reversible causes of cardiac arrest is discussed below.
- Although no randomized, controlled trials have shown improved survival from asystole or PEA following drug administration, the ACLS algorithm recommends epinephrine, 1 mg IV or IO every 3 to 5 minutes, once IV access has been obtained.
- Defibrillation and pacing are not recommended for managing asystole or PEA.
- Do not interrupt CPR for longer than 10 seconds to check for a pulse.
- If asystole is observed on the monitor, check leads and cable connections, assess height of gain on the monitor and confirm rhythm in at least two different leads.

Symptomatic Bradycardia

- Bradycardia may be "absolute" (rate <60 bpm) or "relative" (a heart rate that is less than expected given the patient's clinical condition).
- Bradycardia is considered "symptomatic" if indications of poor perfusion are present and are due to the slow heart rate.
  - Chest pain
  - Shortness of breath
  - Decreased level of consciousness
  - Lightheadedness, dizziness, syncope
  - Hypotension
- If bradycardia is symptomatic:
  - Assess airway and breathing; support as needed
  - Administer supplemental oxygen
  - Obtain IV access and a 12-lead ECG
  - Prepare for transcutaneous pacing (see below)
- Atropine is the drug of choice for acute symptomatic bradycardia. An initial dose of 0.5 mg can be repeated every 3 to 5 minutes for a maximum dose of 3 mg.
- In patients who have undergone heart transplantation, isoproterenol (Isuprel) is the drug of choice for symptomatic bradycardia. Following transplantation, the vagus nerve is not intact and atropine administration will be ineffective.
- If transcutaneous pacing is not available once the maximum dose of atropine has been given, a continuous IV infusion of epinephrine and/or dopamine may be considered.
- Transcutaneous pacemaking
  - Apply pacing electrodes as indicated on the pacing device or the electrode package; placement may be anterior/posterior or anterior/anterior.
  - Set pacemaker rate at 70 bpm.

- Slowly increase the milliamperes (mA) until electrical capture (see below) occurs. Use the lowest level possible that maintains capture.
- Assess pacing activity
  - Electrical capture: Observe the monitor for electrical pacing spikes each followed by a wide QRS complex.
  - Mechanical capture: Present when each pacing spike/QRS complex grouping produces a palpable femoral pulse.
  - Do not use carotid pulse to assess circulation in patient being externally paced as the electrical activity of the pacemaker also causes generalized muscle contraction.
- Once electrical and mechanical capture have been obtained, assess the patient's hemodynamic response to pacing. The pacemaker rate may need to be increased to maintain an adequate cardiac output.
- Sedate the patient if possible due to the pain of concurrent muscle contractions and electrical shock with each paced beat.
- The presence of hypoxemia and acidosis may prevent the heart from responding to pacemaker stimulation. If unable to "capture," assess for and treat these conditions.

TRAUMATIC CARDIOPULMONARY ARREST

- Survival rates from traumatic cardiopulmonary arrest resulting from both blunt and penetrating injuries are poor (0% to 3.7%) and some consider resuscitation of these patients to be futile.[6]
- In trauma patients presenting with VF, consider that this rhythm may be the cause and not the result of trauma.
- Trauma patients experiencing cardiopulmonary arrest should be managed using the ABCDEs of trauma assessment and care as described in Chapter 35, Stabilization of the Trauma Patient.
- Injuries leading to traumatic arrest are generally extensive and often include thoracic trauma such as tension pneumothorax, aortic or ventricular rupture, penetrating chest trauma, or cardiac tamponade.
- Patients with massive hypovolemia, as is often the case in traumatic cardiopulmonary arrest, rarely survive.[6]
- Emergency thoracotomy, particularly in patients with blunt chest trauma, carries an extremely high mortality rate. The American College of Surgeons Committee on Trauma recommends considering emergency department thoracotomy only for patients experiencing cardiopulmonary arrest from penetrating injury if:

- There has been short scene and transport time
- Objective signs of life (pupillary response, spontaneous breathing, palpable carotid pulse, and cardiac electrical activity) were present when the patient arrived at the emergency department.[7]
- Emergency thoracotomy may be helpful in controlling massive intrathoracic hemorrhage leading to pulseless electrical activity (PEA), managing cardiac tamponade, or initiating internal cardiac massage.[7]

CARDIOPULMONARY ARREST IN THE PREGNANT WOMAN

Care of the pregnant woman involves two patients: the mother and her fetus. The best chance for fetal survival is maternal survival, particularly if the mother experiences cardiopulmonary arrest. Management of cardiopulmonary arrest in the pregnant woman should follow the BLS and ACLS treatment algorithms with the additional considerations listed below[8]:

- Administer 100% oxygen and anticipate difficult airway management.
- Perform chest compressions slightly higher on the chest because of the elevated diaphragm and abdominal contents.
- To prevent compression of the inferior vena cava and decreased blood return to the heart by the gravid uterus, manually displace the uterus to the left. If this manual maneuver is unsuccessful, place a firm wedge under the patient's pelvis and chest for a 30-degree left-lateral tilt.
- Obtain IV access above the diaphragm.
- Administer defibrillation and ACLS drugs as usual, without changes in joules or dosage.
- Remove internal or external fetal monitoring devices before defibrillation.
- Search for and treat contributing factors based on the BEAU-CHOPS mnemonic:
  - **B**leeding or disseminated intravascular coagulopathy
  - **E**mbolism: coronary, pulmonary, amniotic fluid
  - **A**nesthetic complications
  - **U**terine atony
  - **C**ardiac disease: myocardial infarction (MI), ischemia, aortic dissection, cardiomyopathy
  - **H**ypertension, preeclampsia, eclampsia
  - **O**thers: consider the H's and T's
  - **P**lacental abruption, placenta previa
  - **S**epsis
- If ROSC does not occur within 4 minutes of resuscitation efforts, consider immediate emergency cesarean section.

PATIENT MANAGEMENT FOLLOWING SUCCESSFUL RESUSCITATION

A major concern is management of the patient once there is ROSC after successful resuscitation from cardiopulmonary arrest. The goals of care during this time are to minimize postarrest brain injury, myocardial dysfunction, and the systemic reperfusion response and to resolve the underlying problem that caused the cardiopulmonary arrest in the first place.[9] Early goal-directed therapy bundles are being developed to improve survival and to promote functional recovery.[10] Two specific interventions that can be initiated in the emergency department are treating the underlying cause of cardiopulmonary arrest through early percutaneous coronary intervention and the induction of hypothermia.

Early Percutaneous Coronary Intervention

- The most common cause of cardiopulmonary arrest is cardiovascular disease and coronary ischemia.[10]
- According to the American Heart Association, patients with ROSC following cardiopulmonary arrest should undergo immediate coronary angiography and percutaneous coronary intervention (PCI) if electrocardiogram criteria for ST elevation myocardial infarction (STEMI) are present or if the presence of acute coronary syndrome is likely.[9]
- If PCI is unavailable, thrombolytic therapy is appropriate for STEMI management in these patients.[9]
- Emergent PCI can be performed in conjunction with therapeutic hypothermia.

Therapeutic Hypothermia

- The main goal of therapeutic hypothermia is to preserve neurologic functioning in patients following cardiopulmonary arrest with ROSC. Therapeutic hypothermia is the only therapy that has been shown to improve neurologic recovery in patients following cardiopulmonary arrest.[10]
- Cooling should begin immediately after ROSC in patients who remain comatose.
  - Cooling can be initiated in the prehospital setting with an IV infusion of iced saline.
  - Other methods of inducing mild hypothermia include ice packs to the groin, axilla, neck, and head and cooling blankets.
  - Commercial devices are available for therapeutic hypothermia and involve either external surface cooling or intravascular methods.
- The temperature and time goals for therapeutic hypothermia are 32° C to 34° C (89.6–93.2° F) for 12 or 24 hours.

- The patient's core temperature must be continuously monitored using an esophageal or bladder catheter thermometer.
  - Axillary, oral, and tympanic temperature monitoring is not appropriate or reliable in these patients.
- Controlling shivering is a priority when caring for a patient undergoing therapeutic hypothermia. Sedation, analgesia, and neuromuscular blockers are given and the patient is intubated and mechanically ventilated.
- Because electrolyte shifts and hyperglycemia are common during the cooling time, baseline laboratory values are obtained. Blood glucose levels are monitored on an hourly basis.
- "Cold diuresis" occurs so an indwelling urinary catheter is needed.
- Once cooling has started, do not interrupt it for diagnostic examinations (computed tomography scan) or other interventions (PCI).

REFERENCES

1. Neumar, R. W., Otto, C. W., Link, M. S., Kronick, S. L., Shuster, M., Callaway, C. W., … Morrison, L. J. (2010). Part 8: Adult advanced cardiovascular life support: 2010 American Heart Association guidelines for cardiopulmonary resuscitation and emergency cardiovascular care. *Circulation, 122*(18 suppl 3), S729–S767.
2. Field, J. M. (Ed.). (2008). *ACLS resource text for instructors and experienced providers.* Dallas, TX: American Heart Association.
3. Turner, M., & Hankins, J. (2010). Pharmacology. In M. Alexander, A. Corrigan, L. Gorski, J. Hankins, & R. Perucca (Eds.), *Infusion nursing: An evidence-based approach* (3rd ed., pp. 263–298). St. Louis, MO: Saunders/Elsevier.
4. Zimmerman, J. L. (2007). *Fundamental critical care support* (4th ed.). Mount Prospect, IL: Society of Critical Care Medicine.
5. Emergency Nurses Association. (2010, September). *Family presence during invasive procedures and resuscitation in the emergency department* [position statement]. Retrieved from http://www.ena.org/SiteCollectionDocuments/Position%20Statements/FamilyPresence.pdf
6. Lockey, D., Crewdson, K., & Davies, G. (2006). Traumatic cardiac arrest: Who are the survivors? *Annals of Emergency Medicine, 48*(3), 240–244.
7. Chalkias, A. (2009). Prehospital thoracotomy: When to do it? *Journal of Emergency Primary Health Care, 7*(4). Retrieved from http://www.jephc.com/full_article.cfm?content_id=548
8. Vanden Hoek, T. L., Morrison, L. J., Shuster, M., Donnino, M., Sinz, E., Lavonas, E. J., … Gabrielli, A. (2010). Part 12: Cardiac arrest in special situations: 2010 American Heart Association guidelines for cardiopulmonary arrest and emergency cardiovascular care. *Circulation, 122*(18 suppl 3), S829–S861.

9. Neumar, R. W., Nolan, J. P., Adrie, C., Aibiki, M., Berg, R. A., Böttiger, B. W., … van den Hoek, T. (2008). Post-cardiac arrest syndrome: Epidemiology, pathophysiology, treatment and prognostication. A consensus statement from the International Liaison Committee on Resuscitation (American Heart Association, Australian and New Zealand Council on Resuscitation, European Resuscitation Council, Heart and Stroke Foundation of Canada, InterAmerican Heart Foundation, Resuscitation Council of Asia, and the Resuscitation Council of Southern Africa); the American Heart Association Emergency Cardiovascular Care Committee; the Council on Cardiovascular Surgery and Anesthesia; the Council on Cardiopulmonary, Perioperative, and Critical Care; the Council on Clinical Cardiology; and the Stroke Council. *Circulation, 118*(23), 2452–2483.

10. Peberdy, M. A., Callaway, C. W., Neumar, R. W., Geocadin, R. G., Zimmerman, J. L., Donnino, M., … Kronick, S. L. (2010). Part 9: Post-cardiac arrest care: 2010 American Heart Association guidelines for cardiopulmonary resuscitation and emergency cardiovascular care. *Circulation, 122*(180 suppl 3), S768–S786.

Intravenous Therapy

Lynn Hadaway

Intravenous (IV) therapy—the delivery of fluids, electrolytes, medications, blood products, and nutritional products into the vascular system—is an essential component of health care. Insertion of some type of vascular access device is often the first line of treatment during emergency care. Insertion and appropriate use of all vascular access devices and safe infusion requires knowledge of anatomy of the vasculature, physiology of blood flow, appropriate application of technology, astute nursing assessment, and strict attention to infection prevention practices and complication prevention.

Site and catheter selection, along with insertion and infusion techniques, are critical to preventing serious life-altering outcomes from the infusion therapy. During emergent situations the need for lifesaving urgency must take precedence over considerations for maximum duration of the catheter, but not all patients in emergency care fall into this group. Patients seen in emergency care may have one of many different types of vascular access devices already in situ. Aging and chronic diseases alter skin and vascular anatomy, enhancing the need for careful attention to the basic principles of infusion therapy.

Infusion nursing is a recognized nursing specialty. This is the most invasive therapy performed by nurses at all levels and settings. Communication between infusion nurse specialists and emergency care specialists is needed to understand the unique perspective of each specialty and work collaboratively to provide safe infusion therapy and vascular access without increasing the risk of serious problems for our patients.

INTRAVENOUS FLUIDS AND MEDICATIONS

Numerous types of IV fluids are currently available, along with hundreds of medications given through this route. The type of IV fluids needed is based on the primary purpose

for treatment, laboratory values, and clinical assessment of the patient and his or her condition. The IV route allows for rapid effect of the medications. Basic principles of fluid compartments, osmosis, and tonicity must be understood to achieve safe outcomes for the patient.

Basic Principles of Fluid and Medication Administration

The human body is about 60% water by weight with about 40% found in the intracellular compartment and the remaining 20% found in the extracellular compartment. Metabolic rate determines the amount of fluid needed in healthy people; however, injury and disease can greatly alter the amount of fluid required. Elevated body temperature increases metabolic rate by 12% for each degree Celsius (7% for each degree Fahrenheit). Decreased intake from fasting or altered consciousness and increased losses from diarrhea and vomiting are other examples leading to fluid and electrolyte imbalances.[1]

- Water moves across semipermeable cellular membranes by the process of osmosis. *Osmolarity* (the osmolar concentration in 1 L of solution) and *osmolality* (the osmolar concentration in 1 kg of water) are often used interchangeably because 1 L of water weighs 1 kg.[1]
- *Tonicity* applies to the solutions being infused and how that solution will affect the size of the cells. Osmotic pressure of a solution causes water to move into or out of cells. Isotonic fluids have the same osmolality as intracellular fluids, between 280 and 295 mOsm/L. Thus isotonic fluids will simply increase the extracellular volume but will not produce any osmotic shifting of fluids into or out of the cell. Hypotonic fluids have an osmolality less than intracellular fluids and hypertonic fluids have an osmolality greater than intracellular fluids. Infusion of hypotonic fluids will cause fluids to move into the cells, resulting in swelling of the cell and possibly causing them to burst. Infusion of hypertonic fluids will cause

fluids to move out of the cells, causing them to shrink.[1] Changes in the cell size from osmotic shifting occur in the venous endothelium, resulting in inflammation and thrombosis at the point where the fluid enters the vein.[2] This process drives the need for a central venous catheter when the required fluids are extremely hypotonic or hypertonic. One example is parenteral nutrition.

> The Infusion Nursing Society Standards of Practice calls for restricting the osmolality of fluids and medications infused through peripheral veins to no more than 600 mOsm/L.[5]

- Another critical factor related to IV fluids and medication is the pH, *the acidity or alkalinity of the solution.* Most IV fluids have a pH of 5, a slightly acidic level that extends their shelf life; however, the pH of fluids ranges from 3.5 to 6.2.[1] The pH of all solutions will affect the integrity of the venous endothelium and extremes will produce inflammation of the vein. An example of an extremely acidic drug is vancomycin and of an extremely alkaline drug is phenytoin.

> The Infusion Nursing Society Standards of Practice states that the pH of fluids and medications infused through peripheral veins should be between 5 and 9.[5]

- Consider the *vesicant or irritating properties* of the solution and medications given intravenously. A vesicant medication will produce tissue damage if it leaks from the vein into the subcutaneous tissue; therefore, the nurse must determine absolute patency of the vein when administering these medications. This means observation of the site condition, palpation for tenderness, aspirating for a positive blood return, and listening to all patient complaints. This level of assessment is necessary with each dose of medication regardless of when the catheter was inserted. Examples of medications in this group are commonly thought of as oncology chemotherapy agents; however, vancomycin, nafcillin, promethazine, high concentrations of dextrose, all calcium preparations, sodium bicarbonate, and potassium solutions are also vesicants.
- Nurses must incorporate the step of checking *compatibility and stability* of fluids and medications as part of safe administration practices. Stability means the amount of time the drug will retain its original characteristics. Drug stability is affected by many factors such as pH, the number of additives in solution, the volume of dilution, time in solution, light, temperature, the sequence of drugs added to solution, and the fluid container. There are three different types of drug incompatibility or undesirable reactions when drugs or

solutions come into contact. Physical incompatibility is seen when there are visible changes such as a precipitate formation, color change, or increased turbidity. Chemical incompatibility is a nonvisible change in the drug's chemical structure. Therapeutic incompatibility occurs after infusion when two drugs have similar effects.[4]

Types of Parenteral Fluids

Intravenous fluids are classified as crystalloids or colloids. Crystalloid solutions contain solutes that mix and readily dissolve in solution. The dissolved electrolytes easily pass between intracellular and extracellular compartments. This group includes dextrose solutions, sodium chloride solutions, balanced electrolyte solutions, and alkalizing and acidifying solutions. (See Table 10-1.)

- Crystalloid solutions are available from a pharmacy compounding service or purchased as premixed solutions. After other medications (e.g., potassium chloride, heparin) have been added the solution is sterilized, providing a safer solution than those prepared by the nurse. While these premixed solutions save nursing time, the available concentrations should be limited to prevent medication errors.[1] (See Table 10-2.)
- Colloid solutions increase the intravascular volume and are also known as plasma expanders. These solutions pull fluid from the interstitial spaces. Albumin, dextran, hetastarch and pentastarch, and gelatins are included in this group. Although frequently used for fluid resuscitation in trauma, there remains controversy over the type and method of fluid to be used.[1] Mannitol, also classified as a colloid, is an intravascular volume expander that acts as an osmotic diuretic.[1] Table 10-1 compares common colloid and crystalloid solutions.

THE INFUSION SYSTEM

When preparing the infusion system, the nurse must make decisions about the fluid container, flow control, and multiple add-on pieces.

Fluid Container

- Glass bottles were the original containers for IV fluids; however, plastic bags are now more common. Glass bottles require venting to allow air to enter and fluid to flow. Administration sets that contain a filtered air vent above the drip chamber are preferred. If vented administration sets are not available, the glass bottle can be vented by inserting a filter needle into the rubber stopper; however, regular needles should not be used for this purpose.[5]
- Plastic bags are collapsible and do not require venting to allow fluid to flow. Polyvinyl chloride (PVC), the

TABLE 10-1   **COMPARISON OF COMMON COLLOID AND CRYSTALLOID SOLUTIONS**

SOLUTION	MOLECULAR WEIGHT	OSMOLALITY	MAX VOLUME EXPANSION* (%)	DURATION OF EXPANSION VOL. (h)	PLASMATIC HALF-LIFE (h)	POTENTIAL FOR ADVERSE REACTIONS	SIDE EFFECTS
Albumin 4%, 5%	69	290	70–100	12–24	16–24	+	Allergic reactions
Albumin 20%, 25%	69	310	300–500	12–24	16–24	+	Allergic reactions
Starches *Hetastarch* 3%, 6%, 10%	450	300–310	100–200	8–36	50	++	Renal dysfunction
Starches *Pentastarch* 10%	280	326	100–200	12–24	2–12	++	Renal dysfunction
Dextrans							
10% Dextran 40	40	280–324	100–200	1–2	4–6	+++	Anaphylactoid
3% Dextran 60	70	280–324	80–140	<8–24	–12	+++	reactions
6% Dextran 70					–12	+++	Anaphylactoid reactions
Gelatins Succinylated and crosslinked: 2.5%, 3%, 4% Urea-linked: 3.5%	30–35	300–350	70–80	<4–6	–2–9	++	High calcium content (urea-linked forms)
Crystalloids 0.9% NaCl	0	285–308	20–25	1–4	0.5	+	Hyperchloremic metabolic acidosis
Crystalloids Ringer's lactate	0	250–273	20–25	1–4	0.5	+	Hyperkalemia

h, Hour; *NaCl*, sodium chloride.
*Max volume expansion is expressed as a percentage of administered volume (Vol.).
Adapted from American Thoracic Society. (2004). Evidence-based colloid use in the critically ill: American Thoracic Society Consensus Statement. *American Journal of Respiratory and Critical Care Medicine, 170*(11), 1247–1259. Retrieved from http://ajrccm.atsjournals.org/cgi/content/full/170/11/1247
Phillips, L. (2010). Parenteral fluids. In M. Alexander, A. Corrigan, L. Gorski, J. Hankins, & R. Perucca (Eds.), *Infusion nursing: An evidence-based approach* (3rd ed., pp. 229–241). St. Louis, MO: Saunders.

original plastic in these containers, requires the addition of chemicals to make them soft and flexible. The chemical di(2-ethylhexyl)phthalate (DEHP) is now the cause of concern as this chemical can leach into the solution and be infused to the patient. Exposure to DEHP carries the greatest risk for male fetuses and infants, along with possible carcinogenic and hepatotoxic effects for others.[5] Plastic fluid containers can have certain drugs adhere to the container's surface. Up to 80% of the dose of insulin and nitroglycerin may adhere to the plastic and not be infused. Plastic containers made of polyolefin may eliminate this problem with many drugs; however, studies have shown that insulin will adhere to this plastic also. Use of glass bottles for infusing insulin may be required or, if plastic bags must be used, the nurse must carefully monitor the patient's response to the infusion.[5]

- Syringes are also considered fluid containers and are used in combination with a syringe-loaded electronic pump. They are used for small volume drugs when the patient's age (e.g., neonates) or condition (e.g., renal failure) cannot tolerate larger volume dilution of the medication.[5]
- Many drugs may be available in a use-activated container where the drug and diluent are in separate chambers. The divider between the chambers must be deliberately ruptured according to the manufacturer's instructions. When the drug and diluent are not properly mixed together, only the diluent may infuse or a delayed rupture of the barrier may result in a rapid infusion of the undiluted drug.
- Some drugs require protection from light during their infusion. No solution containers are available

TABLE 10-2   TYPES OF CRYSTALLOID IV SOLUTIONS

TYPE	CONTENTS	OSMOLALITY	INDICATIONS	COMPLICATIONS
Dextrose solutions	Dextrose, fructose, or invert sugar Dextrose is most commonly used carbohydrate, well metabolized 5% solution = 5 g (20 calories) per 100 mL	2.5%: hypotonic 5%: isotonic in container, hypotonic when infused 10% and up: hypertonic	Provides calories for energy, spares body protein, prevents ketosis Enhances movement of potassium from extracellular to intracellular compartment Helps to excrete solutes, improving kidney and liver function 2.5% and 5% used to treat dehydration and to dilute medications 10% may correct hypoglycemia 20%–70% combined with electrolytes for parenteral nutrition	Overinfusion can lead to electrolyte depletion May produce water intoxication with overinfusion leading to hyponatremic encephalopathy, especially in premenopausal women Hypertonic solutions cause vein irritation and produce thrombosis; sudden discontinuation can create a temporary insulin excess Check compatibility before using as a medication diluent Cannot be used with blood transfusion
Sodium chloride solutions	0.9% (normal saline) contains 154 mEq sodium and 154 mEq chloride; osmotic pressure is similar to body fluids	0.2%: hypotonic 0.45%: hypotonic 0.9%: isotonic 3%: hypertonic 5%: hypertonic	Treatment of shock, hyponatremia, fluid resuscitation, fluid challenges, metabolic alkalosis, hypercalcemia, and fluid replacement in diabetic ketoacidosis. Hypotonic and isotonic as diluent for IV medications. Hypertonic: severe hyponatremia, hypotonic encephalopathy	Use cautiously with congestive heart failure, edema, renal insufficiency, and hypernatremia. More than 1 L of 0.9% per day may produce hypernatremia. May produce acidifying effect due to loss of bicarbonate ions May produce hypokalemia Hypertonic solutions mandate careful monitoring and infusion of only small volumes
Dextrose/ sodium chloride solutions	Combination of various concentrations of dextrose and sodium chloride	2.5% dextrose and 0.45% NaCl: isotonic 5% dextrose and 0.25% NaCl: isotonic 5% dextrose and 0.45% NaCl: hypertonic 5% dextrose and 0.9% NaCl: hypertonic	Hypovolemia in circulatory insufficiency and shock Hydration and diuresis to assess renal function Early treatment of burns	Caution in patients with cardiac, renal, or hepatic disease
Balanced electrolyte solutions	Multiple solutions with a variety of electrolyte combinations; may include sodium, potassium, calcium, lactate, acetate	Lactated Ringer's; isotonic Ringer's: isotonic Some brands are hypertonic depending on the electrolyte concentration	Trauma patients, dehydration, hypovolemia, GI fluid losses, sodium depletion, acidosis, burns	Infusion of excessive amount of electrolytes Calorie deficits Overhydration Metabolic alkalosis with excessive Lactated Ringer's; Contraindicated in hepatic disease.
Alkalizing solutions	Sodium bicarbonate solution	5% solution: hypertonic	Metabolic acidosis Severe hyperkalemia	Metabolic alkalosis, hypocalcemia, hypokalemia

GI, Gastrointestinal; *IV*, intravenous; *NaCl*, sodium chloride.

Phillips, L. (2010). Parenteral fluids. In M. Alexander, A. Corrigan, L. Gorski, J. Hankins, & R. Perucca (Eds.), *Infusion nursing: An evidence-based approach* (3rd ed., pp. 229–241). St. Louis, MO: Saunders.

to solve this problem; however, a simple paper bag placed over the fluid container will protect it from light. The disadvantage is that the fluid level is not easily visible.[5]

All fluid containers must be inspected before use for clarity of the solution and cracks or pinhole leaks, as these small breaks can allow for entry of microorganisms.

Administration Sets

The administration set carries the infusing fluid from the fluid container to the patient. The length of time an administration set can be used depends on its purpose.

- Primary continuous administration sets are used when the infusion is required for multiple hours, days, or weeks. It should be a single device to limit the number of connections. Once attached to the catheter hub, it should remain connected until it is time to be changed, usually no more frequently than 96-hour intervals but at least every 7 days according to the Centers for Disease Control and Prevention (CDC).

> Disconnecting the administration set to change clothing or other patient activities should be discouraged, as it opens the system to contamination.

- Secondary sets are those sets of varying lengths that are used to deliver intermittent medications when continuous fluids are infusing. The secondary set should be attached to the primary continuous set and remain connected. Both the primary and the secondary sets are changed together, usually no more frequently than every 96 hours.
- Primary intermittent sets are those sets used to deliver intermittent medications when there is no primary fluid infusing continuously. These sets are connected and disconnected with each dose, thus increasing the risk of contamination. No studies have established a safe length of time for their use; therefore, the Infusion Nursing Standards of Practice states primary intermittent sets should be changed every 24 hours.[3] The CDC *Guidelines for the Prevention of Intravascular Catheter-Related Infections* now state that the change interval for intermittent sets is an unresolved issue.[6] The male luer end of the set must be maintained in a sterile manner when not connected to the catheter. This is accomplished by placing a new sterile cap securely on the end immediately after it is disconnected from the catheter. If there is any question about the integrity of this covering or the set, it should be discarded and a new set should be used.
- Certain infusions, such as nitroglycerin, fat emulsion, blood products, and arterial pressure monitoring, require special administration sets for safe infusion. The

use of metered-chamber sets has decreased but these still could be useful in some situations. The chamber is located below the fluid container and will hold a small amount of fluid, usually 50 to 150 mL. When this volume has infused, the nurse must return to fill this chamber again. These sets have also been used to deliver intermittent medications; however, there is concern about ensuring that the chamber is properly labeled when the drug is infusing. Some infusion pumps will require a dedicated set while others may accept the general set used for all infusions. Know the specific type of set required for the infusion pump being used.

Flow Control

Accurate control of the fluid flow is critical for many patients. Overinfusion or underinfusion of certain fluids, electrolytes, and medications can produce complications for some patients. Fluid requires a pressure gradient to move from one location to another. Pressure comes from three types of flow control: gravity or manual, mechanical, and electronic.

Gravity

Systems that depend on gravity include the traditional roller clamp and other manual flow regulators. The fluid container must be placed about 3 to 4 feet above the catheter site to create the pressure gradient and produce fluid flow. A standard roller clamp on a standard-bore administration set can be as accurate as plus or minus 10%, but numerous variables are involved. Changes in the distance between the container and the catheter, patient movement, and improperly stabilized catheters can reduce the accuracy to plus or minus 25%. Roller clamps should be placed on the upper third of the set length to allow for easy access and prevent patient manipulation. These clamps should be repositioned on the set periodically as they can produce a permanent kink in the set.[5]

Manual flow controllers are round discs with numbers stamped on the outer side to indicated flow rates. They can be an integral part of the set or added on to the set. The accuracy of this device is plus or minus 10% and can easily be affected by the same movement factors as a roller clamp. This requires close monitoring by the nurse to ensure correct infusion of the fluid as prescribed. One other use for these flow controllers is rate control during magnetic resonance image (MRI). Because of the presence of metal in the electronic infusion pumps, they cannot be placed inside the room; however, these flow controllers may be sufficient to regulate flow during this procedure.

Pressure cuffs are another example of manual flow control and are used for rapid infusion. The cuff is positioned around a plastic fluid container and inflated to exert pressure against the bag. Most systems have a warning on the dial when the maximum of 300 mm Hg or 6 psi has been reached.[5]

Mechanical

Mechanical pumps include elastomeric balloon pumps or spring-based pumps. There is no external power source, and flow is regulated by the size of the opening where the attached administration set joins the housing. Inside the housing is a balloon that has expanded when filled with fluid. When the clamp is opened, the balloon begins to collapse and return to its original size and shape. Commonly used in home care, the emergency nurse may encounter these devices when a patient who uses a home infusion device presents to the emergency department.

Electronic

Electronic infusion pumps come in many varieties, including pole-mounted volumetric pumps, ambulatory infusion pumps, syringe pumps, and patient-controlled analgesia pumps. The industry standard for this group is an accuracy rating of plus or minus 5%, but some may be as accurate as plus or minus 2%. Recent advances in electronic infusion pumps have included dosage error reduction systems and drug libraries. The nurse must understand the specific system in use and know how to operate it properly without bypassing these systems.[5]

Electronic infusion pumps have numerous types of settings including flow rate, volume to be infused, total volume infused, and multiple infusions through one pump. Alarms and safety mechanisms include air in line, occlusion, infusion complete, low battery, low power, door open, and nonfunctional or system error.

With these infusion pumps it is critical to remember that some will continue to pump or force fluid flow regardless of the catheter or vein patency. The alarms are not designed to indicate when an infiltration or flow of fluid into the subcutaneous tissue has occurred.[7] It is imperative that the catheter and infusion site be assessed frequently to avoid serious injury to the patient, especially prior to administering a medication. Many other challenges have been identified with the present design of electronic infusion pumps resulting in serious medication errors.[8,9] It is imperative that nurses thoroughly understand how to operate electronic infusion pumps and that they do not rely totally on the machine to deliver accurate fluid flow constantly. The fluid container should frequently be assessed for fluid level and compared to the total volume infused to ensure that the patient is receiving the prescribed amount.

Other Components

Other components, such as extension sets, filters, and needleless connectors, may be added to the administration set or catheter.

- A short extension set added to a peripheral catheter will facilitate quick attachment of syringes and sets to the catheter without unnecessary pressure or manipulation of the catheter inside the vein. Extension sets may also be necessary to add length to the administration set.

- Filters may be integral to the administration set or be added on to the set. Filters are measured by the size of the opening or pores where the fluid passes. Filters with a 0.22-micron pore size are required on certain solutions such as parenteral nutrition, but other fluids such as fat emulsion are too large to pass through this small filter. When the parenteral nutrition solution is a total nutrient admixture (e.g., all components including the fat emulsion are mixed in one large container), a 1.2-micron filter must be used. Filters remove particulate matter, air, and some microorganisms.[5]

- Needleless connectors, previously called injection or access ports, are devices used to close the catheter hub while allowing for intermittent connection of administration sets and syringes. Needleless connectors are also found on the administration sets. There are multiple ways to categorize all of the devices in this group. Some are clear, allowing the nurse to observe for retained blood or drug precipitate, while others are colored and do not allow for this observation. Some have a straight fluid pathway while others have a complex internal mechanism and fluid pathway.

These devices may also be divided by how they are designed and how they function.[10] Some are designed to use a blunt plastic cannula that is passed through a prepierced split septum. There are now two types of split septum systems that allow the direct attachment of a male luer of the syringe or administration set, thus eliminating the need for the blunt plastic cannula. Others are categorized as mechanical valves that are activated by the connection of the male luer of the set or syringe. The center post is pushed downward, opening the fluid pathway.

Fluid Displacement

Another way to group these devices is by how they function: negative fluid displacement, positive fluid displacement, or neutral fluid displacement.

- Negative fluid displacement devices will allow blood to reflux into the catheter lumen when the syringe or set is disconnected. If the blood is allowed to reside inside the lumen, it can become difficult to flush or become totally occluded.

- Positive fluid displacement devices will hold a small volume of fluid inside the device. Upon syringe disconnection, this small reserved fluid is pushed out to the catheter tip to overcome the blood reflux.

- Neutral fluid displacement devices do not allow blood to move into the catheter lumen on connection or disconnection.[10]

The technique for flushing and clamping these devices must be the correct one for the functionality of the device. Negative displacement devices require flushing the fluid into the catheter lumen, continuing to hold the syringe plunger, closing the clamp before disconnection, and then removing the syringe. This technique in that specific sequence will prevent blood from refluxing into the catheter lumen. This technique cannot be used with a positive displacement device. For those needleless connectors that have a positive displacement mechanism, flush the catheter, disconnect the syringe, and then close the clamp. For those devices with neutral displacement, the disconnection and clamping sequence can be done in either manner.[10]

There is growing concern about the risk of bloodstream infection associated with the use of these needleless devices. Some mechanical valves have been reported to produce an increase in catheter-related bloodstream infection. For this reason many guidelines now recommend the preference for a split septum device instead of some mechanical valves.[6,11] Regardless of the type of needleless connector in use, all require thorough scrubbing with a disinfectant solution such as alcohol or chlorhexadine before each entry, and only sterile devices should be used to access the connector.[6]

VASCULAR ACCESS DEVICES

Access to the vascular system includes devices placed in veins, arteries, and bone marrow. Other catheters are inserted into the spinal column and the peritoneal and pleural cavities. The nurse must know exactly where the catheter tip is located, the relevant anatomy of the catheter pathway, the physiology of blood flow, how the catheter is designed, and the history of how the catheter has performed in each patient.

Catheter Characteristics
Materials

Most catheters used currently are made of polytetrafluoroethylene (Teflon), polyurethane, or silicone. Teflon is relatively rigid, and this characteristic does not change after insertion. Polyurethane is a large family of materials known as thermoplastics. Once inside the body, polyurethane becomes softer because of body heat. While this family of material has superb physical strength, some formulations are limited by their chemical compatibility. Some older formulations do not tolerate contact with alcohol, while newer formulations do not have this same restriction. Silicone is a material widely used in catheters. It is extremely flexible and soft, but these characteristics require special methods for

insertion. All catheter materials are tested for cytotoxicity, allergic reactions, their potential to produce inflammation, and hemocompatibility.[5]

Short peripheral catheters are made of Teflon or polyurethane. Teflon is also used to make introducers for other catheters. Central venous catheters are made of either polyurethane or silicone. Many studies have attempted to discover a difference in thrombogenicity between catheter materials, but one has not been shown to be superior to the other for central venous catheters. For short peripheral catheters, polyurethane is reported to have a longer dwell time with fewer complications.

Diameter

Catheters are measured in several ways. The outer diameter is a measurement from the outside wall through the center of the lumen to the outside wall on the opposite side. This measurement is critical to compare to the internal diameter of the vein lumen. The catheter should not consume more than about a third of the vein lumen. The outer diameter measure is taken in millimeters. Multiplying this measurement times three yields the French size. Thus a 12 French catheter will have an outer diameter of 4 mm.[5]

The internal diameter is measured from the inner wall through the center of the lumen to the inner wall on the opposite side. This measurement produces the internal volume of the catheter, the maximum flow rate through the lumen, and the amount of pressure the catheter can tolerate. The measurement of internal volume applies to the size as it comes from the manufacturer. If the catheter length has been trimmed, the internal volume has changed.[5]

Length

Catheter length is measured in two ways. The total catheter length includes the entire device, including external extension legs and hub. The effective catheter length is the amount of catheter intended for insertion into the vein. When a catheter is trimmed to a patient-specific length, this information should be documented for future reference. Upon removal, the catheter length must be measured and compared to the amount inserted to ensure that the entire length was removed.

Lumens

Many central venous catheters have multiple lumens. These are separate channels throughout the length of the catheter and are used to infuse multiple solutions simultaneously. Some catheters have these lumens exiting into the bloodstream at the same point, while others have staggered lumen exit points. Hemodialysis catheters have the lumen exit points staggered by at least 2 cm, but infusion catheters with staggered lumens may have less than 1 cm of separation.

The tip of all central venous catheters is located in the superior vena cava where the blood flow is approximately 2000 mL per minute. This rapid flow rate will usually provide sufficient hemodilution to prevent mixing of incompatible medications at the catheter tip.[5]

Special Features

Many types of catheters now have integral valves built into the catheter. One type of valve is located on the internal catheter tip, while there are two designs of valves located in the catheter hub. All manufacturers of these valved catheters state that normal saline can be used for flushing and locking these catheters.

> Heparin is not required to flush valved multilumen catheters, although it is not contraindicated and can be used especially if there is a problem with flushing.[4]

- Central venous catheters are now available with anti-infective agents impregnated in the catheter's intraluminal and extraluminal walls. Chlorhexidine and silver sulfadiazine are available for nontunneled central venous catheters. Minocycline and rifampin are available for nontunneled central venous catheters and one brand of peripherally inserted central catheters (PICC) and chlorhexidine is available in another brand of PICC.
- Some catheters are manufactured to withstand the high-pressure injection required to produce accurate pictures from some computed tomography (CT) scans. The pressure used for injection in this situation may reach 300 psi. All catheters used for this purpose must be labeled with this indication. Without this labeling, the catheter may be severely damaged during this procedure.[5]

Considerations Prior to Venous Access

Catheter Selection

Vascular access devices can be divided by their location within the vascular system; however, there are many other aspects to consider. The diameter of the vein lumen is a critical issue when choosing the size of catheter for insertion, especially short peripheral catheters. The basic principle is that the smallest gauge catheter capable of accommodating the prescribed therapy should be chosen.[3] Large gauge catheters (e.g., 14, 16, and 18 gauge) are needed when large quantities and rapid flow rates are required for fluid resuscitation; however, the integrity of the vein must be considered. When a catheter too large for the vein diameter is chosen in emergent situations, the catheter can easily cause rapid vein damage and thus compromise successful patient outcomes. For nonemergent situations, the pH, osmolality, and vesicant nature are the primary factors that must be considered when selecting the catheter and insertion site.

Site Selection

Areas of joint flexion must be avoided as another complication reduction strategy. Catheters inserted in the dorsal venous network of the hand, the cephalic vein at the wrist, and the basilic, median cubital, or cephalic veins of the antecubital fossa are associated with higher complication rates.[12] There are more nerves located in these areas, producing the risk of life-altering damage. Venipuncture techniques should be perfected to avoid excessive probing of subcutaneous tissue and subsequent nerve damage.[13] If veins can be found only in an area of joint flexion, the joint should be supported with an armboard in patients of all ages. This will prevent joint movement from causing the tip of the plastic catheter to erode through the vein wall, producing infiltration or extravasation.[14]

> Armboard use is not considered physical restraint.

Vein Selection

Selecting an appropriate vein is accomplished by practicing good techniques for palpation. After placing the tourniquet several inches above the intended insertion site, palpate venous locations by using the same finger of the same hand each time. Press downward and then slowly release the pressure while you take notice of the elasticity of the vein. Healthy veins will feel soft and bouncy while sclerosed veins will feel hard and ropelike.[2] Lightly rubbing across the skin surface will not produce the same feeling of the vein condition.

Vein Visualization Technology

Use of vein visualization technology, including ultrasound and infrared light devices, is increasing. Patients with difficult venous access will have no visual or palpable veins. This will include those patients with a history of numerous IV infusions resulting from oncology diseases, diabetes, sickle cell disease, and renal or hepatic failure. Ultrasound machines can measure the vein's internal diameter and have been well documented to increase the success with peripheral venipuncture.[15,16] There is a significant learning curve with the ultrasound machines, often requiring dozens of insertions to master the technique. Coupling gel, which could enter the vein, is required and removal of the gel is necessary to ensure adherence of the catheter stabilization device and dressing. Additionally, short peripheral catheters inserted with ultrasound are associated with high rates of catheter complications such as infiltration.[16]

Infrared light devices create an image of the superficial veins that is projected onto the surface of the extremity and offers a hands-free device without requiring application of other substances. While its use is relatively new, one early study has shown promise for this technology to improve venipuncture success in many patients without altering the venipuncture procedure or creating other challenges.[17] Use of both ultrasound and infrared light offers the ability to have technical information about the size of the vein lumen and avoid reliance only on the nurse's ability to palpate the vein size.[5]

Types of Vascular Access Devices

Table 10-3 provides an overview of types of VADs.
- Nontunneled percutaneous central venous catheters are the most common type inserted in emergent situations. This type of catheter can be rapidly inserted into the subclavian or jugular veins.
- Midline catheters and PICCs are not well suited for insertion in the emergency department. The length of the midline catheter requires careful attention to slow advancement into the vein to reduce vein irritation and subsequent thrombosis.

- Tunneled, cuffed catheters and implanted ports (Fig. 10-1) require surgical insertion and are indicated for long-term infusion for patients receiving home or ambulatory care. While these catheters generally would not be inserted in the emergency department, patients with these catheters may often be admitted for emergency care.

Other Access Devices
Winged Devices

Winged metal needles, also known as butterflies or scalp vein needles, have a stainless steel needle with wings extending from each side. The wings are folded together to facilitate venipuncture. The wings also have a device mounted to contain the needle once it is removed from the vein. Extension tubing is attached to the external end of the needle and blood return is easily detected within this tubing. This device is indicated for obtaining blood samples and for direct injection of a one-time dose of medication. Winged devices are not reliable as venous devices and are not suited for infusion for any length of time.[5]

TABLE 10-3   TYPES OF VASCULAR ACCESS DEVICES USED FOR INFUSION

Short Peripheral Catheters

Material used	Teflon®
	Polyurethane
Available sizes	26 gauge to 14 gauge
	$\frac{5}{8}$ inch to $2\frac{1}{4}$ inches
	Safety mechanism is mandatory!
Insertion site(s)	Veins of upper extremity
	Veins of lower extremity for non-ambulating pediatrics and as a very last resort in adults in emergent situations
	Jugular veins in neck for emergent situations
	Avoid areas of joint flexion
Tip location	Close to insertion site
Type of procedure	Clean, no-touch
	Over-the-needle
Indications for use	IV fluids for replacement/hydration
	Most IV medications, although many cause significant local phlebitis; some cause tissue necrosis if extravasation occurs
Contraindications for use	All parenteral nutrition solutions
	Continuous infusion of solution with a dextrose content over 10%, although small quantities (e.g., 50 mL) are given by IV push through peripheral catheters
	Vesicant medications
	Fluid and medications with final osmolarity >600 mOsm/L
	Fluid and medication with pH <5 or >9
	Long-term IV therapy (>5–7 days)
	Repeated intermittent therapy

Continued

TABLE 10-3 TYPES OF VASCULAR ACCESS DEVICES USED FOR INFUSION—cont'd

Limitations for use	Changes in peripheral veins related to age, disease process, nutrition or fluid balance status, and previous use
	Frail elderly patients with poor skin turgor and fragile veins
Special considerations	Decrease vein trauma by choosing the smallest gauge catheter capable of delivering the prescribed therapy (e.g., packed red blood cells can be infused through 22 or 24 gauge)

Midline Catheters

Material used	Silicone elastomer (Silastic®)
	Polyurethane
Available sizes	1.2 Fr (28 gauge) to 6 Fr (10 gauge)
	8 cm (3 in) to 20 cm (8 in)
	Single and dual lumens available
Insertion site(s)	Upper arm insertion into basilic vein is preferred; cephalic and brachial vein may be used
	For neonates, lower extremity and scalp veins may be used
Tip location	Upper arm level with axilla, distal to the shoulder
	Lower extremity is used in neonates and non-ambulating pediatric patients
Type of procedure	Sterile technique
	Through-the-introducer with either a break-away needle or peel-away sheath
Indications for use	IV fluids for replacement and hydration
	IV therapy anticipated to last between 1 and 4 weeks
Contraindications for use	All parenteral nutrition solutions
	Solutions and medications with
	• pH <5 or >9
	• Osmolarity >600 mOsm/L
	• Dextrose content over 10%
	All vesicant medications
Limitations for use	Lack of veins in antecubital region related to disease process, nutritional or fluid balance status, surgery, injury, or multiple previous venipunctures.
	Inability to advance catheter to preferred tip location related to presence of venous valves, scarring, sclerosing
Special considerations	Use of the non-dominant extremity is preferred
	Positive outcome requires proper selection of midline catheter based on characteristics of fluids and medications

Peripherally Inserted Central Catheters (PICC)

Material used	Silicone elastomer
	Polyurethane
Available sizes	1.2 Fr (28 gauge) to 7 Fr (15 gauge)
	25 cm (10 in) to 70 cm (28 in)
	Single, double, and triple lumens
Insertion site(s)	Upper arm insertion into basilic vein is preferred; cephalic and brachial vein may be used
	For neonates, lower extremity and scalp veins may be used
Tip location	Lower superior vena cava near the junction with the right atrium
	Inferior vena cava above the level of the hemidiaphragm when veins of the lower extremity are used in pediatric or neonatal patients
	Radiographic tip confirmation required prior to infusing any solution
Type of procedure	Sterile technique
	Through-the-introducer with a break-away needle or peel-away sheath
	Seldinger or Modified Seldinger technique
Indications for use	All types of IV fluids, medications, and nutrition
	Hemodynamic monitoring in catheters without integral valves
	IV therapy anticipated for up to 1 year

TABLE 10-3	**TYPES OF VASCULAR ACCESS DEVICES USED FOR INFUSION—cont'd**
Contraindications for use	Anomalies of the central venous structure related to disease process
	Thromboses of the subclavian, innominate or superior vena cava
	Avoid placement in extremities with paralysis, AV grafts, lymphedema
Limitations for use	Lack of peripheral veins related to disease, nutritional or fluid balance status, surgery, injury, or previous venipunctures
	Inability to advance catheter to preferred tip location related to venous valves, scarring, sclerosing
	Seldinger technique with fluoroscopy may be necessary in some situations
	Patient preferences
Special considerations	Tips terminating distal to the SVC (also known as midclavicular catheters) are associated with more complications and should be avoided
	Tip termination in the right atrium is a controversial issue and requires a collaborative multidisciplinary decision
	Insertion must be early in the course of therapy to increase insertion success and decrease complications
	Use of the non-dominant extremity is preferred

Nontunneled, Percutaneous Central Venous Catheters

Material used	Polyurethane
	Silicone elastomer
Available sizes	4 to 9.5 Fr
	15 to 30 cm
	Single, dual, or multiple lumens
Insertion site(s)	Subclavian is first choice, followed by internal or external jugular; use of femoral veins is not recommended but may be required during emergent situations
Tip location	Lower third of superior vena cava near the cavoatrial junction
	If femoral vein is used, tip will be in the inferior vena cava above the hemidiaphragm to be considered a central location
Type of procedure	Sterile technique
	Seldinger method
Indications for use	All types of IV fluids, medications, and nutrition
	Hemodynamic monitoring
	Primarily seen in acute care settings
Contraindications for use	Anomalies of the central venous structure related to disease process.
	Thromboses of the subclavian, innominate or superior vena cava
	Burns, radiation, surgeries near insertion site
Limitations for use	Fluid volume deficit prevents satisfactory venous distention
	Respiratory diseases, increased intracranial pressure, and curvatures of the spine make Trendelenburg position difficult or impossible for patient to tolerate
	Tracheotomy increases risk of cross-contamination
Special considerations	Has the highest rate of catheter-related infections

Tunneled, Cuffed Catheters (e.g., Hickman®, Broviac®)

Material used	Silicone elastomer
	Polyurethane
Available sizes	Numerous sizes and lengths available
	Single, dual, and triple lumens
Insertion site(s)	Enters distal subclavian, proximal axillary or internal jugular vein, tunneled in subcutaneous tissue to exit chest wall at a lower site
	Note—subcutaneous tunnels can be used on other small central venous catheters without a cuff
Tip location	Lower third of superior vena cava near the cavoatrial junction
Type of procedure	Sterile technique in a surgical setting

Continued

TABLE 10-3   TYPES OF VASCULAR ACCESS DEVICES USED FOR INFUSION—cont'd

Indications for use	All types of fluids, medications. Long-term, frequent, on-going need for infusion Used when therapy is anticipated to last for months to years
Contraindications for use	Thromboses of the subclavian, innominate or superior vena cava Superior vena cava syndrome Cardiac tamponade
Limitations for use	Patient preferences Septicemia
Special considerations	Subcutaneous tissue grows into the Dacron cuff that encircles the catheter requiring surgical removal. Skin exit site is usually in the mid-chest

Implanted Ports (e.g., Infusa-a-port®, Port-a-cath®)

Material used	Catheter Silicone elastomer or polyurethane Port body Plastic, titanium, or stainless steel
Available sizes	Catheter Numerous sizes and lengths available Single and double lumens Port body Numerous sizes, shapes, and profiles (depth)
Insertion site(s)	Enters distal subclavian, proximal axillary or internal jugular vein with port pocket in the infraclavicular area Upper arm placement in basilic, cephalic vein May be placed in arterial, epidural, intrapleural, or intraperitoneal locations
Tip location	Lower third of superior vena cava near the cavoatrial junction
Type of procedure	Sterile technique in a surgical setting
Indications for use	All types of fluids and medications Long-term, intermittent need Used when therapy is anticipated to last for months to years
Contraindications for use	Thromboses of the subclavian, innominate or superior vena cava Superior vena cava syndrome Cardiac tamponade
Limitations for use	Patient preferences Septicemia
Special considerations	Requires skin puncture with a non-coring needle to access No external catheter is visible Has the least impact on body image; associated with risk for infiltration/extravasation injury if inadequate needle stabilization or improper catheter attachment to port body

AV, Arteriovenous; *IV,* intravenous; *SVC,* superior vena cava.
Used with permission from Lynn Hadaway Associates, Inc.

Hemodialysis and Pheresis Catheters

Catheters used for these procedures must have a large internal diameter to achieve the required high volume and rapid flow rates. These catheters may be designed for short-term or long-term use. After the pheresis procedure is complete, this catheter may be used for routine infusions. Hemodialysis catheters should be reserved for hemodialysis procedures only and should not be used for routine infusion except in emergent situations when no other vascular access can quickly be obtained.[5]

Intraosseous

Intraosseous (IO) devices are designed for rapid insertion into the bone marrow where fluids and medications are quickly absorbed. IO infusion is indicated when therapy is dangerously delayed as a result of difficulty obtaining IV

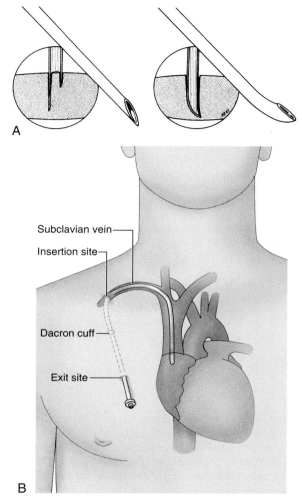

Fig. 10-1 **A,** Cross section of an implanted port. (From Bard Access Systems, Salt Lake City Utah.) **B,** Tunneled catheter. A portion of this catheter lies in a subcutaneous tunnel, separating the point where the catheter enters the vein from where it exits the skin. (From Ignatavicius, Donna, D. *Medical-surgical nursing: Patient-centered collaborative care,* 6th Edition. W.B. Saunders Company, 2009.)

access. For adults, the most common site is the sternum, although this site could be compromised by the need for cardiac compressions during resuscitation. Other sites are the proximal tibia, distal femur, radius, ulna, pelvis, and clavicle. For pediatric patients, the preferred sites include the tibia, femur, and iliac crest.[18]

Subcutaneous

The subcutaneous tissue can be the site of infusion for certain medications and isotonic fluids for hydration. This is most commonly seen in palliative and long-term care and may be seen by the emergency nurse if these patients require transfer to the acute care setting. A winged device has the needle positioned at a right angle and has a short extension set attached. Infusion sites include upper arm, upper and lower back, and anterior thigh. Site selection is determined by the patient's activity level.[18]

Intraspinal Devices

The epidural space is used for infusion of analgesia for both short-term and long-term needs. The medication must diffuse across the dura mater, although a portion of the drug could be absorbed into general circulation because of the vasculature in the epidural space. Intrathecal infusion is directly into the spinal cord. Catheters used for both epidural and intrathecal infusion include short-term externalized catheters and long-term catheters that are tunneled in the subcutaneous tissue and attached to an implanted port.[18]

CATHETER INSERTION

Insertion of all devices into the vascular system mandates careful attention to aseptic technique. Catheter-related bloodstream infection is now regarded as a preventable condition, and hospitals will not receive reimbursement for treatment of these infections acquired while patients are hospitalized. In emergency situations, when strict aseptic technique cannot be followed or confirmed, those catheters must be removed and a new catheter inserted at a new site as soon as the patient is stable or within 48 hours.[6] This recommendation is not restricted to any type of catheter and would apply to both peripheral and central catheters. It also applies to all health care settings, including prehospital emergency care, the emergency department, and any other hospital setting.

Peripheral Venipuncture

The initial site for peripheral catheter insertion should be on the lower forearm, with subsequent sites moving up the arm relative to the original site. Avoid sites of skin infection or irritation, sites near an infiltration or extravasation, and extremities with compromised circulation such as mastectomy with lymph node dissection, paralysis, or dialysis shunt or graft.

For adults, use of veins in the lower extremity should be avoided because of an increased risk of serious complications. If their use is unavoidable, these sites must be changed

TABLE 10-4   PROCEDURE FOR INSERTION OF A PERIPHERAL IV CATHETER

1. Obtain and review order.	15. Perform venipuncture while stabilizing skin with the nondominant hand.
2. Ascertain allergies.	
3. Gather equipment.	16. Enter skin at a 10° to 15° angle. Advance catheter into vein while observing for blood flashback. Slightly advance catheter into vein to ensure that the plastic catheter is inside the vein lumen. Continue to hold skin traction while advancing the catheter off the stylet into the vein lumen.
4. Verify patient's identity using two patient identifiers.	
5. Explain procedure, benefits, care management, and potential complications to patient.	
6. Perform hand hygiene.	
7. Assemble equipment.	17. Release tourniquet and discard.
8. Apply a single-patient use tourniquet. Tourniquets should never be shared between patients.	18. Occlude tip of catheter by pressing finger of nondominant hand over vein to prevent blood spoilage.
9. Assess veins of upper extremity by palpation.	19. Activate needle safety device before removing stylet. Connect IV administration set or injection cap/needleless device. Begin infusing solutions slowly. Observe insertion site for any signs of swelling. If catheter is for intermittent therapy, flush slowly with 3 mL of 0.9% bacteriostatic sodium chloride solution.
10. Apply nonsterile gloves.	
11. Wash intended insertion site with antiseptic soap and water (as needed).	
12. Remove excess hair from insertion site with clippers or scissors (as needed).	
13. Clean intended insertion site with antiseptic solution. Apply skin antiseptic according to the manufacturer's instructions. (Note: CHG now requires a back and forth scrubbing motion.)	20. Stabilize catheter with securement device and/or apply transparent dressing.
	21. Discard stylet into proper receptacle.
	22. Remove gloves. Perform hand hygiene.
14. Allow site to air-dry according to the manufacturer's instruction. (Note: CHG takes 30 seconds while povidone iodine takes 2 minutes.)	23. Label dressing with date, time, gauge and length of catheter, and name of nurse inserting catheter.
	24. Document procedure in the patient's medical record.

IV, Intravenous.
Adapted from Infusion Nurses Society. (2011). *Policies and procedures for infusion nursing* (4th ed.). Norwood, MA: Author.
Perucca, R. (2010). Peripheral venous access devices. In M. Alexander, A. Corrigan, L. Gorski, J. Hankins, & R. Perucca (Eds.), *Infusion nursing: An evidence-based approach* (3rd ed., pp. 456–479). St. Louis, MO: Saunders.

to a more desirable location once the patient is stable. The external jugular vein may also be a choice for insertion of a short peripheral catheter; however, this vein has a tortuous pathway and may not be suitable for procedures such as high-pressure injection because of the risk of infiltration into the area.

Use of a local anesthetic agent may be indicated for pediatric patients, those with a history of vasovagal reactions during venipuncture, and those requesting it for pain prevention. Injection of intradermal lidocaine is one method that is used after skin antisepsis. A very small gauge needle is inserted into the skin at the side of the vein. The site should be aspirated for a lack of blood return. A small amount, usually 0.1 to 0.2 mL, of lidocaine is injected, but care is required to prevent obscuring the vein by the volume of solution. Topical creams are also available for local anesthesia for venipuncture procedures, but they require 30 to 60 minutes to be effective. Other devices are used for accelerated delivery of a local anesthetic employing helium gas or oxygen in a heating element to drive the anesthetic agent into the skin.[5]

Peripheral catheter insertion begins with proper hand hygiene and includes the use of gloves for the procedure.

After selecting the appropriate site for catheter insertion, the patient's skin must be prepared. If visibly dirty, the skin should be washed with soap and water. This is followed by application of chlorhexidine gluconate–alcohol combination agents. Manufacturer's instructions for use of these skin antiseptics state that the site should be scrubbed in a back and forth motion for at least 30 seconds to enhance penetration of the deeper layers of the epidermis. Applying the antiseptic in a circular motion is no longer acceptable practice. The area should be allowed to dry for at least 30 seconds. Alcohol or povidone-iodine antiseptic solutions are only indicated when there is a contraindication for chlorhexidine gluconate–alcohol combination agents.[6] The procedure for making a venipuncture for insertion of a short peripheral catheter is detailed in Table 10-4.[19] According to Infusion Nursing Society Standards of Practice, each nurse should make no more than two venipuncture attempts before calling for assistance.[5]

Central Venous Catheter Insertion

Physicians, nurse practitioners, and physician assistants usually perform venipuncture of the subclavian or jugular veins, although nurses specializing in vascular access are beginning to perform these insertions. The scope of nursing practice is determined by the state board of nursing. Nurses will most frequently be assisting with this procedure.

Current recommendations now include having all supplies and equipment stocked in a dedicated cart or tray. This has been found to facilitate adherence to correct procedure by having all needed supplies in one location. The nurse assisting should have a procedure checklist and be empowered to terminate the procedure if any step on the checklist has not been performed. During emergent situations there may not be time to thoroughly adhere to all steps, but this process should be employed during less critical situations. Remember, when strict aseptic technique cannot be followed for insertion, those catheters must be removed and a new catheter inserted at a new site as soon as the patient is stable or within 48 hours.[6] Insertion of all central venous catheters requires the use of maximum barrier precautions, including sterile gloves, sterile gown, face masks, hair covering, and a large full-body sheet drape.[6,11] Use of this level of barrier precaution has proven to reduce the risk of catheter-related bloodstream infection.

The patient should be positioned with the head down and feet elevated. This encourages the distension of the subclavian and jugular veins. This is more effective in patients who are well hydrated and well nourished. The blind approach or using only anatomical landmarks is no longer recommended. Use of ultrasound provides anatomical information so the operator can guide the needle into the vein and avoid structures such as arteries, nerves, and the apex of the lungs.

A rolled towel may also be placed between the patient's scapulas. This will widen the space between the clavicle and first rib, making it easier to puncture the subclavian vein. Making the venipuncture in a medial location increases the risk of pinch-off syndrome, where the catheter is compressed between these bones. It can produce problems with infusion obstruction or even act as a scissor and completely fracture the catheter, causing part of it to embolize to the right heart. To avoid this problem, the puncture site should be made laterally, which would allow the catheter to enter the proximal axillary vein and then be threaded into the subclavian vein and ultimately to the lower third of the superior vena cava.

The nurse's role is to meet the patient's needs during the procedure while also performing the checklist and assisting with the procedure as required. After insertion the catheter must be stabilized, preferably with a manufactured catheter stabilization device. Sterile tape will not adhere sufficiently to adequately stabilize the catheter. Sutures increase the risk of needlestick injury and the risk of catheter-related infection.

ACCESSING IMPLANTED PORTS

The implanted port is located in a surgically created pocket, usually on the upper chest. The catheter is placed in the vein and then attached to the port body. The right internal jugular is preferred, as it provides a straight pathway to the lower third of the superior vena cava. A needle with a deflected tip is always used to access this device because this type of needle will slice through the dense septum in the port body. If a regular needle is used, the section of the septum can be cored out, resulting in leakage of the infusing fluid.

The port body cannot be seen. Its location and structure must be assessed completely by palpation. A raised area of skin may allow the nurse to locate the port body easily, especially if the patient has lost weight since its insertion. Some ports may be implanted deeply under subcutaneous tissue or located close to breast tissue, making them more difficult to palpate.

Key steps include the following:

- The nurse should pass a competency test for this skill prior to accessing an implanted port.
- Palpate the area and determine the circular area in the center where the dense septum is located. If possible, palpate for the stem and catheter extending from the side of the port body and avoid this area.
- Using sterile gloves and aseptic technique, clean the skin with chlorhexidine gluconate–alcohol by applying in a back and forth scrubbing motion and allow to dry thoroughly.
- Prime the port access needle and extension set with normal saline.
- Place one finger on each side of the circular area of the port body.
- Insert the needle into the septum located between the fingers. Puncture the skin and the dense septum until it stops on the posterior side of the port body.
- Aspirate for a brisk blood return to confirm that the needle is inside the septum.
- Flush the port body and catheter to ascertain if there is any resistance. Do not use the implanted port for infusion of any fluid or medication if there is not a blood return or if resistance to infusion is felt.[3,20]

ASSESSING THE CATHETER

Before each use of the catheter, the nurse must perform an assessment of the patency of the catheter and vein. This is important to prevent serious complications for the patient. Do not rely on the fact that the catheter has been in place only for a few minutes; a complication could still be developing. A convenient way to think about this process is with the OPAL method. (See Table 10-5.)

TABLE 10-5	ASSESSING THE CATHETER AND INFUSION SYSTEM
O = Observe	The fluid container and sets for • Appropriate fluid level • Correct flow rate • Complete connections The insertion site for • All signs for complications • Adherence of dressing
P = Palpate	The insertion site for • Alteration in skin temperature • Induration or cording of the vein
A = Aspirate	The catheter for • A free-flowing blood return, followed by injection of normal saline
L = Listen	The patient for complaints • Pain, burning, and other strange sensations • Along the entire catheter pathway • Chest discomfort with all types of central venous catheters

Used with permission from Lynn Hadaway Associates, Inc.

The presence of a blood return is one component of this assessment, albeit a very critical one. For peripheral catheters, there could be no blood return if the catheter is in a small vein or if the patient is dehydrated. The method of aspirating from the catheter could cause the vein wall or venous valve to occlude the lumen and obstruct the backflow of blood. A large vein could have the catheter erode through the posterior vein wall and then move back into the vein lumen, depending on the movement of the catheter and nearby joint. In this case there would be a blood return yet fluid is leaking from the additional vein damage.

For central venous catheters, there are numerous reasons for no blood return. Fibrin sheath formation can occur at the catheter tip, along part of or the complete catheter length. Fibrin covering the catheter tip occludes blood return. When a complete fibrin sheath is present, the infused fluid cannot flow into the bloodstream. Instead the infused fluid flows backward between the catheter and fibrin and can leak into the subcutaneous tissue around the insertion site, producing risk of tissue damage.

Central venous catheters can be malpositioned by having the tip located in the contralateral subclavian vein, the ipsilateral or contralateral jugular veins, or many small tributary veins that join the subclavian veins, brachiocephalic veins, and superior vena cava. Catheters can also erode through the vein wall into the mediastinum or other intrathoracic spaces, preventing a blood return and causing complications such as vein thrombosis, infiltration, or extravasation.

OBTAINING BLOOD SAMPLES FROM VASCULAR ACCESS DEVICES

Peripheral catheters may be used to obtain a blood sample during the insertion procedure; however, after infusion is started, another venipuncture site is required.

For central venous catheters, consider the types of laboratory tests that are needed. If coagulation tests are needed and the catheter has been heparinized, do not use the central venous catheter for this sample, as heparin is known to interfere with correct coagulation values. For drawing a blood culture from the catheter, the needleless connector must be removed and discarded, a new needleless connector attached, and the sample obtained through the new device. Used needleless connectors contain biofilm and will produce a high rate of false positive results.[21]

Key points include the following:
- The nurse should pass a competency test for this skill prior to drawing blood from an implanted port.
- Gather all needed supplies, including a new needleless connector, a sterile dead end cap if there are infusing fluids, prefilled saline flush syringes, prefilled heparin locking solution, alcohol pads, vacuum laboratory tubes and the tube holder, and the blood transfer device. A sterile empty syringe may be required if there is no blood return with the vacuum laboratory tubes.
- Identify the patient using two methods of identification.
- Perform hand hygiene.
- Don clean exam gloves.
- If a multiple lumen catheter is in use and there is infusion through one or more lumens, turn off but do not disconnect these infusions.
- If a single lumen catheter has fluids infusing and there is no other site for venipuncture, disconnect the administration set and carefully cover the male luer end with a sterile end cap. Do not attach it to a needleless connector higher on the set. Do not leave this male luer tip open. Do not allow it to contact any other surface. If not maintained appropriately, the entire set must be changed.
- Thoroughly scrub the needleless connector, including the connection surface and the luer-locking threads, with alcohol or chlorhexidine gluconate–alcohol pad for at least 15 seconds. Allow to dry thoroughly. Do not allow this connector to come into contact with other items in the environment.

Text continued on page 118.

TABLE 10-6 COMPLICATIONS OF VASCULAR ACCESS DEVICES

COMPLICATION AND DEFINITION	OCCURRING	CAUSE	SIGNS AND SYMPTOMS	TREATMENT	PREVENTION
Infiltration—Leakage of a non-vesicant IV solution or medication into the extravascular tissue	Locally at peripheral or central site At insertion and during dwell	Mechanical— • Puncture of vein at a second location • Dislodgment of catheter or implanted port access needle • Damaged catheter or implanted port septum Blood flow obstruction resulting in fluid overflow from puncture site as a result of: • Thrombosis • Lymphedema • Fibrin sheath encasing catheter Inflammatory process causing fluid leakage at the capillary level	Flow rate reduction Edema at or above the insertion site Changes in color of skin around insertion site, either redness or blanching Changes in skin temperature around insertion site, usually coolness Absence of a blood return from the catheter Fluid leaking from puncture site Complaints of skin tightness, burning, tenderness or general discomfort at the insertion site Complaints of any type of discomfort in shoulder, neck or chest with a CVAD	Stop infusion and remove short peripheral catheter immediately after identification of problem. Apply sterile dressing if weeping from tissue occurs. Apply cold compresses Elevate extremity if it increases patient comfort Insert a new catheter in the opposite extremity For all central venous catheters, obtain a dye study to determine the cause of the problem For implanted port, remove and insert a new port access needle	Stabilize all catheters and implanted port needles, preferably with a manufactured stabilization device Use smallest catheter that will accommodate the infusion Avoid placement in areas of flexion; if unavoidable use armboard to stabilize joint Avoid placing restraints in the area of an IV site Make successive venipunctures proximal to the previous site Assess site frequently, especially before each medication Educate patient about activities and signs and symptoms
Extravasation— Leakage of a vesicant IV solution or medication into the extravascular tissue	Locally at peripheral or central site At insertion and during dwell	Same as infiltration	Same as infiltration Tissue sloughing appears in 1 to 4 weeks	Stop infusion and disconnect administration set. Aspirate drug from short peripheral catheter or port access needle. Administer antidote according to established policy. Apply cold compresses for most drugs Apply heat for vinca alkaloids and vasoconstricting drugs Photograph site Monitor at 24 hours, one week, two weeks, and as needed. Surgical interventions may be required. Provide written instructions to patient and family.	Same as infiltration Know the vesicant potential before giving any IV medication

Continued

TABLE 10-6 COMPLICATIONS OF VASCULAR ACCESS DEVICES—cont'd

COMPLICATION AND DEFINITION	OCCURRING	CAUSE	SIGNS AND SYMPTOMS	TREATMENT	PREVENTION
Nerve damage—Inadvertent piercing or complete transection or compression of a nerve	At insertion During dwell time Local complication that can become a systemic complex regional pain syndrome	Unanticipated nerve locations Excessive subcutaneous probing Compression resulting from large volume infiltration/extravasation	Complaints of numbness, shock-like pain, tingling or feeling pins and needles at, above or below the insertion site.	Immediately stop the insertion procedure if the patient complains of these types of pain. Remove the catheter for signs and symptoms of infiltration/extravasation.	Avoid using the cephalic vein near the wrist. Do not use veins on the palm side of the wrist. Adequately secure the catheter but avoid tape that is too tight Support areas of joint flexion with an armboard
Phlebitis and post-infusion phlebitis Inflammation of the vein occurring during the catheter dwell or after catheter removal.	Local complication during dwell time	Mechanical cause from insertion technique, catheter size, and lack of catheter stabilization Chemical cause from extremes of pH and/or osmolarity of the fluid or medication. Bacterial cause from a break in aseptic technique, poor stabilization, and extended dwell time	Complaints of pain at the IV site; Erythema and edema at or near the insertion site Vein may become hard and cordlike.	Remove short peripheral catheter at the first sign of phlebitis; use warm compresses to relieve pain. Monitor frequently Restart a new catheter using the opposite extremity	Choose the smallest gauge catheter for the required therapy. Avoid sites of joint flexion or stabilize with a handboard. Avoid infusing fluids or medications with a pH below 5 or above 9 through a peripheral vein. Avoid infusing fluids or medications with a final osmolarity above 600 mOsm/L through a peripheral vein. Adequately secure the catheter Use aseptic technique.
Thrombosis and thrombophlebitis—Blood clot inside the vein The presence of a blood clot and vein inflammation	During dwell time at any point along with venous pathway that contains the catheter. May be limited to superficial peripheral veins or associated with large veins of chest	Traumatic venipuncture Multiple venipuncture attempts Use of catheters too large for the chosen vein Contact between the catheter and the vein wall, especially at or near the central venous catheter tip. Suboptimal tip location for central venous catheter Fluid volume deficits in clients with a central venous catheter	Slowed or stopped infusion rate Swollen extremity Tenderness and redness Engorged peripheral veins of the ipsilateral chest and extremity Difficulty moving the neck or jaw	Stop infusion and remove short peripheral catheter immediately Apply cold compresses to decrease blood flow and stabilize the clot. Elevate extremity Surgical intervention may be required For central venous catheters, notify the physician and obtain orders for a diagnostic study. Low dose thrombolytic agents can be used to lyse clot.	Use good venipuncture technique. Make only 2 attempts to perform venipuncture. Choose the smallest gauge catheter in the largest vein possible. Secure catheter adequately Use handboards if short peripheral catheters are placed in areas of joint flexion. Ensure adequate hydration to avoid changes in blood composition and flow.

Complication	Description	Causes	Signs and Symptoms	Treatment	Prevention
Site infection Invasion of microorganisms in the absence of simultaneous bloodstream infection Can be seen at the insertion site Subcutaneous tunnel Implanted port pocket	Local infection within a few days of insertion or at any point during the dwell time	Break in aseptic technique during insertion or the handling of sterile equipment Lack of proper hand hygiene and skin antisepsis Inadequate stabilization of the catheter or implanted port needle	Site appears red, swollen, and warm Complaints of tenderness at the site May observe purulent or malodorous exudate.	Clean exit site with alcohol, expressing drainage if present. Obtain specimen for culture, if ordered. If culture of catheter tip is ordered, remove short peripheral, midline catheter, PICC or nontunneled CVC using sterile technique and avoid contact between skin and catheter. Amputate catheter tip into a sterile container. Tunneled cuffed catheters and implanted ports require surgical removal Clean site with alcohol and cover with dry sterile dressing; physician to evaluate for septic phlebitis and need for antimicrobial therapy or surgical intervention	Use strict aseptic technique when inserting, maintaining or removing catheters. Use only chlorhexidine/alcohol combination for skin antisepsis, unless allergy is present Practice good hand hygiene Ensure dressing remains clean, dry and adherent to skin at all times. Use chlorhexidine dressing at insertion sites for PICC and nontunneled CVC.
Bloodstream infection Invasion of pathogenic organisms enter the client's circulation	Systemic complication occurring at any time during dwell	Inadequate skin antiseptic agents and application techniques. Excessive manipulation of the catheter hub leading to intraluminal contamination Inadequate cleaning of needleless connector before each use Use of contaminated IV administration set Inadequate hand hygiene	Early symptoms include fever, chills, headache, and general malaise; severe or unrecognized infection, which may lead to vascular collapse and death.	Change the entire infusion system from fluid container to VAD Notify physician, obtain blood, catheter or infusate cultures as prescribed, and administer antibiotics prescribed	Same as for site infection above. Change IV sets and needleless connectors according to hospital policy and procedure. Protect the male luer end of intermittent or disconnected IV sets. Use only a sterile device to access a catheter hub or needleless connector. Thoroughly scrub the hub and needleless connector for at least 15 seconds before each entry

Continued

TABLE 10-6 COMPLICATIONS OF VASCULAR ACCESS DEVICES—cont'd

COMPLICATION AND DEFINITION	OCCURRING	CAUSE	SIGNS AND SYMPTOMS	TREATMENT	PREVENTION
Catheter embolism A piece of catheter breaks off and floats freely in the vessel	Systemic event occurring at insertion or during dwell	Reinsertion of needle back into the over-the-needle catheter Improper removal of a needle for a CVC insertion Catheter compression between the clavicle and first rib, known as pinch off syndrome Material fatigue Excessive or forceful pressure for catheter flushing	Hypotension Weak, rapid or thready pulse Cyanosis of nail beds or circumoral area	For any catheter in the extremity immediately apply a tourniquet high on the extremity to possibly trap segment in the extremity Remove remaining catheter Notify physician Obtain radiograph of the chest and extremity, if appropriate. Interventional radiologic or surgical procedure to remove segment.	Follow manufacturer instructions for insertion of all VADs. Never use force when flushing or giving medications through a VAD. Assess patency by aspiration and flushing before each use. For subclavian insertion, medial venipuncture should be avoided.
Catheter migration Movement of a properly placed CVC tip to another vein No change in the external catheter length	Local complication during dwell	Changes in intrathoracic pressure caused by coughing, vomiting, sneezing, heavy lifting and congestive heart failure Rapid, forceful injection techniques Catheter tips allow to reside in the upper portion of the superior vena cava	For migration to the jugular vein—complaints of hearing a running stream or gurgling sound on the side of catheter insertion For migration to the azygos vein—back pain between the shoulder blades Neurologic complications if medications are infused into jugular vein resulting from retrograde infusion into the intracranial	Stop all infusions and flush catheter Notify physician Obtain a chest radiograph to assess tip location Spontaneous repositioning back to the SVC is possible Repositioning by radiology may be required.	Catheter tip properly placed in the lower third of the SVC near the junction with the right atrium. Instruct patient to perform normal activities of daily living but to avoid excessive physical activity Slow gentle technique for flushing catheter

Complication		Cause	Signs and Symptoms	Nursing Interventions	Prevention
Catheter dislodgment	Local complication occurring during dwell	Inadequate catheter stabilization	External catheter length has changed, also changing the internal tip location.	Stop all infusions and flush catheter.	Proper catheter stabilization.
Movement of CVC into or out of the insertion site		Excessive physical activity with a PICC	No other signs or symptoms may be immediately noticed	NEVER readvance the catheter into the insertion site. Determine the amount of external catheter length and compare to the length documented on insertion. Notify the physician or nurse inserting the catheter for further assessment.	Instruct patient to perform normal activities of daily living but to avoid excessive physical activity
Lumen occlusion	Local complication occurring any time during dwell	Thrombotic	Infusion stops and/or pump alarm sounds	Assess history of catheter use.	Always flush with normal saline before and after each medication given through the catheter.
Catheter lumen is partially or totally blocked		• Empty infusion container	Inability or difficulty administering fluids	A suddenly developing problem may indicate contact between incompatible medications. A problem that develops over an extended period may indicate a gradual clot formation.	For intermittent medication, disconnect and flush catheters immediately when medication infusion is complete.
		• Incorrect flushing technique for needleless connector in use	Inability or difficulty aspirating blood	For drug precipitate, determine the pH of the precipitated drug. Use hydrochloric acid for acidic drug. Use sodium bicarbonate for alkaline drugs, according to policy and procedure.	Use correct flushing and clamping technique for the needleless connector in use.
		• Changes in intrathoracic venous pressure	Increased resistance to flushing of the catheter	For thrombotic cause, instill thrombolytic agent according to policy and procedure	
		• Excessive muscular contractions of arm with PICC			
		• Precipitate			
		• Contact between incompatible drugs or mineral			
		• Lipid sludge from long-term infusion of fat emulsion			

CVAD, Central venous access device; *CVC,* central venous catheter; *IV,* intravenous; *PICC,* peripherally inserted central catheter; *SVC,* superior vena cava; *VAD,* vascular access device. Used with permission from Lynn Hadaway Associates, Inc.

- Attach a saline-filled syringe and flush the catheter to remove the heparin locking solution, and then aspirate the volume equal to three times the internal volume of the catheter.
- Attach the vacuum tube holder to the catheter hub or the needleless connector.
- Insert the vacuum tubes into the holder in the proper sequence according to the tests prescribed.
- If unsuccessful with the vacuum tubes, disconnect the tube holder and attach a series of 3-mL or 5-mL syringes. Slowly aspirate blood into each syringe. Smaller syringes produce less pressure on aspiration and may yield a blood return when the vacuum tube will not work. Transfer the blood to the appropriate vacuum tube using a needleless transfer device.
- Flush the catheter with 10 to 20 mL of normal saline, followed by heparin locking solution according to hospital policy.
- Reestablish the flow rate for the other lumens if present.
- Label the vacuum tubes with the patient identification and send them to the lab.

REMOVING CENTRAL VENOUS CATHETERS

Air embolus is a major concern when removing all central venous catheters, especially those inserted through the subclavian and jugular veins. These veins are located above the level of the heart, thus increasing the risk of air entering the veins upon catheter removal. For PICC removal, the same procedure should be used. Although the risk is reduced with a PICC because the exit site is at or below the heart, having the same procedure for removal of all types of central venous catheters will eliminate confusion.

The site of a central venous catheter will have a skin-to-vein tract that does not close quickly. This tract can be firmly attached to an intact fibrin sheath. This will serve as a conduit for pulling air into the circulation.

Key points include the following:
- For subclavian or jugular sites, place the patient in a supine position. For a PICC, place the arm at the patient's side.
- Identify the patient using two identifiers.
- Perform hand hygiene and don clean exam gloves.
- Remove the dressing and catheter stabilization device.
- Withdraw the catheter in short segments. With the last few centimeters of catheter inside the vein, instruct the patient to perform a Valsalva maneuver.
- Withdraw the remaining catheter and immediately place gauze over the site. Hold until bleeding has stopped.

- When hemostasis is achieved, quickly remove the plain gauze and replace with a petroleum gel gauze dressing. Cover with a dry gauze and firmly secure with a transparent membrane dressing or tape sufficient to cover the entire gauze, making an occlusive dressing.
- Instruct the patient to leave this dressing intact for at least 24 hours or until the site has healed.
- The length of time that the patient should remain in a supine position has not been firmly established, but 30 to 60 minutes has been suggested.

VASCULAR ACCESS DEVICES COMPLICATIONS

Complications of vascular access devices can be considered in several ways (see Table 10-6). Some are local complications, occurring only at the insertion site, while others are considered systemic complications. Another approach is to assess those complications that occur at or immediately following insertion versus those that occur later during the dwell time.

REFERENCES

1. Phillips, L. (2010). Parenteral fluids. In M. Alexander, A. Corrigan, L. Gorski, J. Hankins, & R. Perucca (Eds.), *Infusion nursing: An evidence-based approach* (3rd ed., pp. 229–241). St. Louis, MO: Saunders.
2. Hadaway, L. (2010). Anatomy and physiology related to infusion therapy. In M. Alexander, A. Corrigan, L. Gorski, J. Hankins, & R. Perucca (Eds.), *Infusion nursing: An evidence-based approach* (3rd ed., pp. 139–177). St. Louis, MO: Elsevier.
3. Turner, M., Hankins, J. (2010). Pharmacology. In M. Alexander, A. Corrigan, L. Gorski, J. Hankins, & R. Perucca (Eds.), *Infusion nursing: An evidence-based approach* (3rd ed., pp. 263–289). St. Louis, MO: Saunders.
4. Hadaway, L. (2010). Infusion therapy equipment. In M. Alexander, A. Corrigan, L. Gorski, J. Hankins, & R. Perucca (Eds.), *Infusion nursing: An evidence-based approach* (3rd ed., pp. 391–436). St. Louis, MO: Saunders.
5. Infusion Nurses Society. (2011). *Infusion nursing standards of practice*. Norwood, MA: Author.
6. O'Grady N. (2011). *Guidelines for the prevention of intravascular catheter-related infections*. Retrieved from http://www.cdc.gov/hicpac/pdf/guidelines/bsi-guidelines-2011.pdf
7. IV infiltration: Be alarmed even when your infusion pump isn't. (2007). *PA PSRS Patient Safety Advisory, 4*(3), 97–99.
8. Brixey, J. J., Zhang, J., Johnson, T. R., & Turley, J. P. (2009). Legibility of a volumetric infusion pump in a shock trauma ICU. *The Joint Commission Journal on Quality and Patient Safety, 35*(4), 229–235.
9. Nuckols, T. K., Bower, A. G., Paddock, S. M., Hilborne, L. H., Wallace, P., Rothschild, J. M., … Brook, R. H. (2008).

Programmable infusion pumps in ICUs: An analysis of corresponding adverse drug events. *Journal of General Internal Medicine*, 23(Suppl 1), 41–45.

10. Hadaway, L., & Richardson, D. (2010). Needleless connectors: A primer on terminology. *Journal of Infusion Nursing*, 33(1), 22–31.

11. Kagel, E., & Rayan, G. (2004). Intravenous catheter complications in the hand and forearm. *Journal of Trauma*, 56(1), 123–127.

12. Boeson, M. B., Hranchook, A., & Stoller, J. (2000). Peripheral nerve injury from intravenous cannulation: A case report. *AANA Journal*, 68(1), 53–57.

13. Hadaway, L. (2007). Infiltration and extravasation. *American Journal of Nursing*, 107(8), 64–72.

14. Costantino, T. G., Kirtz, J. F., & Satz, W. A. (2010). Ultrasound-guided peripheral venous access vs. the external jugular vein as the initial approach to the patient with difficult vascular access. *Journal of Emergency Medicine*, 39(4), 462–467.

15. Dargin, J. M., Rebholz, C. M., Lowenstein, R. A., Mitchell, P. M., & Feldman, J. A. (2010). Ultrasonography-guided peripheral intravenous catheter survival in ED patients with difficult access. *American Journal of Emergency Medicine*, 28(1), 1–7.

16. Parker, M., & Henderson, K. (2010). Alternative infusion access devices. In M. Alexander, A. Corrigan, L. Gorski, J. Hankins, & R. Perucca (Eds.), *Infusion nursing: An evidence-based approach* (3rd ed., pp. 516–524). St. Louis, MO: Saunders.

17. Hess, H. (2010). A biomedical device to improve pediatric vascular access success. *Pediatric Nursing*, 36(5), 259–263.

18. Perucca, R. (2010). Peripheral venous access devices. In M. Alexander, A. Corrigan, L. Gorski, J. Hankins, & R. Perucca (Eds.), *Infusion nursing: An evidence-based approach* (3rd ed., pp. 456–479). St. Louis, MO: Saunders.

19. Marschall, J., Mermel, L. A., Classen, D., Arias, K. M., Podgorny, K., Anderson, D. J., … Yokoe, D. S. (2008). Strategies to prevent central line-associated bloodstream infections in acute care hospitals. *Infection Control and Hospital Epidemiology*, 29(Suppl 1), S22–S30.

20. Polovich, M., Whitford, J., & Olsen, M. (Eds.). (2009). *Chemotherapy and biotherapy guidelines and recommendations for practice* (3rd ed.). Pittsburgh, PA: Oncology Nursing Society.

21. Sherertz, R., Karchmer, T., Ohl, C., Palavecino, E., & Bischoff, W. (2010). *Blood cultures (BC) drawn through valved catheter hubs have a 10–20% positivity rate with the majority being false positives.* Paper presented at Fifth Decennial International Conference on Healthcare-Associated Infections, Atlanta, GA.

Care of the Patient with Pain

Diana Meyer

Pain is a complex experience for patients. The International Association for the Study of Pain defines pain in the following manner: "An unpleasant sensory and emotional experience associated with actual or potential tissue damage, or described in terms of such damage."[1] McCaffery and Beebe[2] define pain as "whatever the experiencing person says it is, existing whenever he or she says it does." While pain is an event that most humans experience, it is always subjective and each of us experiences pain differently.

Oligoanalgesia, the undertreatment of pain, is the greatest risk to accomplishing pain relief for the patient.[3,4] One of the primary responsibilities to patients in the emergency department (ED) is to assess pain effectively and manage pain to the best of our ability.

TYPES OF PAIN

There are two categories of pain, acute and chronic, which can be further divided into three types: somatic, visceral, and neuropathic (Table 11-1). Noting the type of pain will help in determining the cause and will support choosing an appropriate intervention. More than one kind of pain or mechanism for pain can be present in an individual patient.

PAIN ASSESSMENT

The challenge of assessing a subjective complaint in an objective manner continues to affect the approaches that emergency nurses choose in caring for the patient with pain. Conducting a comprehensive assessment of pain in a nonjudgmental manner creates a trusting relationship and improves communication between the nurse and the patient. Consistent use of pain assessment tools that have been determined to be simple, reliable, valid, population specific, and sensitive to changes in pain intensity is essential to effectively evaluate the patients presenting for care.[5]

Assessment of a patient's pain begins at the time of arrival in the ED and continues throughout the patient's ED stay, with the frequency of reassessment determined by the patient's condition and the interventions provided for pain relief. Each patient should be assessed for the presence and intensity of pain, regardless of the chief complaint and focused on the reason for presenting to the ED for care. The mnemonic PQRST provides the parameters to be assessed (Table 11-2).

Signs that a patient's pain is more serious include:
- Abrupt onset
- Maximum severity at onset
- Awakened patient from sleep
- Has associated vital sign changes
- Describes as a constant ache, pressure, burning, squeezing

Pain Assessment Tools

Assessment tools provide information about the patient's subjective experience with pain. The tools establish a common language to describe the severity of pain and allow the emergency nurse to document pain ratings and compare these ratings over time.

All EDs should establish a standard for pain assessment and response to treatment based the hierarchy of assessment techniques (Table 11-3). No one tool is useful in all populations. Determining which pain assessment tools will be used in the ED supports achieving the goal of evidence-based, consistent pain assessment of the diverse population of patients seen in the ED.

The most reliable of these severity assessment tools are based on patients' self-reporting.[6] The numeric rating scale, the visual analog scale, and picture scales are self-report pain assessment tools (Table 11-4). Some patients have trouble using a horizontal, classic left-to-right pain scale,

TABLE 11-1 TYPES OF PAIN

TYPE OF PAIN	SITES	CHARACTERISTICS
Somatic	Skin and subcutaneous tissues	Localized
	Bone, muscle, blood vessels, and connective tissues	Constant and achy
Visceral	Organs and the linings of the body cavities	Poorly localized
		Diffuse, cramping
Neuropathic	Central and peripheral nervous systems	Poorly localized
		Shooting, burning, sharp, numbness, tingling

TABLE 11-2 PQRST MNEMONIC

P	Palliative or precipitating factors
Q	Quality of pain
R	Region and radiation of the pain
S	Subjective description of pain (use pain rating scale)
T	Temporal nature of the pain

TABLE 11-3 HIERARCHY OF PAIN ASSESSMENT TECHNIQUES

Attempt a self-report from patient.
Identify pathologic conditions or procedures that cause pain.
Use behavioral assessment tools.
Identify behaviors that caregivers and others knowledgeable about the patient think may indicate pain.
Attempt an analgesic trial.

especially if their primary language is read vertically or from right to left. Turn the scale vertically instead. Place the "10" at the top because sequences that progress upward are more universally recognizable than those that progress downward.[7,8]

Younger children may not understand the concept of ranking. Determine the child's ability to use a numerical scale by asking, "Which number is larger, nine or five?" For those who cannot accurately answer that question, use the Finger Span Scale. The child is asked to move the forefinger and thumb apart to report the magnitude. Demonstrate it to the child by using the word for pain, such as "hurt," that is most familiar to the child. Having the thumb and forefinger together represents "no pain," a small distance between fingers represents "tiny" pain, and so on until far apart represents "most possible pain." Estimate based on the finger spread.[9] Using the finger span assessment with FLACC (see Table 11-5) will improve overall assessment.[10]

When patients cannot self-report, using a behavioral tool that results in a numeric rating keeps the documentation of the pain assessment consistent with self-report tools.[11-14]

- PIPP (Premature Infant Pain Profile), for premature and term neonates, uses gestational age, heart rate, oxygen saturation, behavioral state, brow bulge, eye squeeze, and nasolabial furrow.[15-17]
- FLACC (Face, Legs, Activity, Cry, and Consolability) assesses the five categories indicated in the name and assigns a score of 0 to 2 for each category. See Table 11-5.
- PAINAD (Pain Assessment in Advanced Dementia) Scale uses breathing independent of vocalization, negative vocalization, facial expressions, body language, and consolability. See Table 11-6.

Regardless of the pain assessment tools used in the ED, documentation of the patient's pain should be done in a consistent format and include identification of which pain assessment tool is being used.[18]

PROVIDING COMFORT FOR THE PATIENT IN PAIN

The emergency nurse who advocates for the patient's comfort throughout the ED visit supports the ability of the emergency physician to meet the patient's expectation of pain relief. While appropriate management is based on the etiology of the pain, it is important that we begin the treatment of pain while simultaneously exploring the cause of pain. Studies found no difference in physical findings or diagnostic accuracy between patients who received morphine and those who received a placebo.[19-21] The American Pain Society, American College of Emergency Physicians, and Canadian Association of Emergency Physicians recommend that analgesia *not* be withheld during a diagnostic workup.[22-24]

The choice of pain management strategies depends on the etiology and whether the pain condition is solely acute, acute with chronic pain, or a breakthrough chronic pain

TABLE 11-4   SELF-REPORT PAIN ASSESSMENT TOOLS

PAIN SCALE	DESCRIPTION	INSTRUCTIONS	POPULATION
Numeric rating scale (NRS)	Consists of a range of numbers, usually in 0–10 range	Patients are instructed to select the number that is most representative of their pain intensity; 0 is described as no pain and 10 as "worst pain possible"	Pediatric and adult patients able to understand and follow instructions
Visual analog scale (VAS)	Consists of line oriented either horizontally or vertically with verbal descriptors of pain intensity at each end	Patients are asked to place a mark at the point on the line that best represents the pain severity level	Pediatric and adult patients able to understand and follow instructions
Picture scale	A series of facial expressions meant to represent various pain states; each image is assigned a number, which becomes the patient's pain intensity	Images are presented to patients and they are asked to choose the facial expression that best matches their pain intensity	Pediatric, elder, and ethnically diverse versions are available. Patients must be able to follow instructions; however, at times patients who cannot self-report via NRS or VAS are able to report with a picture scale.

TABLE 11-5   FLACC SCALE*

CRITERIA	SCORE = 0	SCORE = 1	SCORE = 2
Face	No particular expression or smile	Occasional grimace or frown, withdrawn, disinterested	Frequent to constant quivering chin, clenched jaw
Legs	Normal position or relaxed	Uneasy, restless, tense	Kicking, or legs drawn up
Activity	Lying quietly, normal position, moves easily	Squirming, shifting back and forth, tense	Arched, rigid, jerking
Cry	No cry (awake or asleep)	Moans or whimpers; occasional complaint	Crying steadily; screams or sobs; frequent complaints.
Consolability	Content, relaxed	Reassured by occasional touching, hugging or being talked to; distractible	Difficult to console or comfort

*Originally validated in pediatric population (ages 2 months to 7 years). The tool has now been validated in adult populations.
From Merkel, S., Voepel-Lewis, T., Shayevitz, J., & Malviya, S. (1997). The FLACC: A behavioral scale for scoring postoperative pain in young children. *Pediatric Nursing, 23*(3), 293–297.

TABLE 11-6   PAIN ASSESSMENT IN ADVANCED DEMENTIA (PAINAD) SCALE*

ITEMS	0	1	2
Breathing independent of vocalization	Normal	Occasional labored breathing. Short period of hyperventilation.	Noisy labored breathing. Long period of hyperventilation. Cheyne-Stokes respirations
Negative vocalization	None	Occasional moan or groan. Low-level speech with a negative or disapproving quality (muttering, mumbling, whining).	Repeated troubled calling out. Loud moaning or groaning. Crying
Facial expression	Smiling or inexpressive	Sad. Frightened. Frown.	Facial grimacing
Body language	Relaxed	Tense. Distressed pacing. Fidgeting.	Rigid. Fists clenched. Knees pulled up. Pulling or pushing away. Striking out
Consolability	No need to console	Distracted or reassured by voice or touch.	Unable to console, distract or reassure

*May also be used with hospice patients.
From Frampton, K. (2004). "Vital sign #5." *Caring for the Ages, 5*(5), 26–35.

TABLE 11-7 CLASSES OF PAIN MEDICATIONS

CLASS	EXAMPLES	PAIN DESCRIPTIONS	CLINICAL EXAMPLES	CAUTIONS
Opioids	Morphine Fentanyl Dilaudid	Stabbing Spasms Shooting Sharp	Kidney stone Gallbladder Pancreatic Bowel obstruction Trauma	Sedation
NSAID	Ibuprofen Ketorolac Acetaminophen	Aching Dull Throbbing	Headache Arthritic Back pain Muscular Menstrual	History of gastrointestinal bleed Taking anticoagulants Thrombocytopenia Renal or hepatic disease
Adjuvant	Corticosteroids Antidepressants Anticonvulsants	Lancinating (piercing) Burning or tingling Shooting Radiculopathy	Neuropathic Phantom limb Peripheral neuropathy (diabetic, peripheral vascular disease)	Related to specific agents used

condition. In most circumstances, using an approach that is multimodal and tailored to the individual is the pathway to success.[25]

Pharmacologic Interventions

Pharmacologic pain management strategies fall into four classes—local, nonopioid, opioid, or adjuvant—and include choosing the right medication (Table 11-7) and route for the patient's problem. Using nonsteroidal anti-inflammatory drugs (NSAIDs) in conjunction with opiates can decrease the dose and frequency of opiates needed.[25] Caution must be taken when using combination products (opiates with acetaminophen or NSAID) because of the risk of exceeding the maximum daily dose of the nonopiate.[26] Whenever possible, administering these medications in their single-ingredient format makes it easier to adjust dosage of the opiate and keep track of the amount of nonopiate being administered.

Studies have found that 1000 mg of acetaminophen (Tylenol) and 800 mg of ibuprofen (Motrin) *at the same time* is effective for mild to moderate pain, especially for musculoskeletal conditions, dental pain, or postoperative pain. The combination of different actions, one central and one peripheral, provides additive pain-relieving activity and is more effective than either drug used alone.[27–30]

> Promethazine (Phenergan) is not recommended to "potentiate" a narcotic.

An underused pain management strategy is nitrous oxide, or Nitronox, which is a premixed combination of nitrous oxide and oxygen that can be self-administered by the patient. Nitronox provides quick pain relief and has a short duration of action and minimal side effects.[27] Figure 11-1 describes the indications and contraindications, precautions, and procedure for administering nitrous oxide in the emergency setting.

> Do not hold the mask on the patient's face when providing self-administered nitrous oxide and oxygen (Nitronox).

For infants up to 4 months, the administration of oral sucrose is known to provide pain relief during procedures such as intravenous line insertion, urinary catheter and nasogastric insertion, and lumbar puncture.[31] The analgesic effect lasts about 5 to 8 minutes and is effective only when administered orally, directly onto the tongue.

In addition to managing pain with a systemic focus, it is often appropriate to treat pain in a more localized method using topical (Table 11-8), aerosolized, and injected agents.[32]

Nonpharmacologic Interventions

In the ED, pain management is primarily grounded in pharmacologic therapy. However, because pain is both a physical and an emotional experience, the addition of nonpharmacologic interventions that address the negative emotions of fear and anxiety should be included to enhance the effectiveness of pharmacologic interventions.[33] Some nonpharmacologic interventions, such as splinting and ice, are effective because of their physiologic impact on the cause of the pain or the pain pathway itself. Examples of nonpharmacologic treatment include the following:

- Place the patient in a position of comfort.
- Immobilize an affected area to minimize further pain.
- Apply superficial heat, such as a warm compress, to relieve the pain of an infiltrated intravenous line.

PeaceHealth St Joseph Medical Center
Nitronox Administration Nurse Initiated Protocol

Utilizing the clinical guidelines from Nurse Initiated Interventions, the EDRN may initiate patient administered nitronox.

- To treat pain associated with fractures and burns
- Prior to painful procedures such as IV insertion and wound care
- To relieve anxiety associated with painful conditions and procedures

General Information

- Nitronox provides rapid onset (2-6 minutes), quickly reversible (2-5 minutes) analgesia
- Children and the elderly may use nitrous oxide as long as they can cooperate and self-administer the nitrous oxide. The nitronox delivery device (mask/mouthpiece) should never be held on the patient's face
- Nitronox causes drowsiness and is not used in patients with an altered LOC, head injuries, or those that are heavily sedated or intoxicated
- Nitronox collects in dead air spaces and can expand the pre-exiting pockets of air associated with pneumothorax, otitis media, perforated viscus, bowel obstruction, air embolus and decompression sickness

Contraindications	Side Effects	Complications
<ul><li>Patient is unable to self-administer and/or understand instructions</li><li>Altered LOC (risk of aspiration)</li><li>Chest injuries (potential of pneumothorax) or COPD patients</li><li>Pregnancy: actual or suspected (associated with fetal defects and SAB)</li><li>Abdominal pain (potential of SBO or perforated viscus)</li><li>Facial injuries where ability to create seal is impaired</li><li>Suspected air embolism or decompression sickness</li></ul>	<ul><li>Vomiting</li><li>Shortness of breath</li><li>Excitement</li><li>Drowsiness</li><li>Confusion</li><li>Light headedness</li></ul>	<ul><li>Propping or holding the mask against the patient's face may result in excessive sedation. The patient must hold the mask to prevent overdosage</li><li>Aspiration may occur if the patient vomits with the mask in place</li></ul>

Patient Preparation

- Assess and document vital signs
- Instruct the patient to do the following:
  - Form a tight seal with the mask or mouthpiece and take slow, deep breaths
  - Exhale into the mask or mouthpiece so that exhaled gas is collected into scavenger and not dispersed into ambient air
  - Avoid unnecessary conversation to limit exhalation of nitrous oxide into the room
  - Discontinue use if nausea, light-headedness or other side effects occur

Procedure

- Allow the patient to inhale the gas for 3 or 4 minutes before beginning any procedures. Some patients may require up to 6 minutes
- As the patient becomes relaxed, he or she will be unable to create an adequate amount of negative pressure to trip the demand value
- Allow the patient to resume gas inhalation when he or she is able to hold the mask or mouthpiece
- Limit nitronox administration to 30 minutes
- Document vital signs, length of gas inhalation and response to medication

Important

- Patient must be able to self administer the nitronox
- Administration of nitronox is discontinued when the acute need for pain and/or anxiety relief has been met
- Consult with physician for additional medications when contraindications exist or pain relief has not been achieved

Patient Sticker

Implemented 7/03 Updated Reviewed: 4/05, 10/07, 9/09

Fig. 11-1 Example of a nurse-initiated nitrous oxide (Nitronox) administration protocol. (Courtesy of PeaceHealth St. Joseph Medical Center.)

TABLE 11-8 **TOPICAL ANESTHETICS**

NAME	INDICATIONS	ADMINISTRATION	SPECIAL CONSIDERATIONS
TAC (tetracaine, adrenaline, cocaine) LET (lidocaine, epinephrine, tetracaine)	Minor wounds that do not involve fingers, toes, penis, or nose	Applied using 4 × 4 held on wound Wear glove while applying so as not to absorb medication yourself	Blanching of skin Infiltration of wound with lidocaine before closure necessary
EMLA (lidocaine, prilocaine)	Cream applied to site before painful procedure (IV start, lumbar puncture)	Place cream on intact skin and cover with occlusive dressing Onset of effect takes 45–60 minutes	Blanching, erythema Length of time to onset may be deterrent to use May require reapplication if first procedure not successful
J-Tip (1% buffered lidocaine)	Used to numb site before IV start	Uses compressed carbon dioxide for needle-free drug delivery into the subcutaneous space	Blanching, erythema Ecchymosis at site "Popping" noise upon administration may frighten patient without preparation Increased risk of ecchymosis in patients ≥65 years of age
Synera (lidocaine, tetracaine)	Used to numb site before IV start	Apply to intact skin for 20 minutes prior to procedure Onset of effect is achieved via a controlled heating mechanism in patch	Blanching, erythema, edema Must be removed before MRI as heating element contains iron powder Do not cut patch as there is risk of thermal injury
Lidocaine 4% solution	To numb naso-oropharynx prior to NG tube insertion	Atomized via mucosal atomization device (MADD) connected to syringe Nebulized	High level of absorption, caution not to exceed maximum dose

IV, Intravenous; *MRI*, magnetic resonance imaging; *NG*, nasogastric.

- Apply superficial cold (an ice pack) to fractures and sprains to reduce pain and swelling.
- Have the patient focus on a stimulus other than the pain. Age-appropriate distraction techniques include:
  - Pediatric: magic wands, bubbles, squeezable balls, stuffed animals, parent reading to child
  - Adolescent and adult: audiotapes, videotapes, games, puzzles, music, engaging in conversation
- Use guided imagery to assist the patient to imagine pleasant images associated with calm, soothing sensations.
- Use relaxation techniques to reduce anxiety. Deep breathing is one technique that can be taught quickly in the ED.

For infants, in addition to sucrose administration the following measures may reduce distress:

- If the infant is able to suck, the addition of nonnutritive sucking provides a calming influence during the procedure.
- Full or partial swaddling to minimize limb flailing and support containment

- Reduction in noxious stimuli (noise and lighting)
- Holding and cuddling

Applying manual pressure for 10 seconds prior to an intramuscular injection minimizes the discomfort of the injection.[8]

Nurse-Initiated Protocols

The availability of nurse-initiated protocols for pain management is an excellent strategy to decrease the time to first intervention for patients. It has been demonstrated that these protocols are safe and significantly decrease the time that patients wait for pain management.[34–37] The use of nurse-initiated protocols can improve patient care and increase patient satisfaction and many organizations are reviewing the effectiveness of implementing these protocols in their ED settings. Nurse-initiated protocols are written in a collaborative manner between nurses and physicians and supported by the ED administrative team. These protocols must clearly state the inclusion and exclusion criteria to be met for implementation and nurses are cautioned to

TABLE 11-9	"DRUG-SEEKING" BEHAVIOR

Goes to different emergency departments
Asks for refill because prescription lost or stolen
Tells inconsistent story about pain
Allergy to everything but certain opioid
States name and dose of the opioid
Prefers needle to a pill
Clock-watcher
Tells nurse where to give drug or how fast
Frequently comes to the emergency department to get opioids

TABLE 11-10	ASSESSING PRESCRIPTION DRUG ABUSE: MODIFIED CAGE PNEUMONIC

FOUR SIMPLE QUESTIONS

C	Have you ever felt the need to **C**ut down on your use of prescription drugs?
A	Have you ever felt **A**nnoyed by remarks your friends or loved ones made about your use of prescription drugs?
G	Have you ever felt **G**uilty or remorseful about your use of prescription drugs?
E	Have you **E**ver used prescription drugs as a way to "get going" or to "calm down"?

follow their own institutional policies, procedures, and protocols carefully. The medication orders must include all necessary parameters, minimally name of medication, dose, and route. If repeat doses are expected, the frequency and indication for repeating the dose must also be included. The Centers for Medicare and Medicaid Services (CMS) also requires that a physician order be signed for the use of these protocols.[38] Fortunately this signature can be obtained after the protocol has been initiated, thereby keeping the benefit of treating the patient's pain prior to seeing the physician intact. An example of a nurse-initiated protocol is provided in Figure 11-2.

Concern-Raising Behaviors

The term "drug-seeking" is frequently used and poorly defined. Most often the term is used to describe patients that present with behaviors that are interpreted by physicians and nurses as indication of addiction or abuse of pain medications or as manipulative (Table 11-9). These behaviors consume scarce resources, particularly the nurse's time, attention, and patience. However, each of these behaviors perceived to be evidence of addiction, abuse, or manipulation may have a legitimate explanation, including unrelieved pain.[39] The term "drug-seeking" has a negative meaning and associating it with patients may create a barrier to compassion and caring. Rather than using language that stigmatizes patients, choosing to use the phrase "concern-raising behaviors" alerts the clinician that something is not right and that careful evaluation is needed.[40,41]

Caring for these challenging patients can lead to frustration unless emergency nurses prepare themselves with knowledge of successful strategies. These strategies include:
- Believe the patient's report of pain.
- Be open to the possibility that the concern-raising behaviors have a legitimate explanation.
- Believing the patient's report of pain does not dictate specific pain interventions.

- Use the Modified CAGE[42] questionnaire (Table 11-10) to screen for the possibility of prescription drug abuse and offer resources and referrals to the patient.
- Abide by pain care management plans if the patient has entered into such a contract for care.
- When patients request opioids that are not in their best interests, practice compassionate refusal[41] by expressing concern for their pain while reinforcing the appropriate pain strategies being offered.
- Develop a care plan for repeating patients so that all staff respond in a consistent manner.[17]
- Accept the possibility that, to avoid failing to treat a patient in pain, you may be giving pain medication to a patient who does not have physical pain.

Sedation for Procedures

The purpose of sedation and analgesia is to decrease anxiety and minimize pain awareness and intensity during procedures that are painful or frightening to patients. In the emergency department, the physician will determine a level of sedation from minimal to deep (Table 11-11) depending on the procedure to be performed.[43–45] For a more detailed discussion of sedation in the emergency department setting, see Chapter 15, Procedural Sedation.

SUMMARY

The importance of assessing, managing, and reassessing a patient's pain while he or she is in the emergency department cannot be overemphasized. Effective tools are available to assess pain and effective therapies are available to treat pain. Emergency nurses play a critical role by providing independent interventions and, with physician colleagues, advocating for appropriate pain relief for the patient. Trust the patient when he or she reports pain and focus on

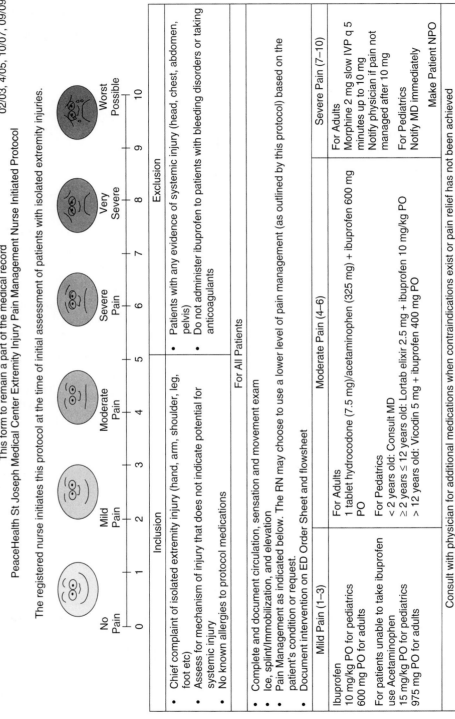

This form to remain a part of the medical record

PeaceHealth St Joseph Medical Center Extremity Injury Pain Management Nurse Initiated Protocol   02/03, 4/05, 10/07, 09/09

The registered nurse initiates this protocol at the time of initial assessment of patients with isolated extremity injuries.

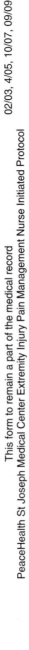

| 0 | 1 | 2 | 3 | 4 | 5 | 6 | 7 | 8 | 9 | 10 |
| No Pain | | Mild Pain | | Moderate Pain | | Severe Pain | | Very Severe | | Worst Possible |

Inclusion	Exclusion
• Chief complaint of isolated extremity injury (hand, arm, shoulder, leg, foot etc) • Assess for mechanism of injury that does not indicate potential for systemic injury • No known allergies to protocol medications	• Patients with any evidence of systemic injury (head, chest, abdomen, pelvis) • Do not administer ibuprofen to patients with bleeding disorders or taking anticoagulants

For All Patients

• Complete and document circulation, sensation and movement exam
• Ice, splint/Immobilization, and elevation
• Pain Management as indicated below. The RN may choose to use a lower level of pain management (as outlined by this protocol) based on the patient's condition or request.
• Document intervention on ED Order Sheet and flowsheet

Mild Pain (1–3)	Moderate Pain (4–6)	Severe Pain (7–10)
Ibuprofen 10 mg/kg PO for pediatrics 600 mg PO for adults For patients unable to take ibuprofen use Acetaminophen 15 mg/kg PO for pediatrics 975 mg PO for adults	For Adults 1 tablet hydrocodone (7.5 mg)/acetaminophen (325 mg) + ibuprofen 600 mg PO For Pediatrics < 2 years old: Consult MD ≥ 2 years ≤ 12 years old: Lortab elixir 2.5 mg + ibuprofen 10 mg/kg PO > 12 years old: Vicodin 5 mg + ibuprofen 400 mg PO	For Adults Morphine 2 mg slow IVP q 5 minutes up to 10 mg Notify physician if pain not managed after 10 mg For Pediatrics Notify MD immediately Make Patient NPO

Consult with physician for additional medications when contraindications exist or pain relief has not been achieved

Patient Sticker

Fig. 11-2 A nurse-initiated protocol for pain management in patients with an isolated extremity injury. (Courtesy of PeaceHealth St. Joseph Medical Center.)

TABLE 11-11   LEVELS OF SEDATION

LEVEL OF SEDATION	DEFINITION	COMMON MEDICATIONS USED
Minimal sedation	Also known as anxiolysis. A drug-induced state during which the patient responds normally to verbal commands. Cognitive function and coordination may be impaired. Ventilatory and cardiovascular functions are unaffected.	Midazolam (Versed) Diazepam (Valium) Lorazepam (Ativan) Fentanyl Morphine
Moderate sedation and analgesia (conscious sedation)	A drug-induced depression of consciousness during which the patient responds purposefully to verbal command, either alone or accompanied by light tactile stimulation. No interventions are necessary to maintain a patent airway. Spontaneous ventilation is adequate. Cardiovascular function is usually maintained.	**Reversal agents** Naloxone (Narcan) for opiates Flumazenil (Romazicon) for benzodiazepines
Deep sedation and analgesia	A drug-induced depression of consciousness during which the patient cannot be easily aroused but responds purposefully following repeated or painful stimulation. Independent ventilatory function may be impaired. The patient may require assistance to maintain a patent airway. Spontaneous ventilation may be inadequate. Cardiovascular function is usually maintained.	Propofol Etomidate Check with your State Board of Nursing to determine if RNs are permitted to administer these medications to unintubated patients.

relieving pain and suffering. While providing pharmacologic interventions to manage pain remains a foundation of therapy for the patient with pain, the emergency nurse's ability to express caring about the patient's pain can be as meaningful as providing pain medication itself.

REFERENCES

1. Classification of chronic pain syndromes and definitions of pain terms. Prepared by the International Association for the Study of Pain, Subcommittee on Taxonomy. (1986). *Pain*, *3*(Suppl), S1–S226.
2. McCaffery, M., & Beebe, A. (1989). *Pain: Clinical manual for nursing practice*. St. Louis, MO: Mosby.
3. Wilson, J. E., & Pendleton, J. M. (1989). Oligoanalgesia in the emergency department. *American Journal of Emergency Medicine*, *7*(6), 620–623.
4. Motov, S. M., & Khan, A. N. (2008). Problems and barriers of pain management in the emergency department: Are we ever going to get better? *Journal of Pain Research*, *2*, 5–11.
5. McCaffery, M., & Pasero, C. (Eds.). (1999). *Pain: Clinical manual* (2nd ed.). St. Louis, MO: Mosby.
6. Acute Pain Management Guideline Panel. (1992). *Acute pain management: Operative or medical procedures and trauma. Clinical practice guideline (AHCRP Publication 92-0032)*. Rockville, MD: Agency for Health Care Policy and Research.
7. McCaffery, M. (2001). Using the 0-to-10 pain rating scale. *American Journal of Nursing*, *101*(81), 81–82.
8. Zimmermann, P. G. (2004). Tips for managing pain more effectively. *Journal of Emergency Nursing*, *30*(5), 470–472.
9. Merkel, S. (2002). Pain assessment in infants and young children: The Finger Span Scale. *American Journal of Nursing*, *102*(11), 55–56.
10. Merkel, S., & Malviya, S. (2000). Pediatric pain, tools and assessment. *Journal of Perianesthesia Nursing*, *15*(6), 408–414
11. Merkel, S., Voepel-Lewis, T., Shayevitz, J., & Malviya, S. (1997). The FLACC: A behavioral scale for scoring postoperative pain in young children. *Pediatric Nursing*, *23*(3), 293–297.
12. Voepel-Lewis, T., Zanotti, J., Dammeyer, J. A., & Merkel, S. (2010). Reliability and validity of the Face, Legs, Activity, Cry, Consolability Behavioral Tool in assessing acute pain in critically ill patients. *American Journal of Critical Care*, *19*(1), 55–61.
13. Warden, V., Hurley, A. C., & Volicer, L. (2003). Development and psychometric evaluation of the pain assessment in advanced dementia (PAINAID) scale. *Journal of the American Medical Directors Association*, *4*(1), 9–15.
14. Herr, K., Coyne, P. J., Key, T., Manworren, R., McCaffery, M., Merkel, S., … Wild, L.; American Society for Pain Management. (2006). Pain assessment in the nonverbal patient: Position statement with clinical practice recommendations. *Pain Management Nursing*, *7*(2), 44–52.
15. Stevens, B., Johnston, C., Petryshen, P., & Taddio, A. (1996). Premature Infant Pain Profile: Development and initial validation. *Clinical Journal of Pain*, *12*, 13–22.
16. Pasero, C. (2002). Pain assessment in infants and young children: Premature Infant Pain Profile. *American Journal of Nursing*, *102*(9), 105–106.

17. Zimmermann, P. G. (2005). Managers forum: Dealing with "drug seekers." *Journal of Emergency Nursing, 31*(1), 97–98.

18. Todd, K. H. (2005). Pain assessment instruments for use in the emergency department. *Emergency Medicine Clinics of North America, 23*, 285–295.

19. Pasero, C. (2003). Pain in the emergency department: Withholding pain medication is not justified. *American Journal of Nursing, 103*, 73–74.

20. Thomas, S. H., William, S., Cheema, F., Reisner, A., Aman, S., Goldstein, J. N., ... Stair, T. (2003). Effects of morphine analgesia on diagnostic accuracy in emergency department patients with abdominal pain: A prospective, randomized trial. *Journal of American College of Surgeons, 196*, 18–31.

21. Vermeulen, B., Morabia, A., Unger, P. F., Goehring, C., Grangier, C., Skljarov, I., & Terrier, F. (1999). Acute appendicitis: Influence of early pain relief on the accuracy of clinical and U.S. findings in the decision to operate—a randomized trial. *Radiology, 210*, 639–643.

22. American Pain Society. (2003). *Principles of analgesic use in the treatment of acute pain and cancer pain* (5th ed.). Glenview, IL: Author.

23. Clinical policy for the initial approach to patients presenting with a chief complaint of nontraumatic acute abdominal pain. American College of Emergency Physicians. (1994). *Annals of Emergency Medicine, 23*(4), 906–922.

24. Ducharme, J. (1994). Emergency pain management: A Canadian Association of Emergency Physicians (CAEP) consensus document. *Journal of Emergency Medicine, 12*(6), 855–866.

25. Gordon, D. B., Dahl, J. L., Miaskowski, C., McCarberg, B., Todd, K. H., Paice, J. A., ... Carr, D. (2005). American Pain Society recommendations for improving the quality of acute and cancer pain management. *Archives of Internal Medicine, 165*(14), 1574–1580.

26. Larson, A. M., Polson, J., Fontana, R. J., Davern, T. J., Lalani, E., Hynan, L. S., ... Lee, W. M.; Acute Liver Failure Study Group. (2005) Acetaminophen-induced acute liver failure: Results of a United States multicenter, prospective study. *Hepatology, 42*(6), 1364–1372.

27. Burton, J. H., & Miner, J. (Eds.). (2008). *Emergency sedation and pain management*. New York, NY: Cambridge University Press.

28. Altman, R. D. (2004). A rationale for combining acetaminophen and NSAIDs for mild-to-moderate pain. *Clinical and Experimental Rheumatology, 22*(1), 110–117.

29. Merry, A. F., Gibbs, R. D., Edwards, J., Ting, G. S., Frampton, C., Davies, E., & Anderson, B. J. (2010). Combined acetaminophen and ibuprofen for pain relief after oral surgery in adults: A randomized controlled trial. *British Journal of Anesthesia, 104*(1), 80–88.

30. Menhinick, K. A., Gutmann, J. L., Regan, J. D., Taylor, S. E., & Buschang, P. H. (2004). The efficacy of pain control following nonsurgical root canal treatment using ibuprofen or a combination of ibuprofen and acetaminophen in a randomized, double-blind, placebo-controlled study. *International Endodontic Journal, 37*(8), 531–541.

31. Harrison, D. M. (2008). Oral sucrose for pain management in infants: Myths and misconceptions. *Journal of Neonatal Nursing, 14*(2), 39–46.

32. Crystal, C. S., & Blankenship, R. B. (2005). Local anesthetics and peripheral nerve blocks in the emergency department. *Emergency Medicine Clinics of North America, 23*, 477–502.

33. Dillard, J. N., & Knapp, S. (2005). Complementary and alternative pain therapy in the emergency department. *Emergency Medicine Clinics of North America, 23*, 529–549.

34. Fry, M., & Holdgate, A. (2002). Nurse-initiated intravenous morphine in the emergency department: Efficacy, rate of adverse events and impact on time to analgesia. *Emergency Medicine, 14*, 249–254.

35. Sequin, D. (2004). A nurse-initiated pain management advanced triage protocol for ED patients with an extremity injury at a level I trauma center. *Journal of Emergency Nursing, 30*(4), 330–335.

36. Fosnocht, D. E., & Swanson, E. R. (2007). Use of triage pain protocol in the ED. *American Journal of Emergency Medicine, 25*, 791–793.

37. Kelly, A. M., Barnes, C., & Brumby, C. (2005). Nurse initiated narcotic analgesia reduces time to analgesia for patients with acute pain in the emergency department. *Canadian Journal of Emergency Medicine, 7*, 149–154.

38. Centers for Medicare & Medicaid Services. (2008, October 24). *"Standing orders" in hospitals—revisions to S&C Memoranda.* Retrieved from https://www.cms.gov/SurveyCertification GenInfo/downloads/SCLetter09-10.pdf

39. McCaffery, M., Grimm, M. A., Pasero, C., Ferrell, B., & Uman, G. C. (2005). On the meaning of "drug-seeking." *Pain Management Nursing, 6*(4), 122–136.

40. Elander, J., Lusher, J., Bevan, D., Telfer, P., & Burton, B. (2004). Understanding the causes of problematic pain management in sickle cell disease: Evidence that pseudoaddiction plays a more important role than genuine analgesic dependence. *Journal of Pain and Symptom Management, 27*(2), 156–169.

41. Hansen, G. R. (2005). The drug-seeking patient in the emergency room. *Emergency Medicine Clinics of North America, 23*, 349–365.

42. Joranson, D. E., Ryan, K. M., Gilson, A. M., & Dahl, J. L. (2000). Trends in medical use and abuse of opioid analgesics. *Journal of the American Medical Association, 283*, 1710–1714.

43. American Society of Anesthesiologists. (2007). *ASA standards, guidelines, and statements.* Park Ridge, IL: Author. Retrieved from http://www.asahq.org/For-Healthcare-Professionals/Standards-Guidelines-and-Statements.aspx

44. Emergency Nurses Association. (2005). *Procedural sedation and analgesia in the emergency department* [position statement]. Retrieved from http://www.ena.org/SiteCollectionDocuments/Position%20Statements/Procedural_SedationENA_PS.pdf

45. Emergency Nurses Association. (2008). *Procedural sedation consensus statement.* Retrieved from http://www.ena.org/SiteCollectionDocuments/Position%20Statements/Procedural_Sedation_Consensus_Statement.pdf

Substance Abuse

Leona Stout-Demps and Darleen A. Williams

The National Institute on Drug Abuse (NIDA) calls drug abuse and addiction "one of America's most challenging public health problems."[1] Substance abuse places a tremendous burden on society, affects every aspect of life, and has been called "an equal opportunity destroyer."[1] It is also an expensive national problem. NIDA estimates that drug abuse and addiction costs the United States more than $500 billion annually.[2] The cost of drug abuse includes the loss of earning potential of those addicted and the loss of wages of those injured by accidents caused by impaired persons. Included in the societal cost of substance abuse are law enforcement salaries, legal fees, and the cost of maintaining federal prison facilities needed for those incarcerated as a result of drug-related offenses. An estimated 31% of America's homeless population have addiction issues.[1] NIDA also notes that 50% to 80% of all child maltreatment cases involve some form of substance abuse by the child's caregivers.[1]

An estimated 19.5 million Americans age 12 years and older are current users of illegal drugs. More than 51% of America's teenagers have at least tried an illegal drug before they leave high school.[1] In 2008 more than 31 million people admitted to driving while under the influence of alcohol at least once in the past year[3] (see Chapter 13, Alcohol Abuse). According to the National Survey on Drug Use and Health (NSDUH), current cocaine use gradually declined between 2003 and 2009 among people age 12 years and older (from 2.3 million to 1.6 million).[16]

Drug abuse and addiction is a preventable disease, and education on the scope of the problem and available resources in individual communities can assist health care providers in dealing with substance abuse.

ANABOLIC STEROIDS

Recent international scandals in professional sports have highlighted the dangers of steroid use. Anabolic-androgenic steroids, sometimes called "roids" or "juice," are synthetic substances similar to testosterone. While anabolic steroids have legitimate medical uses, they should not be used simply to build up muscle bulk. The most common names of abused anabolic steroids are Andro, oxandrolone (Oxandrin), methandrostenolone (Dianabol), stanozolol (Winstrol), nandrolone decanoate (Deca-Durabolin), and boldenone undecylenate (Equipoise).[4]

Signs and Symptoms

There are many consequences for inappropriately taking steroids. As a whole, excess steroids cause alteration in carbohydrate metabolism (elevated glucose), hyponatremia (leading to fluid retention, hypertension), and hypokalemia.

- Cardiovascular effects: Increases in serum low-density lipoprotein and decreases in high-density lipoprotein levels. Steroids increase atherosclerosis, placing the patients who have taken steroids at risk for a heart attack or stroke.
- Skeletal effects: Hypocalcemia, which can lead to osteoporosis. If taken before puberty is completed, the use of these substances can cause early skeletal maturation.
- Feminization or masculinization effects: Males may have decreasing testicular size along with reduced sperm counts. Men taking steroids may also become bald, develop breasts, and potentially develop prostate cancer. Women taking steroids can grow facial hair while becoming bald, stop menstruating, and develop a permanently deeper voice.
- Mood effects: Extreme mood swings that have led to "roid rage" or violent behavior. Users may have feelings of invincibility, jealousy, and depression that can be followed by suicide attempts.
- Cognitive effects: Memory loss and learning disabilities.
- Immunosuppression may occur.

Therapeutic Interventions

The best treatment is prevention and includes education related to the dangers of steroid abuse. Supportive therapy is also used to gain and maintain homeostasis.

COCAINE

Cocaine is a strong central nervous system stimulant that is highly addictive. NIDA reports that, in 2008, 5.3 million Americans age 12 years and older had abused cocaine in some form.[5] There are many street names for cocaine, including blow, bump, C, candy, Charlie, coke, flake, rock, snow, and toot.[5]

"Crack," another street name, is given to the form of cocaine that has been processed to make a rock crystal, which when heated produces vapors that are smoked. The term "crack" refers to the crackling sound produced by the rock as it is heated.

There are three common ways in which cocaine is used.

- Snorting: The powder form of the drug is inhaled through the nose to be absorbed by the nasal membranes
- Smoking: Vapors from burning cocaine are inhaled directly into the lungs for rapid absorption
- Injecting: Drug is put into a syringe and injected directly into the bloodstream

The faster the drug reaches the brain, the more intense the user's high will be; the duration of the high, however, depends on the route administered and the purity of the cocaine used. To maintain their highs, people who take cocaine will frequently "binge," a process of ingesting, inhaling, or injecting cocaine several times in rapid succession. Regardless of the route chosen, the person quickly becomes addicted.

Cocaine dealers frequently dilute their product with other substances, both active and inert, to increase or decrease its potency. This dilution process complicates the patient assessment and treatment, as the substances added to the cocaine may be toxic and contribute to the patient's symptoms.

Signs and Symptoms

Cocaine affects every organ and system in the human body.

- Cardiovascular effects: Constricts blood vessels, elevates blood pressure, and increases heart rate. Acute myocardial infarctions have been reported up to 2 weeks after cocaine use in patients with and without preexisting cardiac disease, some as young as 19 years old.[6]
- Neurotoxicity: Cocaine is the most common stimulant that produces seizures. Other forms of cocaine-induced neurotoxicity include subarachnoid hemorrhage,

cerebral infarction, vasculitis, transient ischemic attacks, and toxic delirium.[7]

- Psychiatric and mood disorders: Causes anxiety, irritability, and restlessness and it is not uncommon for these patients who have taken cocaine to have severe paranoia along with auditory hallucinations.
- Other symptoms:
  - Dilated pupils
  - Increased body temperature
  - Abdominal pain and nausea
  - Poor appetite and associated malnourishment (chronic use)

Cocaine readily crosses the placenta and is excreted in breast milk for up to 36 hours after use.

Therapeutic Interventions

Interventions are dependent on the patient's presenting signs and symptoms. Consuming alcohol along with the cocaine causes a synergistic effect, especially on ventricular contraction.[8] Benzodiazepines are the initial treatment of choice for cocaine-induced chest pain of cardiac origin.

If it is suspected that the patient may have ingested latex packets of cocaine as a "body packer," an immediate abdominal radiograph will be necessary to determine if any packets are present. Administration of activated charcoal with a cathartic may be used as treatment of this patient; however, whole bowel irrigation may be required to remove the packets. Rarely, endoscopy or surgical removal of these packets is necessary; if the packets rupture, the patient may experience sudden severe cocaine toxicity.

A chest radiograph is important for the patient who inhaled cocaine to determine if a pneumomediastinum is present. This condition is caused when the alveoli rupture secondary to the patient taking deep breaths and holding them as long as possible when smoking cocaine; if a pneumomediastinum is present, it is treated with insertion of a chest tube.

> A patient who indicates recent cocaine use and has a fever is at increased risk for complications.

HEROIN

NIDA reported that the number of current heroin users in the United States age 12 years and older rose from 153,000 in 2007 to 213,000 in 2008.[9] In the same year 114,000 first-time heroin users were reported.[9] Heroin's street names include brown sugar, dope, H, horse, junk, skag, skunk, smack, and white horse.[10]

Heroin is an opiate drug synthesized from morphine. It is a naturally occurring substance extracted from the seed pod of the Asian opium poppy plant. Heroin typically comes in a white or brown powder or as a black, sticky substance known as "black tar" heroin. The substance can be injected, snorted, ingested, or smoked. Injected heroin gives the user the most rapid onset of euphoria in as little as 7 to 8 seconds. Although the other routes of administration have slower onset, the effects last longer. Nearly all reported heroin-related fatalities involve the injected route. As with other illegal substances, dealers dilute the heroin with other substances, which can contribute to the patient's symptoms and make the diagnosis more difficult.

Signs and Symptoms

The classic triad of heroin use is central nervous system depression, respiratory depression, and miosis.[9] Assess for any signs and symptoms of chronic abuse. These include redness and swelling of the nares and multiple scars or "track marks" in numerous locations. Drug abuse paraphernalia found among the patient's belongings (i.e., syringes, bent spoons, bottle caps, and rubber tubing) is another indicator of heroin abuse. Heroin addicts, like all drug abusers, are susceptible to multiple infectious diseases and processes, including human immunodeficiency virus (HIV), hepatitis B and C, endocarditis, and multiple skin abscesses.

Therapeutic Interventions

Patients suspected of heroin overdose require close observation and supportive care for 24 to 48 hours. Resuscitation (with a bag-mask) takes priority over administration of naloxone. Naloxone (Narcan) is a rapid acting narcotic antagonist that can be given intravenously, intramuscularly, subcutaneously, intranasally, through the endotracheal tube, or injected sublingually. The duration of the therapeutic effects of naloxone (40 to 90 minutes) may be shorter than the duration of the toxic effects of the offending substance, causing a return of potentially life-threatening symptoms and requiring repeated dosing.

Another similar reversal agent is nalmefene (Revex). Its duration is 4 to 8 hours when given intravenously. It tends not to be used in the emergency department because of the presumption that prolonged withdrawal symptoms would result.

INHALANTS

Inhalants are a group of volatile substances whose vapors are inhaled in order to experience a high or mind-altering reaction. Inhalants, as a rule, can only be inhaled, unlike heroin and cocaine, which are also injected or smoked. Substances used as inhalants are common household items and include paint thinner, gasoline, glues, hair spray, aerosol whipped cream, felt tip markers, spray paint, butane, propane, and nitrous oxide. As it is not illegal to possess these products, they are easily accessible, inexpensive, and found in most homes.

Inhalants are breathed through both the mouth and the nose in several different ways. They are sniffed or snorted directly from the containers or via "bagging," which consists of spraying the substance into a plastic or paper bag and then placing the bag over the head or face to inhale. "Huffing" is a process where a rag or piece of clothing is soaked in the substance and then placed over the nose and mouth to breath in the fumes. Balloons filled with nitrous oxide are also commonly used. As these substances are rapidly absorbed in the lungs, the patient will experience a high usually within 10 to 15 seconds, which can last for several minutes.[11]

Signs and Symptoms

The signs and symptoms seen with each patient depend on the substance abused, duration of exposure, and method used to inhale the vapors. Sudden death is possible regardless of the patient's previous history of inhalant abuse; each and every time fumes are inhaled, damage to brain cells occurs. Signs of chronic abuse include watery eyes, open sores around the mouth and nose, loss of appetite, mood swings, headaches, nausea, vomiting, irritability, poor balance, and possible hallucinations.

> "Huffer rash" is defined as contact dermatitis around the mouth and is the result of inhaling paint fumes from a plastic bag.

Therapeutic Interventions

Provide supportive care as indicated and attempt to determine the substance being abused and the method of inhalation. Education for caregivers and referrals to community resources are also important.

PHENCYCLIDINE

Phencyclidine (PCP) is a synthetic drug manufactured into tablets, capsules, or powder, and in its purest form is crystalline white but can range in color depending on contaminants or additives acquired during processing. Routes of administration depend on the form obtained, so it can be snorted, smoked, or eaten. Initially developed in the 1950s as an intravenous anesthetic, PCP was never approved for use in humans because patients experienced intense psychological effects when waking during the clinical trials. Common street names for PCP include angel dust, ozone, wack, rocket fuel, boat, hog, and peace pill.[12]

Generally it is a traumatic injury that brings the PCP patient to the ED. People who have used PCP experience hallucinations with violent and bizarre psychotic effects. These patients can be extraordinarily strong, have a sense of complete invulnerability, and thereby easily injure themselves or others; they are a threat to caregivers, visitors, and other patients in the ED.

Signs and Symptoms

PCP patients experience agitation with potential for increased physical strength and extreme violence coupled with decreased sensations to pain. They may be hyperthermic, tachycardic, hypertensive, and have rhabdomyolysis. PCP causes hallucinations, nystagmus, and amnesia to events that may have resulted in an ED visit.

Therapeutic Interventions

Physical restraint is necessary and caution must be used to protect everyone involved. Patients may calm down if placed in a low-stimulation environment; however, sedation with a large amount of medications may also be necessary. Frequent assessments are imperative and support measures must be employed to assess and stabilize these patients. Aggressive cooling measures may be required. High-volume fluid loss may be present as the result of violent physical activity, so infusion of crystalloids to maintain urine output is necessary. This may also prevent renal failure associated with rhabdomyolysis.

"CLUB" DRUGS

"Club" drugs are often used by teenagers and young adults at parties, concerts, and bars. Club drugs include MDMA (ecstasy), ketamine, methamphetamine, and lysergic acid diethylamide (LSD), which are central nervous system stimulants and hallucinogens. A subset of these drugs, such as gamma-hydroxybutyrate (GHB) and flunitrazepam (Rohypnol), are central nervous system depressants called "date rape drugs." The effects of these drugs make the person incapacitated and vulnerable to sexual assault. They can easily be added to a drink, which is then consumed by an unknowing person.

Gamma-Hydroxybutyrate

Gamma-hydroxybutyrate (GHB) is a central nervous system depressant that was developed for the treatment of narcolepsy. This drug causes a combination of central nervous system depression, euphoria, and suppression of inhibitions, making GHB an effective date rape drug. GHB usually comes in a liquid form and, because of its salty taste, is commonly hidden in fruity or sweet-tasting drinks.

The onset of GHB can be as little as 15 minutes, with peak effects occurring at 30 minutes and duration of 3 to 6 hours. Respiratory depression and arrest is common in people who have taken of GHB. Street names for GHB include Georgia home boy, grievous bodily harm, and liquid ecstasy.

Signs and Symptoms

GHB, in contrast to other sedative hypnotic intoxications, causes the level of consciousness to fluctuate between mild agitation and severe central nervous system depression. It causes the person to appear drunk (without the smell of alcohol); they can have dizziness, slurred speech, disorientation, and a decreasing level of consciousness resulting in respiratory depression or apnea. Bradycardia, nausea, vomiting, hypothermia, and hypotension may also be present.[13]

Therapeutic Interventions

There is no antidote for GHB; the patient is treated symptomatically. If rape is suspected, the appropriate forensic exam should be performed.

Flunitrazepam

Flunitrazepam (Rohypnol) first appeared in the United States in the early 1990s. Although chemically similar to diazepam (Valium) and alprazolam (Xanax), flunitrazepam is much stronger and is not approved for any medical use in the United States. Therefore its use and import is considered illegal.

Flunitrazepam is commonly found in pill form. Sedation begins affecting the patient within 30 to 60 minutes after ingestion, with peak effects occurring in 2 to 3 hours. It has greater amnesic and hypnotic effects than other benzodiazepines. As with other date rape drugs, flunitrazepam is most commonly mixed into alcoholic beverages consumed by unknowing individuals.[13]

Signs and Symptoms

Patients under the influence of flunitrazepam will experience dizziness, confusion, lack of muscle control, and hypotension. They may also lose consciousness.

Therapeutic Interventions

As with other illicit substances, these patients require basic and advanced supportive care as their condition indicates. The toxicological test for flunitrazepam is not routinely available; however, in cases of suspected criminal activity (e.g., rape), samples should be collected for analysis at a specialized forensic laboratory. Gastric lavage may be helpful only if the patient arrives within 60 minutes of ingestion. If flunitrazepam is suspected, the antidote is flumazenil (Romazicon).

MDMA

MDMA, named for its chemical composition 3,4-methylenedioxymethamphetamine, is most commonly known by the street name "ecstasy" and is a relatively simple chemical classified as an amphetamine. This substance is a stimulant with hallucinogenic properties and is frequently found at "rave" parties. Although people who use ecstasy commonly experience a distorted perception of time, they also feel a sense of emotional warmth and increased physical energy. These sensations generally begin about 30 minutes after ingestion and can last up to 8 to 12 hours. The powdered form of ecstasy can be snorted, resulting in a more rapid onset but shorter duration and lessened effects. Adverse sensations from this drug can cause the user to be nauseated and have chills, sweating, and clenched teeth. In 2008 approximately 894,000 Americans used ecstasy for the first time, which is a significant increase from the 615,000 first-time users reported in 2005.[14]

Signs and Symptoms

Patients who have taken MDMA present confused, agitated, tachycardic, hypertensive, and possibly in pulmonary edema. They can have cardiac dysrhythmias, seizures, and muscle spasms and experience clenched or grinding of teeth.

Therapeutic Interventions

Accurate and ongoing assessments are required, followed by appropriate basic and advanced supportive treatment. If possible, determine the substances involved. Ecstasy can be detected in the urine for up to 72 hours after ingestion but not all laboratories are equipped to perform this qualitative test. Although activated charcoal may be helpful for ecstasy ingestions, there is no known antidote for this drug.

Ketamine

Ketamine was originally developed as a veterinary anesthetic. The injectable form of this drug is currently used routinely in the ED for procedural sedation. Ketamine is also available in both powdered and tablet forms, allowing it to be ingested, smoked, or snorted. Powdered ketamine may be mixed and smoked with marijuana or tobacco. The effects of this drug may last 30 to 60 minutes.

Signs and Symptoms

People who have taken ketamine experience a confused and dreamlike state, which makes this a popular drug both for recreational use and use as a date rape drug. Tachycardia with palpations and hypertension are also possible. Respiratory depression and apnea are the most significant threat to this patient's safety. People who have taken ketamine may also experience flashbacks.

Therapeutic Interventions

There is no specific antidote for ketamine. Patients should be treated symptomatically. If these patients are combative, sedation may be required and must be administered with caution.

PRESCRIPTION DRUG ABUSE

According to the Centers for Disease Control and Prevention, "nonmedical use of opioid analgesics increased 111% during 2004 to 2008 from 144,600 to 305,900 visits. The three most commonly requested drugs were oxycodone, hydrocodone, and methadone."[15] During this same time period, nonmedical prescription use of benzodiazepines increased 89%.[3]

When assessing patients with an altered level of consciousness, emergency health care providers should be aware an underlying prescription substance may be causing life-threatening problems. Access to electronic medical records may help the health care provider gain rapid access to information needed to determine if a prescription medication may be involved.

PREVENTION STRATEGIES AND TREATMENT MODALITIES

There are no easy answers to addiction issues. While education is one valuable component, prevention is key. Treatment for substance abuse is a long-term process, and the ED staff's primary role is to rapidly assess and stabilize these patients. Psychiatric or social services referral upon admission is a critical part of the ED's treatment plan and is important in determining the disposition of these patients once stabilized. Law enforcement may be involved early, as many of these patients require emergency transport for overdose or are in police custody for disruptive or erratic behavior. Follow institutional policy and procedures for reporting suspected or confirmed illegal substance abuse and management of evidence collected during treatment. Long-term mental health and behavioral modification programs are the addicted person's best chance to overcome addiction issues. Substance abuse prevention education, targeted at the elementary and middle school levels, can influence the incidence of future drug use.

REFERENCES

1. National Institute on Drug Abuse. (2005, June). *Drug abuse and addiction: One of America's most challenging public health problems*. Retrieved from http://archives.drugabuse.gov/about/welcome/aboutdrugabuse/index.html

2. National Institute on Drug Abuse. (2008, June). *NIDA Info-Facts: Understanding drug abuse and addiction.* Retrieved from http://www.drugabuse.gov/PDF/InfoFacts/Understanding08.pdf

3. National Institute on Drug Abuse. (2010, January). *NIDA InfoFacts: Nationwide trends.* Retrieved from http://www.drugabuse.gov/infofacts/nationtrends.html

4. National Institute on Drug Abuse. (2009, July). *NIDA InfoFacts: Steroids (anabolic-androgenic).* Retrieved from http://www.drugabuse.gov/PDF/Infofacts/Steroids09.pdf

5. National Institute on Drug Abuse. (n.d.). *Cocaine.* Retrieved from http://www.drugabuse.gov/drugpages/cocaine.html

6. Lange, R. A., & Hillis, L. D. (2001). Cardiovascular complications of cocaine use. *New England Journal of Medicine, 345*(5), 351–358.

7. Kalinski, M. (2006). Seizure, adult. In S. R. Votey & M. A. Davis (Eds.), *Signs and symptoms in emergency medicine* (2nd ed.). St. Louis, MO: Mosby.

8. Hantsch, C. A. E., & Seger, D. L. (2006). Mushrooms, hallucinogens, and stimulants. In V. J. Markovchick & P. T. Pons (Eds.), *Emergency medicine secrets* (4th ed.). St. Louis, MO: Mosby.

9. National Institute on Drug Abuse. (2010, March). *NIDA InfoFacts: Heroin.* Retrieved from http://www.drugabuse.gov/PDF/Infofacts/Heroin10.pdf

10. National Institute on Drug Abuse. (n.d.). *Commonly abused drugs.* Retrieved from http://www.drugabuse.gov/DrugPages/DrugsofAbuse.html

11. National Institute on Drug Abuse. (2010, March). *NIDA Info-Facts: Inhalants.* Retrieved from http://www.nida.nih.gov/infofacts/inhalants.html

12. National Institute on Drug Abuse. (n.d.). *PCP/phencyclidine.* Retrieved from http://www.nida.nih.gov/drugpages/pcp.html

13. Harrison, C. D., & Bebarta, V. S. (2006). Opioids and sedative-hypnotics. In V. J. Markovchick & P. T. Pons (Eds.), *Emergency medicine secrets* (4th ed.). St. Louis, MO: Mosby.

14. National Institute on Drug Abuse. (2010, December). *NIDA InfoFacts: MDMA (ecstasy).* Retrieved from http://www.drugabuse.gov/PDF/Infofacts/MDMA10.pdf

15. Centers for Disease Control and Prevention. (2010). Emergency department visits involving nonmedical use of selected prescription drugs—United States, 2004–2008. *MMWR Morbidity and Mortality Weekly Reports, 59*(23), 705–709. Retrieved from http://www.cdc.gov/mmwr/preview/mmwrhtml/mm5923a1.htm?s_cid=mm5923a1_w

16. National Institute on Drug Abuse. (2011, April). *NIDA Info-Facts: Nationwide trends.* Retrieved from http://drugabuse.gov/infofacts/nationtrends.html

Alcohol Abuse

Dawn M. Williamson

An estimated 7.6 million of the 116.8 million (e.g. 6.5%) emergency department (ED) visits reported in 2010 were related to alcohol use.[1,2]

- Three out of 10 American adults engage in alcohol consumption at a level that puts them at risk for medical or social problems.
- Eighteen percent of those hospitalized after a motor vehicle crash meet the criteria for alcohol dependence.
- Up to 31% of patients treated in EDs and 50% of severely injured trauma patients (i.e., those requiring hospital admission, usually to an intensive care unit) screen positive for alcohol abuse.[3]

ALCOHOL SCREENING

Screening patients in the ED for alcohol use uses the window of opportunity to motivate patients to alter their drinking behavior. Patients treated in EDs are 1.5 to 3 times more likely than those treated in primary care clinics to report heavy drinking, to experience the adverse effects of drinking (e.g., alcohol-related injuries, illnesses, and legal or social problems), and to have been treated previously for an alcohol problem.[4] Of surveyed adults, 15% reported binge drinking and 5% reported heavy drinking, defined as "more than two drinks per day on average for men or more than one drink per day on average for women."[5]

The U.S. Preventive Services Task Force recommends routine screening for alcohol abuse in the outpatient setting.[6] The Emergency Nurses Association (ENA) supports this obligation to screen and provide a brief intervention for underlying alcohol use problems.[7] Screening is cost effective; it is estimated to save $254 per screened person in saving quality life-years and preventing consequences.[8]

Screening, Brief Intervention, and Referral to Treatment

Screening, brief intervention, and referral to treatment (SBIRT) is a framework aimed at providing services for not only those with substance use disorders but also those at risk of developing difficulties with substances.

Implementation involves:
- Screening for severity of use and treatment necessary
- Brief intervention to raise awareness regarding use and enhance motivation for change
- Referral to treatment for specialized care

Screening Tools

- The Alcohol Use Disorders Identification Test (AUDIT) is typically used for inpatients because of its longer length and complexity.[9]
- The Alcohol, Smoking, and Substance Involvement Screening Test (ASSIST) screens for all substances but was designed by the World Health Organization mainly for primary care use.[10]
- CAGE (Table 13-1)[11] and CAGEAID (adapted to include drugs and included the addition of the phrase "or drug use" to each question) is well suited for the ED. However, it does not detect low but risky drinking and does not perform as well among women and minorities.
- T-ACE, based on CAGE, is valuable for identifying a range of use, including lifetime and prenatal use, based on the *Diagnostic and Statistical Manual of Mental Disorders-III-R* criteria (Table 13-2).[11]
- TWEAK was originally designed to screen harmful drinking behavior in pregnant women.
- The Michigan Alcohol Screening Test (MAST) is a 22-question, self-administered test and does not include screening for other drugs.

TABLE 13-1	CAGE ALCOHOL SCREENING TOOL

CAGE

Have you ever felt you should **CUT DOWN** on your drinking?

Have people **ANNOYED** you about your drinking?

Have you ever felt bad or **GUILTY** about your drinking?

Have you ever had a drink first thing in the morning to steady your nerves or get rid of a hangover (**EYE-OPENER**)?

CAGE can identify alcohol problems over the lifetime. Two positive responses are considered a positive test and indicate that further assessment is warranted.

National Institute on Alcohol Abuse and Alcoholism. (2005, April). *Screening for alcohol use and alcohol related problems.* Retrieved from http://pubs.niaaa.nih.gov/publications/aa65/aa65.htm

TABLE 13-2	T-ACE ALCOHOL SCREENING TEST

T **Tolerance:** How many drinks does it take to make you feel high?

A Have people **annoyed** you by criticizing your drinking?

C Have you ever felt you ought to **cut down** on your drinking?

E **Eye-opener:** Have you ever had a drink first thing in the morning to steady your nerves or get rid of a hangover?

A score of 2 or more is considered positive. Affirmative answers to questions A, C, or E = 1 point each. Reporting tolerance to more than two drinks (the T question) = 2 points.

National Institute on Alcohol Abuse and Alcoholism. (2005, April). *Screening for alcohol use and alcohol related problems.* Retrieved from http://pubs.niaaa.nih.gov/publications/aa65/aa65.htm

- HALT
  - "Do you usually drink to get **H**igh?"
  - "Do you drink **A**lone?"
  - "Do you ever find yourself **L**ooking forward to drinking?"
  - "Have you noticed whether you seem to be becoming **T**olerant of alcohol?"
- BUMP
  - "Have you ever had **B**lackouts?"
  - "Have you ever used alcohol in an **U**nplanned way?"
  - "Do you ever drink alcohol for **M**edicinal reasons?"
  - "Do you find yourself **P**rotecting your supply of alcohol?"
- FATAL DT
  - "Is there a **F**amily history of alcoholic problems?"
  - "Have you ever been a member of **A**lcoholics Anonymous?"

TABLE 13-3	SAMPLE QUANTITY AND FREQUENCY ALCOHOL SCREENING QUESTIONS

In the, past 30 days:

- On average, how many days per week do you drink alcohol?
- On a typical day when you drink, how many drinks do you have?
- What is the maximum number of drinks you had on any given occasion during the past month?

TABLE 13-4	STANDARD DRINK EQUIVALENTS

- 12 oz of beer or cooler
- 8–9 oz of malt liquor
- 5 oz of table wine
- 3–4 oz of fortified wine
- 2–3 oz of cordial or liqueur
- 1.5 oz of brandy or spirits

National Institute on Alcohol Abuse and Alcoholism. (n.d.). *What is a standard drink?* Retrieved from http://pubs.niaaa.nih.gov/publications/practitioner/pocketguide/pocket_guide2.htm

- "Do you **T**hink you are an alcoholic?"[3]
- "Have you ever **A**ttempted or had thoughts of suicide?"
- "Have you ever had any **L**egal problems related to alcohol consumption?"
- "Do you ever **D**rive while intoxicated?"
- "Do you ever use **T**ranquilizers to steady your nerves?"
- General questions about quantity and frequency (Table 13-3): One study found that the single question "When was the last time you had more than X drinks in one day?" (where X is 5 for men and 4 for women) was effective. With a threshold value at the past 3 months, this method had a sensitivity and specificity of 85% and 70% in men and 82% and 77% in women. The screening was similar whether screening was conducted in person or by telephone.[12]

Standard Quantities

When discussing quantities, note that a standard drink contains about 0.6 fluid ounces of pure alcohol. Often a mixed drink or full glass of wine is equivalent to more than one drink (Table 13-4). Guidelines from the National Institute on Alcohol Abuse and Alcoholism (NIAAA)[13] make a distinction between low-risk and moderate drinking. Most people do not have a consistent, low-level consumption but drink more heavily on weekends. The weekly total cannot be consumed in 1 or 2 days without consequences.

- Low-risk drinking for healthy men under age 65 years is defined as no more than 4 drinks on any day and 14 per week and for healthy women (and men over 65 years old) is defined as no more than 3 drinks on any day and 7 per week.

GENERAL ASSESSMENT[2]

History

As much as possible, obtain an accurate history of recent alcohol use. History questions can include:
- Time of last drink
- What type of alcohol and amount usually ingested
- Frequency of drinking
- Years of drinking
- History of alcohol-related seizures or delirium tremens
- Prior detoxifications
- Other substance use
- Prescription drug use
- Other medical or psychiatric conditions
- Toxic alcohols

If the patient's answers about consumption seem doubtful, try the following methods in a "matter of fact" manner to get a more forthright answer[14]:
- Start the interview with questions about other non-threatening health behaviors (i.e., whether the individual wears a seat belt or smokes cigarettes) and move to the more sensitive subject of alcohol consumption.
- Frame the questions to take into account a positive response. For example, instead of asking "Do you drink alcohol?" ask "When you drink, how many times a month do you drink four drinks or more?"
- Overestimate and let the individual correct you.
- Feign surprise at a negative or low answer.
- Ask, unexpectedly, a second time later in the interview.

Other assessment and history signs that a patient may have a (denied) problem with excess alcohol include[14]:
- Delay in seeking care for a significant injury.
- Periods of blackout without indication of concern.
- Frequent complaints of gastritis or heartburn.
- A high mean corpuscular volume (MCV) is generally seen with excessive alcohol intake; however, because poor nutrition is often a problem with chronic alcohol abuse, the MCV may be low.
- High gamma-glutamyl transferase (GGT) liver enzyme. There has been regular alcohol consumption in the past 2 months if it is high when the other liver enzymes are normal.

- Elevated carbohydrate-deficient transferring. This is typical early in response to prolonged drinking. Few conditions other than heavy drinking will elevate levels.

> There is no correlation between the strength of alcohol odor on the patient's breath and the level of intoxication.

Consider Other Etiologies and Comorbidities

A coexisting medical condition that is causing the "intoxicated" patient's symptoms must be considered. Intoxicated patients with blood alcohol levels less than 200 to 240 mg/dL and a Glasgow Coma Scale (GCS) of 13 or less should be evaluated for additional causes of altered mental status.[15] Other etiologies and comorbidities can include head trauma, glucose imbalance, sepsis, dehydration, hepatic encephalopathy, or ingestion of other substances that complicate clinical course.

> The mental status of most patients who are intoxicated without complications normalizes 3 to 5 hours from emergency department admission.[31]

Signs and Symptoms

An intoxicated patient should always (Table 13-5):
- Have a physical examination, including inspecting for injury.
- Have a neurologic examination.

TABLE 13-5	BLOOD ALCOHOL LEVELS AND ASSOCIATED SIGNS AND SYMPTOMS	
BLOOD ALCOHOL LEVEL	**ALCOHOL INTAKE**	**SIGNS AND SYMPTOMS**
25–50 mg/dL (0.02–0.05%)	1–2 drinks	Relaxation
80 mg/dL (0.08%)	2–5 drinks	Considered legal intoxication in most states.
150 mg/dL (0.15%)	7–9 drinks	Staggering
250 mg/dL (0.25%)	13–14 drinks	Ataxia, nausea or vomiting
300 mg/dL (0.30%)	15–18 drinks	Stuperous
400 mg/dL (0.40%)	20–24 drinks	Anesthesia
500 mg/dL (0.50%)	25–30 drinks	Lethal in 50%

- Have glucose measured.
- Have temperature checked. (There is a risk for hypothermia from depleted glycogen stores and malnutrition.)

Tolerance

Chronic drinking consistently depresses the central nervous system and the brain compensates and develops tolerance. Tolerance is when a higher dose is required to achieve the same effect. The amount of exposure to alcohol to achieve tolerance varies in individuals.[16] Therefore an individual who develops a high tolerance level, through continual drinking, can survive an alcohol level that would be fatal in a nontolerant individual.

ALCOHOL-RELATED CONDITIONS

Alcohol Intoxication
Signs and Symptoms

- Decreased muscle coordination
- Dehydration
- Hypoglycemia
- Hypotension
- Hypothermia or hyperthermia
- Lactic acidosis
- Nausea, vomiting, and abdominal pain
- Respiratory depression
- Tachycardia

> The three groups vulnerable to alcohol-induced hypoglycemia are chronic alcoholics, binge drinkers, and young children and adolescents.[27]

Therapeutic Interventions

- Ensure that the patient has a secure airway; aspiration is as much of a risk in a patient with an altered level of consciousness from intoxication as from any other cause.
- Administer thiamine 100 mg to prevent Wernicke-Korsakoff syndrome prior to giving dextrose 50% (Table 13-6).
- Administer folic acid and a multivitamin.
- Check magnesium levels. (Chronic alcoholism is the most common cause of hypomagnesemia.[17])
- Infuse 5% dextrose in water, Ringer's lactate solution, or 5% dextrose in normal saline intravenously in patients who are hypovolemic or ketotic.
- Replace electrolytes as needed.
- Monitor for fall risks.

Toxic Ingestion

Ingestion of toxic alcohols requires early diagnosis and treatment to prevent the toxic metabolites resulting in severe metabolic acidosis and end-organ complications.

TABLE 13-6	WERNICKE-KORSAKOFF SYNDROME

Wernicke-Korsakoff syndrome involves two distinct processes. This condition occurs in patients with thiamine deficiency.

Wernicke's Encephalopathy
- Gait ataxia
- Mental confusion
- Nystagmus
- Ophthalmoplegia

Korsakoff's Syndrome
- Confabulation
- Mental confusion

Ethylene glycol is commonly found in antifreeze, coolants, and glass cleaners. Common sources of methanol include antifreeze, windshield washer fluid, and chafing fuel (Sterno). Isopropyl alcohol (isopropanol) is in rubbing alcohol and glass cleaners.

Treatment for methanol and ethylene glycol can include sodium bicarbonate for metabolic acidosis, fomepizole (4-MP) infusion to inhibit metabolism of toxic acid metabolites, vitamins to enhance metabolite elimination, and hemodialysis to rapidly remove the toxic alcohol and its metabolites. Treatment for less toxic isopropyl alcohol is mainly supportive treatment.[18]

Alcohol Poisoning

Enzymes in the liver detoxify alcohol from the body at a rate of 0.5 to 1 ounce per hour, or approximately half of to one standard drink per hour. This means that the blood alcohol level decreases by 15 to 25 mg/dL per hour. When consumption of alcohol exceeds the rate of detoxification it causes alcohol to build up in the bloodstream. Therefore when large quantities are rapidly consumed, death from acute alcohol poisoning can occur.

Medical Complications of Alcohol Abuse

The medical complications of alcohol abuse can be seen in every system of the body. Comorbidities associated with chronic alcohol abuse include:
- Cardiovascular
  - Cardiomyopathy and heart failure
  - Increased systolic and pulse pressure
  - Fluid and electrolyte imbalances
  - Cardiac dysrhythmias
- Respiratory
  - Aspiration and pneumonia
  - Oropharyngeal cancers
  - Respiratory depression

- Hematologic
  - Abnormal red bloods cells, increased MCV
  - Anemia
  - Decreased white blood cells and platelets
- Neurologic
  - Peripheral neuropathy
  - Seizures
  - Hemorrhagic stroke
  - Wernicke-Korsakoff syndrome
  - Cerebellar degeneration
- Metabolic
  - Hypoglycemia
  - Ketoacidosis
  - Electrolyte imbalances
  - Hyperlipidemia
- Gastrointestinal
  - Gastrointestinal bleed
  - Pancreatitis
  - Gastric and duodenal ulcers
  - Acute hepatitis
  - Cirrhosis
  - Liver, esophagus, and pancreatic cancer

Alcohol Withdrawal

The continuum of withdrawal progresses through early withdrawal, withdrawal seizures, alcoholic hallucinations, and delirium tremens. With abrupt cessation of alcohol exposure there is an overreaction of the brain and every mechanism it affects. Excessive drinking even for 1 week can lead to mild withdrawal symptoms with cessation as the brain attempts to regain its chemical equilibrium.[19] The sudden, unplanned withdrawal of alcohol because of an unexpected hospitalization can result in symptoms. Repeated episodes of relapse contribute to worsening of future episodes of withdrawal, termed the "kindling" effect.[20–22] Alcohol withdrawal is affected by the neurochemical balance of glutamate and gamma-aminobutyric acid (GABA). Glutamate is an excitatory neurotransmitter that acts through the N-methyl-D-aspartate (NMDA) neuroreceptors to increase brain activity. The use of alcohol inhibits NMDA neuroreceptors and in chronic use results in compensatory up-regulation of these receptors. At the same time, alcohol enhances the effect of the inhibitory neurotransmitter GABA on GABA-A neuroreceptors, resulting in decreased overall brain excitability. However, long-term exposure to alcohol results in a compensatory decrease of GABA-A neuroreceptors, producing tolerance to the effects of alcohol and an inability to slow brain response to stimuli. Therefore when alcohol intake is decreased drastically it results in brain hyperexcitability without the ability to slow this activity and is manifested clinically in the signs and symptoms of alcohol withdrawal.[23]

Early symptoms can start 6 to 8 hours from the last drink; more serious symptoms appear at 12 to 72 hours afterward.[23] The risk of delirium tremons increases in patients older than age 30 years, in those with prolonged drinking history, with the number of days since the last drink, and with previous episodes of delirium tremons.[24] The condition lasts an average of 2 to 7 days, and up to 2 weeks, while the body readjusts from the hyperstimulated condition of alcohol withdrawal.

> If untreated, the mortality rate for delirium tremens may be as high as 35%, but is less than 5% with early recognition and treatment.[32]

The patient will become more difficult to manage if intervention does not occur in a timely manner. The risk of a complicated withdrawal increases with a comorbid medical disorder.

Consider possible (unknown) alcohol withdrawal for a patient with psychiatric symptoms. Psychiatric conditions rarely present suddenly or with visual, tactile, or olfactory hallucinations.

Table 13-7 outlines the clinical manifestations of alcohol withdrawal.

TABLE 13-7 CLINICAL MANIFESTATIONS OF ALCOHOL WITHDRAWAL

PHASE	SYMPTOMS	ONSET AFTER LAST DRINK
Early withdrawal	Tremulousness Anxiety and uneasiness Labile mood Motor hyperactivity Progresses into hypermetabolic state Tremors Piloerection	6–8 hours
Withdrawal seizures	Generalized Tonic-clonic seizures	6–48 hours
Alcoholic hallucinosis	Hallucinations Visual Tactile Auditory	12–48 hours
Delirium tremens	Tachycardia Hypertension Low-grade fever Diaphoresis Delirium Agitation	48–96 hours

Tetrault, J. M., & O'Connor, P. G. (2008). Substance abuse and withdrawal in the critical care setting. *Critical Care Clinics, 24,* 767–788.

Ongoing Assessment

Ongoing assessment should be done on patients staying in the hospital ED for an extended period of time. The standardized Clinical Institute Withdrawal Assessment of Alcohol Scale, Revised (CIWA-Ar)[25] assesses the presence of 10 symptoms: anxiety, tremor, sweating, auditory disturbances, visual disturbances, tactile disturbances, agitation, nausea and vomiting, headache, and orientation. The higher the score, the more severe the withdrawal symptoms (Table 13-8). The CIWA-Ar has demonstrated reliability, reproducibility, and validity based on use in detoxification, psychiatric, and medical-surgical units.

> Up to 10% of individuals actively withdrawing from alcohol have seizures.[33]

Therapeutic Interventions

The treatment goal with intoxicated patients is to prevent the onset or progression of alcohol withdrawal and treatment consists of benzodiazepines, rest, and seizure precautions. Benzodiazepines differ widely in half-life. Short-acting benzodiazepines, such as lorazepam (Ativan), are preferred in patients who are elderly or who have hepatic disease, delirium, dementia, or cognitive disorders. They are less cumulative in the body, metabolized easier, and are better tolerated by compromised patients. However, short-acting benzodiazepines need to be given more frequently and, for those in severe withdrawal, long-acting agents may be the best choice. Some facilities administer medications by schedule and some administer them by clinical assessment (Table 13-9).

TABLE 13-8   CLINICAL INSTITUTE WITHDRAWAL ASSESSMENT OF ALCOHOL SCALE, REVISED (CIWA-Ar)

Nausea and vomiting: Ask "Do you feel sick to your stomach? Have you vomited?" Observation.
0 No nausea and no vomiting
1 Mild nausea with no vomiting
2
3
4 Intermittent nausea with dry heaves
5
6
7 Constant nausea, frequent dry heaves and vomiting

Tremor: Arms extended and fingers spread apart. Observation.
0 No tremor
1 Not visible, but can be felt fingertip to fingertip
2
3
4 Moderate, with patient's arms extended
5
6
7 Severe, even with arms not extended

Paroxysmal sweats: Observation.
0 No sweat visible
1 Barely perceptible sweating, palms moist
2
3
4 Beads of sweat obvious on forehead
5
6
7 Drenching sweats

Anxiety: Ask "Do you feel nervous?" Observation.
0 No anxiety, at ease.
1 Mild anxious
2
3
4 Moderately anxious, or guarded, so anxiety is inferred
5
6
7 Equivalent to acute panic states as seen in severe delirium or acute schizophrenic reactions

Agitation: Observation.
0 Normal activity
1 Somewhat more than normal activity
2
3
4 Moderately fidgety and restless
5
6
7 Paces back and forth during most of the interview, or constantly thrashes about

Tactile disturbances: Ask "Have you any itching, pins and needles sensations, any burning, any numbness, or do you feel bugs crawling on or under your skin?" Observation.
0 None
1 Very mild itching, pins and needles, burning or numbness
2 Mild itching, pins and needles, burning or numbness
3 Moderate itching, pins and needles, burning or numbness

TABLE 13-8 CLINICAL INSTITUTE WITHDRAWAL ASSESSMENT OF ALCOHOL SCALE, REVISED (CIWA-Ar)—cont'd

4 Moderately severe hallucinations
5 Severe hallucinations
6 Extremely severe hallucinations
7 Continuous hallucinations

Auditory disturbances: Ask "Are you more aware of sounds around you? Are they harsh? Do they frighten you? Are you hearing anything that is disturbing to you? Are you hearing things you know are not there?" Observation.

0 Not present
1 Very mild harshness or ability to frighten
2 Mild harshness or ability to frighten
3 Moderate harshness or ability to frighten
4 Moderately severe hallucinations
5 Severe hallucinations
6 Extremely severe hallucinations
7 Continuous hallucinations

Visual disturbances: Ask "Does light appear to be too bright? Is its color different? Does it hurt your eyes? Are you seeing anything that is disturbing to you? Are you hearing things you know are not there?" Observation.

0 Not present
1 Very mild sensitivity
2 Mild sensitivity
3 Moderate sensitivity

4 Moderately severe hallucinations
5 Severe hallucinations
6 Extremely severe hallucinations
7 Continuous hallucinations

Headache, fullness in head: Ask "Does your head feel different? Does it feel like there is a band around you head?" Do not rate for dizziness or lightheadedness. Otherwise, rate severity.

0 Not present
1 Very mild
2 Mild
3 Moderate
4 Moderately severe
5 Severe
6 Very severe
7 Extremely severe

Orientation and clouding of sensorium: Ask "What day is this? Where are you? Who am I?"

0 Oriented and can do serial additions
1 Cannot do serial additions or is uncertain about date
2 Disoriented for date by no more than 2 calendar days
3 Disoriented for date by more than 2 calendar days
4 Disoriented for place and/or person

The CIWA-Ar is not copyrighted and may be reproduced freely. This assessment for monitoring withdrawal symptoms requires approximately 5 minutes to administer. The maximum score is 67. Patients scoring less than 10 do not usually need additional medication for withdrawal.

From Sullivan J. T., Sykora, K., Schneiderman, J., Naranjo, C. A., & Sellers, E. M. (1989). Assessment of alcohol withdrawal: The revised clinical institute withdrawal assessment for alcohol scale (CIWA-Ar). *British Journal of Addiction, 84*(11), 1353–1357.

TABLE 13-9 COMMON BENZODIAZEPINES FOR ALCOHOL WITHDRAWAL

MEDICATION	DOSE EQUIVALENCY	ABSORPTION RATE AND PEAK	HALF-LIFE	ACTION
Diazepam (Valium) *IV form is a vesicant	5 mg	Rapid PO 1–2 hours IM 1 hour IV 8 minutes	30–100 hours	Long
Lorazepam (Ativan)	1 mg	Intermediate PO 1–4 hours IM/SL 1 hour IV 10 minutes	8–20 hours	Short
Chlordiazepoxide (Librium)	25 mg	Intermediate PO 1–4 hours	30–100 hours	Long
Oxazepam (Serax)	15 mg	Intermediate PO 1–4 hours	3–20 hours	Short

IM, Intramuscular; *IV*, intravenous; *PO*, orally; *SL*, sublingual.

For delirium, delusions, or hallucinations during withdrawal[25,26]:

- Maintain seizure precautions.
- Carbamazepine, beta-blockers, and clonidine can diminish the severity of withdrawal symptoms. However, they do not prevent delirium tremens or seizures. They should be used as an adjunct, not as monotherapy.
- Administer antipsychotic agents as an adjunct to benzodiazepines, particularly haloperidol (Haldol) 5 mg intravenously every 1 to 2 hours. Obtain an electrocardiogram and monitor the QT interval.
- Monitor patient for acute dystonic reaction.

> A potential complication of most typical antipsychotics is QT-interval prolongation, which predisposes to ventricular dysrhythmias.[16]

ALCOHOL AND SPECIAL POPULATIONS

Alcohol and Older Adults

The amount of alcohol that a patient has tolerated throughout his or her lifetime can become an issue with aging. Age-related body changes, such as decreased metabolism, and the interaction of alcohol with medications increase the risk involved with alcohol consumption in the older adult. Also, co-occurring medical conditions and impairment in cognition, memory, and movement with both alcohol use and withdrawal make older drinkers particularly vulnerable for alcohol abuse and withdrawal. The elderly should have only a "small amount" (e.g., no more than one drink per day or two drinks at one time) and only drink occasionally.

Alcohol and Women

Women are at greater risk of developing medical complications from alcohol use. Women have less alcohol dehydrogenase, an enzyme that breaks down alcohol, than men have, thus allowing more alcohol to reach the bloodstream. Also, alcohol is more soluble in water than in fat and, proportionately, women have more body fat and less body water than men. This causes a higher alcohol concentration in women, which in turn causes greater organ damage and places women at greater risk for diseases such as cirrhosis.

College Students

Many college students engage in heavy episodic, or binge, drinking. NIAAA defines binge drinking as consuming enough alcohol to result in a blood alcohol content of 0.08, which for most adults would equal five drinks for men or four for women over a 2-hour period.[27]

According to a national survey on drug use, 85% of college students have tried alcohol.

Approximately 39% to 44% of college students reported binge drinking at least once in the 2 weeks prior to taking a survey.[28,29] Additionally, according to one study, nearly one third of college students met the *Diagnostic and Statistical Manual of Mental Disorders-IV* criteria for alcohol abuse and 6% met the criteria for alcohol dependence.[29]

Addressing alcohol consumption is an important role in treating and promoting the ED patient's health.

> **Referral Options**
> - Alcoholic Anonymous (http://www.aa.org)
> - Moderation Management (http://www.moderation.org)
> - Salvation Army (http://www.salvationarmy.org)
> - Substance Abuse and Mental Health Services Administration (http://www.samhsa.gov)
> - Veterans Health Administration, National Center for Health Promotion and Disease Prevention (http://www.prevention.va.gov)

> **Resources**
> - ENA has developed a free toolkit to implement SBIRT in the emergency department. http://www.ena.org/IQSIP/Injury%20Prevention/SBIRT/ToolKit/Pages/toolkit.aspx
> - The American College of Emergency Physicians (ACEP) has materials, including a brochure that can be customized. http://www.acep.org
> - Rethinking Drinking (from the National Institute on Alcohol Abuse and Alcoholism) is available at http://pubs.niaaa.nih.gov/publications/rethinkingdrinking/rethinking_drinking.pdf

REFERENCES

1. Centers for Disease Control and Prevention. (2010, October 5). *ER visits.* Retrieved from http://www.cdc.gov/nchs/fastats/ervisits.htm
2. The BNI-ART Institute. (n.d.). *SBIRT in health care.* Retrieved from http://www.ed.bmc.org/sbirt/scope.php
3. D'Onofrio, G., & Degutis, L. C. (2002). Preventive care in the emergency department: Screening and brief intervention for alcohol problems in the emergency department: A systematic review. *Academic Emergency Medicine, 9*(6), 627–638.
4. Cherpitel, C. J. (1999). Drinking patterns and problems: A comparison of primary care with the emergency room. *Substance Abuse, 20,* 85–95.
5. Centers for Disease Control and Prevention. (2011, January 13). *Alcohol and public health.* Retrieved from http://www.cdc.gov/alcohol
6. U.S. Preventive Services Task Force. (2004, April). *Screening and behavioral counseling interventions in primary care to reduce alcohol misuse.* Retrieved from http://www.uspreventiveservicestaskforce.org/uspstf/uspsdrin.htm

7. Emergency Nurses Association. (2009). *Alcohol screening, brief intervention, and referral to treatment* [position statement]. Des Plaines, IL: Author.

8. Solberg, L. I., Maciosek, M. V., & Edwards, N. M. (2008). Primary care intervention to reduce alcohol misuse: Ranking its health impact and cost effectiveness. *American Journal of Preventive Medicine, 34*(2), 143–152.

9. Babor, T. F., Higgins-Biddle, J. C., Saunders, J. B., & Monteiro, M. G. (2001). *AUDIT: The alcohol use disorders identification test* (2nd ed.). Geneva, Switzerland: World Health Organization.

10. World Health Organization. (2010). *The Alcohol, Smoking and Substance Involvement Screening Test (ASSIST): Manual for use in primary care.* Geneva, Switzerland: Author. Retrieved from http://whqlibdoc.who.int/publications/2010/9789241599382_eng.pdf

11. National Institute on Alcohol Abuse and Alcoholism. (2005, April). *Screening for alcohol use and alcohol related problems.* Retrieved from http://pubs.niaaa.nih.gov/publications/aa65/aa65.htm

12. Canagasaby, A., & Vinson, D. C. (2005). Screening for hazardous or harmful drinking using one or two quantity-frequency. *Alcohol and Alcoholism, 40*(3), 208–213.

13. National Institute on Alcohol Abuse and Alcoholism. (2005). *Helping patients who drink too much: A clinician's guide.* Washington, DC: Author. Retrieved from http://pubs.niaaa.nih.gov/publications/Practitioner/CliniciansGuide2005/guide.pdf

14. Zimmermann, P. G. (2005). Alcohol use and abuse. In P. G. Zimmermann & R. D. Herr (Eds.), *Triage nursing secrets.* St. Louis, MO: Mosby.

15. Patel, Y., & Garmel, G. M. (2007). Management of intoxicated/violent patients. In A. Mattu & D. Goyal (Eds.), *Emergency medicine: Avoiding the pitfalls and improving the outcomes* (pp. 99–108). Malden, MA: Blackwell Publishing.

16. Bayard, M., McIntyre, J., Hill, K. R., & Woodside, J. Jr. (2004). Alcohol withdrawal syndrome. *American Family Physician, 69*(6), 1443–1550.

17. Metheny, N. M. (2012). *Fluid and electrolyte balance: Nursing considerations* (5th ed.). Sudbury, MA: Jones & Bartlett.

18. Burns, M. J., & Levine, M. (2006). Approach to toxic exposure. In S. R. Votey & M. A. Davis (Eds.), *Signs and symptoms in emergency medicine.* St. Louis, MO: Mosby.

19. National Institute on Alcohol Abuse and Alcoholism. (April, 2009). *Neuroscience: Pathways to alcohol dependence.* Retrieved from http://www.niaaa.nih.gov/Publications/AlcoholAlerts/Documents/AA77.pdf

20. American Society of Addition Medicine. (2001). Addiction medicine essentials: Clinical Institute Withdrawal Assessment of Alcohol Scale, Revised (CIWA-Ar). *ASAM News, 16*(1 Suppl), 1–2.

21. Keys, V. A. (2011). Alcohol withdrawal during hospitalization. *American Journal of Nursing, 111*(1), 40–44.

22. Becker, H. C. (1998). Kindling in alcohol withdrawal. *Alcohol Health and Research World, 22*(1), 25–33.

23. Tetrault, J. M., & O'Connor, P. G. (2008). Substance abuse and withdrawal in the critical care setting. *Critical Care Clinics, 24,* 767–788.

24. Lemon, S. J., Winstead, P. S., & Weant K. A. (2010). Management of alcohol withdrawal syndrome. *Advanced Emergency Nursing Journal, 32*(1), 20–27.

25. Sullivan, J. T., Sykora, K., Schneiderman, J., Naranjo, C. A., & Sellers, E. M. (1989). Assessment of alcohol withdrawal: The revised clinical institute withdrawal assessment for alcohol scale (CIWA-Ar). *British Journal of Addiction, 84*(11), 1353–1357.

26. Marx, J. A. (2006). Alcohol-related disorders. In V. J. Markovchick & P. T. Pons (Eds.), *Emergency medicine secrets* (4th ed.). St. Louis, MO: Mosby.

27. National Institute on Alcohol Abuse and Alcoholism (NIAAA). NIAAA Council approves definition of binge drinking. *NIAAA Newsletter* (3), Winter 2004.

28. Johnston, L. D., O'Malley, P. M., Bachman, J. G., & Schulenberg, J. E. (2004). *Monitoring the future: National survey results on drug use, 1975–2003. Volume II: College students and adults ages 19–45. NIH Pub. No. 04–5508.* Bethesda, MD: National Institute on Drug Abuse.

29. Wechsler, H., Lee, J. E., Kuo, M., Seibring, M., Nelson, T. F., & Lee, H. (2002). Trends in college binge drinking during a period of increased prevention efforts. Findings from 4 Harvard School of Public Health College Alcohol Study surveys: 1993–2001. *Journal of American College Health, 50*(5), 203–217.

30. Reference deleted in proofs.

31. Todd, K., Berk, W. A., Welch, R. D., Williams, J. W., Fisher, J., Wahl, R. P., ... Bock, B. F. (1992). Prospective analysis of mental status progression in ethanol-intoxicated patients. *American Journal of Emergency Medicine, 10*(4), 271–273.

32. Yim, A., & Wiener, S. W. (2009, October 6). *Delirium tremens.* Retrieved from http://emedicine.medscape.com/article/791802-overview

33. Klalinski, M. (2006). Seizures, adult. In S. F. Votey & M. A. Davis (Eds.), *Signs and symptoms in emergency medicine* (2nd ed.). St. Louis, MO: Mosby.

Wound Management

Robert D. Herr

GENERAL PRINCIPLES OF WOUND MANAGEMENT

Wounds can be considered chronic, such as ulcers, or acute, such as wounds from recent trauma. The goals of wound care are the following:

- Identify underlying injury to bones, nerves, vessels, ligaments, tendons, muscles, and other structures.
- Decrease the incidence of infection.
- Promote optimal healing.
- Minimize scarring.
- Manage pain.

> The use of nonsterile but clean gloves show no higher infection rate than sterile gloves and cost less.[1]

Wound care begins with management of the patient, then focuses on the general area of injury, and finally addresses the specific wound. The following principles apply to the management of all wounds, regardless of cause, location, or patient presentation[2,3]:

- Manage the patient through standard primary and secondary assessments and treatments. Specific wound-related care includes the following:
  - Always use standard infection control precautions.
  - Control bleeding with direct pressure, elevation, topical hemostatics, and surgery.
  - Identify and treat hemorrhagic shock. Earliest signs are tachycardia and tachypnea.
  - Assess for hypothermia, particularly when extensive skin loss is present.
  - Expose the patient (as indicated) to identify any other wounds that may warrant intervention.
  - Evaluate the patient's tetanus immunization status.
- Manage the injured area.
  - Assess distal pulses, capillary refill time, skin color, and temperature.
- Check for motor and sensory function distal to the wound.
- Splint fractures.
- Remove rings and other constrictive clothing or objects.
- Identify an open fracture because these require extensive irrigation and the patient should receive intravenous antibiotics as soon as possible. Surgical wound debridement may be required.
- Manage the wound.
  - Remove current dressings. Place dressings where the drainage can be inspected by all caregivers.
  - Obtain radiographs if a fracture or foreign body is suspected.
  - Monitor any wound with copious or pulsatile bleeding since this signifies erosion into blood vessels. In chronic wounds or ulcers this portends worsening bleeding.
  - Remove visible foreign matter.
- According to institutional protocol, perform or assist with the following:
  - Flush abrasions and wounds containing obvious debris.
  - Irrigate puncture wounds and lacerations.
  - Explore the wound for foreign bodies and injury to underlying structures.
  - Debride devitalized tissue.
  - Approximate the wound edges or bandage the wound. If closure is not appropriate, the wound should be packed as discussed later.
  - Notify public health authorities of reportable conditions (e.g., dog bites, gunshot wounds). Refer to local guidelines for mandatory reporting requirements.
  - Collect and preserve forensic evidence from gunshot or stab wounds as per institutional policy.[4]

Suspect an open fracture when there is skin disruption *near* the fracture, not just over the fracture. Bone splinters can pierce skin and retract to centimeters away from the skin opening.

Wound Healing

Wound healing begins immediately after injury. Vasodilatation produces erythema and edema below the epithelial layer that promotes epithelial cell migration within 24 hours of injury. Fibrin is deposited followed by collagen. Epithelialization closes the wound within 48 to 72 hours if skin margins can be approximated and the wound remains uninfected.[4]

Adverse conditions can cause skin ulcers and other chronic wounds that heal slowly and are especially at risk of infection. Epithelialization occurs more slowly in patients with the following situations:

- Poor nutritional status
- Compromised vascular supply, such as in diabetes or severe atherosclerosis or smoking
- Medications that slow collagen formation, such as corticosteroids or phenytoin
- Wounds of the lower legs, feet, or toes
- Advanced patient age
- Low tissue oxygen levels, especially in patients with chronic obstructive pulmonary disease, patients with anemia, and those receiving home oxygen therapy
- Pressure on skin or support tissues

Primary closure of a wound is likely if skin edges can be closed and the wound is not infected. This occurs about 4 days after injury and is enhanced by natural wound contracture. A contracture is hazardous in certain hand wounds where it can limit joint movement.

Secondary closure is needed when wound edges will not approximate or the wound is contaminated. It is standard to let the wound granulate and heal more slowly, often with wound packing. These wounds may require skin grafting if the defect exceeds 1 cm in rough diameter.

Scarring is the cosmetic perception of wound healing that occurs over weeks or months. The scar is a dynamic process of collagen synthesis and lysis. In balance, this "creative destruction" of scar tissue produces a flat scar. Lack of collagen in genetic conditions can cause keloids and hypertrophic scarring; lack of collagen synthesis occurs from wound ischemia, steroid use, and other factors that reduce scarring yet also reduce skin tensile strength.[5]

WOUND ASSESSMENT

Thorough assessment of the wound and the circumstances surrounding the injury can help in prioritizing and developing a plan for wound management:

- Has the patient declined in function or is a limb threatened with loss from sepsis, infection, or allergy?
- What caused the injury? How did it happen? What were the circumstances surrounding the event?
- When did the injury occur? Where was the patient at the time?
- Where is the wound located? What is the condition of the skin and surrounding tissue?
- What care did the wound receive before the patient arrived at the emergency department (ED)?
- Are motor function, sensation, and perfusion intact distal to the wound?
- Can the wound edges be approximated?
- What is the patient's general physical condition? Current medications? Medical history?
- What is the patient's age and occupation?

Additional considerations for existing wounds or ulcers include[6-8]:

- What changes were noted to prompt this evaluation?
- What barriers exist to normal wound healing?

Evaluate all wounds for the presence of foreign bodies:

- Glass and metal objects are identified easily with plain radiographs.
- Matter that has a density similar to that of soft tissue (e.g., wood splinters, thorns, cactus spines, and pieces of plastic) is not found so easily.
- Ultrasound, computed tomography, and magnetic resonance imaging can be used to locate these objects.[4]

TREATMENT CONSIDERATIONS

Wound Preparation

Wound cleansing is customary practice, but there is no strong evidence that it reduces infection. It can be reserved for contaminated wounds for optimal healing and infection prevention. Soaking a wound is not helpful. Surface cleaning is the initial step in wound preparation. Issues to be considered include cleanser selection, hair removal, and wound irrigation.

Tap water from treated sources of water (such as filtered or disinfected water) is as effective as other solutions to cleanse a wound.[9]

Contaminated Wounds

Wounds that are contaminated may be obvious; however, contamination with liquids (such as water) is not always apparent. The potential for contamination should be considered in any open wound.

Determination of contamination is based on historical evaluation and wound inspection. Establish whether the wounding implement was clean or grossly soiled. Common knife contaminants include meat, poultry, and dirt. A laceration over the knuckle that occurred when the fist struck a human mouth is always considered contaminated. Likewise, a retained foreign body may provide a nucleus of infection. Fungal infections may occur in the presence of retained wood fragments. Wound irrigation, debridement, and foreign body removal are critical for healing to occur without infection.[9]

> A laceration on the knuckle from a fist striking a human mouth is always considered contaminated.

Skin Antisepsis and Cleanser

Reducing skin contamination is usually done with chlorhexidine (Hibiclens), a 10% povidone-iodine (Betadine) solution, or hydrogen peroxide. Any benefit may be offset if skin antiseptics spill into the wound because they impair wound defenses, damage delicate tissues, and delay healing. A dilute (1%) povidone-iodine solution is not as toxic to tissue but should be reserved for infection-prone wounds.[10]

> Never put any substance in a wound that should not be put in an eye.

Hair Removal

Wounds in hairy areas heal best without hair in the approximated edges. Unfortunately, shaving abrades the skin, increases wound infection rates, and is cosmetically irritating. Snip hair with scissors or trim it with an electric clipper if removal is necessary. One area that should never be shaved is the eyebrow, as eyebrows provide important landmarks for approximating wound margins and, once shaved, may fail to grow back.[11]

> Moving hair out of the way and securing it in place with a lubricant (e.g., petroleum jelly), a topical ointment, or tape is generally preferable to removal.

Mechanical Irrigation

Irrigation is helpful to wash away small foreign bodies, including soil. Irrigation is essential in wounds caused by bites and in those with fecal contamination.

Remove sand, dirt, and other large particles using low-pressure irrigation with a syringe. However, small particles such as clay and bacteria require higher-pressure irrigation. Forcing fluid through a narrow catheter or needle (e.g., a 19-gauge needle on a 12- or 35-mL syringe) provides an irrigation pressure of 5 to 8 pounds per square inch.

Regardless of the solution or type of irrigation apparatus, place the needle perpendicular to the wound (as close as possible to the surface) and forcefully depress the syringe plunger. Use protective equipment to guard against fluid splatter to the face and eyes and prevent blood-borne pathogen exposure. Splash guards can be attached between the syringe and the catheter to decrease splatter, but they are not a substitute for personal protective equipment.[4]

Tetanus Immunization

Tetanus is caused by *Clostridium tetani*, a gram-positive anaerobic bacillus. Because *C. tetani* forms spores, this organism is highly resistant to measures taken against it. *C. tetani* is present in soil, in garden moss, on farms, and anywhere animal and human excreta can be found. Bacteria enter the circulation through an open wound and attach to cells within the central nervous system. The usual incubation period is 2 days to 2 weeks. However, spores can lie dormant in tissue for years, so scrupulous wound cleansing is crucial. As long as immunizations are current, tetanus is a 100% avoidable condition.

Postexposure immunizations should be given only when needed. Individuals can become sensitized by frequent vaccination, and subsequent injections can cause several days of painful swelling. This type of reaction is the usual source of "tetanus allergy" reported by some patients. Recommendations for tetanus immunization are based on current guidelines from the Centers for Disease Control and Prevention (CDC), which advises that the tetanus vaccine also should contain diphtheria toxin. This combination, dT(Td), is given as a single 0.5-mL intramuscular dose.[12]

- Tetanus vaccination routinely begins in childhood. Properly vaccinated children receive tetanus, diphtheria, and pertussis vaccines at ages 2, 4, 6, and 18 months, as well as at 4 and 6 years of age. A booster is provided at age 16 years.
- To remain vaccinated, adults should have received the initial tetanus series and be revaccinated a minimum of every 10 years.
- If an adult presents to the ED with a wound that has minimal contamination, assure that they have received both the initial tetanus series as well as revaccination within the past 10 years. If it has been longer than 10 years, they should receive dT(Td) as part of their ED visit.
- If an adult presents to the ED with a wound that is grossly contaminated (tetanus prone), assure that they have received both the initial tetanus series as well as revaccination within the past 5 years. If it has been longer than 5 years, they should receive dT(Td) as part of their ED visit.
- Ideally, for patients whose immunization status is outdated, unclear, or unknown, tetanus prophylaxis should be given as soon after the wound is sustained as possible, although, immunization will be effective if given up to 72 hours after the wound occurred. Immunization may

be considered after 72 hours, but there is a risk that tetanus may have become active within the central nervous system at this point and diligent patient follow up should be considered.

- If the patient has not received an initial tetanus series (or has only received one of the series), they should be started on a regimen with 0.5 mL of dT(Td) in the ED. If the patient has a grossly contaminated wound (tetanus prone), simultaneous administration of 250 units of intramuscular antitoxin is recommended.
- Patients with partial immunity, from two or more previous tetanus injections, are considered sufficiently immune. The CDC recommends a booster of 0.5 mL dT(Td), even for patients with grossly contaminated (tetanus prone) wounds.
- Patients over the age of 6 years who have not completed an initial immunization series should be referred to their primary care providers or local health department for a second dT(Td) dose (0.5 mL intramuscularly) in 4 to 6 weeks and a third injection in 6 to 12 months.[11,12] New CDC recommendations suggest the first of these doses should be the tetanus toxoid, reduced diphtheria toxoid, and acellular pertussis (Tdap) vaccine.[13]
- In 2010, the CDC recommended expanded use of Tdap. A single Tdap dose is recommended for adults aged 19 to 64 years and children aged 11 to 18 years who have completed the recommended childhood DTP/DTaP vaccination series.[13]
  - Adults aged 65 years and older who have or will have close contact with an infant younger than 12 months should also receive a single Tdap dose.[13]

Prophylactic Antibiotics

Antibiotics are not indicated for simple open wounds in healthy patients because the wounds rarely become infected. However, they are indicated for wounds with devitalized tissue, contamination with soil or feces, contact with saliva (bites), or patients with lymphoma. Antibiotics should always be considered an adjunct to debridement and irrigation rather than a substitute.[11] The selection of a prophylactic antibiotic depends on many factors, including the location of the wound, the type of pathogens usually encountered with a particular injury, and the fact that most contaminated wounds contain a wide variety of organisms. Little evidence exists to support the routine application of topical antibiotics on simple wounds.[4]

Anesthesia

Routes of anesthesia administration for wound closure include topical, wound infiltration, regional blocks, and intravenous procedural sedation. The methods selected depend on the patient, the wound, and its location.

> Warming lidocaine to 37° C (98.6° F) can minimize the pain during its injection.[11]

Anesthetic Agents

The most common anesthetic for local infiltration or regional use is lidocaine, primarily because of its low tissue toxicity. Additionally, lidocaine has a short duration of action, which is desirable for repairs of areas such as the mouth or lip, where recovery of sensation reduces the incidence of unintentional biting of the wound. Likewise, prompt return of sensation to a finger prevents further injury as the patient begins to use the hand.

One disadvantage of lidocaine is the pain associated with injection. Warming the solution to 37° C (98.6° F) can minimize this effect. Sodium bicarbonate also reduces the pain associated with lidocaine injection. Buffer lidocaine by adding one part 8.4% sodium bicarbonate (1 mEq/mL) to 10 parts 1% lidocaine (i.e., add 1 mL of sodium bicarbonate to 10 mL of lidocaine). However, this mixture reduces the shelf life of lidocaine from 3 years to a few days, after which the solution will precipitate in the bottle.[12]

Preparations of lidocaine with epinephrine are also available. Epinephrine increases the duration of anesthesia and decreases bleeding. Use of this combination is contraindicated in heavily contaminated wounds or those with a tentative blood supply such as avulsions. Adverse effects of epinephrine include an increased rate of infection and ischemia when lidocaine with epinephrine is injected into the ear, tip of the nose, digits, or penis.

Another anesthetic agent used for infiltration is bupivacaine (Marcaine, Sensorcaine). The effects of this drug last four times longer than lidocaine. This makes bupivacaine ideal for situations in which wound closure will require longer than 2 hours or when prolonged local anesthesia is desirable.

Anesthetic Allergy

Patients frequently report an allergy to lidocaine; however, true allergy to injected anesthetics is uncommon.[12] Many reported allergies are actually adverse reactions such as hyperventilation, vasovagal syncope or light-headedness, cardiovascular stimulation from epinephrine, and various idiosyncratic reactions to the injury and subsequent wound repair. Contact dermatitis, caused by topical local anesthetics, also has been reported. This type of reaction is not immunoglobulin E–mediated and poses little risk. If a true allergy is suspected, an anesthetic from a different chemical class can be used. Sterile saline infiltration, guided imagery, and hypnosis are nonpharmacological options. If local anesthesia is not possible, needleless wound closure techniques such as tying hair on the scalp or applying adhesive closure strips (e.g., Steri-Strips) or wound glue should be considered.

Infiltration Anesthesia

Direct injection of an anesthetic agent into the wound is the most common anesthetic technique used in the ED. Infiltration of lidocaine along wound edges anesthetizes subcutaneous nerves. Some have recommended injecting through intact, antiseptically cleansed skin at the periphery of the wound to prevent spread of contamination. However, injecting through the edge of the wound is less painful. Several methods are available to reduce discomfort from anesthetic infiltration:

- Use the thinnest possible needle, 30 gauge or smaller.
- Minimize the number of skin punctures; a longer needle, inserted to the hub, can cover most of the edge of a wound.
- Perform subsequent needlesticks through already anesthetized skin.
- Inject into the subdermal area rather than into the dermis; raising a wheal is painful.
- Anesthetic agents injected slowly (longer than 10 seconds) are more comfortable than those injected quickly (<2 seconds).

Digital Block

Digital blocks can be used when the nerve supply to the wound is superficial. This technique is particularly superior to infiltration anesthesia in regions where the skin is sensitive, especially the digits, palms, soles, and face. Another advantage of digital or other regional nerve blocks is that they do not distort the wound or interfere with approximation.

Topical Anesthesia

Topical anesthetics reduce the pain associated with injection, prevent tissue swelling, and cause vasoconstriction, which limits bleeding. TAC (0.5% tetracaine, 0.5% epinephrine [adrenaline], and 11.8% cocaine), the traditional topical anesthetic agent, has been replaced by newer combinations such as LET (4% lidocaine, 0.1% epinephrine, and 0.5% tetracaine) and XAP (xylocaine-adrenaline-pontocaine). These solutions are applied topically 20 minutes before wound repair and are left until the skin blanches around the application site. Absence of blanching indicates incomplete anesthesia.[14]

Topical anesthesia also can be achieved by applying a mixture of 5% lidocaine and prilocaine (EMLA) for 60 minutes. However, EMLA cream is designed for use on intact skin. Use on lacerations is not recommended because it causes inflammation, which increases infection rates.

Procedural Sedation

Procedural sedation can be used to facilitate wound care and for anxiety management in pediatric and adult patients who are unable to cooperate because of underlying physical, emotional, or developmental challenges. Procedural sedation commonly is used for reduction of fractures and dislocations but is also a valuable adjunct when extensive cleansing, irrigation, and wound debridement are required. See Chapter 15, Procedural Sedation, for further information.

Wound Closure

The goal of wound repair is rapid healing without infection. As a rule, healing occurs faster in wounds that are primarily closed with sutures, staples, tape, or cyanoacrylate glue. However, bites, other punctures, and contaminated wounds are so prone to infection that irrigation, debridement, and prophylactic antibiotic therapy take priority over closure.[9]

Every attempt should be made to close wounds as soon as possible. Common belief is that clean wounds become infected after 8 hours, but some older wounds can be closed days later without resulting in infection. Signs of infections can be seen within 8 hours in skin with poor blood supply resulting from crush injury, smoking, or location distal to the heart. The face has such an effective blood supply that infection is less likely and clean closure is more cosmetically desirable. Primary closure of wounds on the face may be attempted regardless of wound age.

Wound Closure Materials

Materials for wound closure include sutures, staples, tape, and adhesive bonding agents. The choice of material and technique depends on the preference of the health care provider, the amount of tension at the wound edges, the probability of infection, and the availability of closure materials.

Absorbable sutures, such as catgut, work well for pediatric facial wounds because removal is not needed as sutures dissolve within 3 to 5 days. Nonabsorbable sutures retain their strength for 60 days; nonetheless, they are slowly absorbed over a period of months to years, can leave their own scars, and should be removed as soon as epithelialization occurs to minimize scarring. Epithelialization takes the shortest time in facial lacerations and the longest time in the legs and feet. Table 14-1 lists optimal times for suture removal by various body locations. Leave sutures in place longer in patients with delayed healing caused by debilitation or the use of medications such as corticosteroids. Because the wound does not regain full tensile strength for

TABLE 14-1 **GUIDELINES FOR SUTURE REMOVAL**

LOCATION	TIME FOR REMOVAL
Face, eyelid, lip	3–5 days
Eyebrow	4–5 days
Ear	4–6 days
Scalp	5–8 days
Back, chest, trunk, arm, hand, thigh	7–10 days
Lower leg, foot	10–14 days

Modified from Denke, N. J. (2010). Wound management. In P. K. Howard & R. A. Steinmann (Eds.), *Sheehy's emergency nursing: Principles and practice* (6th ed., pp. 111–126). St. Louis, MO: Mosby.

several weeks, apply tape strips across newly removed suture sites to reduce tension.[9]

Closure Techniques

Tape Closure. Closure with a sterile, microporous tape (e.g., Steri-Strips) is appropriate for wounds with well-approximated edges in areas with minimal skin tension. Tape strips commonly are used for transverse lacerations over the brow, under the chin, or across the malar prominence of the cheek (Fig. 14-1). This technique is not recommended for wounds that may become edematous. Taping avoids the pain of anesthesia and later suture removal. Tape adheres poorly to wet skin, but adherence can be increased by applying tincture of benzoin to the area around the wound.[9]

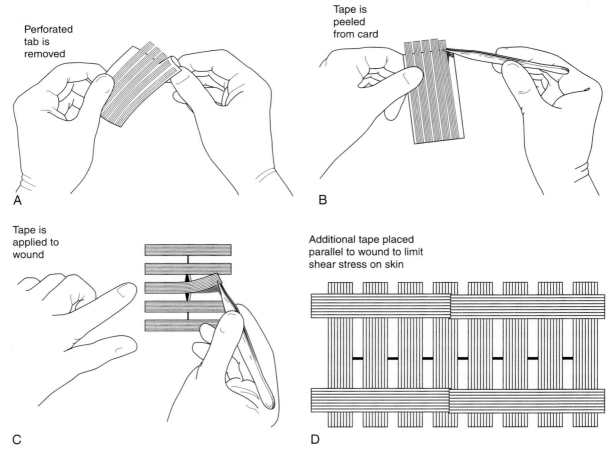

Perforated tab is removed

A

Tape is peeled from card

B

Tape is applied to wound

C

Additional tape placed parallel to wound to limit shear stress on skin

D

Fig. 14-1 Tape closure. (From Rothrock, J. C. [2007]. *Alexander's care of the patient in surgery* [13th ed.]. St. Louis, MO: Mosby.)

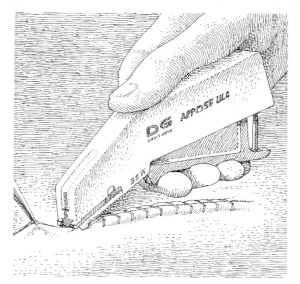

Fig. 14-2 Application of skin staples. Staples are centered over incision line, using locating arrow or guideline, and placed approximately 0.25 inch apart. (From Rothrock, J. C. [2007]. *Alexander's care of the patient in surgery* [13th ed.]. St. Louis, MO: Mosby.)

Suture. Suture is available in absorbable and nonabsorbable material. A synthetic monofilament, such as nylon, is associated with the fewest wound infections and can be used safely in all types of skin closures. Contrary to popular belief, nylon is absorbed but usually over a period of a year or more; therefore, nylon is reserved for skin use where it can be removed as soon as the wound has healed sufficiently. A variety of stitches are used to close different skin lesions. The type of stitch is based on the wound size, depth, and site. Skin heals at different rates depending on body location and heals more slowly in patients with underlying conditions that retard repair.[12]

Staples. Stapling the skin (Fig. 14-2) is faster than suturing and is associated with lower rates of tissue reactivity and wound infection.[2] Unfortunately, stapling cannot align the wound margins as neatly as suturing because edges must be prepositioned and held in place while the staple is inserted. Invariably, the margins are slightly malpositioned. Therefore stapling is most appropriate in locations where scarring can be tolerated, such as on the scalp. Stapling does not provide the same degree of hemostasis that is possible with sutures.[7]

Wound Glue. Adhesive bonding is the latest approach to wound repair. One such wound glue is n-butyl cyanoacrylate monomer (Dermabond). Contact with an alkaline pH causes the glue to polymerize and form a thin, waterproof bandage. This requires 1 second on moist skin and several seconds on dry skin. Adhesive bonding is most effective on wounds that have little tension.[9]

Wound Drainage Devices

Wound drainage devices include gauze packing, soft rubber drains, and closed systems that drain to a reservoir. Gauze packing is the most common way to drain pus from a wound such as an abscess cavity after incision and draining. This allows for infection to heal before skin edges close and is the method of choice for infected skin lacerations. A wound is packed by inserting gauze into the wound cavity using an instrument to break up loculated pus at the deep edge of the wound. This may require thin-width gauze such as $\frac{1}{4}$–inch Iodoform, but it must be a continuous strip and sufficient width to pack the center of the wound as well. A common error is to inadequately drain loculated pus in order to avoid causing pain. Analgesic can be given during packing but rarely alleviates the pain. The wound packing should be replaced each day until the wound stops producing pus. Then the wound is managed with dressing changes while pink granulation tissue forms.

Wound Dressing and Aftercare

- Dressings are applied to wounds to absorb drainage, protect the site from contamination, and hold antibiotic ointments in place. The choice of dressing materials depends on the wound type and the purpose of the dressing. Bulky dressings are used to provide additional protection and can absorb the significant amount of drainage associated with some wounds in the initial phase of healing. Other wounds, particularly those on the face, may be left uncovered.
- Generally, a dry sterile dressing is applied for 2 days unless the area is a gingival surface or is too hairy to accommodate a dressing. These wounds should be left without a dressing.
- Wounds closed with tape have a lower risk of infection than those closed with suture. Do not put topical antibiotics on taped wounds as these can weaken the adhesive property of the type.
- Patients may shower following wound closure without increasing the incidence of infection.

> Infection incidence is not increased by showering after wound closure.

Removal of Glue, Sutures, and Staples

Wound glue will slough 5 to 10 days after application, but it can be removed by applying antibiotic ointments. Sutures and staples should be exposed for removal by applying hydrogen peroxide to adhering blood or scab. Sutures should be cut and pulled out in such a way as to avoid shear forces that could reopen the wound. Staples are removed using staple removers that apply a downward force to the center that crimps the staple and an upward force that frees the tips from the skin. These staple removers tend to be flimsy, and staple removal can be difficult. A tip is to take extra care and expect to be humbled.

> Hyperpigmentation can occur in abraded skin after sun exposure. Sunscreen should be used for 6 months after injury.

Aftercare Instructions

Home care advice should incorporate the following:
- Essential wound care follow-up instructions, including the anticipated removal date for sutures or staples
- Any activity restrictions
- Signs of wound infection and indications of circulatory compromise
- Specific reasons to contact a primary care physician or return to the ED
- The need for sunscreen use for 6 months after injury (abraded skin is sensitized and hyperpigmentation can occur after sun exposure)
- Elevation of an injured extremity to limit edema formation[2]

WOUND MANAGEMENT BY TYPE

Basic wound types include abrasions, abscesses, avulsions, contusions, incisions, lacerations, and punctures. Although each wound is distinct and warrants different treatment, it is important to remember that any number of wound types may occur simultaneously in a patient. Additional considerations related to specific wounds include their size, location, and cause. Bites from animals and human beings cause a constellation of injuries commonly involving a combination of contusions, crush injuries, puncture wounds, and lacerations.

Abrasions

Rubbing skin against a hard surface removes the epithelium and exposes the dermis or subcutaneous layer. The resulting abrasion, or friction burn, initially may appear yellow, white, pink, or bloody depending on the tissue exposed. Abrasions can be superficial or can involve multiple skin layers. Embedded foreign bodies, such as gravel or asphalt, may cause permanent tattooing if not removed. Abrasions have the same physiologic effect as a partial thickness burn. Large abrasions—and their associated disruption of protective outer skin layers—may precipitate significant fluid loss and hypothermia because of evaporation.[2]

Therapeutic interventions include the following:
- Provide pain control through the use of topical anesthetics or parenteral pain medication before cleaning, particularly when wounds are extensive or contain a large amount of embedded foreign material.
- Cleanse the wound with irrigation and gentle scrubbing.
- Remove all foreign material.
- Apply an antibiotic ointment and a sterile dressing.

Abscesses

An abscess forms when pus does not drain through the skin. The underlying infection may arise from inoculation by an insect bite or sting, a puncture wound, an infected hair follicle, or any injury that has closed without proper drainage. An abscess typically is recognized when it enlarges sufficiently to distend the skin and produce pain. Underlying pus causes the skin to become tense and discolored. When pus makes the skin tent, the abscess is said to "point" and is ready to be drained. Abscesses that point eventually will drain spontaneously. However, these wounds are treated optimally before this time. Therapeutic draining in the ED decreases pain, allows wound packing, and helps prevent the development of cellulitis. Abscesses in the perirectal area are usually much deeper than they initially appear, and drainage may require general anesthesia. Antibiotic therapy is indicated for patients with concurrent cellulitis, immunosuppression, endocarditis, or a facial abscess that is draining into the sinuses.[2]

Therapeutic interventions include the following:
- Premedicate the patient with analgesics; use procedural sedation for patients experiencing severe discomfort.
- A local anesthetic is injected around the abscess to dull pain.
- A scalpel is used to make an incision in the tense, overlying skin to drain a pointing abscess. Needle drainage will not adequately prevent rapid abscess recurrence. Pus initially is allowed to drain spontaneously; any remaining pus is expressed by pressing on the wound edges.
- The abscess cavity is packed with iodinated gauze to prevent premature closure of the skin and to facilitate further pus drainage. See "Wound Drainage Devices."

Avulsions

An avulsion involves peeling of the skin from underlying tissues. Peeling compromises the blood supply to the site and can lead to further tissue devitalization. Avulsions are described as proximal-based or distal-based.

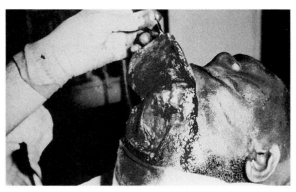

Fig. 14-3 Degloving injury of the scalp. (From Auerbach, P. [2001]. *Wilderness medicine* [4th ed.]. St. Louis, MO: Mosby.)

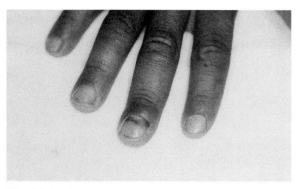

Fig. 14-4 This 25% subungual hematoma is enough to cause intense pain and pressure. (Courtesy James R. Roberts, MD.)

Proximal-based avulsions in general have better circulation. Nonetheless, wound edges may look gray or dusky, indicating the tenuous nature of the blood supply. An avulsion injury is called a degloving injury when skin is separated completely from underlying tissue (Fig. 14-3). Degloving injuries typically involve the hand or foot. However, scalp-degloving incidents can occur.[2]

Therapeutic interventions include the following:

- Clean, irrigate, and debride the wound of devitalized tissue.
- Avoid lidocaine with epinephrine because its vasoconstrictive properties can further compromise blood supply to the avulsed fragment.
- Sometimes, avulsed skin that is crinkled or folded can be extended to cover the entire wound and then can be sutured into place (unless contraindicated by wound age, contamination, or other factors).
- Even skin that appears gray or dusky may heal surprisingly well. Such skin edges should be approximated, not trimmed. If necessary, the edges can be debrided on the following day.
- Avulsions are common in patients with thin skin caused by age or long-term corticosteroid therapy. In such cases the skin may be too thin to suture; approximate wound edges with adhesive strips. In patients with extremely thin skin, even these strips can cause tearing. An occlusive dressing such as Tegaderm can be used to hold avulsed tissue in place.

If the skin is too thin to tolerate sutures or adhesive strips, use an occlusive dressing such as Tegaderm to hold avulsed tissue in place.

Contusions

Contusions (bruises, hematomas) occur when blunt trauma causes extravasation of blood into subcutaneous tissue. When viewed through the skin, such blood classically looks black and blue. After about 2 days, breakdown of blood pigments changes the color to yellow. Although most contusions are minor and resolve with little or no treatment, large hematomas are painful and can cause tissue swelling in fascial compartments.[2] Continued subfascial swelling will lead to compartment syndrome because fascia does not stretch well enough to accommodate the increase in volume. Rising pressure within a muscle compartment compromises blood supply to nerves and other tissues.

Therapeutic interventions include the following:

- Provide ice, elevation, and systemic analgesia with nonsteroidal, antiinflammatory agents. Stronger analgesia with narcotics may be required for some patients.
- No dressing is necessary.

Subungual Hematoma

In this condition, a direct blow to the fingertip ruptures vessels and blood collects below the nail (Fig. 14-4). The resulting hematoma makes the nail appear black or blue. The patient experiences significant pain as pressure builds in the subungual region. A widespread hematoma can lift the entire nail off of its bed. This actually provides significant pain relief because pressure is substantially reduced.[11]

Therapeutic interventions include the following:

- Initial treatment involves ice, elevation, and analgesia to minimize the painful throbbing.
- Obtain a radiograph of the digit to rule out a tuft fracture of the distal phalanx.

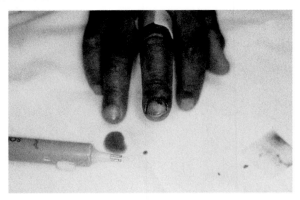

Fig. 14-5 Pressure was relieved by repeated application of electrocautery filament to bore a hole down to the trapped blood. (Courtesy James R. Roberts, MD.)

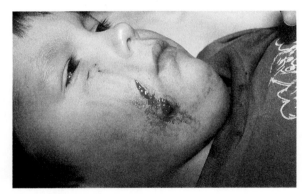

Fig. 14-6 Superficial laceration. (Courtesy Thomas Lintner, MD.)

- If the nail is intact, a hole is drilled through it directly over the hematoma. The nail itself has no nerve endings, so no anesthesia is required. A small battery-powered electrocautery can be used to drill through the nail or the nail can be trephined slowly away with a scalpel (Fig. 14-5).
- If the nail is loose, it may be removed entirely.

Incisions and Lacerations

Incisions are produced when tissue is sliced with a sharp object, whether it is a scalpel, a kitchen knife, a metal edge, or a piece of glass. In contrast, a laceration results when blunt trauma causes tissue tearing or crushing. These wounds may penetrate only the top layer of skin or can extend well beyond the dermis into deeper structures. Incisions are relatively resistant to infection, and the margins usually can be approximated. Lacerations can be linear (Fig. 14-6) or stellate, with jagged or smooth edges.

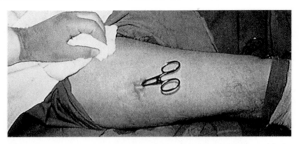

Fig. 14-7 An unintentional stab wound of the thigh. (From Newberry, L. [Ed.]. [2003]. *Sheehy's emergency nursing: Principles and practice* [5th ed.]. St. Louis, MO: Mosby.)

Therapeutic interventions include the following:
- Determine the age of the wound.
- Anesthetize the wound.
- Cleanse the wound using irrigation.
- Explore the wound for bone exposure and damage to underlying structures.
- Remove any foreign bodies.
- Excise necrotic tissue.
- Approximate the wound edges. Consider tissue adhesive.
- Apply a sterile dressing.

Punctures

A puncture occurs when a sharp object penetrates the skin (Fig. 14-7). A depth that is greater than the diameter of the entry hole characterizes these wounds. Because the ability to explore a puncture is limited, a high index of suspicion is needed to predict associated injury. Missiles can cause extensive tissue damage, whereas puncture wounds from nails, glass, pins, and other foreign bodies tend to move vessels and nerves aside, rather than sever the structures. Punctures can introduce bacteria deep into wounds that are inherently difficult to clean and tend to close early.[12]

Evaluate puncture wounds for the presence of foreign bodies. Determine what caused the puncture and investigate whether a foreign body (or some portion of it) may still remain in the wound. Ask the patient or the person who removed the object whether it appeared to be intact. Inspect the wound for contaminants such as clothing, rust, or dirt.[15]

Punctures into joint spaces can lead to septic arthritis; punctures into cartilage, bone, and periosteum are associated with osteomyelitis. Such wounds warrant exploration in the operating room. Radiographic evaluation is recommended for any puncture wound near a bone or joint. Specific types of punctures that merit separate discussion are bites, gunshot wounds, punctures of the plantar area of the foot, and high-pressure injuries.

Therapeutic interventions include the following:

- Obtain a plain radiograph of all infected puncture wounds and those with a possible retained foreign body.
- Inspect the entrance site and explore the wound for obvious contaminants.
- Irrigate and clean uncomplicated, uncontaminated puncture wounds that are less than 6 hours old.
- Routine use of prophylactic antibiotics is not recommended for uncomplicated puncture wounds in healthy individuals.[16] Use actually can predispose a patient to a secondary infection with *Pseudomonas*. Prophylactic antibiotics, such as first-generation cephalosporins (e.g., Ancef, Kefzol), are recommended for contaminated puncture wounds, wounds on the plantar area of the foot, or in patients with immunocompromising conditions such as diabetes mellitus, peripheral vascular disease, or systemic immunodeficiency.[12]
- All puncture wounds are considered tetanus-prone and require prophylactic vaccination in inadequately immunized individuals.
- Observe for complications such as cellulitis, abscess formation, joint infection, or osteomyelitis.

> Routine use of prophylactic antibiotics in uncomplicated puncture wounds in healthy individuals can predispose a patient to a secondary infection.[16]

Plantar Puncture Wounds

Wounds over the metatarsal-phalangeal joints require special attention because the injury is usually caused by deep penetration as a result of weight bearing on a sharp object. Penetration to bone is frequent. Such penetration may lead to osteomyelitis in adults or osteochondritis in children. Suspect these conditions when a patient reports pain 4 to 7 days after injury and the wound is red or swollen. *Pseudomonas aeruginosa* has been cultured from the inner soles of tennis shoes and sneakers. Wound inoculation with *Pseudomonas* occurs when a sharp object penetrates the shoe, sole, and skin and contacts bone or cartilage. About half the time, an infected plantar puncture wound contains a foreign body—usually a piece of fabric. For this reason, careful inspection of any puncture wound is essential. Antibiotic prophylaxis is recommended for contaminated puncture wounds.[12]

> An infected plantar puncture wound contains a foreign body about half of the time.[12]

Gunshot Wounds

In contrast to other punctures, gunshot wounds cause extensive damage to underlying tissues and organs. The amount of damage has no relationship to the size of the entrance or exit wounds. Bullets can shatter bone and cause further injury as bone fragments become secondary projectiles. A gunshot wound forms a negative pressure cavity that can pull overlying clothing and debris into the wound in the wake of the bullet. Bullets from rifles have a higher velocity than those from handguns and are associated with greater tissue damage.[17] High-velocity and high-energy missiles cause shock waves to travel through the tissues, shearing and crushing nerves, vessels, muscles, and organs several centimeters (or more) from the actual missile path. At close range, shotgun wounds can embed wadding and other debris (as well as pellets) in the tissues.

- Notify law enforcement agencies according to local reporting requirements.[18]
- Document the exact location of the wounds. Photographs and diagrams can be helpful.
- Record the number of wounds. Note that distinguishing entrance from exit wounds is an important forensic task but does not affect how the wounds are managed.
- Place paper bags over the patient's hands to protect evidence such as gunpowder residue.
- Cut around (not through) bullet holes, powder marks, and other possible evidence when removing clothing. (Not all jurisdictions encourage this practice.)
- Place clothing in a paper bag and give it to the police. Some agencies accept clothing in plastic bags, so consult local authorities to determine the procedure in the geographic area.[18]

See Chapter 6, Forensics, for more information on documentation and evidence collection.

High-Pressure Injuries

Paint guns and grease guns are designed to inject these substances into hard-to-reach places. When forced against the skin, such guns inject paint or grease for several centimeters, typically following tissue planes. In the volar aspect of the hand, paint or grease can travel down tendon sheaths and along the digits. These wounds are serious, and immediate surgical intervention is required to drain the paint or oil and to preserve tissue.[11]

> Wounds from paint guns or grease guns require surgical intervention to drain the paint or oil.[11]

Ulcers

Pressure Ulcers

Pressure ulcers consist of local damage to the skin and underlying tissue caused by compression between a bony prominence and an external surface.[7] Pressure ulcers are classified along a four-grade scale (Table 14-2). They derive from factors such as:

TABLE 14-2 CLASSIFICATION OF PRESSURE ULCERS BY GRADE*

Grade 1—Non-blanchable erythema of intact skin. Discoloration, warmth, induration, or hardness of skin may also be used as indicators, particularly in people with darker skin

Grade 2—Partial-thickness skin loss, involving epidermis, dermis, or both. The ulcer is superficial and presents clinically as an abrasion or blister

Grade 3—Full-thickness skin loss involving damage to or necrosis of subcutaneous tissue that may extend down to, but not through, underlying fascia

Grade 4—Extensive destruction, tissue necrosis or damage to muscle, bone, or supporting structures, with or without full-thickness skin loss

*As defined by the European Pressure Ulcer Advisory Panel and National Pressure Ulcer Advisory Panel. (2009). *Prevention and treatment of pressure ulcers: Quick reference guide.* Washington, DC: National Pressure Ulcer Advisory Panel.

- Sensory deficits in individuals who cannot detect local persistent pressure and who neglect to reposition themselves
- Debility or paralysis so repositioning is not possible
- Medications that reduce tissue blood flow such as sedatives, analgesics, and other medication
- Malnutrition that increases extent and severity

Facility-based caregivers have reporting requirements for such ulcers under the Centers for Medicare and Medicaid Services (CMS).

Interventions include the following:

- Assess and document risk factors in the individual and environment including observations on caregiver's ability and how safe discharge can be done.
- Assess surfaces for softness, such as wheelchairs, prosthetics, or bed coverings that you see.
- Assess nutritional and metabolic status by including serum albumin and other testing.
- Patients with ulcers tend to have allergies to certain dressings and topical medications, which should be considered prior to wound care.
- CMS reporting means that facility records should reveal ulcer size and location on admission.
- Assess the wound for infection, drainage, contaminants, perspiration, and other contributing factors.
- Remove any drainage devices such as packing and examine wound depth and condition.
- Surgical debridement may be needed, especially for extensive grade 3 or 4 ulcers. Wounds cannot be staged with an eschar present.

- Aside from local care, patient may require higher care level for ulcers that are infected, worsening, or new.
- Surgical consult may be indicated.
- Discharge teaching should include how pressure is being relieved on pressure points, including the ulcer.

Consider osteomyelitis when any of the following is present: ulcer down by the bone, fevers, high white blood cell count, or high sedimentation rate.

Venous Ulcers

Venous ulcers are defined as local damage to the skin and underlying tissue of the leg caused by chronic venous insufficiency, age, and limited mobility. Symptoms include aching, heaviness, itching, swelling, and skin breakdown. Most can be managed by compression bandaging.[6]

Therapeutic interventions include the following:

- Leg elevation.
- Improve mobility.
- Improve nutrition.
- Surgery in selected cases. In the United States, venous surgery is becoming more common not only as a last resort in treating varicose veins, but also as an option from the beginning.
- Dress with simple low adherence dressings under multilayer compression bandage.
- Four-layer compression bandaging.
  - Compression treatment heals ulcers at 12 to 15 weeks, and high compression is significantly better than low compression.
  - Applying these bandages takes some expertise and referral should be made to someone skilled in this area.

Diabetic Foot Ulcers

Diabetic foot ulcers occur from neuropathy that affects more than half of diabetics and cause loss of the sensations of temperature and pain from trauma. Diabetics are prone to infection from reduced white cell responses. Most cellulitis and fasciitis occurs from these ulcers. Osteomyelitis is common and commonly requires amputation if it does not heal.[7]

Therapeutic interventions include:

- Identification of new necrotic tissue or unhealthy tissue for debridement.
- Documentation of the degree of neuropathy and mechanism of trauma, if any.
- Antibiotics and close observation or admission for infected wounds.
- Appropriate wound care, proper footwear, instruction to patient or caregiver in foot assessment, and return instructions for early infection in noninfected ulcers.

- Off-load pressure with total contact casting, removable cast walkers, and ambulatory braces, splints, half shoes, and sandals.
- Good glycemic control results in faster healing and reduced infection. Assess home glucose monitoring and HgA1c level along with plan to have patient optimize medication through his or her supervising clinician.

Bites

All bites from human beings or animals introduce bacteria into the wound, which predisposes it to infection. These wounds are considered tetanus-prone. Patients may require prophylaxis for viral infections such as hepatitis or rabies as well. Most clinicians elect to immediately close bites on the face but not those on the hand. Hand wounds are closed after 3 to 5 days or are packed and left open. Bites to the torso, arms, and legs are managed in a variety of ways to minimize infection and scarring. All puncture wounds from bites are closed by secondary intention.

For all bites, therapeutic interventions include:
- Document the circumstances surrounding the bite, the source of the bite, signs of infection, number of bites, and the wound type, location, and depth.
- Assess for damage to underlying bone, muscle, tendons, and nerves.
- Irrigate and debride wounds to minimize bacterial contamination.[5]

Dog Bites

Dog bites are grouped roughly into two categories: provoked and unprovoked. Provoked bites are incurred while petting, teasing, or reaching for the dog or entering the animal's territory. Unprovoked attacks occur without warning or provocation and are more likely to be associated with rabies.[19] Actual tissue damage from a dog bite depends on the size and general state of the animal.[19] The wound may consist of multiple punctures, caused by the animal's teeth, or major tissue loss (avulsion) can result if flesh is torn away from underlying structures. Significant crush injuries occur if the animal bites down on a limb.

The dog bite infection rate for patients not receiving antibiotics is 6% to 16%.[12] The most common pathogens in the animal's saliva include *Staphylococcus aureus* and *Pasteurella multocida*.[2] Prophylaxis with amoxicillin/clavulanate potassium (Augmentin) is recommended.

If evidence of infection is present, culture the wound and begin antibiotic therapy. Progressive infection and sepsis warrant intravenous antibiotics, hospital admission, and (in some cases) operative debridement.

Cat Bites

Cats have long, slender fangs that cause puncture wounds rather than lacerations. Cat bites show signs of infection within 12 hours, and need treatment for *P. multocida*. The antibiotic of choice for these infections is penicillin. Prophylaxis with amoxicillin/clavulanate potassium (Augmentin) is recommended, especially for bites on the hand. Wounds are left open unless they are located on the face.[12]

Rabies Prophylaxis

Rabies is introduced into bites from an infected animal. Theoretically, any mammal can be a carrier of rabies. Common carriers are bats, raccoons, foxes, and wild dogs. Herbivores, such as rodents, also can transmit the disease, although this is unlikely. Local animal control offices can provide information about rabies carriers in the area.

Bites from dogs that have been vaccinated, or from any animal that can be observed for 2 weeks, usually do not require rabies prophylaxis. If the animal dies within the 2-week observation period, the brain is autopsied to look for signs of rabies infection. This allows prompt prophylaxis for the victim if disease is detected.

Rabies has a minimum incubation period of 2 weeks in which the virus migrates along the nerves to the brain. Consequently, extremity bites have a longer incubation than face or head wounds. Rabies prophylaxis must be administered before symptoms begin. The disease is fatal in human beings.

TABLE 14-3	**CDC AND PREVENTION RECOMMENDATIONS FOR RABIES PROPHYLAXIS**

Passive Immunity
- Rabies immune globulin (RIG)
  - 20 units/kg
  - Give half the dose intramuscularly and inject the other half locally into the wound.
  - Inject in the deltoid for adults and in the anterolateral thigh in children.

Active Immunity
- Human diploid cell vaccine (HDCV)
  - Give 1 mL intramuscularly on days 0, 3, 7, 14, and 28.
  - Give 1 mL intramuscularly only on days 0 and 3 if the patient had been immunized preexposure.

Data from Denke, N. J. (2010). Wound management. In P. K. Howard & R. A. Steinmann (Eds.), *Sheehy's emergency nursing: Principles and practice* (6th ed., pp. 111–126). St. Louis, MO: Mosby.

Rabies prophylaxis is initiated routinely if a bat, wild animal, or domestic animal that cannot be observed adequately caused the wound. Table 14-3 provides current guidelines for rabies prophylaxis.

Many states require that all animal bites be reported. Refer to local guidelines to determine requirements in your practice area.[20]

REFERENCES

1. Perelman, V. S., Francis, G. J., Rutledge, T., Foote, J., Martino, F., & Dranitsaris, G. (2004). Sterile versus nonsterile gloves for repair of uncomplicated lacerations in the emergency department: A randomized controlled trial. *Annuals of Emergency Medicine, 43*, 362–370.
2. Denke, N. J. (2010). Wound management. In P. K. Howard & R. A. Steinmann (Eds.), *Sheehy's emergency nursing: Principles and practice* (6th ed., pp. 111–126). St. Louis, MO: Mosby.
3. Grey, J. E., Enoch, S., & Harding, K. G. (2006). Wound assessment. *BMJ, 332*(7536), 285–288.
4. Roberts, J., & Hedges, J. (Eds.). (2009). *Clinical procedures in emergency medicine* (4th ed.). Philadelphia, PA: Saunders.
5. Hardy, M. A. (1989). The biology of scar formation. *Physical Therapy, 69*(12), 1014–1024.
6. Simon, D. A., Dix, F. P., & McCollum, C. N. (2004). Management of venous leg ulcers. *BMJ, 328*(7452), 1358–1362.
7. Grey, J. E., Harding, K. G., & Enoch, S. (2006). Pressure ulcers. *BMJ, 332*(7539), 472–475.
8. Bader, M. S. (2008). Diabetic foot infection. *American Family Physician, 78*(1), 71–79.
9. Lammers, R. (2010). Methods of wound closure. In J. Roberts & J. Hedges (Eds.), *Clinical procedures in emergency medicine* (5th ed., pp. 592–633). Philadelphia, PA: Saunders.
10. Gabriel, A. (2011, May 19). *Wound irrigation.* Retrieved from http://emedicine.medscape.com/article/1895071-overview
11. Tintinalli, J., Gabor, D., & Stapczynski, J. (2004). *Emergency medicine: A comprehensive study guide* (6th ed.). New York, NY: McGraw-Hill.
12. Simon, B., & Hern, H. (2010). Wound management principles. In J. Marx, R. Hockenberger, & R. Walls (Eds.), *Rosen's emergency medicine concepts and clinical practice* (7th ed.). St. Louis, MO: Mosby.
13. Centers for Disease Control and Prevention. (2011). Updated recommendations for use of tetanus toxoid, reduced diphtheria toxoid and acellular pertussis (Tdap) vaccine from the Advisory Committee on Immunizations Practices, 2010. *Morbidity and Mortality Weekly Report, 60*(1), 13–15.
14. Windle, M. L. (2011, January 31). *Topical anesthesia.* Retrieved from http://emedicine.medscape.com/article/109673-overview#al
15. Betts, J. (2003). Review: Wound cleansing with water does not differ from no cleansing or cleansing with other solutions for rates of wound infection or healing. *Evidence-Based Nursing, 6*(3), 81.
16. Hiller, K. M., & Li, J. (2011, February 15). *Antibiotics—a review of ED use.* Retrieved from http://emedicine.medscape.com/article/816704-overview
17. University of Utah. (n.d.). *Ballistics.* Retrieved from http://library.med.utah.edu/WebPath/TUTORIAL/GUNS/GUNBLST.html
18. Smock, W. (2010). Forensic emergency medicine. In J. Marx, R. Hockenberger, & R. Walls (Eds.), *Rosen's emergency medicine concepts and clinical practice* (7th ed.). St. Louis, MO: Mosby.
19. Denke, N. (2009). Wound management. In P. K. Howard & R. A. Steinmann (Eds.), *Sheehy's emergency nursing: Principles and practice* (6th ed., p 111–126). St. Louis, Mo: Mosby.
20. Schaider, J., Hayden, S. R., Wolfe, R., Barkin, R. M., & Rosen, P. (Eds.). (2006). *Rosen and Barkin's 5-minute emergency medicine consult* (2nd ed.). Philadelphia, PA: Lippincott Williams & Wilkins.

Procedural Sedation

Lauren Wheatley McCauley

Concern for comfort and alleviating pain and suffering are fundamental to emergency nursing practice and emergency department (ED) care. Sedation is used in the ED setting when the patient's condition is urgent or emergent, requiring the use of one or more drugs to relieve anxiety and pain.[1] Sedation is also used to induce central nervous system depression (resulting in a decreased level of consciousness) to achieve the intervention or to perform a diagnostic procedure.[1] Procedural sedation consists of the use of sedatives or dissociative agents to allow a patient tolerate an unpleasant procedure. The emergency nurse's goal is to minimize anxiety and pain during the interventions or diagnostic procedures.[2] Using moderate sedation, previously known as conscious sedation, prior to procedures is becoming commonplace in the ED; however, it is not without risks. Specialized knowledge of sedation techniques and interventions is critical. This chapter defines and discusses implications for procedural sedation in the ED setting. Safe nursing care and practice before, during, and following the procedure (including medication administration, pharmacology, definitions for levels of anesthesia, regulatory guidelines, and age-specific indications) will be addressed.

The steps of sedation in the ED setting are:
- Presedation assessment and patient and family education
- Ongoing assessments during sedation and the procedure
- Postprocedure recovery and assessments
- Postprocedure discharge instructions and education

The emergency nurse's primary focus is to ensure patient safety through safe medication administration, anticipation of untoward events, airway management, patient education, and discharge instructions. Table 15-1 explains the different levels of sedation used for procedural sedation.[3]

Following institutional policies and procedures surrounding sedation is necessary. Procedural sedation policies and procedures should include the regulatory, state, and licensing specifics. The use of anesthetic pharmacological or dissociative agents for procedural sedation or analgesia in the ED setting is governed by nationally recognized guidelines as well as institutional policies and procedures that include identification of clinical indications; medical staff and allied health staff credentialing; and emergency nurse education, training, and competencies. State law and nursing scopes of practice dictate nursing administration of anesthetic or dissociative agents.[1]

USE OF PROCEDURAL SEDATION IN THE EMERGENCY DEPARTMENT

A variety of procedures that occur in the ED setting have the potential to increase pain, discomfort, and anxiety in patients. Procedural sedation can alleviate pain and anxiety in the ED setting. The emergency nurse must have special knowledge, skills, and competencies to administer medications for procedural sedation. Nurses who meet the competencies are able to manage procedural sedation within their institutional guidelines. This task is performed under the direct supervision of a physician credentialed by the institution. Compliance with regulatory, legislative, institutional, and professional standards of care is required.[2]

Therapeutic, diagnostic, or surgical procedures that may require procedural sedation include[4]:
- Laceration repair
- Invasive procedures
- Burn or abrasion debridement
- Cardioversion
- Fracture reduction or dislocation
- Imaging procedures
- Interventional imaging procedures
- Lumbar punctures

TABLE 15-1 SEDATION DEFINITIONS

Minimal Sedation (Anxiolysis)
- Normal response to verbal commands
- Coordination and cognitive function may be impaired
- Airway reflexes intact; no effect on cardiac or ventilations

Moderate Sedation (Conscious Sedation)
- Decreased level of consciousness that is drug-induced
- Purposeful response to verbal and/or light touch
- Airway reflexes intact, spontaneous respirations are normal, and no airway adjuncts needed
- Cardiac function not usually affected

Deep Sedation
- Drug-induced depression of consciousness
- Patient is not easily aroused to verbal or light touch, but will respond following repeated stimulation
- Airway reflexes may not be intact, ventilatory function may not be able to be independently maintained, and airway adjuncts may be needed to maintain ventilations
- Cardiac function not usually affected

General Anesthesia
- Drug induced loss of consciousness
- Patient not arousable
- Unable to maintain independent ventilatory function. Airway adjuncts such as positive pressure ventilation needed to maintain open airway.
- Cardiac function may be affected and impaired

Dissociative Sedation[9]:
- Trance-like catatonic state
- Profound analgesia
- Amnesia
- Airway reflexes intact; no effect on cardiac or ventilations

Data from American Society of Anesthesiologists. (2009, October 21). *Continuum of depth of sedation definition of general anesthesia levels of sedation/analgesia.* Retrieved from http://www.asahq.org/For-Members/Clinical-Information/~/media/For%20Members/documents/Standards%20Guidelines%20Stmts/Continuum%20of%20Depth%20of%20Sedation.ashx

The goals of procedural sedation include:
- Decreasing the patient's fear, anxiety, and pain related to the procedure
- Maintaining spontaneous ventilation, airway patency, and reflexes
- Maintaining a level of sedation where patient remains arousable, can cooperate, and can follow verbal commands
- Reducing the patient's recall of procedures

Registered Nurse Competencies

The emergency nurse managing the care of the patient receiving moderate sedation or assisting with procedural sedation must be able to monitor and respond appropriately to possible adverse reactions to medications administered, changes in vital signs, level of consciousness, airway management, and oxygen saturation. Recommended preparations include:
- Proficiency in airway management
- Advanced cardiac life support (ACLS)
- Pediatric advanced life support (PALS), if caring for pediatric patients
- Knowledge of medications administered, including actions, side effects, half-life, pharmacological dosages and routes of administration, antagonists, and reversal agents for the type of sedation administered
- Ability to identify and manage cardiac dysrhythmias[5]
- Institutional competency for moderate sedation

It is the position of the Emergency Nurses Association that a registered nurse may administer sedation medications in the presence of a physician, advanced practice registered nurse, or other health care professional credentialed and privileged for procedural sedation.[2] The state where the nurse is licensed and working defines the scope of nursing practice. As each state has varying scopes of practice, know your state's scope of practice, as well as institutional guidelines, policies, and procedures on procedural sedation. Each institution has different guidelines to credential medical staff, allied health providers, and advanced practice nurses. Also ensure that the physician or practitioner ordering the moderate sedation is credentialed and has the privileges to manage moderate sedation.

Staffing Requirements

The Joint Commission Standard PC.03.01.01 requires that there be a sufficient amount of staff to ensure patient safety before, during, and following the procedure.[6] According to The Joint Commission's minimum requirements, the person performing the sedation procedure must be a nurse who is competent to administer the medications and to monitor and recover the patient.[6] When the condition of the patient or the complexity of the procedure requires the diversion of the designated individual from monitoring the patient, provisions for additional personnel must be made.[6]

Preprocedure Assessment

An assessment of the patient's general health assists clinicians in determining which patients are appropriate for sedation. A documented history and physical assessment by a physician or licensed independent practitioner[1] and immediate reassessment including an American Society of Anesthesiologists (ASA) score are standard practice. The patient's oral intake status, anesthesia plan, and postsedation plan of care should be documented as well.[6]

American Society of Anesthesiologists Physical Status Classification System

The ASA developed a system for scoring the fitness of patients prior to surgery, commonly known as the ASA score. The ASA classifications are as follows[7]:

- Class 1: A normal healthy patient
- Class 2: A patient with mild systemic disease
- Class 3: A patient with severe systemic disease
- Class 4: A patient with severe systemic disease that is a constant threat to life
- Class 5: A moribund patient who is not expected to survive without the operation

Not all patients will fall neatly into just one class. Patients who are Class 3 or higher are considered to be at increased risk for complications compared to healthier patients.[8] Being aware of the ASA classification helps the emergency nurse anticipate potential adverse events with procedural and moderate sedation, such as decreased level of consciousness and inability of the patient to independently manage airway patency. Proactive planning and being aware of the anesthesia plan ensures that appropriate staffing and necessary emergency equipment are readily available. In addition to determining the ASA score, the health care provider should perform a complete history and physical and the nurse should review this information prior to the procedure.

Informed Consent

Informed consent is required for the procedure and may include separate consent for moderate sedation depending on institutional policy. Awareness of institutional policy and procedure regarding informed consent and moderate sedation is necessary.

Time-Out Procedures

Patient safety is of utmost importance and is the goal of the emergency nurse as a patient advocate. Each institution has specific guidelines that encompass these requirements. The "time-out" or procedural pause is meant to be a deliberate interaction and collaboration between the patient, provider, and staff involved in the patient's procedural care. It is meant to occur immediately prior to the procedure. It is vital for the emergency nurse and physician to follow the institutional policy and procedure for time-out, ensuring the correct patient, the correct procedure, and the correct location and laterality.

ASSESSMENT, PREPARATION, AND CONTINUOUS MONITORING FOR PROCEDURAL SEDATION

During procedural sedation the emergency nurse is responsible for the assessment, preparation, and continuous monitoring of the patient. The individual components of this process are discussed below.

Patient Identification

- Use two patient identifiers, such as full patient name and patient's date of birth.

Verification of Order

- Review written or electronic physician order, including medications ordered and that proper consent has been obtained.

History and Physical Assessment

- Review medications
  - Home medications
  - Herbal and over-the-counter preparations
  - Medications received in the ED
- Allergies
  - Review, validate, and update
- Obtain accurate height and weight
  - Weight should be actual, not stated
  - Document patient's weight in kilograms, as most medications ordered will be based on the patient's weight
- Obtain baseline vital signs including:
  - Temperature
  - Heart rate
  - Cardiac rhythm
  - Blood pressure
  - Respiratory rate and effort
  - Pulse oximetry

Vascular Access

- Maintained throughout procedure.
- Do not discontinue vascular access until immediately prior to discharge.

Last Oral Intake or Fasting Status

- The combination of vomiting and loss of protective airway reflexes is rare during procedural sedation, resulting in a low risk for aspiration.[1]
- Follow institutional guidelines for fasting prior to procedural sedation.
- General guidelines are as follows:

- If the patient has recently eaten and the sedation may pose significant risk for aspiration, consider airway protection.
- For nonemergent procedures, adults and children over 3 years old should be nothing by mouth (NPO) for 8 hours after any heavy or fatty meal and for 6 hours after a light meal.
- Children under 3 years old should be NPO for solid food for 4 to 6 hours but may have clear liquids up to 2 hours prior to the procedure and breast milk up to 4 hours prior to procedure.[8,9]

Emergency Supplies and Equipment

- Emergency crash cart with emergency medications and supplies
- Monitor and defibrillator
- Airway equipment
  - Alternative advanced airway device in addition to an endotracheal tube in the event of a difficult airway
  - Appropriate-sized oral airway and nasal airway
  - Bag-mask
  - Administer oxygen to the patient and set up suction in the room

Reversal Agents

- Reversal agents must be immediately available, preferably at the bedside.

Continuous Monitoring

- Continuously monitor the patient (have an unobstructed view of the patient and monitoring equipment) throughout the procedure and recovery period.
- Observe for respiratory depression, ischemia, and deepening levels of sedation.
- Follow institutional policy and procedures related to frequency of monitoring and documentation before, during, and after sedation and procedure.
- Monitor the patient's heart rhythm, blood pressure, respiratory rate, pulse oximetry, and exhaled carbon dioxide (CO_2).
- Document the patient's level of sedation. The Ramsay sedation scale is a useful tool for this documentation (Table 15-2).
- Postanesthesia recovery (PAR) score or Aldrete score (institutional policy governs whether this is done by the health care provider or nurse):
  - Assess score immediately following the procedure and prior to discharge.
  - PAR score includes:
    - Patient's ability to move extremities to commands

TABLE 15-2	**RAMSAY SEDATION SCALE**

Light Sedation
1 = patient is anxious, agitated, or restless
2 = patient is cooperative, orientated, and tranquil

Moderate Sedation
3 = patient is drowsy
4 = patient is asleep, but responds when stimulated verbally or with light tactile stimuli

Deep Sedation
5 = patient is asleep with a slow response (not easily aroused), retains purposeful response to repeated or painful stimuli

Anesthesia
6 = Patient has no response

- Respiratory evaluation that addresses the patient's ability to cough and deep breathe
- Circulation (measured by blood pressure)
- Level of consciousness
- Oxygen saturation on oxygen or room air
- Each aspect of the PAR score has a numeric value. If patient is unimpaired, the score equals 10. Use the PAR score to determine patient's status to baseline before discharge.[2]

The benefit of exhaled carbon dioxide monitoring is that it can be an early detector of hypercapnia, which often precedes hypoxia.

CONSIDERATIONS IN PEDIATRIC SEDATION

Three categories of indications for pediatric sedation are minor trauma (e.g., laceration repair, fracture relocations or reductions), instrumentation, and imaging studies.[9] Medications used are sedatives, analgesics, and dissociative drugs. Caregiver involvement in understanding the anesthesia plan and postprocedure instructions should be primary considerations.

In addition to routine assessment, in the pediatric population additional considerations include[9]:

- Time of day:
  - If it is close to the patient's nap time, less sedation may be indicated.
- Fasting prior to the procedure may increase irritability or lack of cooperation.
- Previous experiences with hospitals, medical professionals, diagnostic procedures, or treatments may heighten fear and anxiety.

- Anxiety of caregivers.
- Age-specific developmental awareness:
  - Infants: absent cooperation
  - Toddlers: variable cooperation
    - Distractible: offer distractions such as reading stories or guided imagery
  - Older children: may have good cooperation

Pediatric patients may be more agitated during sedation, which may lead to complications including the inability to proceed with the procedure, the possibility of the patient waking during the procedure, or the need for additional sedating medications that can compromise patient safety. Developmentally, pediatric patients may not understand how the pharmacological agents will make them feel or medications effects. This fear of the unknown may increase resistance or agitation.[10]

PHARMACOLOGICAL OPTIONS FOR MODERATE SEDATION

A variety of pharmacological options induce moderate sedation. Benzodiazepines, such as midazolam (Versed) and lorazepam (Ativan) may be given alone or in conjunction with an opiate, such as morphine or fentanyl (Sublimaze). The synergistic dynamics when benzodiazepines are given with opiates may increase the risk for respiratory depression. Always have reversal agents at the bedside. Etomidate and propofol (Diprivan) have the potential to result in deep sedation, requiring additional monitoring and staffing. Ketamine, a dissociative agent, is often used in the pediatric population, as the emergence phenomenon is generally milder than in adults.[11]

The goal of administering these medications is to adequately sedate a patient. This is achieved when a patient has one or more of the following characteristics:

- Appearance of being visibly relaxed
- Patient report of feeling relaxed
- Slurred speech
- Exhibition of arousable sleep

Oversedation

Reversal agents must be immediately available. Despite diligence in monitoring a sedated patient and because moderate sedation is a component of the sedation continuum, patients may unintentionally become oversedated. Patients may be too deeply sedated when:

- They are asleep and respond slowly to stimulation.
- They are not easily aroused but retain purposeful response to repeated or painful stimulation.
- They have difficulty maintaining their airways.

Follow institutional policy and procedure for dosing and reporting use of reversal agents. A minimum of 2 additional hours of monitoring is required following the use of a reversal agent.

Other pharmacological agents are available to achieve sedation; they have not been discussed here but are gaining popularity in emergency care settings and procedural areas because of their rapid onset and short duration of action.[12] Some examples include:

- Propofol
- Ketofol (a combination of ketamine and propofol)
- Brevital
- Etomidate

These drugs are intended to produce a level of sedation beyond moderate sedation, and studies show they can be used safely in the ED setting.[6] As the use of pharmacological anesthetic agents becomes more commonplace in the ED setting for procedural sedation, the importance of knowing and following safe practice and careful preparation, administration, and monitoring is vital to prevent respiratory depression and harmful sequelae.[1]

POSTSEDATION RECOVERY AND DISCHARGE

Document the PAR score immediately following procedure completion and again at the end of the recovery period. Monitoring during the recovery period includes heart rate, cardiac rhythm, blood pressure, oxygen saturation, Ramsay sedation scale, and a pain scale if appropriate.[11] Continuously observe and record these per the institution's policy. Do not leave a sedated patient alone until the recovery period is complete. There should be specific criteria for discontinuing sedation monitoring and discharging the patient.

Discharge Planning

Planning for the patient's discharge begins when planning for the procedure. Patients receiving procedural sedation require a responsible adult to take them home at discharge and, if necessary, to care for them while the drugs remain in their system. Medications may impair the patient's memory. Provide discharge instructions to patients and their caregivers *prior* to the procedure to help with compliance following the directions after the procedure.

Sedation discharge instructions often include the following:

- Do not drive or operating any equipment
- Do not cook
- Do not sign any legal papers
- Do not drink any alcoholic beverages, including beer and wine
- Do not take any sedatives, tranquilizers, or pain medications unless prescribed

- Common side effects of the medications administered
- Medication reconciliation

Provide written and verbal instructions and have the patient and caregiver repeat back the information to establish understanding.

Procedural sedation in the ED setting is becoming commonplace as more procedures and diagnostics are being done in the outpatient arena. The use of moderate sedation for procedural sedation is a high-risk procedure and requires specialized skill, training, and annual competencies by the emergency nurse and credentialing of the medical staff to supervise and order the sedation. Knowledge of evidence-based practice standards, research, emergency procedures, medication effects, reversal agents, and indications for adults and pediatrics is vital for safe patient care in patients undergoing moderate sedation in the ED setting.[2]

REFERENCES

1. Godwin, S. A., Caro, D. A., Wolf, S. J., Jagoda, A. S., Charles, R., Maret, B. E., & Moore, J. (2005). Clinical policy: Procedural sedation and analgesia in the emergency department. *Annals of Emergency Medicine, 45*(2), 177–196.
2. Emergency Nurses Association. (2005). *Procedural sedation and analgesia in the emergency department* [position statement]. Retrieved from http://www.ena.org/SiteCollection Documents/Position%20Statements/Procedural_Sedation ENA_PS.pdf
3. American Society of Anesthesiologists. (2009, October 21). *Continuum of depth of sedation definition of general anesthesia levels of sedation/analgesia.* Retrieved from http://www. asahq.org/For-Members/Clinical-Information/~/media/For %20Members/documents/Standards%20Guidelines%20Stmts /Continuum%20of%20Depth%20of%20Sedation.ashx
4. Sheta, S. A. (2010). Procedural sedation analgesia. *Saudi Journal of Anesthesia, 4*(1), 11–16.
5. Air & Surface Transport Nurses Association; American Academy of Emergency Medicine; American Association of Critical Care Nurses; American College of Emergency Physicians; American Nurses Association; American Radiological Nurses Association; American Society for Pain Management Nursing; Emergency Nurses Association; National Association of Children's Hospitals and Related Institutions. (2008, March 20). *Procedural sedation consensus statement.* Retrieved from http://www.ena.org/SiteCollectionDocuments/Position%20 Statements/Procedural_Sedation_Consensus_Statement.pdf
6. The Joint Commission. (2008). *Comprehensive accreditation manual for hospitals: The official handbook.* Oakbrook Terrace, IL: Author.
7. American Society of Anesthesiologists. (n.d.). *ASA physical status classification.* Retrieved from http://www.asahq.org/ clinical/physicalstatus.htm
8. Kost, M. (2004). *Moderate sedation/analgesia: Core competencies for practice* (2nd ed.). St. Louis, MO: Saunders.
9. Krauss, B., & Green, S. M. (2006). Procedural sedation and analgesia in children. *The Lancet, 367,* 766–780.
10. Lightdate, J. R., Valim, C., Mahoney, L. B., Wong, S., DiNardo, J., & Goldman, D. A. (2010). Agitation during procedural sedation and analgesia in children. *Clinical Pediatrics, 49*(1), 35–42.
11. Windle, M. L. (2011, April 5). *Procedural sedation.* Retrieved from http://emedicine.medscape.com/article/109695-overview
12. Holder, A. (2010, October 25). *Sedation.* Retrieved from http:// emedicine.medscape.com/article/809993-overview

Laboratory Specimens

Linda K. Cook and Polly Gerber Zimmermann

Laboratory results establish a baseline, identify trends, diagnose a particular condition, and monitor the treatment plan.

GENERAL PRINCIPLES OF SPECIMEN COLLECTION

The following are general principles for all specimen collection:
- Identify the patient with two unique identifiers, such as name and date of birth. See institutional policy regarding which identifiers should be used.
- Prepare the site antiseptically.
  - Do not use alcohol to prepare the skin if an alcohol level is to be drawn.
  - When using ChloraPrep® for cleaning a puncture site, use a vigorous up and down motion and allow the site to air-dry.
- Observe standard precautions and hand hygiene.
- Label the specimen collection tubes and bottles at the patient's bedside after specimens are collected as per institutional policy.
- Avoid drawing excessive amounts of blood, especially from critically ill patients. The volume of blood collected often exceeds the need and can contribute to anemia. Consider pediatric tubes for fragile veins or an anemic patient.[1]

Use the following procedures to prevent hemolysis of blood specimens[1]:
- Promptly transport the specimen to the laboratory.
- Use a properly sized syringe (no larger than 20 mL) to prevent excessive suction.
- If transferring blood from the syringe into blood collection tubes, allow the vacuum of the tubes to facilitate the transfer of the blood specimen. Do not exert pressure to force blood through the needle into the tubes. Use a needleless transfer device, if available, to decrease the risk of needlesticks and spray.
- Drawing blood specimens through a small needle or catheter can rupture the blood cells and potentially cause inaccurate results that require recollection of blood specimens.
- Gently invert the tube approximately five times to mix the blood specimen with any preservative that may be present in the tube.[2] Do not invert tubes without additives to reduce the incidence of hemolysis.
- Release the tourniquet as the final tube is filling. See Chapter 10, Intravenous Therapy, for more information.

> Hemolyzed specimens can occur in as many as 3.3% of all routine samples, nearly five times higher than other causes for unsuitable blood specimens.[3] Hemolysis is less likely when blood is collected in evacuated tubes rather than with a syringe.[2]

Order of Specimen Tube Draws

Proper tube order prevents cross-contamination of preservatives that are found in specimen collection tubes. The Clinical and Laboratory Standards Institute (CLSI) indicates the order should be as follows[4]:
- Blood cultures: This minimizes potential contamination.
- Light blue: This tube contains sodium citrate, which removes calcium. This prevents contamination of the clot activator and interference with coagulation cascade.
- Red: This tube has no additive and is for the collection of serum.
- "Tiger" or Yellow: These serum separator tubes contain a polymer gel and clot activator in order to separate the serum with centrifuge.
- Green: This tube contains lithium heparin.
- Lavender: This tube contains ethylenediaminetetraacetic acid (EDTA), an anticoagulant additive that chelates calcium.

- Gray: This tube contains sodium fluoride and potassium oxalate anticoagulant to inhibit glycolysis.

BLOOD COLLECTION PROCEDURES

Venous Blood Samples

The larger median cubital and cephalic veins are the usual choice for venous access, but the basilic vein on the dorsum of the arm or dorsal hand veins are also acceptable. Foot or ankle veins are to be used as a last resort because of the higher probability of complications to the site.

Use the following techniques to find a good site for venous access:

- Lower the extremity so that the site is below the level of the heart.
- Apply a warm compress to the area.
- Use good, direct lighting.
- Palpate for a vein using fingertips. Some large veins are deep and cannot be visualized but can be palpated. If available, use an ultrasound vein finder to assist in locating veins.

> Using your nondominant hand will sometimes enhance sensitivity with palpation for vein location.

Once access is established, to obtain the best specimen follow these guidelines:

- Avoid having the patient repeatedly clench and unclench his or her fist when blood is being draw for potassium; making a single fist is acceptable. Fist exercises, with excessive tourniquet use, before venipuncture may cause an elevation of potassium as high as 1 mEq/L.[1,5]
- Limit the use of a tourniquet to no more than 2 minutes (1 minute is optimal) during specimen collection.
- Avoid using a site that is heavily scarred, is excessively swollen, has a hematoma, is on the affected side after a mastectomy, is an extremity affected by stroke or neurological injury, or has a fistula in the same extremity.
- Do not use a pulsating, thick-walled vessel (classic for an artery) or a cordlike, easily rolled vessel (classic for thrombosed vein) for blood specimen collection.
- Avoid drawing a blood specimen from a vein above the site of an infusing intravenous solution since this can lead to false results.

Venous Access Procedure

- Perform hand hygiene. Don clean examination gloves and prepare the site with available antiseptic.
- Palpate the site above the proposed needle entry point; do not touch the actual site.

- Stabilize the vein with the thumb of the nondominant hand.
- Draw the skin taut below the site to prevent the vein from moving when punctured.
- Insert the needle at a 30-degree angle with the bevel facing up (downward in small children). An angle steeper than this increases the risk of passing through the vein.
- Draw blood into specimen tubes in the order established by facility policy. See "Order of Specimen Tube Draws" which begins on page 167.
- Remove gloves, dispose of supplies, and perform hand hygiene.

Peripherally Inserted Central Catheter, Central Line, or Port

In preparing to collect blood specimens, it is important to review what laboratory tests have been ordered to ensure gathering of the appropriate supplies. It is important when using an established intravenous (IV) or central line for blood collection that the nurse clears the IV or central line from potential contamination from recently administered IV fluids or other medications. For additional information, see Chapter 10, Intravenous Therapy.

General principles for clearing the IV or central line include the following:

- Gather required supplies, such as the following:
  - Clean examination gloves
  - Three to four prefilled 10-mL normal saline flushes
  - Alcohol wipes and/or chlorhexidine
  - Replacement IV adaptor hub as needed
  - 10-mL syringes and blood transfer device
  - Blood collection tubes (types depend on specimens being collected)
  - Heparin flush per institution policy
- Inform the patient of the need to obtain blood specimens.
- Perform hand hygiene. Don clean examination gloves.
- Stop the infusion for at least 2 minutes prior to the blood specimen draw. If the central line has multiple lumens, stop all infusions and clamp the lumens not being used for the specimen collection.
- Aggressively cleanse the hub of the IV adaptor with an alcohol wipe or chlorhexadine.
- Flush the peripheral line or lumen being used with 10 mL of normal saline.
- Attach a 10-mL syringe and withdraw 8 to 10 mL of blood from the lumen and discard.
- Attach a 10-mL syringe and withdraw 10 mL of blood and transfer to the blood collection tubes until all specimens are collected.

- Flush the lumen with 10 mL of normal saline or heparin as per institutional protocol.
- Replace the hub of the IV adaptor used for the blood draw.
- Unclamp any lumens currently in use and clamped and resume all infusions.
- Label all blood collection tubes per institutional policy and send to the laboratory for processing.
- Discard supplies and perform hand hygiene.

Additional tips for specimen collection with a peripheral line or port:

- When using a peripheral line, slight manipulation of the catheter (pull back slightly on the catheter, move catheter from left to right) may be required to facilitate withdrawal of the blood.
- Do not use a peripheral line for blood specimen collection if there is a risk of compromising the integrity of the site when completed. Perform a venipuncture instead.
- Do not leave the tourniquet on for prolonged periods of time, especially if drawing a lactate or potassium level.
- Turn off IV infusion and discard an adequate amount of blood to ensure accuracy of the results.
- If collecting the blood specimen from a saline lock or unused port of a multiple lumen central line, flush with saline or heparin lock solution per institutional policy.
- If available, use needleless blood collection systems when collecting blood specimens from a peripheral IV line or central line to reduce the risk of needlestick and exposure to blood.

Arterial Puncture for Blood Gas Collection

Prior to the collection of an arterial blood gas (ABG) specimen from a radial artery, perform an Allen test to ensure adequate collateral circulation from the ulnar artery in the event that postcannulation circulation is compromised in the radial artery. Follow institutional policies regarding who can and how ABG specimens are collected.

General principles guiding collection of an arterial blood sample include the following:

- Gather the appropriate supplies. Inform the patient of the need to obtain the ABG specimen.
- Perform hand hygiene. Don clean examination gloves.
- Perform an Allen test. The modified Allen test is an option for the radial site to check the collateral ulnar circulation.[4]
  - Apply pressure to the radial and ulnar arteries simultaneously.
  - Have the patient open and close his or her hand repeatedly. The hand should blanch.
  - Release the pressure on the ulnar artery while maintaining the pressure on the radial artery.
  - Pinkness should return in 6 to 7 seconds.

- If the hand remains pale, use another site for the arterial stick.
- Prepare the arterial site by cleansing the site following hospital protocol.
- Immobilize the artery between two fingers of the non-dominant hand (be careful not to contaminate the puncture site).
- Hold the syringe like a pencil, needle bevel up. Access the artery at a 30- to 45-degree angle for radial or brachial artery (90 degrees for the femoral artery).
- Watch for spontaneous filling of the syringe (with the plunger moving). This usually indicates that the needle is in the artery. If the syringe does not fill spontaneously, reposition the needle.
- Use dry gauze to apply direct manual pressure to the puncture site for at least 5 minutes after withdrawing the needle. Longer periods of direct manual pressure may be required in patients receiving thrombotic or anticoagulation therapy.
- Apply a pressure dressing to the site.
- Care of the specimen includes the following steps:
  - Expel all air bubbles from the sample syringe.
  - Remove the needle and cap the syringe with the rubber cap.
  - Place the syringe in a container of ice unless the sample will be analyzed immediately. If an i-STAT system is used, directly apply the specimen to the cartridge and process.
  - Immediately send the specimen for testing.

> In patients with a systolic blood pressure less than 100 mm Hg, the syringe for an ABG specimen may not fill spontaneously. Manually withdraw the plunger to collect the specimen.

Interpretation of ABG Values

Once ABG results are received, interpretation of the results will influence additional interventions and facilitate in determining the medical diagnosis of the patient.

What are considered normal ABG values may vary slightly depending on the institution's range of normal values. Typical normal values are as follows:

- pH: 7.35 to 7.45
- $PaCO_2$: 35 to 45 mm Hg
- PaO_2: 80 to 100 mm Hg
- HCO_3: 22 to 26 mEq/L

Steps for Interpreting ABG Results

- Evaluate the pH result.
  - Is it acidotic, alkalotic, or normal?
  - Low values of pH indicate acidosis; high levels indicate alkalosis.

- Determine the primary cause of the pH disturbance by evaluating the $PaCO_2$ and HCO_3 results in relation to the pH.
  - Is it respiratory or metabolic?
  - Overall, primary alterations in respiratory function are relatively fast while alterations in metabolic function occur over hours to days.
  - In respiratory changes, $PaCO_2$ usually goes in the opposite direction as the pH abnormality.
  - In metabolic changes, the HCO_3 usually goes in the same direction of the pH abnormality.
- When analyzing the pH result, evaluate for compensation.
  - A normal pH level in the presence of other abnormal results often indicates compensation. Look at the values that would respond and compensate in the presence of the primary disorder. For example, if the patient has a normal range pH with an elevated $PaCO_2$ (respiratory acidosis), consider the HCO_3 level.

If compensation is present as evident by the pH result, determine if it is partial or complete. See Chapter 18, Respiratory Emergencies, for more information.

Heel Stick[6]

In children younger than 1 year, blood specimens are often best obtained by using the heel-stick method. Use the outside plantar surface; do not use the center of the heel. The heel-stick method is not appropriate for blood cultures.

General principles of the heel-stick method include the following:
- Place the infant supine and allow the foot to dangle lower than the torso.
- Warm the foot for 3 to 5 minutes using a warm, moist cloth or chemical warmer to promote blood flow to the area.
- Avoid repuncture of an old puncture site.
- Use appropriate puncture depth to avoid inadvertently striking the calcaneus and causing osteomyelitis. Premature infants should have a puncture depth of 0.65 to 0.85 mm. In larger infants the puncture depth should be 1 mm. Never puncture deeper than 2 mm.[6]
- Do not use a scooping motion against the surface of the skin to move the blood into the collection container. This can activate platelets and may cause hemolysis.
- Maintain adequate blood flow to obtain the entire specimen by intermittently releasing the pressure on the foot or by lowering the foot.

OTHER SPECIMEN COLLECTION

Blood Cultures

Collect blood specimens for culture and sensitivity using a sterile (rather than a clean) technique to avoid contamination with skin's normal flora, which can lead to false-positive results. Careful skin preparation and sterile specimen handling are essential. Larger amounts of blood (8–10 mL per bottle) are desired when obtaining blood cultures, although most laboratories can perform blood cultures on much less than the recommended volumes if no more blood is available. Please consult your institutional guidelines to confirm the amount of blood needed. It is best to draw cultures before initiation of antibiotic therapy. In cases of suspected sepsis (e.g., suspected meningococcemia), do not allow difficulty obtaining blood cultures to delay administration of lifesaving medications.

Procedure for Blood Culture Specimen Collection

To obtain blood culture specimens, perform the following steps:
- Gather equipment
  - Sterile 20-mL syringe (or two 10-mL syringes) and needle for each set of cultures to be drawn
  - Alcohol wipes
  - Chlorhexidine for skin antisepsis
  - Tourniquet
  - Blood culture vials (aerobic and anaerobic) in the age-appropriate size; one or two sets as ordered
  - 2 × 2 inch gauze pad
  - Adhesive strip
  - Sterile gloves
- Inform the patient of the need to collect blood cultures.
- Perform hand hygiene.
- Prepare the venipuncture site by scrubbing the site with alcohol followed by chlorhexidine. Let the area dry before proceeding.
- Allow the site to air-dry. Do not touch the site after cleansing.
- Remove the caps of the blood culture vials and cleanse rubber stoppers with alcohol wipes (not povidone-iodine).
- Don sterile gloves.
- Perform the venipuncture. Withdraw 18 to 20 mL of blood in adults and 1 mL of blood for each bottle in pediatric patients.
- Release the tourniquet. Place a dry, sterile 2 × 2 inch gauze over the venipuncture site and withdraw the needle. Apply pressure to the venipuncture site and then cover site with an adhesive strip.

- Inject 8 to 10 mL of blood into each adult blood culture bottle and 1 mL into each pediatric bottle (refer to your institutional guidelines to confirm the amount of blood needed). Fill the aerobic blood culture vial, then the anaerobic vial.
- Remove gloves and perform hand hygiene.
- Label samples and transport the specimens to the laboratory.

Urine Specimens

Urine specimens are collected in the emergency department for a variety of common diagnostic procedures such as urinalysis, culture and sensitivity, toxicology screening, pregnancy determination, and electrolyte levels. Urine specimens should be collected using a midstream, clean-catch technique, or by bladder catheterization.

Procedure for Urine Specimen Collection

To collect a urine specimen, perform the following steps:
- Gather the supplies (clean-catch kit, in-and-out catheter kit, or urinary catheter kit).
- Inform the patient of the need for a urine specimen.
- Identify the patient using two identifiers.
- When obtaining a clean-catch specimen, instruct the patient to do the following:
  - Cleanse the urethral opening using appropriate materials.
  - Start the urine flow, stop the flow of urine, and then collect a midstream (not the first, not the last) urine specimen in a sterile container.
- If the specimen must be sterile or the patient is unable to perform a clean-catch procedure, a catheterized specimen is required. Use the following:
  - An indwelling urinary catheter if the catheter will be left in place for ongoing urine drainage or output monitoring
  - A straight catheter for a simple in-and-out procedure
- Send the labeled specimen to the laboratory for processing.

Cerebrospinal Fluid (Lumbar Puncture)[7]

Lumbar puncture is performed to remove samples of cerebrospinal fluid (CSF) in order to evaluate the presence of infection, such as meningitis, or bleeding or to measure CSF pressure. Normal CSF is clear and looks like water. Abnormal CSF may be bloody, cloudy, or yellow. Elevated intracranial pressure is a contraindication to lumbar puncture, as cerebellar herniation can occur. Never delay administration of antibiotics to obtain a lumbar puncture or perform other diagnostic procedures when there is suspected overwhelming infection (sepsis, meningitis, etc.).

Patient Positioning for Lumbar Puncture

- If supine, the patient should be in the tightest fetal position possible, with the shoulders and hips in a straight plane perpendicular to the floor. The patient must be lying down for a valid opening pressure.
- If sitting up, the upper body should rest on a bedside table with the patient's legs supported on a stool or on the floor. Have the patient push his or her lumbosacral spine back toward the practitioner performing the lumbar puncture.
- Avoid excess neck flexion, as it may cause respiratory compromise. The risk is highest in pediatric and sedated patients.[8]

Collection of Cerebrospinal Fluid

- Observe the characteristics of the CSF; it should be clear like water.
- Drain approximately 1 to 1.5 mL of CSF into each tube. Sequentially number the tubes as they are filled. Typical orders for the tubes are:
  - Tube 1: Cell count and differential
  - Tube 2: Gram stain, culture and sensitivities, and other special diagnostic procedures
  - Tube 3: Glucose and protein
  - Tube 4: Cell count and differential
- In pediatric patients, three tubes are usually collected.
- Transport specimens to the laboratory immediately.

Complications of Cerebrospinal Fluid Collection

- Headache is the most common complication, occurring in 5% to 30% of patients, and is most common in younger, thinner females. It is thought to be a result of leakage of fluid through the dural puncture site.[9]
  - To reduce headaches[8,9]:
    - Use smaller needles that split rather than transecting the dural fibers
    - Lay the patient prone for at least 2 hours postprocedure
    - Increase the patient's fluid intake
  - Treatment for a headache can include a blood patch (e.g., autologous blood into the epidural space).
- CSF leakage at the puncture site.
- Change in level of consciousness.
- Signs of infection.

Joint Aspiration

Monitor patients with bleeding disorders and those taking anticoagulants carefully during and after the procedure. General principles for joint aspiration include the following:

- Use sterile technique.
- The joint is positioned in full extension or in 1- to 20-degree flexion to open the joint space.
- After the procedure, apply direct pressure at the puncture site for 2 minutes.
- Aftercare includes the following:
  - Apply an elastic bandage to help stabilize the joint if a large amount of fluid was aspirated.
  - Ice and elevation can help prevent swelling.
  - Avoid excess use of the joint for the next few days.
  - Monitor for signs of infection.

COMMON LABORATORY RESULTS

Complete Blood Count

A complete blood count (CBC) is a routine hematological screening study performed to evaluate a patient's status and can facilitate diagnosis of disease states. Components of a CBC include hemoglobin, hematocrit, total red blood cell count, white blood cell count (with or without a differential), platelet level, mean corpuscular cell volume, mean cell hemoglobin concentration, and mean cell hemoglobin.

Sodium Abnormalities[1]

Approximately 2% to 2.5% of hospitalized patients have alterations in serum sodium levels, with a 15% incidence in critical care patients.[1] Cellular swelling or shrinking occurs depending on whether the sodium level is low or elevated. Primary manifestations of sodium level abnormalities are neurological in nature. Acute mental status changes—ranging from headache and lethargy to confusion and coma—occur in 95% to 100% of patients depending on the rapidity (hours or days) and severity of the alteration in sodium level.[10]

Hyponatremia results from excessive water gain, such as in heart failure, or excessive renal sodium loss. Treatment of hyponatremia caused by heart failure includes fluid restriction and reduction of fluid volume through the use of diuretics. In severe cases of hyponatremia due to sodium loss, infusion of 3% saline may be required.

Hypernatremia results from a water deficit or, less often, excessive gain of sodium. A contributing factor is inability of the patient to obtain adequate fluids as a result of health issues or the unavailability of fluids. Failure to replenish fluid loss during extreme heat or severe vomiting or diarrhea is another factor in developing hypernatremia. The most common cause of hypernatremia in children is diarrhea (40% to 90%).[1] Half of elderly patients with hypernatremia live in nursing homes.[1]

Clinical signs of sodium abnormalities vary but generally depend on the following factors:

TABLE 16-1	SYMPTOMS OF SODIUM ABNORMALITIES	
	EARLY SYMPTOMS	**LATE SYMPTOMS**
Hyponatremia	Malaise, nausea, progression to headache, lethargy, confusion, and obtundation	Stupor, seizures, and coma
Hypernatremia	Altered mental status, weakness, neuromuscular irritability, thirst, dry mucous membranes, poor skin turgor	Severe neurological compromise

- Magnitude of the serum sodium decrease or increase.
- Speed of development (acute versus chronic).
- Cause of abnormality.
- Age. Those most susceptible for hyponatremia are prepubescent children (because of the discrepancy between skull size and brain size) and women who are of menstruating age (estrogen has been shown to impair brain adaptation).[11]

Table 16-1 illustrates early and late symptoms of hyponatremia and hypernatremia.

Potassium Abnormalities[1]

Potassium affects the normal function of muscle cells. Skeletal muscles, especially the large muscles of the legs, are sensitive to hypokalemia, resulting in muscle cramping. The cardiac muscle is most significantly affected. On the electrocardiogram, the T-wave is generally peaked in hyperkalemia and flattened in hypokalemia. Cardiac sensitivity to digitalis is heightened in the setting of hypokalemia. Most clinical signs are not present until the potassium falls below 3.0 mEq/L or rises above 6.0 mEq/L.

Patients with hypokalemia are also at risk for hypomagnesia; the combination of both imbalances increases cardiac irritability and risk for ventricular dysrhythmias. Replacement of potassium is accomplished via the oral or IV route.

The major cause of hyperkalemia is decreased renal excretion (normally 80% is excreted through the kidney). Patients may require education regarding salt substitutes, as their content is mostly potassium. Treatment of hyperkalemia includes loop diuretics and oral or rectal administration of cation exchange resins such as sodium polystyrene (Kayexelate). Severe hyperkalemia can be treated with the IV administration of calcium gluconate, regular insulin, 50% dextrose, and sodium bicarbonate. The combination of these medications temporarily forces potassium back into the cells, allowing time to initiate other treatments including hemodialysis.

> Hypokalemia has been estimated to occur in as many as 75% of cancer patients at some point in their illness.[1]

> Angiotensin-converting enzyme (ACE) inhibitor medications predispose individuals to hyperkalemia.

Magnesium Abnormalities

Those at risk for developing hypomagnesemia are patients with chronic alcoholism, patients with cirrhosis, patients taking diuretics or laxatives, and patients who are malnourished. Magnesium depletion is almost always associated with hypocalcemia and hypokalemia and acid–base abnormalities are common.[10] Correction of hypomagnesemia is done through the use of oral or IV supplements.

> Hypomagnesemia may be present in as many as 7% to 10% of hospitalized elderly patients.[12]

Elevation of serum magnesium levels, hypermagnesemia, can occur as a result of the use of large quantities of magnesium-containing laxatives or antacids and may be seen in patients with tissue lysis syndrome, diabetic ketoacidosis, or end-stage renal disease. In patients with severe hypermagnesemia, mechanical ventilation to manage respiratory failure or a temporary pacemaker in symptomatic bradycardia may be required.

Calcium Abnormalities

Patients at risk for hypocalcemia include those with chronic renal failure, malnutrition, and alcoholism. Development of symptoms of hypocalcemia are related to severity of calcium deficit and rapidity of onset.[13] Signs and symptoms of hypocalcemia include wheezing, bronchospasm, and cardiac dysrhythmias.[12]

Hypercalcemia can be seen in patients with bone metastasis from breast or non-small cell lung cancer and primary hyperparathyroidism.[13] Patients may present with nonspecific complaints of bone pain, anorexia, lethargy, headache, and confusion.[13]

REFERENCES

1. Metheny, N. M. (2010). *Fluid and electrolyte balance: Nursing considerations* (5th ed.). Sudbury, MA: Jones & Bartlett.
2. Baer, D. M., Ernst, D. J., Willeford, S. I., & Gambino, R. (2006). Investigating elevated potassium values. *Medical Laboratory Observer, 38*(11), 24, 26, 30–31.
3. Lippi, G., Blanckaert, N., Bonini, P., Green, S., Kitchen, S., Palicka, V., Plebani, M. (2008). Haemolysis: An overview of the leading cause of unsuitable specimens in clinical laboratories. *Clinical Chemistry and Laboratory Medicine 46*(6), 764–772.
4. Clinical and Laboratory Standards Institute. (2010). *Procedures for the handling and processing of blood specimens for common laboratory tests; approved guideline* (4th ed.) (CLSI document H18-A4). Wayne, PA: Author.
5. McPherson, R. A., & Pincus, M. R. (2007). *Henry's clinical diagnosis and management by laboratory methods* (21st ed., p. 158). Philadelphia, PA: Saunders.
6. Barone, J. A., & Madlinger, R. V. (2006). Should an Allen test be performed before radial artery cannulation? *Journal of Trauma, 61*(2), 468–470.
7. Moreira, M. E. (2006). Meningitis. In V. J. Markovchick & P. T. Pons (Eds.), *Emergency medicine secrets* (4th ed., pp. 152–153). St. Louis, MO: Mosby.
8. Stacey, J. F. (2009). Lumbar puncture. In J. A. Proehl (Ed.), *Emergency nursing procedures* (4th ed., pp. 466–472). St. Louis, MO: Saunders.
9. Goldsetin, H. N., & Edlow, J. A. (2006). Headache. In S. R. Votey & M. A. Davis (Ed.), *Signs and symptoms in emergency medicine* (2nd ed., p. 215). St. Louis, MO: Mosby.
10. Ayus, J. C., Achinger, S. G., & Arieff, A. (2008). Brain cell volume regulation in hyponatremia: Role of sex, age, vasopressin, and hypoxia. *American Journal of Physiology: Renal Physiology, 295*(3), F619–F624.
11. Lerma, E. V. (2009). Anatomic and physiologic changes of the aging kidney. *Clinics in Geriatric Medicine, 25*(3), 325–329.
12. Beach, C. B. (2010, March 29). *Hypocalcemia in emergency medicine.* Retrieved from http://emedicine.medscape.com/article/767260-overview
13. Hemphill, R. R. (2010, September 1). *Hypercalcemia in emergency medicine.* Retrieved from http://emedicine.medscape.com/article/766373-overview

End-of-Life Issues for Emergency Nurses

Tina D. Cronin

Emergency clinicians are frequently involved with deaths that occur suddenly and unexpectedly as a result of motor vehicle crashes, penetrating trauma, massive cerebrovascular events, or myocardial infarction. With today's medical advances in treating chronic diseases, emergency nurses are just as likely to care for a significant number of patients with terminal illnesses for whom death is expected. As illness progresses, visits to the emergency department (ED) often become more frequent. Nurses play a unique and vital role in caring for—and advocating on behalf of—these patients and their families, as the focus of intervention shifts from curative to palliative. The end of life is defined as the period in which:

- There is little likelihood of cure.
- Further aggressive therapy is considered futile.
- Patient comfort becomes the primary goal.

The trend toward offering patients in-home palliative care earlier in the end-of-life process is having an impact on how patients die in today's society. Palliative care focuses on the physical, psychological, social, spiritual, and existential needs of the patient and family. The goal of palliative care is to help the patient achieve the best quality of life by relieving uncomfortable symptoms while respecting religious and cultural practices.[1] Palliative care is often provided through hospice services or palliative care services. Nonetheless, emergency providers still have many opportunities to improve care by helping to provide a dignified end of life for patients and their families and supporting cultural and religious practices.[2]

END-OF-LIFE DECISIONS

Advance Directives

An advance directive is a means of documenting an individual's wishes regarding future health care if he or she is unable to make medical decisions because of reasons such as coma or cognitive impairment.

- An advance directive may include a living will or health care proxy and is based on the belief that patients have a right to make their own treatment decisions.
- An advance directive is not the equivalent of a Do Not Resuscitate (DNR) order.
- The purpose of an advance directive is to encourage patients and their families (or significant others) to understand, reflect on, and discuss desired treatment options before the need for resuscitation or other emergency interventions.[3]
- Although state law (usually a Natural Death Act) is the legal basis for advance directives, laws differ in respect to format, forms, witness requirements, and the need for a notary public.

Statements made in an advance directive typically reflect the values and beliefs of the individual and may change over time as an illness progresses or an emergency arises. Discussion and formal documentation before such a crisis is more likely to ensure that a patient's wishes are respected and carried out. Two possible components of an advance directive are the following:

- A living will allows individuals to specify whether they would accept or refuse particular life-sustaining interventions such as dialysis, mechanical ventilation, cardiopulmonary resuscitation (CPR), tube feeding, intravenous (IV) hydration, and blood transfusions.[4]
- A health care proxy (or durable power of attorney for health care) identifies a specific individual who can make medical decisions on behalf of the patient once the patient is unable to make decisions for himself or herself.[1]

Living wills and health care proxies are flexible documents that can be changed easily or revoked. This can be done in a variety of ways, including by simply telling a health care provider. In the emergency setting, emergency providers must exercise care to make sure the latest version of these documents is available.

> Living wills and health care proxies can be revoked or changed by the patient at any time. If the documents are changed, make sure to completely document the time, date, and who requested the changes and ensure that this information is witnessed.

The Patient Self-Determination Act of 1990 is a federal law that requires all health care agencies that receive federal funding to recognize advance directives. Under the law, hospitals must do the following:[5]

- Ask patients if they have an advance directive.
- Offer patients and families information about advance directives.
- Inform patients of state laws that pertain to advance directives.
- Notify patients about any hospital policies that affect advance directives.

Standards may differ from state to state and from institution to institution. Patients are never required to have advance directives, and facilities may not discriminate against patients who have or do not have one.

- Most hospitals attempt to honor a patient's wishes, but specific exceptions may exist and institutional policies must identify these situations clearly.
- In the event that a health care provider is not willing or able to honor an advance directive, the provider should inform the patient and family of this and arrange for transfer of care to a new practitioner.
- Hospitals need a clear method for identifying patients with advance directives and must have a plan for making these documents readily available to guide treatment decisions.

If a patient does not have an advance directive and is unable to make his or her own medical decisions, then clinicians must seek guidance from a spouse, adult child, parent, or friend or they must pursue appointment of a legal guardian.

- In some situations, consultation with the ethics committee for the hospital can guide care decisions. Unfortunately, ethics committee consultations are usually difficult or impossible in emergent situations.
- Potential problems should be identified proactively and addressed with any patient nearing the end of life who uses the ED frequently.
- Consult the ethics committee or risk management department if there appears to be a misunderstanding or disagreement about patient preferences and treatment options.

Table 17-1 provides a list of Internet resources related to advance directives.

Do Not Resuscitate

"Do Not Resuscitate," "No Cardiac Resuscitation," and "Do Not Attempt Resuscitation" are terms that refer to patients for whom life-sustaining efforts are limited at the request

TABLE 17-1	**INTERNET RESOURCES RELATED TO ADVANCE DIRECTIVES**
ORGANIZATION OR GROUP	**INTERNET ADDRESS**
American Association of Retired Persons	http://www.aarp.org/index.html
Aging with Dignity— Five Wishes	http://www.agingwithdignity.org/5wishes.html
American Bar Association (ABA Network)	http://www.abanet.org/home.cfm
American Medical Association	http://www.ama-assn.org
Compassion & Choices	http://www.compassionandchoices.org

of the patient, family, or health care team. Other variations of DNR include "Do Not Intubate" and "Do Not Defibrillate." Some institutions may prefer to use the phrases "Allow for Natural Death" or "Comfort Care Only" to reduce fears that DNR means no care will be given. Positively worded phrases help to emphasize that care will be continued (e.g., pain control and comfort measures) and that the patient is not being abandoned.

A problem unique to the emergency setting is the patient who presents in a state of crisis, requiring an immediate decision to act or not act. Initial information is frequently limited or confusing depending on the presenting situation. Therefore emergency providers are justified in starting or continuing care that may later be determined to be contrary to patient or family wishes.

Out-of-Hospital Do Not Resuscitate Orders

Many states in the U.S. have passed legislation allowing out-of-hospital DNR orders. These laws go by a variety of names, including portable DNR, community-based DNR, and physician order for life-sustaining treatment (POLST). These laws require the following:

- If an individual with an out-of-hospital DNR order experiences a cardiac or respiratory arrest, emergency medical services personnel should not initiate CPR. However, they can provide the following:
  - Assessment
  - Assistance if the patient is choking (airway clearance, oxygen, and medications for dyspnea)
  - Aggressive pain management
  - Grief counseling
  - Other appropriate services for the patient and family
- Some states limit access to out-of-hospital DNR orders to patients who are terminally ill or elderly, whereas other states make them available to any competent adult.

TABLE 17-2	CLINICAL AND LEGAL DISTINCTIONS BETWEEN ADVANCE DIRECTIVES AND DO NOT RESUSCITATE ORDERS		
COMPONENT	**ADVANCE DIRECTIVE**	**INSTITUTION-BASED DNR**	**OUT-OF-HOSPITAL DNR**
How do you obtain one?	From many sources including the Internet, hospitals, physicians, or clinics	The physician writes a DNR order in the medical record.	Forms can be obtained only from a licensed, independent health care provider.
Who signs the document?	Only the person for whom it applies (witness required)	The physician	The physician and the patient or a legal surrogate
When does it apply?	Only when the patient is unable to speak for himself or herself. Some state laws specify certain conditions (e.g., permanent vegetative state or coma)	Immediately	Immediately
What should occur if the person suffers cardiopulmonary arrest?	Start CPR. When patient is stabilized evaluate the situation and communicate with the patient or legal surrogate	Do not begin CPR.	Do not begin CPR.
Does the document represent informed consent?	No. The document is a written statement of a person's wishes. It does not require disclosure of specific information by a health care provider, so it does not represent an informed decision.	Yes. The order results from a discussion between the physician (or team) and the patient or legal surrogate. Like any other order for treatment, informed consent should be part of the process.	Yes. The form is signed by the physician and the patient or legal surrogate. The form is written evidence that informed consent has occurred.

CPR, Cardiopulmonary resuscitation; *DNR,* Do Not Resuscitate.
From Wilkie, D. J. (2001). *Toolkit for nursing excellence at end of life transition* [CD-ROM]. Seattle, WA: University of Washington.

- To be valid, an out-of-hospital DNR order requires the health care provider's signature and the patient's or surrogate's signature.
- To avoid potential confusion, patients should have a copy of the original order and some form of wearable identification such as a medical alert bracelet.
- Most states include a provision allowing emergency medical services personnel to perform CPR if the family persistently and strongly requests it, even if the patient has an out-of-hospital DNR order. However, in these difficult situations, emergency medical services personnel are trained to counsel families to forgo CPR.
- Ideally, medical facilities will have a policy that defines the circumstances under which an out-of-hospital DNR order will be honored within the health care facility. These policies should address care of the person with an out-of-hospital DNR in the ED, clinic, or inpatient setting. In addition, discussion regarding out-of-hospital DNR orders should be part of the physician and nursing discharge plan for all appropriate patients.
- Many states are working to make out-of-hospital DNR orders the standard for nursing homes and other community-based care facilities so that emergency medical services personnel responding to these facilities can honor DNR requests.

Importantly, an out-of-hospital DNR order is not an advance directive. The out-of-hospital DNR order is a physician's order to withhold life-sustaining therapy, and it requires a patient's or surrogate's signature as evidence that informed consent occurred, similar to consent for a surgical procedure. Table 17-2 summarizes specific differences between advance directives, institution-based DNR orders, and out-of-hospital DNR orders.

COMMON MEDICAL EMERGENCIES AT THE END OF LIFE

Patients with a terminal illness may present to the ED with a problem that requires rapid intervention. Examples include conditions such as uncontrolled pain, delirium, hemorrhage, bowel obstruction, and spinal cord compression. Emergency personnel should attempt to determine the wishes of the patient and family as well as explore other possible alternatives.

Uncontrolled Pain

Patients with chronic illness often present with moderate to severe pain related to their diagnosis and disease trajectory. Effective pain control is possible for the vast majority of patients at the end of life. (See Chapter 11, Care of the Patient with Pain, for more information.)

- If the patient is comatose or unable to verbalize pain status, closely monitor the patient's vital signs and facial expressions, and note any guarding and increased restlessness. Clinicians should provide pain medication when indicated.
- The doses of analgesics and routes may be different from those used in routine practice. Patients at the end-of-life often receive drugs through transdermal patches, intrathecal infusions, or continuous IV drips at doses many times greater than those used for standard therapy. Careful assessment of patients with transdermal patches is necessary to maintain patient safety when additional pain medications are indicated.

Delirium

Delirium is defined as an acute change or fluctuation in mental status accompanied by inattention and the presence of disorganized thinking or altered level of consciousness.[6] Essential criteria for the diagnosis of delirium are:

- Disordered attention and cognition
- Disturbances of psychomotor behavior

Behavioral disturbances may have an acute or subacute onset and include:

- Agitation
- Hallucinations
- Paranoia

Distinguishing between pain, dementia, and delirium can be very difficult. The patient with delirium may moan, groan, and be restless in the absence of pain. Conversely, delirium can limit a patient's perception of and ability to express pain.

Preexisting cognitive problems, such as dementia and Alzheimer's disease, may become more evident at the end of life. Delirium can be distinguished from dementia in that dementia is more likely to have a gradual onset, exist as a chronic condition, and coexist without alteration in level of consciousness. The underlying cause of delirium must be identified to assure optimal treatment. Table 17-3 lists potential causes of delirium and their appropriate therapeutic interventions.

Agitation and hallucinations can be managed with orally or subcutaneously administered haloperidol (Haldol) to prevent patient and family distress. Doses range from 1 mg (orally or subcutaneously) every 8 to 12 hours to 2 mg every 30 minutes in severe cases. The maximum dose of 20 to 30 mg per day may be necessary.

If haloperidol is not effective, alternatives include low-dose antipsychotic medications. Discussion with the patient and family should emphasize that confusion and agitation are expressions of brain malfunction and that the aim of

TABLE 17-3	CAUSES AND TREATMENT OF DELIRIUM IN PATIENTS AT THE END-OF-LIFE
CAUSE	**TREATMENT**
Opioid toxicity	Switch to another opioid.
Sepsis	Start antibiotic therapy (with the approval of the patient or family).
Drugs	Discontinue drugs that aggravate delirium such as tricyclic antidepressants and benzodiazepines.
Dehydration	Consider intravenous hydration after consultation with the patient and family. This intervention can have undesired side effects such as increased urine output, decreased catecholamine release, increased pressure from tumors, and increased pulmonary congestion.
Metabolic disorders (hypercalcemia, uremia, hepatic failure, hyponatremia)	Correct the underlying problem when possible.
Hypoxia	Provide supplemental oxygen. This may involve simply blowing oxygen across the face.
Brain metastases	Consider corticosteroid therapy, which may provide temporary improvement.

controlling symptoms is not to prolong life but to provide comfort.

Some common pitfalls in delirium management include failure to do the following:

- Recognize depression as a variant of delirium and provide antidepressants.
- Distinguish between delirium and poor pain management, to avoid aggravating the problem by giving more opioids.
- Identify urinary retention or constipation, easily treated problems that can mimic some signs of delirium.

Bowel Obstruction

A large number of patients on high-dose opioid therapy experience constipation if a prophylactic bowel regimen is not started. Untreated constipation can progress to incomplete or complete bowel obstruction. Metastases are another common cause of bowel obstruction. Findings associated with bowel obstruction include:

- Nausea
- Vomiting
- Abdominal pain
- Distension
- High-pitched or absent bowel sounds
- Tympanic sounds on percussion
- History of infrequent bowel movements
- Absence of flatus

Management of constipation is a preventive measure for bowel obstruction. Subcutaneous methylnaltrexone reverses opioid-induced constipation without affecting the analgesic properties of the opioid. For a limited number of patients, surgical intervention (bowel resection, gastrostomy tube insertion) may be an option. Gastric or duodenal (Miller-Abbott) tubes can provide temporary relief.

Spinal Cord Compression

Patients with end-stage cancer may experience spinal cord compression. Treatment delays can lead to paralysis and loss of bowel and bladder control.

- Central back pain worsened by movement, coughing, and straining is the usual initial symptom and may be present for days to weeks before the onset of neurologic symptoms.
- Back pain is followed by progressive sensory loss, motor weakness, incontinence, reduced muscle tone, and diminished reflexes.
- Plain radiographs have limited diagnostic value; magnetic resonance imaging (MRI) or computed tomography (CT) scans are preferred methods of diagnosis.
- The initial treatment of choice is steroid therapy but radiation or surgery may be needed.

Seizures

Seizures are common in patients with cerebral tumors or meningeal involvement but may also be related to metabolic disturbances, infection, toxicity, drug withdrawal, metastases, intracerebral hemorrhage, or acute ischemic stroke. First seizures are upsetting to patients and families. If the patient is not going to be admitted to the hospital, educational information about seizure management and safety should be initiated.

- Active seizures may be controlled with lorazepam (Ativan).
- To prevent future seizures, prophylactic treatment with antiepileptic drugs may be started.

Massive Hemorrhage

Tumors (especially of the head and neck) can infiltrate large vascular structures, producing catastrophic bleeding. Other causes of end-of-life hemorrhage include thrombocytopenia, liver failure, massive gastrointestinal bleeding, and disseminated intravascular coagulation. Few treatment options may be available once such bleeding has started; the bleeding is a preterminal event.

- Application of direct pressure can minimize external bleeding.
- Turning the patient to the side may prevent aspiration in those with hemoptysis or hematemesis.
- Reducing or stopping vasopressor agents can decrease blood loss.
- The presence of bleeding is often distressing to the patient and the use of sedation with midazolam may reduce anxiety over the event. Providing the patient and family with compassion and support in the event of hemorrhage may help lessen fears and assist with coping. This can be a traumatic event for the family to witness, so it is important that the family be supported during this time and measures be taken to reduce the trauma of this experience on the patient and family.

ORGAN AND TISSUE DONATION

Interest in organ transplantation can be traced to 2500 to 3000 B.C., when ancient Hindu text described skin graft techniques.[7] Today, organ donation and transplantation have proven to be therapeutic and effective lifesaving management strategies for individuals with organ failure. In the past 20 years, important medical breakthroughs such as tissue typing and immunosuppressant drugs have lengthened survival and increased the number of transplants performed. The most notable development was the discovery of the immunosuppressant cyclosporine, which was approved for commercial use in 1983.

In early 2011 more than 110,000 people were listed with the Organ Procurement and Transplantation Network (OPTN) as awaiting an organ for transplantation.[8] According to the US Department of Health and Human Services, approximately 20 people die daily awaiting for organ transplants.[9] Most organ donors are individuals who have sustained a traumatic brain injury, anoxic event, or stroke that causes brain death. Emergency nurses are in a key position to identify potential organ donors.[10] Federal law mandates that health care professionals offer the option of organ and tissue donation to all who qualify. Although an individual can make his or her wishes concerning organ donation known on a driver's license or donor card, in practice family members should always be consulted before the donation process begins.

General Tissue and Organ Donor Criteria

Tissue and organ donations are derived from individuals who are brain dead and from those without a beating heart (donation after cardiac death). Almost anyone who dies can

TABLE 17-4	**CRITICAL PATHWAY FOR ORGAN DONATION**

PHASE	ACTION
I	Referral of potential donor
II	Declaration of brain death; obtain consent for donation
III	Donor evaluation by organ procurement personnel
IV	Donor management
V	Recovery of organs

donate tissue such as corneas, bone, skin, and heart valves. Donor requirements change frequently; consult the local organ and tissue bank for current criteria. Procurement specialists are always available to assist with evaluation of potential donors and in many cases are called for all imminent deaths. These trained individuals talk to family members who are considering donating the "gift of life." The procurement specialist can anticipate and answer most questions or concerns related to donation. Table 17-4 highlights the critical pathway for organ donation.

When caring for a potential organ donor, health care providers must consider the family's cultural, religious, and emotional situation. Contrary to widely held beliefs, the majority of major religions approves of organ and tissue donation and considers donation a great gift. All families of potential organ donors should be offered the option of donating organs. In August 1998 the Centers for Medicare and Medicaid Services published its final rule on organ donation. This rule contains two key provisions:

- Hospitals must contact their organ procurement organization in a timely manner about any individual who dies in the hospital or whose death is imminent.
- Only organ procurement organization staff or trained hospital staff members may approach the patient's family about organ donation.

Determination of Death for Organ Donation

The Uniform Determination of Death Act (1978) plays an integral role in identifying criteria to determine brain death. Table 17-5 lists criteria for the determination of brain death. It is important that emergency nurses help family members understand that patients who are brain dead are not in a potentially recoverable state.

- Once brain death is determined, the date and time of brain death must be documented in the medical record.
- The physician notifies the family of death and many facilities allow the family to be present during brain death testing.
- Upon brain death, the organ procurement coordinator obtains signed consent from the family and reviews the patient's medical and social history.

TABLE 17-5	**CRITERIA FOR DETERMINATION OF BRAIN DEATH**

1. A person with irreversible cessation of circulatory and respiratory function is dead.
   a. Cessation is recognized by clinical examination and criteria.
   b. Irreversibility is recognized by persistent cessation of all functions during a period of observation, trial of therapy, or both.
2. A person with irreversible cessation of all functions of the entire brain, including the brainstem, is dead.
   a. Cessation is recognized when evaluation discloses the following:
      i. Cerebral functions are absent.
      ii. Brainstem reflexes (papillary, corneal, gag) are absent.
   b. Irreversibility is recognized when evaluation discloses the following:
      i. Reversible conditions such as hypothermia and hyponatremia have been corrected and the vital signs are hemodynamically stable.
      ii. The cause of the coma is established and is sufficient to account for loss of brain function.
      iii. The possibility of brain function recovery is excluded.
      iv. Cessation of all brain functions persists for an appropriate period of observation, trial of therapy, or both.

From Uniform Determination of Death Act, 1978.

- Conditions that require medical examiner notification vary by state but commonly include:
  - Homicide
  - Suicide
  - Unintentional injury death
  - Death within 24 hours of admission
  - Patients admitted in a comatose state
  - Death of a minor
- These conditions do not necessarily exclude donation, and many medical examiners will act quickly to release the body. Many organ procurement organizations prefer notification of an impending death to help ensure that a potential donor is not lost. It is also important to notify the medical examiner of the potential of donation so he or she is aware of the time sensitivity involved.

Donor Management

In most settings, donor management occurs in the intensive care unit. However, there will be times and situations when the emergency nurse must initiate the process. Because these patients are considered deceased, their care and management does not have to be directed by a physician.

Orders written by authorized transplant coordinators are valid and should be followed. Emergency departments should establish guidelines for the role of the emergency nurse in coordination with the organ procurement organizations (OPOs).

> The Uniform Anatomical Gift Act[11] recommends the following order of priority for relatives asked to consent to donation:
> * Spouse
> * Adult child
> * Either parent
> * Adult sibling
> * Grandparent
> * Legal guardian

The Procurement Process

One organ donor can save eight lives, so careful management is needed. Tissue procurement (eyes, corneas, bone, heart valves, and skin) can occur up to 10 hours following asystole, but shorter intervals are preferable. Ideally, the body should be kept in a refrigerated room.

If the eyes are to be donated:
* Elevate the patient's head 20 degrees and tape the eyelids shut with paper tape.
* Ice applied to the eyelids reduces edema and facilitates the recovery process.
* Enucleation is performed as a clean procedure using sterile technique.
* Corneas are usually transplanted within 24 to 48 hours.[12]

Recovery of solid organs (patients with beating-hearts or donation immediately after cardiac death) occurs in the operating room and can require multiple teams, depending on how many organs will be recovered. Follow institutional policy and procedures regarding organ procurement.

> The donor's family will not be billed for any medical costs related to donation or recovery. Once the patient becomes an organ donor candidate, the recipient, the recipient's insurance, Medicaid, or Medicare pays all costs.

DEATH NOTIFICATION AND POSTMORTEM CARE

A majority of patients who die in the ED have family members (or other significant persons) present at the time of death or shortly thereafter. In such instances, notification of death is given face to face. Depending on the circumstances, the family may or may not be prepared to receive this information. In cases of chronic, progressive, or terminal illnesses, families may have had time to prepare for such news and may be further along in the bereavement process than the family

of a patient whose death was unexpected. Witnessing the actual events and observing prehospital care may or may not provide loved ones with insight into what has happened.

Ideally, families are given the opportunity to be with the patient before death is pronounced. This practice has been shown to be a beneficial part of the bereavement process. With proper support and information before entering the room, family members typically do not become disruptive. Consider the following measures to support the family during this difficult time:
* Before they view the patient, provide families with information about what they are likely to see: tubes, activities, medications, and the condition of the patient.
* The accompanying staff member can be a role model for families by speaking directly to and touching the patient who is dying.

The Emergency Nurses Association recommends family presence during these times and suggests that the emergency nurse follow the institution's policy and procedures regarding family presence.

When family members must be notified of a death, certain steps should be taken. A physician-and-nurse team approach works well.
* The health care providers who approach the family should be free of other distractions (e.g., pagers or wireless phones turned off) and should sit down, introduce themselves, and identify the family members.
* The team should briefly ascertain what the current understanding of the situation is, then provide a synopsis of what occurred and describe the result of these actions.
* Simple words, including "died" or "dead," are appropriate. Use of euphemisms and medical jargon ("didn't respond," "coded," "flatlined," and "failed resuscitative efforts") may be confusing to the family.

If family members were not present at the death, the nurse should offer the family an opportunity to see their deceased loved one. For families that choose cremation, this may be the last time they will see their loved one. If the family accepts the offer, the nurse should excuse herself or himself to ensure that the body is presentable. The following preparations may be necessary:
* The body may need to be moved to another room to allow the ED to continue to function. This also applies in situations in which family members wish to view the body but will be delayed in arrival.
* Although certain tubes must remain in place in medical examiner cases, IV catheters, indwelling urinary catheters, and chest tubes can be plugged and made less obvious.
* Except in medical examiner cases, blood should be washed off. In some cultures and religions, the family (or other designated party) may wish to perform this activity.

- Large wounds should be covered.
- Place clean sheets and a clean gown on the body and tidy the room as much as possible.
- Dimming the lights, or aiming mobile lights away from the deceased, makes the dead person's skin appear more lifelike.
- Arms should be at the side, the jaw shut, dentures in the mouth, and eyes closed.
- The nurse should prepare the family for what they will see. If the nurse touches the deceased, he or she models that touching is acceptable.
- Lower the stretcher height or the gurney side rails and provide chairs.
- Determine from the family's nonverbal cues whether to stay in the room or to give them privacy.
- If the family prefers to be alone, check frequently to offer assistance and answer any questions they may have.

Before the family's departure, certain formalities are usually necessary, such as completion of demographic or contact information and transfer of valuables and clothing (in non–medical examiner cases). Provide the family with instruction sheets containing information related to funeral arrangements and who to contact about the death. Any interaction with the family should be done with great sensitivity and support. A friend, neighbor, taxi driver, or even the police may be needed to help get the family members home.

PEDIATRIC DEATH

It is estimated that around 53,000 children die each year in the United States.[13] Although it is estimated that 17,000 of the pediatric deaths in the ED are a result of trauma, many may be a result of chronic illness.[13] The death of a child is an extremely emotional event, and families may need to spend a lot of time with the deceased child. The following are examples of things that can be done to help the family:

- Wrap small infants and children snugly so that parents can hold their child.
- Provide a rocking chair if possible.
- An offer to snip a lock of hair for the parents to keep may be appreciated. (This should be documented clearly in the medical record.)
- Some families may ask that photographs be taken and imprints be made of the hands and feet.

Fetal Loss

The legal differentiation between "products of conception" and a "fetus" typically is based on weight or gestational age. Individual states may have more specific parameters. However, it is important to remember that gestational age does not predict the degree of loss experienced by the parents. Parents may request a photograph, a lock of hair (if available), and imprints of the hands or feet and may wish to hold funeral services. These physical reminders give the parents something to look at, hold, and touch to aid in the grieving process. If the family wishes to hold funeral services, follow institutional policy and procedures regarding the transfer of the "products of conception" or "fetus."

REFERENCES

1. Chan, G. K. (2004). End-of-life models and emergency department care. *Academic Emergency Medicine, 11*(1), 79–86.
2. Emergency Nurses Association. (2010). *End-of-life care in the emergency department* [position statement]. Retrieved from http://www.ena.org/SiteCollectionDocuments/Position%20 Statements/EndofLifeCareintheEmergencyDepartment.pdf
3. American Hospital Association. (2010). *Put it in writing.* Retrieved from http://www.putitinwriting.org/putitinwriting_app/index.jsp
4. Mappes, T. A., & DeGrazia, D. (2005). *Biomedical ethics* (6th ed.). New York, NY: McGraw-Hill.
5. *Federal patient self determination act 1090.* (n.d.). Retrieved from http://www.fha.org/acrobat/Patient%20Self %20Determination%20Act%201990.pdf
6. Thomason, J. W. W., Shintan, A., Peterson, J. F., Pun, B. T., Jackson, J. C., & Ely, E. W. (2005). Intensive care unit delirium is an independent predictor of longer hospital stay: a prospective analysis of 261 non-ventilated patients. *Critical Care, 9*(4), R375–R381. doi: 10.1186/cc3729.
7. Linden, P. K. (2009). History of solid organ transplantation and organ donation. *Critical Care Clinics, 25*(1), 165–184, ix.
8. United Network for Organ Sharing. (n.d.). *Home/transplant trends.* Retrieved from http://www.unos.org
9. US Department of Health and Human Services. (n.d.). *Statistics and facts.* Retrieved from http://www.organdonor.gov/ aboutStatsFacts.asp
10. Emergency Nurses Association. (2004). *Role of the emergency nurse in tissue and organ donation.* Retrieved from http://www.ena.org/SiteCollectionDocuments/Position%20 Statements/OrganDonation.pdf
11. National Conference of Commissioners on Uniform State Laws. (1987). *Uniform anatomical gift act.* Retrieved from http://www.law.upenn.edu/bll/archives/ulc/fnact99/uaga87. htm
12. Bonalumi, N. (2010). Organ and tissue donation. In P. K. Howard & R. A. Steinmann, (Eds.), *Sheehy's emergency nursing: Principles and practice* (6th ed., pp. 155–163). St. Louis, MO: Mosby.
13. Friebert, S. (2009). *NHPCO facts and figures: Pediatric and palliative and hospice care in America.* Alexandria, VA: National Hospital and Palliative Care Organization. Retrieved from http://www.nhpco.org/files/public/quality/Pediatric_Facts- Figures.pdf

Common Non-Traumatic Emergencies

Respiratory Emergencies

Robin Walsh

Respiratory emergencies, ranging from simple to complex, account for many presentations to the emergency department (ED). Some patients respond well to medications and therapy while others require more extensive interventions and nursing care. The respiratory system functions to supply oxygen to the blood for delivery throughout the body. The purpose of a respiratory assessment is to determine the adequacy of gas exchange. An across-the-room assessment is the beginning of the nurses' patient evaluation and may rapidly determine the acuity level and triage designation. Rapid and accurate assessment of these patients can prevent potentially life-threatening complications. As with all emergencies, the first priority is to evaluate the patient's airway, breathing, circulation, and disability (ABCD) status.

RESPIRATORY ASSESSMENT

Physical Assessment

- Vital signs—including a pulse oximetry (SpO_2) level and temperature
- Level of consciousness
  - **A**lert
  - **V**erbal
  - **P**ain
  - **U**nresponsive
- Skin color, moisture, and temperature
- Breath sounds
  - Present, absent, or diminished
  - Symmetrical
  - Adventitious
- Respiratory pattern and rate
  - Fast or slow
  - Regular or irregular
- Work of breathing
  - Quality
  - Degree of effort

- Presence of pursed-lip breathing
- Use of accessory muscles
  - Intercostal
  - Suprasternal
  - Supraclavicular
- Position of comfort
  - Can the patient tolerate a supine position?
  - Does the patient assume a "tripod" position?
- Speech pattern
  - Is the patient able to speak in full sentences?
- Presence of indicators of a chronic respiratory problem
  - Increased anterior-posterior (AP) diameter of the chest ("barrel chest")
  - Clubbing of the fingers
  - Nicotine stains on fingers
  - Portable oxygen tank
  - Thoracotomy scar
  - Kyphosis

History

- Determine onset, duration, and quality of the symptoms
- Obtain medical history, including previous hospitalizations and prior intubations for respiratory problems
- Document smoking history of patients or persons living with patient and any occupational risk factors
- Inquire about recent infectious disease exposure
- Additional factors that may influence the patient's respiratory status include:
  - Abdominal distention or enlargement
    - Pregnancy
    - Obesity
    - Ascites
    - Peritonitis

185

- Circulatory problems, especially any history of:
  - Pulmonary edema
  - Anemia
  - Thrombophlebitis
- Environmental influences
  - Air pollution
  - Seasonal allergies
  - Temperature changes
- Trauma (current or past)
- Known food and drug allergies

Diagnostic Procedures

Pulse Oximetry

Pulse oximetry is a noninvasive method of measuring oxygenation of the patient's hemoglobin. Normal values are 95% to 100%; readings of 85% or less may indicate inadequate tissue oxygenation. Pulse oximetry is useful in many situations, including[1]:
- Monitoring patients during a procedure (e.g., conscious sedation, surgery)
- Continuous monitoring of a patient's respiratory status
- Monitoring patients at risk for desaturation and hypoxia
- Evaluating response to an intervention (pain medication)

Pulse oximetry readings may not be reliable in:
- Cardiopulmonary arrest
- Shock states
- Use of vasoconstrictive medication
- Use of diagnostic intravenous dyes
- Anemia
- High carbon monoxide levels

Capnography

Capnography, noninvasive monitoring of exhaled carbon dioxide (ECO_2), is useful in evaluating ventilation. Traditionally used to verify endotracheal tube placement, it measures exhaled carbon dioxide at the end of each breath. Other uses for capnography monitoring include[2]:
- Monitoring for tube displacement or obstruction while transporting a patient
- Assessing adequacy of chest compressions during cardiopulmonary resuscitation
- Monitoring ventilation during procedural sedation
- Assessing perfusion in mechanically ventilated patients
- Determining the severity of an asthma exacerbation and assessing the effectiveness of interventions
- Verifying correct gastric tube placement

TABLE 18-1	ASTHMA MANAGEMENT BASED ON PEAK EXPIRATORY FLOW RATES	
ZONE	**READING**	**DESCRIPTION**
Green	71%–100% of the usual or normal peak flow readings	Readings in the green zone indicate that the asthma is under good control.
Yellow	50%–70% of the usual or normal peak flow readings	Indicates caution. Respiratory airways are narrowing and additional medication may be required.
Red	<50% of the usual or normal peak flow readings	Indicates a medical emergency. Severe airway narrowing may be occurring and immediate action needs to be taken.

Data from American Lung Association. (n.d.). *Measuring your peak flow rate.* Retrieved from http://www.lungusa.org/lung-disease/asthma/living-with-asthma/take-control-of-your-asthma/measuring-your-peak-flow-rate.html

Peak Flow Measurement

A peak flow meter measures the patient's maximum speed of expiration or peak expiratory flow rate (PEFR or PEF). It is a measurement of airflow through the bronchi and indicates the degree of obstruction in the airways. Peak flow readings are often classified into three zones of measurement[3] (green, yellow, and red) and can be used to develop an asthma management plan (Table 18-1).

Arterial Blood Gases

Arterial blood gas (ABG) values are useful in assessing respiratory status and acid-base balance; they are a measurement of systemic gas exchange. By comparing the pH, $PaCO_2$, and HCO_3, the body's ability to compensate an acid-base imbalance can be assessed; PO_2 values indicate the presence or absence of hypoxemia. Table 18-2 lists normal and abnormal ABG values.

Interpreting ABG values involves three steps:
- Step 1: Assess the pH to determine the presence of acidosis or alkalosis.
- Step 2: Assess $PaCO_2$ to determine if the cause of the acid-base imbalance is respiratory or metabolic. If the

TABLE 18-2　NORMAL AND ABNORMAL VALUES FOR ARTERIAL BLOOD GASES

VALUE	DEFINITION	NORMAL RANGE	ABNORMAL VALUES
pH	Indication of hydrogen ion concentration	7.35–7.45	<7.35 = acidosis >7.45 = alkalosis
$PaCO_2$	Respiratory parameter; indication of adequacy of ventilation and carbon dioxide elimination	35–45	<35 = alkalosis >45 = acidosis
PaO_2	Reflects the body's ability to use and transport oxygen through the system	80–100	<80 = hypoxemia
HCO_3 level	Metabolic parameter; assesses the kidney's ability to retain or excrete HCO_3	22–26	<22 = acidosis >26 = alkalosis

HCO_3, Bicarbonate; $PaCO_2$, partial pressure of arterial carbon dioxide; PaO_2, partial pressure of arterial oxygen.
Data from Selfridge-Thomas, J., & Hoyt, K. S. (2007). Respiratory emergencies. In *Emergency nursing core curriculum* (6th ed., pp. 685–720). Philadelphia, PA: Saunders Elsevier.

TABLE 18-3　ACID-BASE ABNORMALITIES DETERMINED BY ARTERIAL BLOOD GAS VALUES

	PH	$PaCO_2$	HCO_3	POSSIBLE CAUSES
Respiratory acidosis	Decreased	Increased	Normal	CNS depression resulting from drugs, injury, or disease; asphyxia; hypoventilation
Respiratory alkalosis	Increased	Decreased	Normal	Hyperventilation; respiratory stimulation (drugs, disease, infection, fever); gram-negative bacteria
Respiratory acidosis with metabolic compensation	Decreased	Increased	Increased	
Metabolic acidosis	Decreased	Normal	Decreased	Diarrhea, inadequate excretion of acids in renal disease; hepatic disease; endocrine disorders, shock
Metabolic alkalosis	Increased	Normal	Increased	Prolonged vomiting or gastric suction; potassium loss from renal disease or steroids; excessive alkali ingestion
Metabolic alkalosis with respiratory compensation	Increased	Increased	Increased	

CNS, Central nervous system; HCO_3, bicarbonate; $PaCO_2$, partial pressure of arterial carbon dioxide.

pH and $PaCO_2$ are moving in opposite directions (the pH is elevated and the $PaCO_2$ is decreased, or the pH is decreased and the $PaCO_2$ is elevated), the imbalance is respiratory in nature.

- Step 3: Assess HCO_3 to determine if the cause of the acid-base imbalance is metabolic. If the pH and the HCO_3 are moving in the same direction (the pH is elevated and the HCO_3 is elevated, or the pH is decreased and the HCO_3 is decreased), the imbalance is metabolic in nature.

When an acid–base imbalance exists, the body will attempt to compensate and normalize the pH. The result of these efforts can be uncompensated, partially compensated, or fully compensated. Table 18-3 defines various acid-base abnormalities based on ABG values.

ASTHMA EXACERBATIONS

Asthma affects millions of adults and children and is considered to be the most prevalent chronic childhood disease. Annually, asthma is responsible for almost 2 million ED visits, 500,000 hospital admissions, 400 deaths, and 100 million days of restricted activity.[4] Asthma is a chronic disease characterized by airway hyperreactivity, inflammation, and reversible airflow obstruction (bronchospasm). Exacerbations of this common disease can become life-threatening.

Asthma severity is classified as:[4]
- Intermittent
  - Symptoms twice a week or less and nighttime symptoms twice a month or less

- Symptoms do not interfere with normal activity
- Use of a short-acting beta-agonist (SABA) inhaler 2 days or less a week
- Mild persistent
  - Symptoms more than twice a week but less than once a day with nighttime symptoms three to four times a month
  - Minor limitations to normal activities because of symptoms
  - Use of SABA inhaler more than 2 days a week but not daily
- Moderate persistent
  - Daily symptoms and nighttime symptoms more than once a week but not daily
  - Some limitations to normal activity because of symptoms
  - Daily use of SABA inhaler
- Severe persistent
  - Continual daytime symptoms with frequent nighttime symptoms, often daily
  - Extreme limitations to normal activities because of symptoms
  - Poor to no control of symptoms

Asthma Triggers

A wide variety of stimulants can precipitate an asthma exacerbation. Specific individuals tend to have particular triggers. Common triggers include:

- Allergies to food or inhalants (e.g., pollen, latex, mold, animal dander)
- Exercise
- Cold exposure (breathing cold air, eating ice cream)
- Tobacco smoke
- Strong smells
- Upper respiratory infections
- Air pollutants
- Sinusitis, rhinitis
- Medications, especially aspirin and nonsteroidal anti-inflammatory drugs
- Food additives

Signs and Symptoms

- Wheezing—most commonly expiratory, but may also be inspiratory or absent
- Cough—may be present without wheezing, especially in children
- Use of accessory muscles of respiration, especially sternocleidomastoid muscles in adults
- Chest tightness and hyperresonance on percussion (resulting from hyperinflation)
- Anxiety or restlessness
- Halting speech (inability to speak in full sentences)

Diagnostic Procedures

- Routine laboratory tests and chest radiograph not usually necessary; do not delay initiation of treatment to obtain these[5]
- Arterial blood gases to determine degree of hypoxemia
- Peak expiratory flow rate less than 50% of predicted value
  - As a measure of airflow limitation, PEFR is a more reliable indicator of severity of exacerbation than degree of symptoms[6]
- Pulse oximetry—value less than 92% indicates probable need for hospitalization[5]

Therapeutic Interventions

- Allow the patient to maintain a position of comfort.
- Assess duration and severity of symptoms; document medications already taken in an attempt to manage the exacerbation.
- Obtain intravenous access for medication administration and hydration; dehydration can contribute to mucus plugging and catecholamine release.[7]
- Provide continuous cardiac and pulse oximetry monitoring.
- Administer supplemental oxygen to keep pulse oximetry greater than 90%.
- Administer inhaled SABA such as albuterol (Proventil) via nebulizer or metered dose inhaler (MDI), preferably with a spacer.
- Anticholinergics such as ipratropium bromide (Atrovent) are frequently combined with SABA.
- Measure PEFR before and after interventions. Serially measure PEFR as long as the patient is able to cooperate. A patient's inability to perform PEFR testing is an indicator of severe disease.
- Corticosteroids may be given to treat the inflammatory component of asthma.
- Magnesium sulfate may be considered if other interventions are ineffective; magnesium relaxes bronchial smooth muscles by an uncertain mechanism.[5]
- Heliox, a mixture of helium and oxygen, may improve gas exchange because of the low density of helium.
- Endotracheal intubation and intensive care unit admission is often necessary with imminent respiratory failure or arrest.

Status asthmaticus is a severe asthma exacerbation that does not respond to therapy. Ominous signs indicating a need for endotracheal intubation include:
- "Silent chest," indicating minimal airflow
- Fatigue and decreasing level of consciousness
- Hypoxemia, hypercapnia, or metabolic acidosis

ACUTE BRONCHITIS

Acute bronchitis is a self-limiting respiratory infection characterized by cough with or without sputum production.[8] It is most often the result of a virus such as influenza A or B or the respiratory syncytial virus (RSV); less than 10% of cases are bacterial in nature.[8] The diagnosis of acute bronchitis is made after ruling out other causes of cough such as:

- Pneumonia
- Acute exacerbation of chronic bronchitis in the patient with chronic obstructive pulmonary disease (COPD)
- Acute asthma
- Angiotensin-converting enzyme inhibitor–induced cough[9]
- Gastroesophageal reflux disease (GERD)
- Infection with *Bordetella pertussis* (whooping cough)

Signs and Symptoms

- Cough is always the predominant symptom and may last up to 3 weeks
- Sputum may or may not be present
- Wheezing
- Pleuritic chest pain
- Cold-like symptoms

Diagnostic Procedures

- Diagnosis is based on clinical presentation and history
- No acute findings on chest radiograph

Therapeutic Interventions

- Symptomatic treatment, including rest and oral hydration.
- Dextromethorphan (Benylin, Delsym) or codeine may be given for short-term relief from coughing.
- Bronchodilators may be useful if wheezing is present.
- Research does not support the use of expectorants or mucolytics.[8]
- Antibiotics are not effective or appropriate for treating acute bronchitis. Patient education related to overuse of antibiotics and the development of antibiotic-resistant organisms is an important aspect of care for these patients.

ACUTE EXACERBATION OF CHRONIC OBSTRUCTIVE PULMONARY DISEASE

Chronic obstructive pulmonary disease is defined as a preventable and treatable disease, characterized by progressive airflow limitation. It is associated with an abnormal inflammatory response of the lungs that is not fully reversible.[10] Traditionally, COPD is described as consisting of chronic bronchitis (defined as cough and sputum production for at least 3 months during 2 consecutive years) or emphysema (which involves destruction of the alveoli); most patients have some degree of both components. Asthma is characterized by reversible airflow limitations and is not included in the definition of COPD.

Chronic obstructive pulmonary disease is a progressive and irreversible disease; there is no cure and the goal is to manage the symptoms and limit disease progression. Patients often present to the ED with acute exacerbations or when their current level of therapy is no longer adequate.

Signs and Symptoms

- Acute onset, more common in winter months, often precipitated by viral respiratory infection
- Increasing dyspnea, tachypnea, and hypoxemia
- Change in sputum amount and color
- Distant breath sounds, scattered rhonchi, wheezes, and crackles
- Hyperresonance on percussion
- Pursed-lip breathing, use of accessory muscles of respiration
- Fatigue
- Possible cor pulmonale (right-sided heart failure resulting from respiratory disease)
  - Characterized by jugular venous distention, hepatomegaly

Diagnostic Procedures

- Arterial blood gases may be obtained but the clinical picture is the most important guide to management[10]
- Complete blood count to check for erythrocytosis
  - Secondary erythrocytosis or polycythemia can occur as the body produces more erythrocytes in an attempt to compensate for the decreasing level of oxygen in the blood
- Chest radiograph to rule out pneumothorax

Therapeutic Interventions

- Pulse oximetry to monitor response to therapy.
- Supplemental oxygen to maintain oxygen saturation of 90% to 92%.
  - Patients with COPD normally operate on a minimally acceptable PaO_2 level; however, never withhold oxygen from a patient who is hypoxic. Monitor the patient for a decrease in respiratory rate, which signals increasing serum oxygen levels.
  - The most severe life-threatening problem for these patients is hypoxemia.
  - Observe the patient carefully for decreased mental status that may signal hypercapnia.

- Bronchodilators—inhaled SABA such as albuterol (Proventil) and nebulized anticholinergics such as ipratropium bromide (Atrovent).
- Bed rest in a high Fowler's position. Alternatively, these patients frequently prefer to sit at the side of the stretcher, legs dangling, leaning forward, with elbows propped on a bedside table.
- Initiate and maintain vascular access and provide adequate hydration.
- Monitor for cardiac dysrhythmias.
- Noninvasive positive pressure ventilation in an attempt to prevent endotracheal intubation, as it is often difficult to wean patients with COPD from mechanical ventilation.
- Intravenous corticosteroids and antibiotics are often considered.

> Patients with COPD often present with numerous comorbidities that further stress the respiratory system and require additional assessment and management.

COMMUNITY-ACQUIRED PNEUMONIA

Community-acquired pneumonia (CAP) is an acute infection of the alveoli, distal airways, and lung interstitium. Most frequently, pneumonia is caused by a bacterial infection resulting from the *Streptococcus pneumoniae* or *Haemophilus influenzae* organism; less common causes include viral, mycoplasmal, fungal, or protozoal infection.[11] Aspiration of oropharyngeal secretions or stomach contents can also lead to pneumonia. Risk factors for CAP include:

- Extremes of age
- Alcohol dependence
- Smoking
- Coexisting heart or lung disease
- Immunosuppression
- GERD

Signs and Symptoms

- Dyspnea, tachypnea
- Varying degrees of fever
- Dry or productive cough; sputum may be purulent or blood-tinged
- Pleuritic chest pain
- Crackles, rhonchi, or wheezes on auscultation
- Dullness to percussion if consolidation or pleural effusion is present
- Fatigue
- In elderly patients, new onset of or increased confusion

Diagnostic Procedures

- Chest radiograph demonstrating lobar infiltrates and consolidation; may be negative early in course of disease
- Sputum for gram stain and culture

- Complete blood count to assess for leukocytosis
- Diagnostic bronchoscopy with bronchoalveolar lavage (BAL)
- Arterial blood gases are necessary only in severe cases
- Blood cultures prior to antibiotic administration

Therapeutic Interventions

- Administer supplemental oxygen; monitor oxygen saturation levels.
- Provide oral or intravenous hydration.
- Consider symptomatic management including nebulized bronchodilators and expectorants.
- Administer the first antibiotic dose while the patient is still in the ED.[12]
- Assess risk for unusual pathogens (e.g., tuberculosis, fungi, methicillin-resistant *Staphylococcus aureus*) and treat appropriately.
- Patient may require mechanical ventilation or management of severe sepsis.
- Use the Pneumonia Severity Index (scoring system based on patient demographics, comorbidities, physical examination, and laboratory and radiographic findings) to determine need for hospitalization.[13]

PLEURAL EFFUSION

A pleural effusion is an abnormal collection of fluid in the pleural space. Pleural effusion is not a disease but a clinical manifestation of an underlying problem that may originate in the pleural space, the pulmonary system, or an extrapulmonary site. The pleural effusion may be the result of the following pathophysiology:

- Increased hydrostatic pressure in the pulmonary vasculature (e.g., heart failure)
- Decreased oncotic pressure resulting from hypoalbuminemia (e.g., nephritic syndrome, malnutrition)
- Increased capillary permeability secondary to inflammation (e.g., pneumonia, infected wound, lung abscess)
- Impaired or blocked lymphatic drainage (e.g., tumor, fibrosis, trauma, infection)

Pleural effusions can be classified based on the composition of the accumulated pleural fluid. Table 18-4 notes the pathophysiology and examples of various pleural effusions.

Signs and Symptoms

- Dyspnea
- Cough—productive or nonproductive
- Chest pain
  - Mild or severe
  - Sharp, stabbing, or pleuritic
- Dullness to percussion over effusion
- Decreased breath sounds on affected side

TABLE 18-4   **CLASSIFICATION OF PLEURAL EFFUSIONS BASED ON TYPE OF FLUID IN THE PLEURAL SPACE**

	PATHOPHYSIOLOGY	EXAMPLES
Transudate	Water, protein-free fluid leaks from capillaries because of increased intravascular hydrostatic pressure or decreased oncotic pressure	Left ventricular failure Cirrhosis of liver Hypoalbuminemia (nephritic syndrome, malnutrition) Constrictive pericarditis
Exudate	Protein-rich fluid leaks from the capillaries because of increased capillary permeability	Inflammation Infection Malignancy Pulmonary embolism Pancreatitis Postcardiac surgery (Dressler syndrome)
Pus (empyema)	Pus or debris secondary to infection accumulates in pleural space	Pneumonia Lung abscess Infected wound
Lymphatic fluid (chylothorax)	Milk-colored fluid from blocked lymphatic drainage	Malignancy Trauma Infection Tuberculosis

- Pleural friction rub
- Decreased chest expansion on side of effusion
- Egophony—increased resonance of voice auscultated near the top of fluid line

Diagnostic Procedures

- Anterior-posterior and lateral chest radiograph—as little as 50 mL in the pleural space can be detected by posterior or costophrenic blunting on the lateral film[14]
- Chest computed tomography (CT) or transthoracic ultrasonography to identify or rule out possible causes
- Pleural aspiration to examine pleural fluid

Therapeutic Interventions

- Administer supplemental oxygen.
- Provide analgesia.
- Identify and treat underlying disease process.
- If effusion is large and compromising respiration, needle thoracentesis may be indicated. Large and rapidly accumulating effusions may require chest tube insertion.

SPONTANEOUS PNEUMOTHORAX

Pneumothorax refers to the accumulation of air in the pleural space. As air accumulates the increased pressure (or the loss of negative pressure) causes a partial or complete collapse of the lung. Spontaneous pneumothorax occurs in the absence of traumatic cause. It may occur in individuals without lung disease (primary) or in those with underlying pulmonary disease (secondary). Table 18-5 shows a comparison of primary and secondary spontaneous pneumothoraces.

> Regardless of the cause, the development of a tension pneumothorax is a concern following spontaneous pneumothorax.

Signs and Symptoms

- Sudden onset of pleuritic chest pain (often localized on the side of the pneumothorax)
- Dyspnea and tachypnea
- Cough
- Decreased breath sounds over the affected side
- Hyperresonance to percussion
- Less commonly, subcutaneous emphysema and asymmetrical chest movement

Diagnostic Procedures

- Chest radiograph for definitive diagnosis

Therapeutic Interventions

- Position patient in high Fowler's position.
- Monitor vital signs, including oxygen saturation.
- Administer supplemental oxygen to improve hypoxia.
- Initiate and maintain vascular access.
- Provide analgesia.

TABLE 18-5	COMPARISON OF PRIMARY AND SECONDARY SPONTANEOUS PNEUMOTHORACES	
	PRIMARY SPONTANEOUS PNEUMOTHORAX	**SECONDARY SPONTANEOUS PNEUMOTHORAX**
Underlying Disease Risk Factors	No apparent lung disease Patient is typically a healthy young man of taller than average height Cigarette smoking Changes in atmospheric pressure Mitral valve disease Marfan syndrome Possible familial propensity	Presence of underlying lung disease Incidence higher in men COPD accounts for nearly 70% of cases Acquired immunodeficiency syndrome Lung malignancy Tuberculosis Lung abscess
Causes	Rupture of bleb, usually at the lung apex	Underlying pulmonary disease weakens the alveolar-pleural interface

COPD, Chronic obstructive pulmonary disease.
Data from Kosowsky, J.M. (2009). Pleural disease. In J. A. Marx (Ed.), *Rosen's emergency medicine: concepts and clinical practice* (7th ed.), Philadelphia, PA: Mosby Elsevier.

- Chest tube placement in the fifth or sixth intercostal space in the midaxillary line to re-expand the lung
- Needle thoracostomy is indicated only for emergency treatment of tension pneumothorax.

PULMONARY EMBOLISM

A potentially lethal condition, pulmonary embolism (PE) occurs when foreign material occludes one or more pulmonary blood vessels. Most often the embolus results from a venous thrombus that breaks loose and travels through the right side of the heart and into the pulmonary circulation. Pulmonary emboli can arise from anywhere in the body, but most commonly come from the deep veins of the lower extremities. Other sources include:

- Pelvic, renal, or upper extremity vessels
- Mural thrombi in the right side of the heart
- Fat, amniotic fluid, or air embolus
- Intravenous injection of particulate matter associated with intravenous drug use
- Foreign bodies such as a bullet

The incidence of pulmonary embolism is difficult to determine. The average annual incidence in the United States is estimated at 1 per 1000 patients. An additional equal number are diagnosed at autopsy.[15]

Virchow's triad describes the three major risk factors for thromboemboli formation, which are:

- Venous stasis
  - Caused by heart failure, venous insufficiency, limb immobilization, prolonged bed rest, obesity, or pregnancy

- Endothelial injury
  - Caused by intimal damage from trauma, burns, surgery, or infection
- Hypercoagulable states
  - Caused by postpartum period, major surgery, malignancy, contraceptive use, polycythemia vera, and other disease states

The diagnosis of pulmonary embolism is difficult to make and often missed because the signs and symptoms may be vague and nonspecific and are similar to those of several other conditions. A high index of suspicion is necessary, particularly when the patient presents with significant risk factors.

Significant Risk Factors

- Previous venous thromboembolism
- Surgery within the previous 4 weeks
- Current estrogen use
- Active or metastatic cancer
- Recent travel with relative immobility
- Intravenous drug use
- Advanced age

Signs and Symptoms

- Symptoms of PE are often nonspecific and may mimic other conditions, including pleuritis, myocardial infarction, and panic attacks. Patients may experience vague, nagging symptoms for weeks prior to presenting to the ED.
- Dyspnea with tachypnea, possibly hemoptysis.
- Pleuritic chest pain (usually with a sudden onset).

- Tachycardia.
- Anxiety, apprehension, restlessness.
- Pleural friction rub may occasionally be auscultated.
- Clinical signs and symptoms of deep vein thrombosis.
- Atypical symptoms may include:
  - Seizures
  - Abdominal, flank, or shoulder pain
  - Syncope
  - Wheezing
  - Fever
  - New onset of atrial fibrillation

Diagnostic Procedures

- Anterior-posterior and lateral chest radiographs are not very sensitive for PE but may rule out other conditions such as pneumothorax
- Arterial blood gas determinations generally demonstrate hypoxemia
- D-dimer measurement elevation over 500 ng/mL
- Ultrasound of the leg and pelvic veins to detect venous thrombosis as source of embolus
- Helical (spiral) CT scan
- Magnetic resonance imaging or magnetic resonance angiography
- 12-lead electrocardiogram to rule out acute myocardial infarction
- Baseline coagulation panel

Therapeutic Interventions

- Administer supplemental oxygen and obtain intravenous access.
- Monitor vital signs and continuous oxygen saturation levels.
- Initiate heparin therapy (weight-based bolus followed by a continuous infusion); check partial thromboplastin time every 6 hours.
- Consider intravenous thrombolytic (rt-PA) therapy, particularly if patient is hemodynamically unstable.

NONCARDIOGENIC PULMONARY EDEMA

Pulmonary edema refers to the accumulation of fluid in the extravascular spaces of the lungs. It is classified as cardiogenic or noncardiogenic based on the underlying cause. The main pathophysiological alteration in noncardiogenic pulmonary edema is an increase in pulmonary capillary permeability rather than an increase in pulmonary vascular pressures as seen in cardiogenic pulmonary edema.[16] Cardiogenic pulmonary edema is discussed in Chapter 20, Shock.

Common causes of noncardiogenic pulmonary edema include:

- Acute respiratory distress syndrome (ARDS)
- Kidney failure resulting in fluid overload
- Submersion injury
- Head trauma or seizures (neurogenic pulmonary edema)
- Rapidly re-expanding lung (following thoracentesis or chest tube placement for pneumothorax)
- High altitude pulmonary edema
- Inhalation of toxic gases (chlorine, anhydrous ammonia)[17]
- Heroin, cocaine, or methadone overdose[17]

Regardless of the etiology of pulmonary edema, accumulation of fluid in the alveoli and interstitial space inhibits the exchange of oxygen and carbon dioxide and leads to tissue hypoxia.

Signs and Symptoms

- Shortness of breath
- Tachypnea
- Anxiety, agitation
- Sensation of suffocation
- Orthopnea
- Tachycardia
- Cough
- Crackles, wheezes
- Diaphoresis
- Pink, frothy sputum

Diagnostic Procedures

- Chest radiograph finding similar to those of cardiogenic pulmonary edema

Therapeutic Interventions

- Administer high-flow oxygen.
- Establish intravenous access for careful fluid administration.
- Noninvasive positive pressure ventilation may be attempted.
- Mechanical ventilation with low tidal volumes (lung protective strategy) is often necessary.
- Specific supportive treatment will vary depending on specific cause.

ACUTE RESPIRATORY DISTRESS SYNDROME

Acute respiratory distress syndrome, a form of noncardiogenic pulmonary edema, is an inflammatory syndrome characterized by diffuse alveolar injury.[18] The increase in permeability of the alveolar-capillary barrier allows protein-rich fluid to pass into the alveoli.[19] The result is severe hypoxemia often refractory to high concentrations of

TABLE 18-6 CAUSES OF ACUTE RESPIRATORY DISTRESS SYNDROME

DIRECT MECHANISMS	INDIRECT MECHANISMS
Aspiration of gastric contents	Sepsis
Pneumonia	Multiple trauma
Toxic inhalation (such as smoke inhalation)	Massive transfusions
Pulmonary contusion	Severe pancreatitis
Submersion injury	Drug overdose
Oxygen toxicity	Burns
Reperfusion injury post–lung transplant	Disseminated intravascular coagulopathy (DIC)
Radiation	Shock

inspired oxygen (FiO_2) associated with loss of surfactant, alveolar collapse, and decreased lung compliance ("stiff" lungs).

The precipitating event can be either direct injury to the lungs or an indirect injury resulting from a systemic illness. Table 18-6 describes both direct and indirect causes of ARDS.

Signs and Symptoms

- Dyspnea
- Tachypnea
- Tachycardia
- Cyanosis
- Anxiety, restlessness, agitation
- Accessory muscle use
- Fever or hypothermia

Diagnostic Procedures

- Chest radiograph will demonstrate bilateral pulmonary infiltrates.
- Arterial blood gases will indicate severe hypoxemia.
- PaO_2: FiO_2 ratio less than 200.
- Complete blood count may indicate leukocytosis or leukopenia.
- Bronchoscopy with bronchoalveolar lavage
- Chest CT is of questionable benefit.

Therapeutic Interventions

- Endotracheal intubation and critical care unit admission.
  - Mechanical ventilation with positive end expiratory pressure (PEEP).

- For more specific information, see Mechanical Ventilation in the Emergency Department later in this chapter.
  - Lower tidal volumes (6 to 8 mL/kg) as lung protective strategy.
  - Sedation and neuromuscular blockade is often required.
- Identify and treat the underlying cause, particularly infection, as sepsis is the major precipitating event.
- Careful fluid management.
  - The patient that is hemodynamically unstable and septic may require aggressive fluid resuscitation.
  - Use of a pulmonary artery catheter may assist in fluid management in selected patients.
- Careful and frequent assessment for complications of ARDS and of treatment modalities.
  - Addition of PEEP may increase intrathoracic pressure and decrease venous return to the heart, resulting in hypotension and hemodynamic instability.
  - Acute renal failure is a common complication; monitor intake and output and laboratory values carefully.
  - Assess for and treat hypoglycemia and hyperglycemia.

SUBMERSION INJURY

The World Health Organization (WHO) defines drowning as "the process of experiencing respiratory impairment from submersion/immersion in liquid."[20] WHO further discourages the use of the terms "wet" or "dry" drowning and "near-drowning." In 10% to 20% of drownings, laryngospasm prevents the aspiration of water.[21] If aspiration occurs, the amount is generally less than 4 mL/kg; as little as 1 to 3 mL/kg can alter surfactant function and interfere with gas exchange.[21] Lung damage is increased by contaminants such as mud, algae, and chlorine in the water. Although salt water and freshwater differ significantly in composition, these differences do not affect patient management.

The faster that resuscitation efforts are begun and that hypoxia, hypercarbia, and acidosis are resolved, the better the chance for survival. At least one third of drowning survivors experience moderate to severe neurologic sequelae.[21] Submersion in cold (below 32° F [0° C]) water may slow the progression of hypoxic brain injury, but these victims may also require treatment for hypothermia.[21]

Risk Factors

- Lack of supervision
- Inability to swim
- Risk-taking behaviors
- Alcohol or drug intoxication

- Underlying medical conditions such as seizures, hypoglycemia, cardiac arrhythmias, and stroke

Signs and Symptoms

- Clinical presentations vary widely and are directly related to the extent of hypoxic injury
- History of immersion
- Respiratory or cardiopulmonary arrest
- Dyspnea that may worsen over several hours
- Cyanosis
- Crackles, wheezing
- Cough (sometimes with pink, frothy sputum)
- Tachycardia
- Mental confusion, coma

Diagnostic Procedures

- Diagnosis based on history of event and clinical presentation

Therapeutic Interventions

- Initiate basic and advanced life support measures, including endotracheal intubation, as necessary.
- Consider concurrent neck and spinal injuries.
- Establish vascular access.
- Monitor ABGs and oxygen saturation.
- Check core body temperature; warm the patient as needed.
- The addition of positive airway pressure (BiPAP or PEEP) will help recruit collapsed alveoli.
- Correct acid–base imbalances.
- Consider prophylactic antibiotics.
- Insert a gastric tube to decompress the stomach, as gastric distension and vomiting is common.
- Admit for a minimum of 24 hours of observation; ARDS is a serious complication of drowning.

CARBON MONOXIDE POISONING

Carbon monoxide is a colorless, tasteless, odorless gas with an affinity for hemoglobin 200 to 250 times that of oxygen; in its presence, hemoglobin molecules quickly become saturated with carbon monoxide and cannot transport oxygen. Carbon monoxide also shifts the oxyhemoglobin dissociation curve to the left, impairing the ability of hemoglobin to release the oxygen that has attached. These two factors result in tissue hypoxia.

Carbon monoxide poisoning is especially harmful to a developing fetus. Fetal hemoglobin has an even greater affinity for carbon monoxide and the fetus can have a carboxyhemoglobin level approximately 30% higher than that of its mother.[22]

Carbon monoxide poisoning comes from the inhalation of combustible fumes such as those produced by generators, small gasoline engines, or a malfunctioning furnace. Exposure often occurs in an enclosed or confined space. Carbon monoxide may be a component of inhalation injury; see Chapter 42, Burns, for more specific information. Additionally, chronic carbon monoxide poisoning exposure can occur from automobile exhaust, tobacco smoke, or industrial sources.[22]

Signs and Symptoms

- Nausea
- Headache
- Dizziness
- Impaired judgment
- See Table 18-7 for symptoms of carbon monoxide poisoning based on carboxyhemoglobin (COHb) level

Diagnostic Procedures

- Elevated COHb.
- Pulse oximetry (SpO$_2$) is *not* useful in carbon monoxide poisoning. Pulse oximetry measures the *percent* of hemoglobin saturated, not whether oxygen or carbon monoxide is the saturating molecule.
- Obtain arterial blood gases to check a *measured* saturation level (SaO$_2$).

Therapeutic Interventions

- Administer 100% oxygen. Oxygen is the antidote for carbon monoxide; begin its administration immediately.
- Monitor cardiac rhythm and COHb level.
- Hyperbaric oxygen therapy (HBO) involves breathing oxygen under increased atmospheric pressure.[23] It can be highly effective but logistically complicated. Few facilities have an HBO chamber available so interfacility transfer may be required. Breathing 100% oxygen decreases the half-life of CO; because of this, COHb may actually be lowered to acceptable levels in less time than it would take to complete a transfer to a hyperbaric unit.

MECHANICAL VENTILATION IN THE EMERGENCY DEPARTMENT

Frequently, emergency nurses care for critically ill patients who require mechanical ventilation. Several essential concepts are important in providing skilled care for these patients. This section reviews modes of ventilation, common ventilator settings, troubleshooting alarms, and basic caring principles for the patient on ventilation.

TABLE 18-7	SYMPTOMS OF CARBON MONOXIDE POISONING BASED ON CARBOXYHEMOGLOBIN LEVEL			
CARBOXYHEMOGLOBIN (COHb) LEVEL				
5%–10%	10%–20%	20%–40%	40%–60%	≥60%
Headache Dizziness	Headache Nausea, vomiting Loss of coordination Flushed skin Dyspnea	Confusion Lethargy Visual disturbances Angina	Dysrhythmias Seizures Coma	Cherry-red skin Death

Mode of ventilation refers to the method of inspiratory support provided by the ventilator. Ventilation can be volume-controlled or pressure-regulated.

- With volume ventilation, a preset tidal volume is delivered during the inspiratory phase; the pressure required to deliver that preset tidal volume will vary depending on lung compliance and resistance.
- Pressure ventilation ensures a constant inspiratory pressure; however, tidal volume varies with lung compliance and resistance.
- Table 18-8 reviews commonly used modes of mechanical ventilation.[24]

Additional ventilator settings will be determined by the patient's clinical status. Table 18-9 lists various ventilator settings and their definitions.

Nursing Care of the Mechanically Ventilated Patient

Care of the mechanically ventilated patient requires frequent assessment of vital signs, mental status, sedation, and pain control. Additional information related to airway management and mechanical ventilation can be found in Chapter 8, Airway Management.

- Assess endotracheal tube placement frequently, particularly after moving the patient.
- To prevent aspiration, elevate the head of the bed to 30 degrees unless contraindicated.
- Reposition patient, side-to-side if possible, every 2 hours or more often if needed for comfort.
- Suction mouth and posterior pharynx as needed.
- Auscultate lungs frequently; suction endotracheal tube only as needed, not routinely.
  - Use sterile technique and a closed suction system.
  - Hyperoxygenate the patient prior to suctioning.
  - Suction only the length of the endotracheal tube to prevent trauma to the lower airways.
- Communicate frequently with the intubated patient to ensure his or her understanding of interventions and to determine his or her needs.

- If neuromuscular blockade is necessary, ensure adequate sedation and analgesia for the patient; monitor level of sedation and muscular blockade.
- *Never* turn off or disable ventilator alarms. Table 18-10 lists various alarms and their potential causes.
  - If cause of ventilator alarm cannot be immediately determined, remove patient from the ventilator and begin manual ventilation.
- Consider restraints according to the facility's policies for patient safety and airway protection.
- Provide oral care every 2 to 4 hours, including brushing teeth every 12 hours.
- Consider peptic ulcer and deep vein thrombosis prophylaxis.

The DOPE mnemonic is helpful in troubleshooting ventilator alarms:
- **D:** Displacement of endotracheal tube
- **O:** Obstruction of tube or circuitry
- **P:** Check the patient and consider pneumothorax
- **E:** Equipment failure

PREVENTION OF RESPIRATORY CONTAMINATION

In the ED, respiratory etiquette is necessary to prevent the spread of respiratory illnesses. Multiple patients and visitors come to the ED throughout the day, creating the possibility and probability of the spread of respiratory pathogens. From triage to discharge, ED staff members are challenged to keep themselves, their patients, and department visitors safe from respiratory contamination. Recommendations from the Centers for Disease Control and Prevention (CDC) highlight strategies to protect ED staff, patients, and visitors through respiratory etiquette.[25] Issues of crowding, boarding, and inadequate staffing all have an impact on this public health concern. All ED staff, including physicians, need to partner in these initiatives to protect themselves and their patients. Policies, planning, and communication are

TABLE 18-8 MODES OF VENTILATION

MODES	DESCRIPTION	INDICATIONS
Assist control (AC)	Delivers a pre-set tidal volume for every breathe whether initiated by the patient or by the ventilator	Apneic patients, patients on neuromuscular blockade agents or sedation, or patients who require a greater tidal volume than they can take on their own
Synchronized intermittent mandatory ventilation (SIMV)	Delivers a pre-set tidal volume and allows the patient to breathe at his or her own pace and tidal volume; synchronized with the patient's own ventilatory efforts	Allows the patient to breathe at his or her own rate and tidal volume in addition to the pre-set rate and tidal volume of the ventilator
Continuous positive airway pressure (CPAP)	Delivers constant positive pressure to the airway	Allows the patient to breathe at his or her own pace while providing constant positive pressure
Pressure control ventilation	Delivers a pre-set pressure, selected inspiratory time and rate; tidal volume is dependent on inspiratory time, pressure and lung compliance	Allows the patient to breathe spontaneously although the pre-set inspiratory time will remain constant; patient may need sedation
Pressure Support Ventilation (PSV)	Select amount of inspiratory pressure that is maintained throughout the inspiratory cycle; used to overcome endotracheal resistance or to assist with weaning	Allows the patient to initiate each ventilator cycle at his or her own rate, timing and tidal volume; can be used with SIMV or CPAP
Inverse ratio ventilation	Ventilation is accomplished during a brief expiratory phrase after a prolonged inspiratory phase; helps open collapsed lungs using higher stabilizing pressures during inspiration	Acute lung injury; acute respiratory distress syndrome
Positive End Expiratory Pressure (PEEP)	Delivers positive pressure to the airway at the end of expiration	Prevents alveolar collapse, improves oxygenation; at high pressure levels can potentially decrease cardiac output, increase the work of breathing and increase the potential for barotrauma

Reprinted with permission from McCorstin, P., Cottrell, D. B., Rose, M., & Dwyer, G. (2008). Management of the mechanically ventilated patient in the emergency department. *Journal of Emergency Nursing, 34*(2), 121–125.

TABLE 18-9 VENTILATOR SETTINGS

Respiratory rate	The number of breaths that the ventilator will deliver per minute
Tidal volume	The amount of air inhaled and exhaled with each breath
Flow rate	Rate at which the tidal volume is delivered
Fraction of inspired oxygen (FiO$_2$)	Percentage of oxygen delivered
Inspiratory-expiratory ratio	Amount of time for inspiration compared to the amount of time required for expiration
Pressure limit	Maximum amount of pressure generated by the ventilator to deliver the tidal volume

important components of the process.[26] Examples of actions that can be taken to minimize the spread of respiratory contaminates include:

- Early identification, isolation, and interventions are keys in managing risk from both traditional and emerging respiratory infections.
- Hand washing remains the single most effective measure to limit the spread of infection.
- Alcohol hand wash, tissues, and masks should be made available to all visitors.
- Patients identified with a possible respiratory illness at triage should be given a surgical mask immediately and placed in a private room.
  - If private rooms are not available, patients with respiratory illnesses should be cohorted.
- Patients should wear face masks during transport to other areas of the hospital.

TABLE 18-10   FREQUENT MECHANICAL VENTILATOR ALARMS

ALARM	POSSIBLE CAUSES	INTERVENTIONS
High pressure alarm	Decreased lung compliance from pneumothorax, atelectasis, ARDS, pulmonary edema	Assess changes in lung sounds, vital signs, and pulse oximetry
	Kinks in endotracheal tube	Assess tube for kinks, reposition as needed, assess need for bite block
	Obstruction of ventilator tubing or secretions in airway	Assess breath sounds and suction as needed
	Bronchospasm/cough	Check endotracheal tube position, reposition, and secure as needed
		Consider bronchodilators
	Patient-ventilator asynchrony	Assess patient for anxiety, oxygenation status, vital signs
		Provide emotional support
		Sedatives may be required
Low pressure alarm	Disconnection or endotracheal tube leak	Check all ventilator connections; check endotracheal tube for placement or cuff leak
Apnea alarm	Patient not breathing within pre-set ventilator settings	Assess for sleep apnea, oversedation, neurologic changes
		Assess for need to change ventilator mode/settings

ARDS, Acute respiratory distress syndrome.
Reprinted with permission from McCorstin, P., Cottrell, D. B., Rose, M., & Dwyer, G. (2008). Management of the mechanically ventilated patient in the emergency department. *Journal of Emergency Nursing, 34*(2), 121–125.

- Surge planning during peak seasons for respiratory illnesses should be ongoing.
- Staff must care for themselves by staying home when ill, performing meticulous hand washing, and receiving annual flu vaccination.

REFERENCES

1. Valdez-Lowe, C., Ghareeb, S. A., & Artinian, N. T. (2009). Pulse oximetry in adults. *American Journal of Nursing, 109*(6), 52–59.
2. Gilboy, N., & Hawkins, M. R. (2006). Noninvasive monitoring of end-tidal carbon dioxide in the emergency department. *Advanced Emergency Nursing Journal, 28*(4), 301–313.
3. American Lung Association. (n.d.). *Measuring your peak flow rate*. Retrieved from http://www.lungusa.org/lung-disease/asthma/living-with-asthma/take-control-of-your-asthma/measuring-your-peak-flow-rate.html
4. Corbridge, S., & Corbridge, T. C. (2010). Asthma in adolescents and adults. *American Journal of Nursing, 110*(5), 28–38.
5. House, D. T., & Ramirez, E. G. (2008). Emergency management of asthma exacerbations. *Advanced Emergency Nursing Journal, 30*(2), 122–138.
6. Bateman, E. D., Hurd, S. S., Barnes, P. J., Bousquet, J., Drazen, J. M., FitzGerald, M., ... Zar, H. J. (2008). Global strategy for asthma management and prevention: GINA executive summary. *European Respiratory Journal, 31*(1), 143–178.
7. Oman, K. S., & Koziol-McLain, J. (2006). *Emergency nursing secrets* (2nd ed.). St. Louis, MO: Mosby.
8. Bramann, S. S. (2006). Chronic cough due to acute bronchitis: ACCP evidence-based clinical practice guidelines. *Chest, 129* (1 Suppl), 95S–103S.
9. Hart, A. M. (2009). Treatment strategies for cough illness in adults. *The Nurse Practitioner, 34*(11), 26–33.
10. Kosowsky, J. M. (2009). Pleural disease. In J. A. Marx (Ed.), *Rosen's emergency medicine: concepts and clinical practice* (7th ed.), Philadelphia, PA: Mosby.
11. Goss, L. K. (2008). The essentials of hospital-acquired pneumonia. *Nursing Made Incredibly Easy, 6*(5), 32–43.
12. Mandell, L. A., Wunderink, R. G., Anzueto, A., Bartlett, J. G., Campbell, G. D., Dean, N. C., ... Whitney, C. G., Infectious Diseases Society of America; American Thoracic Society. (2007). Infectious Diseases Society of America/American Thoracic Society consensus guidelines on the management of community-acquired pneumonia in adults. *Clinical Infectious Diseases, 44*(Suppl 2), S27–S72.
13. Cunha, B. A. (2011, March 29). *Community-acquired pneumonia*. Retrieved from http://emedicine.medscape.com/article/234240-overview
14. Mertin, S., Sawatzky, J. V., & Diehl-Jones, W. L. (2009). Getting to the heart of pleural effusions: A case study. *Journal of the American Academy of Nurse Practitioners, 21*(9), 509–512.
15. Ouellette, D. R., Setnik, G., Beeson, M. S., Garg, K., Amorosa, J. K., Stern, E. J., & Harrington, A. (2011, July 27). *Pulmonary embolism*. Retrieved from http://emedicine.medscape.com/article/759765-overview
16. Khan, A. N., Irion, K. L., Kasthuri, R. S., & MacDonald, S. (2011, May 27). *Noncardiogenic pulmonary edema imaging*. Retrieved from http://emedicine.medscape.com/article/360932-overview

17. Mullen, W. H. (2007, May 15). *Toxin-related noncardiogenic pulmonary edema.* Retrieved from http://www.chestnet.org/accp/pccsu/toxin-related-noncardiogenic-pulmonary-edema?page=0,0

18. Gallagher, J. J. (2009). Taking aim at ARDS. *Nursing 2009, 39*(11), 49–54.

19. Harman, E. M. (2011, July 26). *Acute respiratory distress syndrome.* Retrieved from http://emedicine.medscape.com/article/165139-overview

20. van Beeck, E. F., Branche, C. M., Szpilman, D., Modell, J. H., & Bierens, J. J. (2005). A new definition of drowning: Towards documentation and prevention of a global public health problem. *Bulletin of the World Health Organization, 83*(11), 853–856.

21. Verive, M. J. (2011, July 18). *Near drowning.* Retrieved from http://emedicine.medscape.com/article/908677-overview

22. Goldstein, M. (2008). Carbon monoxide poisoning. *Journal of Emergency Nursing, 34*(6), 538–542.

23. Latham, E., Hare, M. A., & Neumeister, M. (2010, May 19). *Hyperbaric oxygen therapy.* Retrieved from http://emedicine.medscape.com/article/1464149-overview

24. McCorstin, P., Cottrell, D. B., Rose, M., & Dwyer, G. (2008). Management of the mechanically ventilated patient in the emergency department. *Journal of Emergency Nursing, 34*(2), 121–125.

25. Centers for Disease Control and Prevention. (2010, September 20). *Prevention strategies for seasonal influenza in healthcare settings.* Retrieved from www.cdc.gov/flu/professionals/infectioncontrol/healthcaresettings.htm

26. Rothman, R. E., Irvin, C. B., Moran, G. J., Sauer, L., Bradshaw, Y. S., Fry, R. B. Jr., ... Hirshon, J. M. (2007). Respiratory hygiene in the emergency department. *Journal of Emergency Nursing, 33*(2), 119–134.

Cardiovascular Emergencies

Belinda B. Hammond

Chest pain is the chief complaint of many patients presenting to the emergency department (ED). If the chest pain is a result of cardiac problems, time to treatment is important, and management may be initiated before a complete medical history and full diagnostic workup have been completed. Because of the life-threatening nature of these emergencies, assessing airway, breathing, and circulation (ABC) is always given priority.

This chapter assumes that the reader possesses a basic knowledge of risk factors for cardiac disease, basic life support and cardiopulmonary resuscitation (BLS/CPR), and dysrhythmia detection.

ASSESSMENT OF CHEST PAIN

- The PQRST mnemonic (Table 19-1) is useful in assessing the characteristics of chest pain and may be used to gather comprehensive information about the nature of the pain.
- Patients often deny "pain" but complain of burning, pressure, or tightness. Describe the patient's pain or discomfort using his or her own words in the documentation.
- Assess for "anginal equivalents," particularly in women, diabetics, and the elderly.
  - Patients with anginal equivalents may report shortness of breath, fatigue, palpitations, near-syncope, and nausea and vomiting.
  - These symptoms may be more bothersome to the patient than any chest discomfort.[1]
  - Discomfort is more likely to be localized outside the chest area.
  - If angina is present, it is often precipitated by mental stress rather than physical exertion.
- Have the patient rate the pain or discomfort on a scale of 1 to 10.

- Obtain a 12-lead electrocardiogram (ECG) within 10 minutes of patient arrival; assess for dysrhythmias and ST segment elevation or depression.
- There are many possible etiologies for chest pain (Table 19-2); therefore it is important to rule out the most serious or life-threatening causes immediately.
- Document current medications, including prescriptions, over-the-counter medications, and herbal therapies.
  - Determine compliance with prescribed medications.
  - Specifically question the patient about recent use of phosphodiesterase inhibitors for erectile dysfunction.
- Recent cocaine use is a common cause of ischemic chest pain resulting from coronary vasospasm. It is important to ask the patient about recreational drug use.
- Document positive and negative risk factors for cardiovascular disease, including those for previous cardiac disease such as prior myocardial infarction (MI), coronary interventions such as stent placement, and presence of a pacemaker or implantable cardioverter defibrillator (ICD).

> Cocaine stimulates both alpha- and beta-adrenergic receptors. Use of beta-blockers in the patient who has recently used cocaine leaves alpha activity unopposed, resulting in additional coronary vasoconstriction and systemic hypertension.[1]

DIAGNOSTIC PROCEDURES

- 12-lead ECG
  - Records the heart's electrical activity from twelve different views
  - Determines rate, rhythm, and presence of dysrhythmias
  - Examines contiguous leads for ST segment depression or ST segment elevation
- Continuous bedside ST monitoring

TABLE 19-1 THE PQRST MNEMONIC

P	What things **p**rovoke or **p**recipitate or **p**alliate or alleviate the pain or discomfort?
Q	What is the **q**uality of the pain or discomfort? Document this characteristic in the patient's own words.
R	Does the pain or discomfort **r**adiate? If so, to what locations? What is the location or **r**egion of the pain or discomfort?
S	Rate the **s**everity of the pain or discomfort. Are there associated **s**ymptoms?
T	What are the **t**ime elements of the pain or discomfort? When did it start? How long did it last? Did the pain or discomfort begin suddenly or gradually?

TABLE 19-2 LIFE-THREATENING AND NON–LIFE-THREATENING CAUSES OF CHEST PAIN

LIFE-THREATENING	NON–LIFE-THREATENING
Acute coronary syndrome	Pericarditis
Pulmonary embolism	Esophageal reflex (GERD)
Aortic dissection	Pneumonia
Tension pneumothorax	Spontaneous pneumothorax
Acute myocardial infarction	Costochondritis
	Pancreatitis
	Herpes zoster infection
	Cocaine use

GERD, Gastroesophageal reflux disease.

- Serum electrolytes, complete blood count, clotting times, and cardiac biomarkers
- Chest radiograph
- Cardiac catheterization with angiography
- Echocardiogram to determine left ventricular (LV) ejection fraction (EF); presence of hypertrophy, dyskinetic, or akinetic areas; structural abnormalities such as LV aneurysm or valvular dysfunction; and pericardial effusion
- Doppler studies of peripheral blood flow
- Stress testing

Contiguous leads are those leads that "look at" the same area of the heart.	
Anterior left ventricle (LV)	Leads V1–V4
Ventricular septum	Leads V1 and V2
Inferior surface of LV	Leads II, III, aVF
Lateral LV wall	Leads I, aVL, V5, V6
Posterior LV	Leads V1 and V2

TABLE 19-3 DIAGNOSTIC DIFFERENCES BETWEEN TYPES OF ACUTE CORONARY SYNDROME

	12-LEAD ECG FINDINGS	CREATINE KINASE TROPONIN TEST
Unstable angina	Normal or nondiagnostic changes such as ST depression and T wave inversion	Negative
Non-STEMI	ST depression or T wave changes	Positive
STEMI	ST elevation >1 mm in two contiguous leads New or presumably new LBBB	Positive

ECG, Electrocardiogram; *LBBB*, left bundle branch block; *STEMI*, ST segment elevation myocardial infarction.

SPECIFIC CARDIAC EMERGENCIES

Acute Coronary Syndrome

Acute coronary syndrome (ACS) refers to the clinical presentations of acute myocardial ischemia. This continuum includes unstable angina, non–ST segment elevation myocardial infarction (non-STEMI), and ST segment elevation myocardial infarction (STEMI). These presentations represent varying degrees of myocardial oxygen supply and demand imbalance and refer to different stages of myocardial ischemia. Table 19-3 summarizes the characteristics of these three problems.

- Unstable angina—a change in the patient's usual pattern of angina
  - Ischemic chest pain becomes unpredictable, more intense, and more difficult to relieve. Unstable angina may occur at rest, even awakening the patient from sleep. It occurs more frequently and is longer in duration than the patient's usual angina.
  - Indicates an unstable atherosclerotic plaque with the potential for rupture.
  - Transient (ST segment depression or T wave inversion) or negative ECG changes; negative cardiac biomarker results.
- Non-STEMI
  - Ischemic chest pain or anginal equivalent associated with ST segment depression and positive cardiac biomarkers.
  - Indicates rupture of unstable atherosclerotic plaque and intermittent coronary occlusion.[2]

- STEMI
  - Associated with complete occlusion of a coronary artery by a thrombus superimposed on a ruptured plaque.
  - ECG shows 1-mm (or more) ST segment elevation in two or more contiguous leads or new (or presumed new) left bundle branch block (LBBB) pattern.
  - Cardiac biomarkers will be positive.

Signs and Symptoms

- Chest pain or discomfort unrelieved by rest.
  - Pain or discomfort may be described as burning, crushing, tightness, pressure, or aching.
  - Patient may deny chest pain and complain of a toothache, pain in the jaw or elbow, or indigestion-like discomfort.
  - Discomfort is often substernal.
  - Radiation of pain to arm, neck, jaw, back, or shoulder is not uncommon.
  - Associated with nausea, vomiting, shortness of breath, diaphoresis, weakness, dizziness, syncope, and palpitations.
- Patient may experience a sense of impending doom.
- Sign of LV failure (crackles, S_3 heart sound, respiratory distress) if infarct involves a large portion of the anterior left ventricle.
- Tachycardia may be the result of sympathetic stimulation; bradycardia or varying degrees of atrioventricular (AV) block often seen with inferior MI.

Diagnostic Procedures

- 12-lead ECG.
  - Non-STEMI: ST depression.
  - STEMI: 1-mm or more ST segment elevation in two or more contiguous leads. See Table 19-4 for localization of MI and potential complications associated with MI location.
- LBBB on the 12-lead ECG distorts the ST segment. In the presence of new or presumed new LBBB and ischemic chest discomfort, manage the patient as though STEMI is present.
- If initial ECG is nondiagnostic, repeat the 12-lead ECG in 1 hour; if the patient remains symptomatic or experiences new symptoms, obtain repeat ECGs at 5- to 10-minute intervals or initiate continuous ST segment monitoring.
- If inferior wall MI is present, obtain right-sided V-leads to detect possible right ventricular infarct (Fig. 19-1A).
  - Patients experiencing right ventricular (RV) infarction are "preload dependent."
    - Administer nitroglycerin with caution because of potential for worsened hypotension.
    - May require volume administration.
  - The classic triad of RV failure because of RV infarct.
    - Severe systemic hypotension.
    - Absence of pulmonary congestion.
    - Increased central venous pressure (CVP) and jugular venous distension.
- If inferior MI is associated with ST depression in V2 and R wave larger than S wave in leads V1 and V2, obtain posterior ECG to detect possible posterior wall MI (Fig. 19-1B).
- Cardiac biomarkers.
  - Troponin I elevates 3 to 12 hours after infarct; level peaks between 10 and 24 hours.
  - Creatine kinase-MB elevates 4 to 12 hours after infarct; level peaks between 10 and 24 hours.
- Chest radiograph to detect pulmonary congestion or cardiac enlargement.
- Complete blood count, blood chemistries, and coagulation studies.

TABLE 19-4 DIFFERENCES BETWEEN TYPES OF MYOCARDIAL INFARCTION

OCCLUDED CORONARY ARTERY	AREA OF HEART AFFECTED	LEADS SHOWING CHANGES	POTENTIAL COMPLICATIONS
Left anterior descending	Anterior wall of LV	V1, V2, V3, V4	Left ventricular failure
		Reciprocal changes II, III, aVF	Cardiogenic shock
Circumflex	Lateral wall of LV	I, aVL, V5, V6	
		Reciprocal changes II, III, aVF	
Right coronary artery (posterior descending)	Inferior and/or posterior LV	II, III, aVF	Bradycardia
	AV node (95%)	Reciprocal changes I and aVL	Varying degrees of heart block
Right coronary artery (proximal)	Right ventricle	V4R	Right ventricular failure
	Inferior LV	II, III, aVF	
	Posterior LV wall	R>S in V1 and/or V2	

AV, Atrioventricular; *LV,* left ventricle.

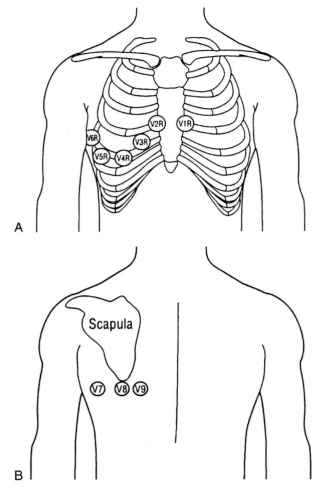

Fig. 19-1 A, Right precordial leads. **B,** Posterior chest leads. (From Moser, D., & Reigel, B. [2008]. *Cardiac nursing: A companion to Braunwald's heart disease.* Philadelphia, PA: W.B. Saunders.)

Creatine kinase-MB (CK-MB) levels return to normal within approximately 72 hours; on the other hand, troponin values remain elevated up to 9 days. This is significant in the patient who "infarcts at home" and comes to the ED several days after experiencing chest pain or angina equivalents; the troponin remains elevated but the CK-MB has returned to normal.

Therapeutic Interventions

- Administer supplemental oxygen to maintain oxygen saturation above 92%.
- Maintain intravenous (IV) access.

- Give non–enteric coated aspirin, 162 to 325 mg; have patient chew and swallow aspirin if possible. Administer aspirin as rectal suppository if necessary.
- Administer nitroglycerin sublingual tablet or spray if systolic blood pressure greater than 90 mm Hg and heart rate greater than 50 beats per minute. If the patient experiences no relief from pain, the emergency nurse may repeat nitroglycerin every 5 minutes up to three doses.
- The American Heart Association does not recommend the routine use of IV nitroglycerin in patients with STEMI.[2] If it is used, monitor the patient closely for drug-induced hypotension that can decrease coronary perfusion and worsen myocardial ischemia.
  - If the patient has used a phosphodiesterase inhibitor within the past 24 hours, nitroglycerin administration may result in severe hypotension refractory to vasopressors.
  - Nitroglycerin must be administered with caution in patients with inferior wall MI and possible RV involvement. These patients are often highly dependent on RV filling pressures; venodilation and decreased preload can precipitate a dramatic and irreversible decrease in cardiac output.
- Use of morphine is indicated for STEMI when chest discomfort is unresponsive to nitrates. It should be used with caution in unstable angina and non-STEMI because of an association with increased mortality.
- Medications to limit platelet aggregation are important treatment modalities.
  - Aspirin (see above)
  - Clopidogrel (Plavix) or prasugrel (Effient)
- In STEMI, early reperfusion of the myocardium, by pharmacologic or mechanical means, has been shown to reduce mortality.
  - Opening the infarct-related artery restores myocardial perfusion and therefore limits infarct size and reduces complications (including death) associated with acute MI.
  - The goal for "total ischemic time" (from time of symptom onset to intervention) is under 90 minutes.
  - Percutaneous coronary intervention (PCI) is the preferred method of reperfusion.[3]
    - Bivalirudin (Angiomax), a direct thrombin inhibitor, can be used for anticoagulation in patients undergoing primary PCI.[3]
    - Glycoprotein IIb/IIIa inhibitors are antiplatelet agents that may be considered at the time of PCI.[3]
      - Abciximab (ReoPro)
      - Eptifibatide (Integrilin)
      - Tirofiban (Aggrastat)
  - If the patient is unable to undergo primary PCI within 90 to 120 minutes of first medical contact,

immediate fibrinolytic therapy should be administered.

- Patients who receive fibrinolytics as primary reperfusion therapy should be transferred as soon as possible to a PCI-capable facility.[3]
- Prehospital administration of half-dose fibrinolytics, followed by urgent PCI, is being implemented in some areas of the country.
- Medical management.
  - Beta-blockers—oral beta-blockers are recommended for all types of ACS unless contraindicated by signs of heart failure or low output states.
    - Beta-blockers decrease myocardial oxygen demand by decreasing heart rate, contractility, and blood pressure.
    - Early administration should be considered in patients with STEMI who are hypertensive.
  - Angiotensin-converting enzyme (ACE) inhibitors (capotopril, enalapril, lisinopril) are generally started after reperfusion therapy has been completed.
    - The use of ACE inhibitors has been shown to improve survival in patients with MI.
    - ACE inhibitors reduce infarct size and improve ventricular remodeling.
- Consider transfer of patient with STEMI due to large anterior MI, signs of heart failure, or pulmonary edema to a facility with interventional (PCI, coronary bypass grafting) capabilities. The goal for door-to-transfer time is less than 30 minutes.

Acute Decompensated Heart Failure

Heart failure is the result of inadequate cardiac output and oxygen delivery to the tissues. It can be caused by an inability of the heart to pump effectively (systolic failure) or by an inability of the heart to fill adequately (diastolic failure). Furthermore, heart failure can primarily affect the left ventricle, resulting in pulmonary venous congestion and respiratory symptoms, or the right ventricle, resulting in circulatory congestion.

Acute decompensated heart failure usually occurs in the setting of chronic failure; symptoms worsen, requiring additional and often emergent interventions.

Common Precipitating Conditions

- ACS, particularly with ischemia or necrotic damage to the ventricles
- Uncontrolled hypertension
- Cardiomyopathies
- Valvular dysfunction
- Cardiac infections such as myocarditis or endocarditis
- Noncompliance with medications and diet

TABLE 19-5	SIGNS AND SYMPTOMS OF RIGHT-SIDED AND LEFT-SIDED HEART FAILURE	
RIGHT-SIDED HEART FAILURE		**LEFT-SIDED HEART FAILURE**
Peripheral edema		Shortness of breath
Jugular venous distension		Dyspnea
Ascites		S_3 heart sound
Nausea because of venous congestion of abdominal viscera		Crackles
		Pulmonary edema

Signs and Symptoms

Table 19-5 provides a comparison of signs and symptoms of right- and left-sided heart failure. Patients may have symptoms of both right- and left-sided failure.

Diagnostic Procedures

- Chest radiograph to evaluate chamber size and assess for pulmonary congestion
- Echocardiogram to determine ejection fraction and detect possible structural abnormalities
- 12-lead ECG
- B-type natriuretic peptide (BNP) greater than 100 pg/mL
- Complete blood count and metabolic panel
- Cardiac biomarkers to rule out acute MI

Therapeutic Interventions

- Assessing and managing the patient's airway, breathing, and circulation are always the first priority.
- Administer supplemental oxygen to maintain oxygen saturation above 90%.
- Obtain IV access; administer fluids with caution to prevent fluid overload.
- Noninvasive positive ventilation (BiPAP) may improve pulmonary congestion by forcing alveolar fluid back into the pulmonary capillaries.
- Administer a loop diuretic. Furosemide (Lasix) causes an almost immediate venous dilation (decreasing preload) followed by diuresis within 10 minutes of IV administration. However, many patients with chronic heart failure may have become resistant to loop diuretics.
- Morphine also causes venous dilation and a decrease in preload. By decreasing the patient's anxiety, morphine diminishes sympathetic stimulation and decreases the workload of the heart.

- IV nitroglycerin dilates the venous capacitance vessels to further decrease preload. Nitroglycerin is contraindicated if the patient's blood pressure is less than 90 mm Hg.
- Nitroprusside (Nipride) causes both arteriolar and venous dilation thus decreasing both preload and afterload and the myocardial oxygen demands.
- Nesiritide, a recombinant BNP, is another potent vasodilator that is administered by continuous IV infusion.
- Both nitroprusside and nesiritide administration require close patient monitoring, particularly of the patient's blood pressure, as response to these medications can be immediate and unpredictable. Blood pressure monitoring with an arterial line is recommended.
- Randomized, controlled trials do not support the use of positive inotropic drugs in heart failure unless the patient is experiencing cardiogenic shock.[4] In that situation, the patient will need admission to the intensive care unit (ICU) for administration of dobutamine, dopamine, or milrinone.
- ACE inhibitors should be considered to interrupt the renin-angiotensin cycle and minimize fluid retention. Angiotensin receptor blockers (ARBs) may be used if the patient is unable to tolerate ACE inhibitors.
- Closely monitor the patient's response to treatment. In particular, assess:
  - Breath sounds, respiratory rate, and oxygen saturation
  - Shortness of breath and work of breathing
  - Arterial blood pressure and heart rate
  - Level of consciousness
  - Jugular venous distension
  - Urine output—an indwelling urinary catheter may be necessary

Acute Aortic Dissection

Acute aortic dissection is a life-threatening condition that occurs when a tear in the intimal (or innermost) layer of the aorta allows blood flow to enter the aortic media. Propelled by the pulsatile flow and high pressures with the aorta, this column of blood produces a "false channel" for antegrade or retrograde blood flow. Pressure within this false channel can compress the true aortic lumen and reduce blood flow through aortic branch vessels. The result is ischemia of distal tissues and organs. Aortic dissections are classified based on their location and potential complications can be anticipated based on that location.

> The most important aspect of diagnosing acute aortic dissection is a high index of suspicion; consider aortic dissection in all patients presenting with chest pain.

Risk Factors for Aortic Dissection

- Hypertension is the most common risk factor
- Atherosclerosis
- Age 60 years or older
- Previous cardiovascular surgery[5]
- Bicuspid aortic valve[5]
- Marfan syndrome—a genetic syndrome characterized by:
  - Cystic medial necrosis leading to intimal weakness
  - Very long arms (arm span may exceed height of body); long, "spiderlike" fingers (arachnodactyly) and toes
  - "Pigeon chest" or pectus exacavatum
  - Dislocated optic lenses
- Iatrogenic or traumatic intimal tear
- Cocaine use
- Syphilis

Signs and Symptoms

- Severe ripping, tearing pain in the chest
  - Pain may radiate to back, flank, or shoulders
  - Acute onset
  - Pain difficult to relieve
- Difference in blood pressure of 20 mm Hg between arms
- If aortic arch is involved:
  - Altered level of consciousness
  - Signs and symptoms of stroke
  - Cardiac tamponade
    - Muffled heart sounds
    - Jugular venous distension
    - Hypotension
  - Acute MI
  - Acute aortic valvular insufficiency
    - Dyspnea
    - Sudden onset LV failure
    - New systolic murmur
- If descending aorta is involved:
  - Anuria and renal failure
  - Paraplegia
  - Loss of distal pulses

Diagnostic Procedures

- Chest radiograph—often normal but may reveal widened mediastinum or pleural effusion.
- 12-lead ECG may be compatible with acute MI if dissection compromises coronary blood flow.
- Transthoracic echocardiogram (TTE) or transesophageal echocardiogram (TEE) to visualize dissection
- Chest computed tomography (CT), magnetic resonance imaging or angiography, or spiral CT angiography

- Aortogram is no longer a first-line diagnostic study but may be used to determine exact anatomy of dissection.

Therapeutic Interventions

- Administer supplemental oxygen; obtain IV access with two large-bore catheters.
- Assess blood pressure in both arms.
- Continually assess vital signs, neurologic status, status of peripheral pulses, movement and sensation, and urinary output.
- Medical management consists of maintaining systolic blood pressure between 100 and 120 mm Hg and decreasing the force of myocardial contraction.
    - Nitroprusside or nitroglycerin.
        - These agents cause vasodilation and decrease blood pressure and the resistance to LV ejection (afterload).
        - Anticipate arterial line placement with nitroprusside administration.
        - Do not use alone because of possible reflex tachycardia.
    - IV beta-blockers, such as labetalol, esmolol, or propranolol, to decrease contractility in an attempt to limit propagation of the dissection.
- Administer opiates for analgesia to further decrease sympathetic stimulation and blood pressure.
- Surgical repair will be required for aortic dissections involving the aortic arch. Anticipate transfer to tertiary center with cardiopulmonary bypass capabilities if necessary.

Hypertensive Emergency

Hypertensive emergency, or crisis, is present in a patient with a systolic blood pressure over 180 mm Hg or a diastolic blood pressure over 120 mm Hg and evidence of impending or progressive end-organ damage. It is this major organ dysfunction, rather than a specific blood pressure value, that makes this a life-threatening emergency. Acute end-organ damage can be evident as encephalopathy, ischemic or hemorrhagic stroke, or heart or renal failure.[6]

Table 19-6 lists possible causes of hypertensive emergencies.

Signs and Symptoms

- Cerebrovascular impairment
    - Headache
    - Altered level of consciousness
    - Drowsiness, stupor, or coma
    - Confusion
    - Seizures

TABLE 19-6 POSSIBLE CAUSES OF HYPERTENSIVE EMERGENCIES

Essential hypertension	Noncompliance with antihypertensive medications
Preeclampsia or eclampsia	Cocaine or amphetamine use
Acute aortic dissection	Renal artery stenosis
Pheochromocytoma	Hyperaldosteronism
Glomerulonephritis	Alcohol withdrawal

- Cardiovascular compromise
    - Chest pain, ischemic changes on ECG
    - Presence of S_3 and S_4, signs and symptoms of heart failure
- Retinopathy
    - Retinal hemorrhage and exudates
    - Papilledema
- Renovascular impairment
    - Hematuria
    - Decreased urine output
- Others
    - Epistaxis
    - Blurred vision

Diagnostic Procedures

- Urinalysis
- Blood urea nitrogen and creatinine to assess for kidney damage secondary to elevated blood pressure
- 12-lead ECG—ischemic changes
- Chest radiograph—LV enlargement
- Computed tomography of head to rule out intracranial bleeding

Therapeutic Interventions

- Administer supplemental oxygen; obtain IV access
- Continuous blood pressure monitoring (at least every 5 minutes)
    - Use appropriately sized blood pressure cuff
    - Compare blood pressure measurements in both arms
    - May require arterial line insertion
- Sublingual or continuous IV nitroglycerin, particularly if patient has history of coronary artery disease (CAD)
- Continuous IV infusion of nitroprusside (Nipride)
    - Very rapid onset
    - Titrate slowly because of risk for sudden hypotension
    - Anticipate arterial line insertion
    - Rapid reduction of blood pressure slows the progression of end-organ damage[6]

- Limit decrease in blood pressure to 25% in the first 2 hours of treatment
- IV labetalol—onset of action is slower than that of nitroglycerin or nitroprusside but is safe and effective in pregnancy
- Continuously monitor response to therapy, particularly level of consciousness

Pericarditis

The pericardium is a fibrous sac surrounding the heart; it normally contains 15 to 50 mL straw-colored fluid to "lubricate" the heart as it contracts and relaxes. Acute pericarditis is an inflammation of the pericardium and may be an isolated condition or the result of systemic disease. Possible complications of pericarditis include cardiac tamponade, recurrent pericarditis, and pericardial constriction. Causes of pericarditis include:

- Idiopathic
- Viral
- Infections, including tuberculosis
- Acute MI
- Neoplastic invasion of the pericardium
- Inflammation following radiation therapy to the chest
- Following cardiac or thoracic surgery
- A complication of cardiac or thoracic trauma
- Aortic dissection
- Uremic syndrome in renal failure
- Autoimmune disorders

Signs and Symptoms

- Chest pain
  - Onset is generally sudden
  - Pain is severe, may be sharp or dull, often pleuritic in nature
  - Increases with activity, lying flat, and inspiration
  - Occasional radiation to neck, back, or arm
  - Decreased by sitting up and leaning forward
  - Unrelieved by rest or nitroglycerin
- Possible pericardial friction rub
  - "Leathery," grating quality on auscultation
  - May be transient
  - Best heard at the left sternal border with the patient leaning forward
  - Not associated with respiration but may be best heard at end-expiration
- Tachycardia, tachypnea
- Possible elevated body temperature

Diagnostic Procedures

- Cardiac biomarkers to rule out MI; however, troponin may be elevated in some patients
- 12-lead ECG

- Widespread ST segment elevation
- Tall, peaked T waves (usually present in all leads except aVR and V1)
- PR segment depression in Lead II
- No reciprocal changes in opposite leads
- Chest radiograph to rule out other causes
- Echocardiogram to detect possible pericardial effusion

Therapeutic Interventions

- Because patient presentation can mimic ACS, obtain a 12-lead ECG within 10 minutes of patient arrival.
- Administer supplemental oxygen, establish IV access, and monitor oxygen saturation and cardiac rhythm.
- Allow patient to assume position of comfort; provide overbed table to support patient as he or she leans forward.
- Administer anti-inflammatory medications.
  - Ibuprofen
  - Aspirin
  - Indomethacin
  - Colchicine
  - Corticosteroids if symptoms are resistant to non-steroidal anti-inflammatory drugs
- Pericardiocentesis may be needed if large pericardial effusion is present.

Acute Arterial Occlusion

Acute arterial occlusion can result from thrombosis, generally secondary to atherosclerotic lesions, or from an embolism that has detached from a thrombus. Patients often have a history consistent with atherosclerosis such as previous MI, stroke, or transient ischemia attack. A less common cause of occlusion is arterial injury from IV drug use. The vessels most commonly affected are the aortoiliac, femoral, and popliteal arteries resulting in limb-threatening ischemia.

Signs and Symptoms

- The signs of acute arterial occlusion are often referred to as the "5 P's"
  - Pain—may be severe and sudden in onset, particularly if collateral circulation has not developed
  - Pallor—delayed return of color after blanching skin. If the occlusion results from embolism, there may be a sharp demarcation between the ischemic (white) and nonischemic tissue.
  - Pulselessness—compare quality of pulse to contralateral limb
  - Paresthesia
  - Paralysis—indicates limb-threatening ischemia

- Evidence of underlying chronic arterial insufficiency from atherosclerosis
  - Muscle atrophy of lower extremity
  - Loss of hair on toe and foot
  - Thickened nail bed
  - Shiny, scaly skin
- Identifiable source of embolus such as atrial fibrillation or mitral valve disease

Diagnostic Procedures

- Doppler ultrasonography to detect peripheral circulation
- Ankle-brachial index (ABI)—the ratio of the systolic blood pressure of the ankle to the systolic blood pressure of the arm
  - Normal value is 0.9 to 1.3
  - ABI less than 0.9 indicative of peripheral arterial disease

Therapeutic Interventions

- Protect ischemic limb from injury.
- Initiate anticoagulation with IV heparin.
- Anticipate surgical intervention and embolectomy.
- Low-dose intraarterial fibrinolytic may be used if occlusion is not immediately limb-threatening.

Supraventricular Tachycardia

Supraventricular tachycardia (SVT) refers to any rapid rhythm that originates above the ventricles and includes sinus tachycardia, atrial flutter, atrial fibrillation with a rapid ventricular response (RVR), multifocal atrial tachycardia, and AV nodal reentrant tachycardia. The consequences of SVT are related to the decreased diastolic time associated with tachycardia (see Fig. 19-2). Decreased diastole limits the filling time of the ventricles and thus decreases cardiac output. The coronary arteries also fill during diastole, so a decrease in diastole can potentially lead to inadequate coronary perfusion. In addition, the rapid rate of ventricular contraction increases the workload and oxygen demands of the heart. Therefore patients with excessive heart rates may experience significant decreases in cardiac output and be highly symptomatic.

Signs and Symptoms

- Palpitations
- Chest pain
- Shortness of breath
- Diaphoresis, pallor
- Poor peripheral pulses
- Anxiety
- Syncope, near-syncope
- Hypotension

Effects of SVT on Coronary Perfusion

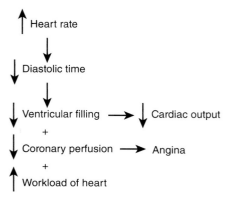

Fig. 19-2 Effects of supraventricular tachycardia on coronary perfusion.

Diagnostic Procedures

- 12-lead ECG
  - Ventricular rate 150 to 300 beats per minute
  - QRS complex narrow (less than 0.12 seconds) unless there is aberrant ventricular conduction
  - P waves often difficult to discern, as they may be buried in the preceding QRS complex
- Chest radiograph

Therapeutic Interventions

- Vagal maneuver is an effective means of terminating SVT in adults, particularly if attempted soon after onset.
- If QRS is narrow and rhythm is regular, adenosine, administered by rapid injection, is the drug of choice. Because its administration is followed by a period of asystole, have resuscitative equipment readily available.
- If the rhythm is irregular, consider diltiazem or beta-blockers. Use caution with beta-blockers for patients with pulmonary disease or heart failure.
- Synchronized cardioversion is indicated if the patient is hemodynamically unstable because of the arrhythmia.

Symptomatic Bradycardia

Bradycardia is generally defined as a heart rate less than 60 beats per minute. However, it is not unusual for young healthy people or patients taking beta-blockers to present to the ED with slow heart rates. The important determination to make in these patients is whether the heart rate is adequate for systemic perfusion. Treatment is necessary only if signs and symptoms of poor perfusion are present and result from the slow heart rate; asymptomatic patients do not require treatment.

Signs and Symptoms of Poor Perfusion

- Ischemic chest pain
- Acute alteration in level of consciousness
- Hypotension or signs of shock
- Syncope
- Acute heart failure
- Seizure

> Always consider symptomatic bradycardia as a possible cause of syncope or seizure.

Diagnostic Procedures

- 12-lead ECG to determine bradycardic rhythm, which may include but is not limited to:
  - Sinus bradycardia
  - Sinus node dysfunction (sick sinus syndrome)
  - Mobitz type II block
  - Complete heart block
- Other diagnostic procedures to rule out other causes of poor perfusion

Therapeutic Interventions

- Assess and manage airway, breathing, and circulation.
  - Administer supplemental oxygen; monitor pulse oximetry.
  - Obtain IV access.
  - Initiate continuous cardiac monitoring.
- Initiate transcutaneous pacemaking.
  - Apply pacing electrodes as indicated on the pacing device or the electrode package; placement may be anterior-posterior or anterior-anterior.
  - Set pacemaker rate at 70 beats per minute.
  - Slowly increase the milliamperes (mA) until electrical capture (see below) occurs. Use the lowest level possible that maintains capture.
  - Assess pacing activity.
    - Electrical capture—observe the monitor for electrical pacing spikes, each followed by a wide QRS complex.
    - Mechanical capture—present when each pacing spike–QRS complex grouping produces a palpable femoral pulse.
    - Do not use carotid pulse to assess circulation in a patient being externally paced, as the electrical activity of the pacemaker also causes generalized muscle contraction.
  - Once electrical and mechanical capture has been obtained, assess the patient's hemodynamic response to pacing. Pacemaker rate may need to be increased to maintain an adequate cardiac output.

- Sedate the patient if possible because of the pain of concurrent muscle contractions and electrical shock with each paced beat.
- The presence of hypoxemia and acidosis may prevent the heart from responding to pacemaker stimulation. If unable to "capture," assess for and treat these conditions.
- Administer atropine 0.5 mg intravenously every 3 to 5 minutes to maximum total dose of 3 mg.
  - Use atropine with caution in patients with known coronary artery disease, as an increase in heart rate will increase myocardial oxygen demand and may worsen ischemia.
  - Atropine will likely be ineffective in a patient following heart transplantation, as the transplanted heart lacks vagal innervations. Atropine is not recommended for bradycardia caused by second and third degree heart blocks.

Firing of an Implanted Cardioverter Defibrillator

ICDs are becoming the standard of care for many cardiovascular patients. Indications for their use include the following:
- Ventricular tachyarrhythmias and reduced ejection fraction after MI
- Ventricular resynchronization in advanced heart failure or cardiomyopathies
- Congenital long QT syndrome.
The ICD has three functions:
- Sensing—detection of tachyarrhythmias.
- Pacing—for bradyarrhythmias. Newer ICDs attempt to convert dysrhythmias by rapid pacing before delivering a shock.[7]
- Defibrillation—delivery of shock to terminate ventricular tachycardia (VT) or ventricular fibrillation (VF). The delivered shock is typically between 1 and 50 joules.

Patients may present to the ED for several problems related to their ICDs. Most often these visits result from firing of the device; the firing may be an appropriate firing to terminate a dysrhythmia or an inappropriate firing, which may indicate a change in the sensing threshold or a fractured lead. Intermittent beeping of the device can signal a low battery.

> Repetitive shocks by an ICD, or more than three shocks in a 24-hour period, are considered a medical emergency.

Signs and Symptoms

- Palpitations, syncope or near-syncope, or chest pain.
- Patient is generally anxious and fearful of additional shocks. Although the energy level delivered by an ICD is

considerably less than that of external defibrillation, it is nonetheless painful.
- Subcutaneous pulse generator often located in left upper chest.

Diagnostic Procedures
- 12-lead ECG to determine underlying rhythm.
- Chest radiograph may show fractured lead.
- Complete metabolic panel to detect possible electrolyte imbalance as cause of dysrhythmia.
- Patient should not undergo magnetic resonance imaging (MRI).

Therapeutic Interventions
- If patient is experiencing chest pain, manage patient as any other patient with ischemic chest pain (aspirin, supplemental oxygen, IV access, sublingual nitroglycerin).
- Monitor patient through defibrillation or pacing pads.
- Obtain patient's ICD information card, which lists type of device, manufacturer and model number, name of electrophysiologist, and contact telephone numbers.
- Contact the device representative to interrogate the ICD to obtain rhythm and shock history.
- Placing a magnet over the ICD will disable the delivery of shocks in response to VT or VF but will not disable the pacemaker function.[7]
  - Tape the magnet to the patient's chest to prevent its displacement during movement.
  - Monitor patient with defibrillation pads while magnet is in place.
- If manual defibrillation is required in a patient with an ICD, the defibrillation paddles or patches should be placed 10 cm away from the ICD to reduce the chance of damaging the electronic components of the device.

- If the ICD fires appropriately during the ED visit, allow the ICD to fire. If the ICD is unsuccessful in converting the rhythm, place a magnet over the ICD as above and wait 30 seconds before manually defibrillating the patient.

REFERENCES

1. McCord, J., Jneid, H., Hollander, J. E., de Lemos, J. A., Cercek, B., Hsue, P., ... Newby, L. K. (2008). Management of cocaine-associated chest pain and myocardial infarction. *Circulation*, *117*, 1897–1907.
2. Field, J. M. (Ed.). (2008). STEMI provider manual. Dallas, TX: American Heart Association.
3. Kushner, F. G., Hand, M., Smith, S. C., King, S. B., Anderson, J. L., Antman, E. M., ... Williams, D. O. (2009). 2009 focused updates: ACC/AHA guidelines for the management of patients with ST-elevation myocardial infarction (updating the 2004 guideline and 2007 focused update) and ACC/AHA/SCAI guidelines on percutaneous coronary intervention (updating the 2005 guideline and 2007 focused update): A report of the American College of Cardiology Foundation/American Heart Association Task Force on Practice Guidelines. *Circulation*, *120*, 2271–2306.
4. Ezekowitz, J. A., Hernandez, A. F., Starling, R. C., Yancy, C. W., Massie, B., Hill, J. A., ... Fonarow, G. C. (2009). Standardizing care for acute decompensated heart failure in a large megatrial: The approach for the Acute Studies of Clinical Effectiveness of Nesiritide in Subjects with Decompensated Heart Failure (ASCEND-HF). *American Heart Journal*, *157*(2), 219–228.
5. Golledge, J., & Eagle, K. A. (2008). Acute aortic dissection. *Lancet*, *372*, 55–65.
6. Hays, A. J., & Wilkerson, T. D. (2010). Management of hypertensive emergencies: A drug therapy perspective for nurses. *AACN Advanced Critical Care*, *21*(1), 5–14.
7. Graffeo, C. S., & Krygowski, J. D. (2007). When your patient has an implantable cardioverter-defibrillator. *Emergency Medicine*, *39*(3), 30–37.

Shock

Shelley A. Calder

No matter the cause, shock can be defined as a clinical syndrome resulting from inadequate tissue perfusion. Despite clinical advancements in diagnostic methods and treatment, mortality from shock remains high; as many as 115,000 deaths annually in the United States can be attributed to shock.[1] Emergency nurses play an essential role in the early recognition, diagnosis, and timely delivery of interventions for patients presenting to the ED in shock.

PATHOPHYSIOLOGY

Shock can be classified according to the cause of inadequate tissue perfusion:
- Hypovolemic shock: inadequate tissue perfusion resulting from inadequate circulating volume
- Cardiogenic shock: inadequate tissue perfusion resulting from pump failure
- Distributive shock: inadequate tissue perfusion resulting from abnormal distribution of blood
- Obstructive shock: inadequate tissue perfusion resulting from obstruction of blood flow

The cascade of physiologic events and the progression of clinical decline are remarkably similar in all types of shock. The imbalance between the body's demand for oxygen and the actual delivery of oxygen to the tissues results in impaired metabolism at the cellular level. A deadly cascade ensues, resulting in the following[1]:
- Accumulation of toxins and waste products within the cells leading to cell injury, inflammation, and death.
- Anaerobic metabolism leading to the production of lactic acid and the production of only 8 molecules of adenosine triphosphate (ATP) (as opposed to the production of 30 molecules of ATP with aerobic metabolism).
- Microvascular thrombosis and depletion of clotting factors

The end result is multiple organ failure and inevitable death of the patient.

STAGES OF SHOCK

The physiologic progression of shock can be categorized into three stages: compensated, uncompensated (progressive), and irreversible (refractory) shock.[1]

Compensated Shock

In the compensated stage, the clinical presentation of shock reflects the sympathetic nervous system's response to decreased tissue perfusion. These compensatory mechanisms are generally quite effective and the clinician may not recognize the development of shock. Table 20-1 describes the physiologic responses seen during the compensated stage of shock.

Uncompensated Shock

When the compensatory mechanisms are no longer able to maintain adequate tissue perfusion, the patient's clinical situation begins to deteriorate. Signs and symptoms demonstrate the failure of compensatory mechanisms and the progression of the shock state. These changes are described in Table 20-2.

Irreversible (Refractory) Shock

The irreversible, or refractory, phase of shock indicates progression to cellular, tissue, and organ death. The patient in irreversible shock experiences multiple organ dysfunction, is unresponsive to even aggressive treatment, and will inevitably die.

MONITORING THE PATIENT IN SHOCK

- The initial interventions to stabilize the patient in shock focus on insuring adequate airway, breathing, and circulation.
- Identifying the etiology of the shock state will help determine the most appropriate course of treatment.

TABLE 20-1 PHYSIOLOGIC RESPONSES DURING COMPENSATED SHOCK

PHYSIOLOGY	RESPONSE
Sympathetic nervous system (SNS)	
• Baroreceptors activate the SNS triggered by a decrease in blood pressure	• Increased heart rate
• Release of epinephrine and norepinephrine	• Increased cardiac contractility
• Vasoconstriction redistributes blood to the heart and brain	• Increased blood pressure
Renin-Angiotensin-Aldosterone System	
• Decreased blood flow to the kidneys activates secretion of angiotensin I	• Decreased urinary output
• Angiotensin I is converted to angiotensin II in the lungs	• Increased vascular tone and volume
• Angiotensin II causes vasoconstriction and release of aldosterone from the adrenals	• Increased blood pressure
• Aldosterone increases sodium and water reabsorption in the tubules	• Increased blood return to the heart
	• Increased cardiac output
Antidiuretic Hormone (ADH) Release	
• ADH is secreted by the posterior pituitary in response to hypovolemia	• Increased blood pressure
• Triggers renal reabsorption of sodium and water	• Increased cardiac output
	• Decreased urinary output
Intracellular Fluid Shift	
• Intravascular volume depletion causes fluid to shift from intracellular to the intravascular space	• Increased blood pressure
• Increased intravascular volume, blood return to heart, cardiac output, and blood flow	• Increased cardiac output

TABLE 20-2 PHYSIOLOGIC RESPONSES DURING UNCOMPENSATED SHOCK

PHYSIOLOGY	RESPONSE
Altered Capillary Permeability	
• Leakage of fluid and protein out of the vascular space into the interstitial space	• Edema
	• Decreased intravascular volume leading to decreased blood pressure and tissue perfusion
Respiratory Insufficiency	
• Pulmonary interstitial edema	• Increased respiratory rate or tachypnea
• Ventilation and perfusion mismatching	• Crackles throughout lung fields
	• Dyspnea
Cardiac Depression	
• Decreased venous return to the heart	• Decreased blood pressure
• Decreased cardiac output and ischemia of nonvital organs	• Increased heart rate
	• Decreased peripheral pulses
	• Cardiac dysrhythmias
Tissue hypoperfusion	
• Intense vasoconstriction leads to ischemia of nonvital organs, kidney, intestines, and skin	• Decreased urine output
	• Elevated serum lactate level
	• $SvO_2 < 65\%$
	• Increasing base deficit level
	• Skin cool, diminished quality of peripheral pulses, delayed capillary refill
Neurological Response	
• Blood flow to the brain diminished	• Altered mental status

- Ongoing assessment of cardiac rhythm, pulse oximetry, respiratory rate, and arterial blood pressure is essential in all patients suspected of a shock diagnosis.
- Trending of vital signs is crucial and identifies early physiologic changes.
- Mean arterial pressure (MAP) may provide a better indication of perfusion than either systolic or diastolic pressures. In the shock state, the goal is to maintain the MAP above 60 mm Hg.[2]
- Insertion of an arterial line is often necessary to accurately track BP measurement; the nurse needs to initially correlate the intraarterial pressure with a cuff pressure.

> Formula for manually calculating mean arterial pressure (MAP): (Systolic pressure + 2[diastolic pressure])/by 3

- Urine output is a reliable indicator of vital organ perfusion in the ongoing assessment of the shock patient.[3]
- Skin perfusion is assessed through pulse quality, skin temperature and moisture, and capillary refill.
- Level of consciousness is continually monitored as an indicator of cerebral perfusion.
- Invasive hemodynamic monitoring may be initiated in the ED.
- Central venous pressure (CVP) gives an indication of right-sided preload; pulmonary artery pressures reflect left-sided preload.
- Additionally, mixed venous saturation levels, drawn from either a central line ($ScvO_2$) or the pulmonary artery catheter (SvO_2) can be obtained to assess the amount of oxygen extracted from the blood by the tissues—an SvO_2 of less than 60% indicates hypoperfusion.
- Measurements of base deficit and a lactate level are also important parameters to monitor.

> A base deficit greater than −4 mEq/L or a serum lactate level greater than 4.0 mmol/L indicates widespread tissue hypoperfusion.[3]

TYPES OF SHOCK

Hypovolemic Shock

Hypovolemic shock refers to a condition in which blood, plasma, or fluid loss causes a decrease in circulating blood volume and cardiac output. This results in multiorgan failure because of inadequate tissue perfusion.

Etiology

The common causes of hypovolemic shock include the following:
- Penetrating trauma
- Internal solid organ injury and hemorrhage

- Ruptured abdominal aneurysm
- Severe gastrointestinal bleeding
- Placenta previa and abruption of the placenta
- Ruptured fallopian tube secondary to ectopic pregnancy
- Acute pancreatitis
- Ascites
- Extensive burns
- Severe vomiting or diarrhea

Signs and Symptoms

In hypovolemic shock, the size of the vascular compartment remains unchanged while the fluid volume diminishes. Reduced intravascular volume results in decreased venous return to the heart (preload) followed by a decrease in stroke volume and cardiac output. This series of events results in decreased tissue perfusion and impaired cellular metabolism. Figure 20-1 illustrates the pathway of hypovolemic shock development.

The body responds to acute hemorrhage by activating all major physiologic systems. The severity of clinical presentation and the interventions required are largely determined by the amount of fluid lost or shifted from the intravascular space because of injury. Fluid loss can be estimated by the type of injury. Table 20-3 lists estimated blood loss by site of injury.

An estimation of volume loss and an assessment of vital signs, urine output, and mental status will assist the health care provider in determining the severity of hypovolemic shock. Age and preexisting medical conditions also play a role in the severity of the physiologic response to blood. Table 20-4 describes a classification of hypovolemic shock based on the amount of blood loss and the physiologic response.[4]

Additional points to consider when assessing the potentially hypovolemic patient include the following:
- The expected increase in heart rate (due to sympathetic stimulation) may be absent or diminished in patients who are taking beta-blocker medications.
- The blood pressure value is not a reliable indicator of shock. Vasoconstriction and increased myocardial contractility (additional responses to sympathetic stimulation) can maintain the blood pressure for some time.
- Pulse pressure (the difference between the systolic and diastolic pressures) is an indicator of stroke volume; pulse pressure drops as the patient's shock level progresses.

Therapeutic Interventions

Management of the patient in hypovolemic shock is directed toward preventing further fluid loss and restoring circulating volume. Hemorrhage contributes to the largest percentage of mortality in the first hour and 50% of deaths in the first day following trauma.[4]

- Interventions for hypovolemic shock include aggressive airway management. The patient may require endotracheal intubation and mechanical ventilation. Excessive positive pressure ventilation should be avoided as it may further decrease venous return to the heart.[5]
- Control of hemorrhage is a priority in the actively bleeding patient. Direct pressure to the bleeding site remains an important initial intervention.
- Circulatory support requires fluid resuscitation with two large-bore intravenous (IV) catheters and the infusion of warmed crystalloid solutions.
  - Initiate warmed IV isotonic crystalloids, usually a 1- to 2-liter bolus for adults or 20 mL/kg for pediatric patients.[6]
  - Intraosseous access may be indicated if peripheral access cannot be established or if the patient is in cardiopulmonary arrest or severe shock.
- Place the patient on a cardiac monitor and assess for dysrhythmias.

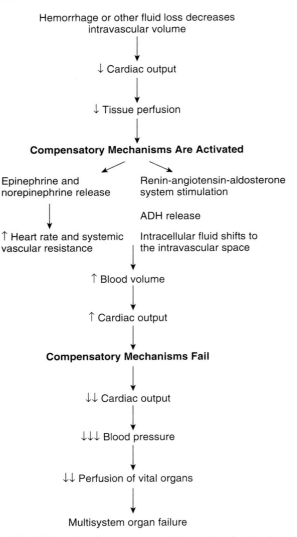

Fig. 20-1 The development of hypovolemic shock.

TABLE 20-3	ESTIMATED BLOOD LOSS BY SITE OF INJURY
INJURY	**ESTIMATED BLOOD LOSS**
Pelvis fracture	3000 mL
Femur fracture	1000 mL
Tibia fracture	650 mL
Intra-abdominal injury	2000 mL
Thoracic injury	2000 mL

Data from Emergency Nurses Association. (2009). *Sheehy's emergency nursing: Principles and practice* (6th ed.). St. Louis, MO: Mosby.

TABLE 20-4 CLASSIFICATIONS OF HYPOVOLEMIC SHOCK

	CLASS I	CLASS II	CLASS III	CLASS IV
Blood loss (mL)	<750	750–1500	1500–2000	>2000
Blood loss	<15%	15%–30%	30%–40%	>40%
Pulse (beats per minute)	<100	100–120	120–140	>140
Blood pressure	Normal	Normal	Decreased	Decreased
Respiratory rate (breaths per minute)	14–20	20–30	30–40	>35
Urinary output (mL/hour)	>30	20–30	5–20	Negligible
Central nervous system	Slightly anxious	Mildly anxious	Anxious, confused	Confused, lethargic
Fluid replacement	Crystalloid	Crystalloid	Crystalloid and blood	Crystalloid and blood

Data from American College of Surgeons Committee on Trauma. (2008). *ATLS: Advanced trauma life support for doctors student course manual* (8th ed.). Chicago, IL: Author.

- Prepare the patient for diagnostic procedures and possible surgical interventions. Diagnostic procedures routinely performed may include:
  - Serial hemoglobin and hematocrit levels
  - Urine specific gravity
  - Serum electrolytes
  - Lactic acid levels (>4 mmol/L)
  - Increasing base deficit (normal level is −2 mEq/L)
  - Computed tomography
  - Radiographs as indicated to determine source of bleeding
- Insert an indwelling urinary catheter and monitor hourly urine output.
- Prevent hypothermia by using warm blankets, warming lights, or convection heaters.
- Splint large bone injuries for stability and comfort (e.g., femur, pelvis).
- Insert a gastric tube to reduce gastric distension, which is associated with vomiting and aspiration.

> Consider placing patients in shock in supine position with the legs elevated; this position may facilitate venous return to the heart. Do not place the patient in the Trendelenburg position. It does not improve cardiac performance, may worsen gas exchange, and may predispose the patient to aspiration.[3]

Crystalloids and Colloids

The debate concerning the most appropriate fluid for resuscitation of the hypovolemic patient continues. No indisputable advantages of colloids over crystalloids has been demonstrated.[5,7] Crystalloids restore volume quickly, are easily obtained and inexpensive, and have a low incidence of adverse reactions; for these reasons crystalloids are generally the preferred choice for initial fluid resuscitation.[8] Normal saline (NS) and Lactated Ringer solution are the most commonly used crystalloids. Lactated Ringer solution should be used judiciously, however, as it may result in elevated lactate levels, which could mask inadequate perfusion.[8] Adults may receive 1 to 2 liters rapidly and pediatric patients should receive boluses of 20 mL/kg.[6]

> Do not use dextrose 5% in water for fluid resuscitation. Because it is quickly distributed throughout the body compartments, it does not contribute to expansion of intravascular volume.[9]

Colloids may be used after initial fluid resuscitation to maintain intravascular volume.[10] Colloid products are classified as protein based (albumin) or non–protein based (hetastarch and dextran). Because of their oncotic pressure,

colloids remain in the intravascular space longer than crystalloids and thus expand intravascular volume to a greater degree. Their cost is much higher than that of crystalloids and their use in fluid resuscitation has not been shown to improve mortality.[5]

Blood Replacement

Blood volume replacement with whole blood, packed red blood cells (PRBC), fresh frozen plasma, and blood substitutes, is an important part of the management of hemorrhagic hypovolemic shock. Type-specific and crossmatched blood is preferred if time allows for matching. In cases of severe hemorrhagic hypovolemia, O-negative blood may be used until a type and crossmatch are complete. Male patients and women beyond childbearing age may be given O-positive blood. In cases of thoracic trauma, consider autotransfusion if large blood loss is present or if more than 500 mL of blood is collected. Autotransfusion is contraindicated in cases of severe trauma with potential for contamination with bowel contents.[3] (See Chapter 35, Stabilization of the Trauma Patient, for more information.)

Massive Transfusion

A standard definition of massive transfusion has not been established. However, most definitions refer to replacing a large percentage of the patient's blood volume within a relatively short period of time (generally <24 hours). Because PRBCs lack sufficient clotting factors, it is recommended that 1 unit of fresh frozen plasma be given for each 1 or 2 units of PRBCs that the patient receives to prevent coagulopathies.[3]

All fluids and blood products administered during resuscitation should be warmed to minimize hypothermia and subsequent metabolic acidosis. While receiving blood products, the patient should be routinely assessed for response to treatment and complications associated with infusion of blood products. Table 20-5 summarizes complications associated with blood product replacement.

> If the patient is not responding to interventions, consider that possibly *not enough treatment* was given or that this is *not the correct* treatment.

Cardiogenic Shock

Cardiogenic shock is the result of myocardial pump failure, decreased cardiac output, and inadequate tissue perfusion in the presence of adequate intravascular volume.[11] Because the heart is no longer an effective pump, it is unable to maintain a cardiac output sufficient to meet the body's needs.

TABLE 20-5	COMPLICATIONS ASSOCIATED WITH BLOOD PRODUCT ADMINISTRATION	
PROBLEM	**CAUSE**	**COMMENTS**
Hypothermia	Crystalloids and banked blood transfused without warming.	Hypothermia inhibits efforts to reverse metabolic acidosis and slows the clotting cascade.
Hyperkalemia	Intracellular potassium released from lysed RBCs. Potassium levels are particularly high in banked blood.	Monitor serum potassium levels. Observe for dysrhythmias and peaked T waves.
Hypocalcemia	The citrate anticoagulant used in banked blood binds free serum calcium.	Check serum calcium level after infusion of about 10 units of blood. Replace calcium with calcium chloride or calcium gluconate as needed.
Acidosis	The pH of banked blood is 7.1	Monitor arterial pH. Observe for dysrhythmias.
Alkalosis	The citrate in banked blood is converted by the liver to bicarbonate	Monitor arterial pH, especially in patients with hepatic dysfunction.
Coagulopathies	PRBCs contain few clotting factors. Hemodilution further decreases available clotting factors	Monitor coagulation parameters. Transfuse fresh frozen plasma, platelets, and cryoprecipitate as needed.
Intravascular debris	Banked blood contains debris as a result of processing.	Always infuse blood through a blood filter.

PRBCs, packed red blood cells; *RBCs*, red blood cells.

Etiology

Causes of cardiogenic shock include the following:
- Myocardial infarction (MI) or ischemia
  - MI is the most common cause of cardiogenic shock, particularly with involvement of the anterior wall of the left ventricle
  - Generally cardiogenic shock is the result of loss of more than 40% of functional myocardium.
  - Papillary muscle rupture or ventricular septal rupture are possible sequelae of acute MI that lead to cardiogenic shock
  - Right ventricular infarction may lead to cardiogenic shock in which volume replacement is essential. Usual therapeutic interventions for cardiogenic shock will often contribute to rather than resolve the shock state in this situation. See Chapter 19, Cardiovascular Emergencies, for a more in-depth discussion of the management of RV MI.
- Blunt cardiac trauma
- Sustained cardiac dysrhythmias
- Acute valvular dysfunction
- End-stage cardiomyopathy

Signs and Symptoms

Most patients presenting with cardiogenic shock do so in conjunction with acute MI. Clinical manifestations of cardiogenic shock reflect heart failure and inadequate tissue perfusion and are often associated with symptoms of acute cardiac ischemia.

- Ischemic chest pain or anginal equivalents
- Pulmonary congestion including tachypnea, crackles, and possible frank pulmonary edema
- Sinus tachycardia and other cardiac dysrhythmias
- S_3 heart sound
- Altered level of consciousness
- Pale, cool, clammy skin with delayed capillary refill time
- Minimal urine output
- Hypotension (systolic BP <90 mm Hg or a decrease in MAP by 30 mm Hg)[11]

Diagnostic Procedures

- Electrocardiogram (ECG) may show changes indicative of myocardial ischemia, injury, or infarction
- Chest radiograph reveals pulmonary congestion; may also detect other possible causes of shock
- Arterial blood gases to identify hypoxia or acidosis
- Echocardiogram to identify structural causes of cardiogenic shock
- Complete blood count (CBC) and platelet count to rule out anemia and to identify possible coagulopathy
- Routine laboratory blood studies (electrolytes, renal and liver function tests) to assess function of vital organs
- Serum lactate level—elevated in presence of tissue hypoperfusion
- SvO_2 level <65%
- Elevated left sided heart pressures (PAP, PAOP) if pulmonary artery catheter is inserted

Therapeutic Interventions

Management of the patient in cardiogenic shock focuses on reducing cardiac workload and improving myocardial contractility. Specific interventions include the following:

- Airway management, including possible endotracheal intubation and mechanical ventilation
  - Positive end-expiratory pressure (PEEP) may be used if patient is in pulmonary edema
- Reduce cardiac workload by optimizing preload
  - Most often, workload of the heart can be minimized by *decreasing* preload (venous return to the heart) using the following:
    - Position the patient in semi-Fowler's or Fowler's position
    - Administer vasodilating agents such as nitroglycerin or diuretics.
    - Morphine sulfate administration results in vasodilation.
  - In some instances, preload may need to be cautiously *increased* with an IV fluid challenge.
    - Patients who experience right ventricular infarction are preload dependent and will need fluid administration to increase venous return to the right side of the heart.
- Reduce cardiac workload by decreasing the resistance that the ventricle must overcome to eject its volume of blood (afterload).
  - Continuous IV infusion of nitroglycerine results in vasodilation, decreased systemic vascular resistance (afterload), and arterial BP.
  - Nitroprusside (Nipride) is a potent arteriolar dilating medication that can be used to decrease afterload.
- Improve myocardial contractility with positive inotropic agents such as dobutamine.
- Support cardiac function and improve contractility and coronary artery perfusion with the intraaortic balloon pump (IABP).
- Cardiac catheterization and angioplasty may be necessary to improve myocardial perfusion and improve contractility.
- Treat cardiac dysrhythmias.

Distributive Shock

Distributive shock is characterized by an abnormal distribution of intravascular volume as a result of decreased sympathetic tone, increased vascular permeability, and pooling of blood in venous and capillary beds. Signs and symptoms may mimic those of hypovolemic shock; however, the mechanism is very different. The three categories of distributive shock are:

- Septic
- Anaphylactic
- Neurogenic

This chapter describes anaphylactic and neurogenic shock. Because of the high incidence and mortality of septic shock, it is discussed separately in Chapter 21, Sepsis.

Anaphylactic Shock

Anaphylactic shock is an acute, life-threatening hypersensitivity (allergic) reaction to a sensitizing substance. Common allergens include certain foods (such as shellfish and peanuts), food additives, insects (hymenoptera stings), drugs (particularly antibiotics such as penicillins), latex, and iodine contrast dyes.

Etiology

In a sensitized individual (someone who has experienced previous exposure), antigen exposure triggers the release of a variety of mediators that exert their effects on the vascular and pulmonary systems. Massive vasodilation and increased capillary permeability redistribute fluid into the interstitial space, causing profound hypovolemia and vascular collapse. Fluid leaking into the alveoli produces pulmonary congestion. Angioedema causes progressive airway obstruction and subsequent respiratory arrest. Figure 20-2 outlines the development of anaphylactic shock.

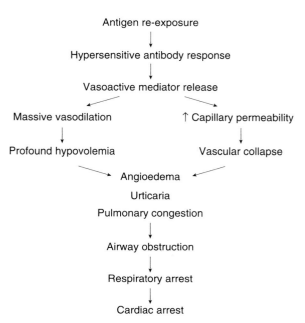

Fig. 20-2 The development of anaphylactic shock.

Signs and Symptoms

Symptoms of anaphylaxis are acute and rapidly progressive. In 60% of cases, initial symptoms, particularly hives and flushing, are related to the skin.[12] Observe for the following signs of a multiple system reaction:

- Dyspnea
- Cough, tightness in throat
- Stridor
- Wheezing
- Bronchospasm
- Airway obstruction resulting from upper airway edema
- Uticaria
- Erythema
- Pruritus
- Angioedema, particularly of the tongue and lips
- Syncope
- Chest tightness, palpitations
- Hypotension
- Tachycardia
- Respiratory and cardiopulmonary arrest

Therapeutic Interventions

Management of the patient in anaphylactic shock is directed toward maintaining a patent airway and counteracting the anaphylactic reaction. General interventions include the following:

- Ensure a patent airway; emergent endotracheal intubation may be necessary.
- Administer high-flow oxygen.
- Obtain IV access for medication administration and fluid resuscitation.
- Remove the causative agent if possible.
- Intravenous administration of epinephrine promotes vasoconstriction, dilates the bronchioles, and inhibits further release of mediators.[12]
- If the IV route is not available, intramuscular (IM) administration is preferable to the subcutaneous route because of more rapid and reliable absorption[13,14]
- Epinephrine administration may be repeated in 15 to 20 minutes as needed.[12]
- Inhaled beta-2 adrenergic agonists such as albuterol promote bronchodilation.
- Antihistamine therapy is an adjunct to epinephrine administration.
  - H1 blockers: diphenhydramine (Benedryl)
  - H2 blockers: cimetidine, ranitidine, famotidine
- Corticosteroids have no immediate effect but may be administered to prevent a possible late biphasic reaction[14]

- The patient may require hospital admission for observation
- Prior to the patient's discharge, note the allergy in all of the patient's medical records.
- Teach patients and families about the need for medical alert bracelets and how to use an EpiPen.

Neurogenic Shock

Neurogenic shock is classified as distributive shock because of the massive vasodilation that results from the loss of sympathetic output. Without the vasoconstrictive effects of the sympathetic nervous system, there is a decrease in systemic vascular resistance (afterload), decreased cardiac output, and inadequate tissue perfusion. Without the sympathetic response, the body is unable to compensate for the drop in cardiac output with an increase in heart rate or by peripheral vasoconstriction.

Etiology

Common causes of neurogenic shock include the following:

- Spinal cord injury, particularly involving the cervical or high thoracic vertebrae
- Spinal anesthesia
- Vasomotor center depression from head trauma

Signs and Symptoms

- Bradycardia
- Hypotension (systolic blood pressure <90 mm Hg or 30 mm Hg less than baseline)
- Skin may be warm, dry, and flushed with full pulses

Therapeutic Interventions

- Addressing the ABCs is a priority in the patient with a spinal cord injury and subsequent neurogenic shock in order to prevent secondary cord injury due to hypoperfusion and tissue hypoxia.
- Fluid resuscitation to expand intravascular volume.
- Administration of vasopressors to constrict the vasculature and increase BP.
- Atropine may be needed to increase heart rate.
- Use of high-dose corticosteroids is no longer recommended.

Obstructive Shock

In obstructive shock, cardiac output and thus tissue perfusion are inadequate because of resistance to ventricular filling. An obstruction, generally external to the heart itself, limits venous return during the diastolic filling time of the heart. If the obstruction is extreme, systolic function may also be impaired.

Etiology

Causes of obstructive shock include the following:

- Pericardial tamponade
- Tension pneumothorax
- Pulmonary embolism

Please see relevant chapters for more information on these life-threatening conditions.

Therapeutic Interventions

Management of obstructive shock focuses on addressing the ABCs, identifying the cause of shock, and relieving the source of obstruction.

- Pericardial tamponade (See Chapter 38, Chest Trauma)
  - Immediate pericardiocentesis
  - Surgical intervention for cardiac repair
- Tension pneumothorax (See Chapter 38, Chest Trauma)
  - Immediate needle thoracostomy
  - Chest tube placement
- Pulmonary embolism (See Chapter 18, Respiratory Emergencies)
  - Intravenous anticoagulation
  - Thrombolytics in selected situations

END POINTS OF SHOCK RESUSCITATION

Regardless of the type of shock, the goal of management is to restore adequate tissue perfusion. End points of successful shock resuscitation include but are not limited to the following:

- MAP greater than 60 to 70 mm Hg
- CVP of 8 to 12 mm Hg
- Urine output of 0.5 mL/kg per hour or 30 to 60 mL per hour
- Normalization of serum lactate levels
- SvO_2 65% to 75%
- Systolic blood pressure greater than 90 mm Hg

REFERENCES

1. Wilmot, L. A. (2010). Shock: Early recognition and management. *Journal of Emergency Nursing, 36*(2), 134–139.

2. Ferns, T., Harris, G., McMahon, T., & Wright, K. (2010). Mean arterial blood pressure and the assessment of acutely ill patients. *Nursing Standard, 25*(12), 40–44.

3. Jones, A. E., & Kline, J. A. (2010). Shock. In J. A. Marx (Ed.), *Rosen's emergency medicine: Concepts and clinical practice* (7th ed., p. 41). St. Louis, MO: Mosby.

4. Cocchi, M. N., Kimlin, E., Walsh, M., & Donnino, M. W. (2007). Identification and resuscitation of the trauma patient in shock. *Emergency Medicine Clinics of North America, 25*(3), 623–642

5. Kolecki, P. (2010, March 11). *Hypovolemic shock.* Retrieved from http://emedicine.medscape.com/article/760145

6. Emergency Nurses Association. (2007). *Trauma nursing core course* (6th ed.) Des Plaines, IL: Author.

7. Gross, E., & Martel, M. (2010). Multiple trauma. In J. A. Marx (Ed.), *Rosen's emergency medicine: Concepts and clinical practice* (7th ed., p. 248). St. Louis, MO: Mosby.

8. Gonzalez, E. A. (2008). Fluid resuscitation in the trauma patient. *Journal of Trauma Nursing, 15*(3), 149–157.

9. McLean, B., & Zimmerman, J. L. (Eds.). (2007). *Fundamental critical care support* (4th ed., p. 77). Mount Prospect, IL: Society of Critical Care Medicine.

10. Emergency Nursing Association. (2009). *Sheehy's emergency nursing: Principles and practice* (6th ed.). St. Louis, MO: Mosby.

11. Lenneman, A. (2011). *Cardiogenic shock.* Retrieved from http://emedicine.medscape.com/article/152191-overview

12. Martelli, A., Ghiglioni, D., Sarratud, T., Calciani, E., Veehof, S., Terracciano, L., & Fiocchi, A. (2008). Anaphylaxis in the emergency department: A paediatric perspective. *Current Opinion in Allergy and Clinical Immunology, 8*(4), 321–329.

13. Lieberman, P., Nicklas, R. A., Oppenheimer, J., Kemp, S. F., Lang, D. M., Bernstein, D. I., . . . Wallace, D. (2010). The diagnosis and management of anaphylaxis practice parameter: 2010 update. *Journal of Allergy and Clinical Immunology, 126*(3), 477–480.e1–e42.

14. Kemp, S. F. (2011). *Anaphylaxis treatment and management.* Retrieved from http://www.emedicine.medscape.com/article/135065-treatment

Sepsis

Bethany Chimento Jennings and Fiona Winterbottom

Sepsis is a progressive syndrome that leads to dysfunction and dysregulation of the body. Despite early identification, treatments, and aggressive interventions, mortality remains 20% to 50% for those patients who progress to severe sepsis or septic shock.[1,2] Sepsis has no boundaries and can affect any age, gender, or race.[3] Severe sepsis and septic shock are responsible for one in four deaths internationally and the incidence is increasing.[1-7]

Deaths resulting from sepsis exceed those from myocardial infarction, breast cancer, and stroke.[8] Evidence-based studies indicate that early recognition, diagnosis, and treatment of sepsis in the emergency department (ED) will improve patient outcomes and decrease mortality. Early goal-directed therapy is a protocol that has been standard care in the intensive care setting. Research indicates that patients may benefit from starting this protocol when they present to the ED rather than waiting until they get to the intensive care unit (ICU).[9,10] While not all patients with sepsis enter the hospital through the ED, timely initiation of care can have a positive impact on outcomes.

DEFINITIONS[11]

Through the years attempts have been made to define sepsis and sepsis-related terms to help understand the syndrome and accurately diagnose patients. However, efforts have not always been met with universal support.[12] In 1991 the American College of Chest Physicians (ACCP) and the Society of Critical Care Medicine (SCCM) met with the goal of agreeing on sepsis definitions.[13] In 2001 ACCP, SCCM, the European Society of Intensive Care Medicine (ESICM), the American Thoracic Society (ATS), and the Surgical Infection Society (SIS) revisited the 1991 definitions and found that they still had merit and should remain as described 10 years prior. The following list contains definitions of common terms used in the diagnosis and classification of sepsis[13]:

- Infection: Microbial phenomenon characterized by an inflammatory response to the presence of microorganisms or the invasion of normally sterile host tissue by those organisms.
- Bacteremia: Presence of viable bacteria in the blood.
- Systemic inflammatory response syndrome (SIRS): Systemic inflammatory response to a variety of severe clinical insults, manifested by two or more of the following conditions:
  - Temperature greater than 38° C (100.4° F) or less than 36° C (96.8° F)
  - Heart rate greater than 90 beats per minute
  - Respiratory rate greater than 20 breaths per minute or $PaCO_2$ greater than 32 mm Hg
  - White blood cell count greater than 12,000/mm³, less than 4000/mm³, or more than 10% immature (band) forms
- Sepsis: Presence of infection or suspicion of infection, with two or more of the SIRS criteria.
- Severe sepsis: Sepsis associated with organ dysfunction, hypoperfusion, or hypotension. Hypoperfusion and perfusion abnormalities may include, but are not limited to, lactic acidosis, oliguria, or an acute alteration in mental status.
- Septic shock: Sepsis-induced shock with hypotension despite adequate crystalloid resuscitation, along with the presence of perfusion abnormalities that may include, but are not limited to, lactic acidosis, oliguria, or an acute alteration in mental status. Patients receiving inotropic or vasopressor agents may not be hypotensive at the time that perfusion abnormalities are measured.
- Sepsis-induced hypotension: A systolic blood pressure less than 90 mm Hg, mean arterial pressure (MAP) less than 65 mm Hg, or a reduction of 40 mm Hg from baseline in the absence of other causes for hypotension.

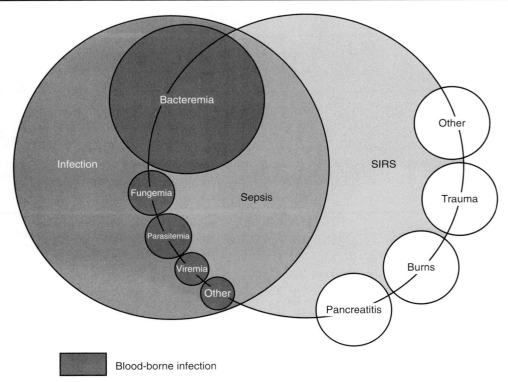

Fig. 21-1 Interrelationships among systemic inflammatory response syndrome (SIRS), sepsis, and infection. (From American College of Chest Physicians & Society of Critical Care Medicine Consensus Conference Committee. [1992]. American College of Chest Physicians/Society of Critical Care Medicine Consensus Conference: Definitions for sepsis and organ failure and guidelines for the use of innovative therapies in sepsis. *Critical Care Medicine, 20*[6], 864–874.)

- Multiple organ dysfunction syndrome: Altered organ function in an acutely ill patient such that homeostasis cannot be maintained without intervention

Figure 21-1 shows the interrelationships among SIRS, sepsis, and infection.

IDENTIFYING SIRS OR SEPSIS

The pathophysiology of sepsis is a complex set of events that involves innate immune response, inflammatory cascades, procoagulant and antifibrinolytic pathways, alterations in cellular metabolism and signaling, and acquired immune dysfunction.[14]

SIRS is a dynamic state that starts when a major insult to the body (Fig. 21-1) progresses to an overwhelming *systemic* inflammation. When infection is the cause of that insult, the systemic inflammatory response can quickly transition into severe sepsis or septic shock. Prompt identification of the patient with potential sepsis is crucial in the ED setting. While nearly 30% of all patients diagnosed with sepsis enter the hospital through the ED, it is also known that these patients may not fit neatly into the definitions described in the literature.[11]

General assessment of the patient during triage, coupled with a thorough history and physical assessment is crucial in identifying sepsis. Patients with sepsis may present with fever, chills, shortness of breath or tachypnea, tachycardia, rash, or confusion. These symptoms can mimic other disease processes making it difficult to diagnose sepsis in the early stages.[15] In the triage process it is important to consider the age and history of the patient. The elderly, children, and infants have a higher incidence of sepsis than young adults.[5] It is also essential to determine whether the patient is immune-compromised or if he or she has had any recent surgery, urinary tract infections, respiratory infections, skin infections, or invasive medical procedures.

Medical history, such as diabetes, should also be factored into triage decisions.

Patients with a suspected infection should be immediately assessed for signs and symptoms of SIRS. Treatments and medications taken by the patient should be considered when analyzing SIRS criteria; for instance, a patient who is taking prescribed beta-blockers may not have an elevated heart rate. Further laboratory testing can also provide more information about the patient's condition.

If the patient history is suspicious for a new infection *and* if any two of the following signs or symptoms of infection are present and new for the patient, there is a high index of suspicion for sepsis:

- Fever higher than 38° C (100.8° F)
- Hypothermia: temperature less than 36° C (96.8° F)
- Tachycardia: heart rate greater than 90 beats per minute
- Tachypnea: respirations greater than 20 breaths per minute
- Acutely altered mental status
- Abnormal lab values
  - Leukocytosis: white blood cell count greater than 12,000/mm³
  - Leukopenia: white blood cell count less than 4000/mm³
  - Hyperglycemia: serum glucose greater than 120 mg/dL in the absence of diabetes

If there is suspicion of infection *and* any of the following signs of new-onset organ dysfunction are present, the patient meets criteria for severe sepsis:

- Systolic blood pressure (SBP) less than 90 mm Hg or MAP less than 65 mm Hg
- SBP decrease greater than 40 mm Hg from baseline
- Respiratory insufficiency
- Creatinine greater than 2.0 mg/dL or urine output less than 0.5 mL/kg per hour for more than 2 hours
- Bilirubin greater than 2 mg/dL
- Platelet count less than 100,000/mm³
- Coagulopathy
- Lactate greater than 4 mmoL/L

If the patient meets the criteria for severe shock *and* is hypotensive with a SBP less than 90 mm Hg, which has not been reversed with fluid resuscitation, the patient meets the criteria for septic shock.

The Surviving Sepsis Campaign and the Institute for Healthcare Improvement recommend that facilities consider evaluating high-risk patients for sepsis or severe sepsis.[16,17] These groups have developed a tool that can be implemented in the ED setting and provides an algorithm for decision making using SIRS criteria. This screening tool is shown in Figure 21-2.

According to the Surviving Sepsis Campaign, patients with SIRS and an identified source of infection are considered to have sepsis.[16] If a patient presents with two or more of the SIRS criteria and new-onset organ dysfunction, the patient meets criteria for *severe* sepsis. Patients in septic shock present with severe sepsis along with hypoperfusion, which is recognized by a MAP of less than 65 mm Hg or a measured lactate level of greater than 4 mmoL/L.[2] In septic shock, hypoperfusion will continue despite fluid resuscitation. The patient's SBP will remain less than 90 mm Hg or the patient's SBP will drop more than 40 mm Hg.[18]

The PIRO model of sepsis identification uses **p**redisposition, **i**nfection or insult, **r**esponse, and **o**rgan dysfunction to stage sepsis and predict mortality (Table 21-1).[19] A PIRO score can be calculated within each category:

- Predisposition includes such risk factors as age, history of malignancy, liver disease, or chronic obstructive pulmonary disease as well as residency in a nursing home.
- Infection or insult is measured based on the presence of pneumonia, skin infection, or other infection risk.
- Response is measured in terms of respiratory rate, heart rate, or presence of bands (immature cells) in the white blood cell count.
- Organ dysfunction is scored based on blood urea nitrogen, presence of hypoxemia, lactate levels, platelet count, and SBP.[20]

Another method of identifying potential sepsis patients is the Mortality in Emergency Department Sepsis (MEDS) score (Table 21-2). It takes into account some of the variables of PIRO. This score combines such variables as the patient's age, mental status, tachypnea or hypoxemia, and platelet count along with risk factors such as being a nursing home resident or having a lower respiratory infection or terminal illness. There is evidence that this is a reliable means of risk stratification in SIRS or sepsis patients in the ED.[21,22]

EARLY GOAL-DIRECTED THERAPY: INITIAL RESUSCITATION AND THE FIRST SIX HOURS

According to the Surviving Sepsis Campaign guidelines, resuscitation goals should be achieved during the first 6 hours.[16] For this to occur, early recognition and implementation of treatment toward specific targets or goals are crucial. Goals established in studies and by the Surviving Sepsis Campaign are listed in Table 21-3. Volume resuscitation and antibiotic administration should be priorities of care after airway and breathing. Depending on the status of the patient, therapies may be instituted simultaneously.

Chart record – use patient label. Do not remove from chart

Evaluation for Severe Sepsis Screening Tool

Instructions: Use this optional tool to screen patients for severe sepsis in the emergency department, on the wards, or in the ICU.

1. Is the patient's history suggestive of a new infection?

    ☐ Pneumonia, empyema   ☐ Bone/joint infection   ☐ Implantable device
    ☐ Urinary tract infection   ☐ Wound infection   infection
    ☐ Acute abdominal infection   ☐ Bloodstream catheter   ☐ Other _____
    ☐ Meningitis   infection
    ☐ Skin/soft tissue infection ☐ Endocarditis

    ___ Yes ___ No

2. Are any two of following signs and symptoms of infection both present and new to the patient? **Note:** laboratory values may have been obtained for inpatients but may not be available for outpatients.

    ☐ Hyperthermia >38.3° C   ☐ Tachypnea >20 bpm   ☐ Leukopenia (WBC count
      (101.0 °F)   ☐ Acutely altered mental   <4000 µL −1)
    ☐ Hypothermia <36° C   status   ☐ Hyperglycemia (plasma
      (96.8°F)   ☐ Leukocytosis (WBC count   glucose >120 mg/dL) in
    ☐ Tachycardia >90 bpm   >12,000 µL −1)   the absence of diabetes

    ___ Yes ___ No

    If the answer is yes to both question 1 and 2, suspicion of infection is present:

    ✓ Obtain: lactic acid, blood cultures, CBC with differential, basic chemistry labs, bilirubin.
    ✓ At the physician's discretion obtain: UA, chest x-ray, amylase, lipase, ABG, CRP, CT scan.

3. Are any of the following organ dysfunction criteria present at a site remote from the site of the infection that are not considered to be chronic conditions? **Note:** the remote site stipulation is waived in the case of bilateral pulmonary infiltrates.

    ☐ SBP <90 mm Hg or MAP <65 mm Hg
    ☐ SBP decrease >40 mm Hg from baseline
    ☐ Bilateral pulmonary infiltrates with a new (or increased) oxygen requirement to maintain SpO_2 >90%
    ☐ Bilateral pulmonary infiltrates with PaO_2/FiO_2 ratio <300
    ☐ Creatinine >2.0 mg/dl (176.8 mmol/L) or Urine Output <0.5 ml/kg/hour for >2 hours
    ☐ Bilirubin >2 mg/dl (34.2 mmol/L)
    ☐ Platelet count <100,000
    ☐ Coagulopathy (INR >1.5 or aPTT >60 secs)
    ☐ Lactate >2 mmol/L (18.0 mg/dl)

    ___ Yes ___ No

    If suspicion of infection is present **AND** organ dysfunction is present, the patient meets the criteria for **SEVERE SEPSIS** and should be entered into the severe sepsis protocol.

Date: ____/____/____ (circle: dd/mm/yy or mm/dd/yy)   Time: ____:____ (24 hr. clock)

Version 7.12.2005   © 2005 Surviving Sepsis Campaign and the Institute for Healthcare Improvement

Fig. 21-2 Sample screening tool for severe sepsis. (From Surviving Sepsis Campaign. [2005]. *Individual chart measurement tool.* Retrieved from http://ssc.sccm.org/files/Tools/individualchartmeasurementtool.pdf. Reproduced with permission. Copyright 2005. European Society of Intensive Care Medicine, International Sepsis Forum, and Society of Critical Care Medicine.)

TABLE 21-1 PIRO SCORE

PREDISPOSITION	INFECTION/INSULT	RESPONSE	ORGAN DYSFUNCTION
Years of Age <65 = 0	Pneumonia = 4	RR >20 = 3	BUN >20 = 2
65–80 = 1	Skin or soft tissue = 0	Bands >5% = 1	Respiratory failure/hypoxemia = 3
>80 = 2	Any other = 2	HR > 120 = 2	Lactate >40 = 3
COPD = 1			SBP <70 = 4
Liver disease = 2			70–90 = 2
Malignancy			>90 = 0
w/o metastases = 1			Platelets <150k = 2
w metastases = 2			

BUN, Blood urea nitrogen; *COPD*, chronic obstructive pulmonary disease; *HR*, heart rate; *SBP*, systolic blood pressure; *RR*, respiratory rate.
From Howell, M. D., Talmor, D., Schuetz, P., Hunziker, S., Jones, A. E., & Shapiro, N. I. (2011). Proof of principle: The predisposition, infection, response, organ failure sepsis staging system. *Critical Care Medicine, 39*(2), 322–327; Rubulotta, F., Marshall, J. C., Ramsay, G., Nelson, D., Levy, M., & Williams, M. (2009). Predisposition, insult/infection, response and organ dysfunction: A new model for staging severe sepsis. *Critical Care Medicine, 7*(4), 1329–1335.

TABLE 21-2 MEDS SCORING AND PREDICTED MORTALITY

Meds Scoring

CHARACTERISTIC	POINTS ASSIGNED
Predisposition	
Age >65 years	3
Nursing home resident	2
Rapidly terminal comorbid illness	6
Infection	
Lower respiratory infection	2
Response	
Bands >5%	3
Organ dysfunction	
Tachypnea or hypoxemia	3
Septic shock	3
Platelet count <150,000/mm³	3
Altered mental status	2

Meds Predicted Mortality

POINT RANGE	MEDS GROUP	28-DAY PREDICTED MORTALITY
0–4	Very low	1.1%
5–7	Low	4.4%
8–12	Moderate	9.3%
13–15	High	16.1%
>15	Very high	39.0%

From Shapiro, N. I., Howell, M. D., Talmor, D., Donnino, M., Ngo, L., & Bates, D. W. (2007). Mortality in Emergency Department Sepsis (MEDS) score predicts 1-year mortality. *Critical Care Medicine, 35*(1), 192–198.

TABLE 21-3 END POINTS OF RESUSCITATION

ADULT	PEDIATRIC
Central venous pressure = 8–12	Normalization of heart rate
Mean arterial pressure ≥65 mm Hg	Capillary refill ≤2 seconds
ScvO₂ ≥70% or SvO₂ ≥65%	Equalization of central and peripheral pulses
Urine output ≥0.5 mL/kg/h	Urine output >1 mL/kg/h

Data from Dellinger, R. P., Levy, M. M., Carlet, J. M., Bion, J., Parker, M. M., Jaeschke, R., … Vincent, J. L. (2008). Surviving sepsis campaign: International guidelines for management of severe sepsis and septic shock: 2008. *Critical Care Medicine, 36*(1), 296–327.

Diagnostic Procedures

Obtain laboratory tests, including the following:
- Serum lactate—measures cellular level perfusion; an elevated serum lactate level can identify occult hypoperfusion.[8]
- Procalcitonin—a prohormone of calcitonin; plasma concentrations are very low in healthy individuals. Studies show that plasma levels increase in sepsis.[23]
- Basic metabolic panel.
- Complete blood count, including hemoglobin and hematocrit.
- Blood type and crossmatch.
- Cultures:
  - These may include sputum, cerebral spinal fluid, urine, blood, and wound cultures; obtain at least one blood culture from peripheral circulation.
  - If the patient has a venous access device, obtain culture from this source as well.[9]

Imaging studies should include the following:

- Chest radiograph.
- Computed tomography scan and/or ultrasound.
- Depending on the patient's clinical condition, portable bedside studies may be best if the patient has severe sepsis or septic shock.

Communicate any abnormal assessment or laboratory findings to the emergency physician.

Therapeutic Interventions

Begin resuscitation immediately in patients with hypotension or elevated serum lactate greater than 4 mmoL/L. This may mean establishing central venous access and hemodynamic monitoring in the ED pending ICU admission.

Specific therapy guidelines include:

- Oxygen
  - Septic patient should receive supplemental oxygen with the goal of maintaining pulse oximetry readings of greater than 93%.[8]
  - Anticipate advanced airway management and possible rapid sequence intubation.
    - Intubation and mechanical ventilation may reduce the work of breathing, which reduces oxygen demand.
  - Measurement of venous oxygenation saturations may be accomplished via central line or pulmonary artery catheters.
    - SvO_2 measures oxyhemoglobin in the pulmonary artery whereas $ScvO_2$ is obtained from the right atrium via triple lumen catheter.[24]
- Large-bore intravenous catheter for fluid resuscitation
  - 250 to 1000 mL boluses of crystalloid solution (normal saline) every 15 minutes for hypotension.[18]
  - Maintain MAP of 65 mm Hg.
  - If MAP is less than 65 mm Hg, administer vasopressors (dobutamine, norepinephrine, or dopamine).
- Insertion of a central venous pressure (CVP) line
  - CVP pressures can guide resuscitation, with the goal being to maintain CVP of 8 mm Hg.
  - During insertion, ensure "time-out" documentation, proper infection prevention precautions, and draping of the patient and personal protective equipment for all staff involved in the procedure according to hospital policy.
- Source identification and control
  - Establish the source or site of infection as rapidly as possible (within first 6 hours of presentation) and evaluate the amenability for source control (e.g., abscess drainage, tissue debridement, indwelling line or catheter removal).
- Transfusion with red blood cells may be considered if the hemoglobin is less than 7 g/dL, the $ScvO_2$ is less than

70%, or the hematocrit is less than 30%. Because the shock state results in inadequate tissue perfusion, interventions should focus on restoring oxygen-carrying capability.

- Antibiotic administration within 1 hour of arrival[27,28]
  - Timely administration of antibiotics is crucial and affects outcomes.
  - A 1-hour delay may reduce survival by almost 8%.[8]
- Consider administration of vasopressors to maintain MAP greater than 65 mm Hg.
  - The *Surviving Sepsis Campaign Guidelines for Management of Severe Sepsis and Septic Shock*[9] recommend norepinephrine and dopamine as the initial vasopressors of choice to increase vascular tone and blood pressure.
  - Optimize fluid replacement before starting vasopressors.
- Inotropic therapy, such as dobutamine, may be initiated to increase cardiac output in patients with myocardial dysfunction.[30–32] Available data do not support the use of low-dose dopamine for renal protection.[33]
- Consider hydrocortisone when hypotension is refractory to fluid resuscitation and vasopressors.[9]

> Maintain CVP of 8 to 12 mm Hg. Colloids have not been shown to be of more benefit than crystalloids for fluid resuscitation.[25,26]

> Early administration of appropriate antibiotics decreases mortality in patients with gram-positive and gram-negative bacteremias. Initiate empiric broad-spectrum antibiotics before identification of the infecting organism and reassess after 48 to 72 hours based on culture results and clinical data.[29]

GOALS OF CONTINUING THERAPY

According to the Surviving Sepsis Campaign, patients requiring continued support should be managed with the following strategies for optimal outcomes. These strategies may be implemented in the ED or upon transfer to the intensive care setting.

- Mechanical ventilation of sepsis-induced acute lung injury or acute respiratory distress syndrome
  - Use of target tidal volumes of 6 mL/kg (predicted) body weight
  - Target plateau pressure of less than 30 cm H_2O
  - Permissive hypercapnia ($PaCO_2$ may increase above normal)
  - Use positive end expiratory pressure (PEEP) to avoid alveolar collapse at end expiration

- Maintain head of bed raised at 30 degrees or more unless contraindicated
- Glucose control
  - Use intravenous insulin to control hyperglycemia
  - Aim to keep blood glucose less than 150 mg/dL (8.3 mmol/L)
  - Monitor blood glucose values every 1 to 2 hours in patients with intravenous insulin
- Deep vein thrombosis prophylaxis
  - Use low-dose heparin unless contraindicated
  - Use compression stockings or an intermittent compression device
- Stress ulcer prophylaxis
  - Provide stress ulcer prophylaxis using H2 blockers or proton pump inhibitor

ONGOING EVALUATION

During the initial acute phase of sepsis and septic shock, the patient's condition is dynamic and interventions must be assessed rapidly to direct further care initiatives. Closely monitor the patient's global condition data accumulated to provide a full picture of the patient's condition. Closely follow institutional protocols for vital sign assessment and document patient response monitoring. It is important to look at trends, especially in vital signs.

PEDIATRIC CONSIDERATIONS

While sepsis mortality in the pediatric population is declining, sepsis remains a major cause of death in children.[34] Early recognition of pediatric sepsis is crucial and should be based on clinical presentation and history. It is essential for the emergency nurse to know normal vital signs for neonates, infants, and children. The following may be present before hypotension, which is an ominous sign:

- Hypothermia or hyperthermia
- Altered mental status
- Peripheral vasoconstriction with capillary refill greater than 2 seconds ("cold shock") or peripheral vasodilation ("warm shock")

SIRS criteria do apply to pediatrics, with several exceptions[34]:

- Either temperature or leukocyte abnormalities must be present.
- Bradycardia may be a sign of SIRS in the neonate but not necessarily in older children.
- Relying solely on blood pressure may be misleading, as children often maintain a blood pressure while they are in a shock state.

Fluid resuscitation is a priority for the pediatric sepsis patient. The pediatric patient in severe sepsis may require up to 40 to 60 mL/kg of crystalloids.[9] Inotropes may be added after fluid therapy to maintain heart rates and blood pressures that are normal for age as well as capillary refill times of less than 3 seconds. It is recommended that central circulation access be obtained before giving inotropes to children. In cases where multiple organ failure is present, be cautious to avoid fluid overload.[35]

Blood pressure is not a reliable end point to resuscitation. Measure responses in terms of capillary refill, normalization of heart rate, and evaluation of central and peripheral pulses.

PATIENT AND FAMILY SUPPORT

Patient and family education and support is critical during the initial phase of treatment. Health care professionals are often busy providing care to reach therapeutic goals in a specific window of time, leaving families excluded. Frequent brief updates from members of the multidisciplinary team can be helpful in keeping families informed, leading to decreased anxiety.

CONSIDERING LIMITATION OF SUPPORT

Early goal-directed therapy has improved outcomes for patients with sepsis and septic shock; however, mortality remains high in this patient population. Provide patients and families with factual information, realistic expectations, and likely outcomes of care. Conversations regarding limitation of life support may be necessary if patient conditions do not improve or deteriorate despite therapy. Palliative care teams and chaplains can be particularly helpful in these situations and often are able to assist nurses by spending time with patients and families as the nurse attends to basic patient care needs.

Early goal-directed therapy is based on early recognition and identification of infection, hypoperfusion, and organ dysfunction that can trigger the initiation of specific pathways of care. Interventions are frequently assessed and reassessed in a timely fashion to direct further therapy. Following established protocols can lead to decreased mortality in the patient with severe sepsis or septic shock.

REFERENCES

1. Angus, D. C., Linde-Zwirble, W. T., Lidicker, J., Clermont, G., Carcillo, J., & Pinsky, M. R. (2001). Epidemiology of severe sepsis in the United States: Analysis of incidence, outcome, and associated costs of care. *Critical Care Medicine*, 29(7), 1303–1310.
2. Martin, G. S., Mannino, D. M., Eaton, S., & Moss, M. (2003). The epidemiology of sepsis in the United States from 1979

through 2000. *New England Journal of Medicine, 348*(16), 1546–1554.

3. Martin, J. B., & Wheeler, A. P. (2009). Approach to the patient with sepsis. *Clinics in Chest Medicine, 30*(1), 1–16.

4. Ahrens, T., & Tuggle, D. (2004). Surviving severe sepsis: Early recognition and treatments. *Critical Care Nurse, 24*(Suppl), 2–13.

5. Rivers, E., Nguyen, B., Havstad, S., Ressler, J., Muzzin, A., Knoblich, B., … Tomlanovich, M. (2001). Early goal-directed therapy in the treatment of severe sepsis and septic shock. *New England Journal of Medicine, 345*(19), 1368–1377.

6. Rivers, E. P., McIntyre, L., Morro, D. C., & Rivers, K. K. (2005). Early and innovative interventions for severe sepsis and septic shock: Taking advantage of a window of opportunity. *Canadian Medical Association Journal, 173*(9), 1054–1065.

7. McIntyre, L. A., Fergusson, D. A., Herbert, P. C., Cook, D. J., Magder, S., Dhingra, V., & Bell, D. R. (2003). Are delays in the recognition and initial management of patients with severe sepsis associated with hospital mortality? *Critical Care Medicine, 31*(Suppl. 12), A75.

8. Frakes, M. A. (2007). Emergency department management of severe sepsis. *Advanced Emergency Nursing Journal, 29*(3), 228–238.

9. Dellinger, R. P., Levy, M. M., Carlet, J. M., Bion, J., Parker, M. M., Jaeschke, R., … Vincent, J. L. (2008). Surviving sepsis campaign: International guidelines for management of severe sepsis and septic shock: 2008. *Critical Care Medicine, 36*(1), 296–327.

10. Rivers, E. P. (2006). Early goal-directed therapy in severe sepsis and septic shock: Converting science to reality. *Chest, 129*(2), 217–218.

11. Nguyen, H. B., Rivers, E. P., Abrahamian, F. M., Moran, G. J., Abraham, E., Trzeciak, S., … Talan, D. A. (2006). Severe sepsis and septic shock: Review of the literature and emergency department management guidelines. *Annals of Emergency Medicine, 48*(1), 28–54.

12. Vincent, J. L., Martinez, E. O., & Silva, E. (2009). Evolving concepts in sepsis definitions. *Critical Care Clinics, 25*(4), 665–675.

13. Bone, R. C., Balk, R. A., Cerra, F. B., Dellinger, R. P., Fein, A. M., Knaus, W. A., … Sibbald, W. J. (1992). Definitions for sepsis and organ failure and guidelines for the use of innovative therapies in sepsis. The ACCP/SCCM Consensus Conference Committee. American College of Chest Physicians/Society of Critical Care Medicine. *Chest, 101*(6), 1644–1655.

14. O'Brien, J. M., Ali, N. A., Aberegg, S. K., & Abraham, E. (2007). Sepsis. *American Journal of Medicine, 120*(12), 1012–1022.

15. National Institute of General Medical Sciences. (2009, October). *Sepsis fact sheet. Taking aim at sepsis: Progress from the National Institute of General Medical Sciences.* Retrieved from http://www.nigms.nih.gov/Publications/factsheet_sepsis.htm

16. Society of Critical Care Medicine. (n.d.). *Surviving sepsis campaign.* Retrieved from http://ssc.sccm.org/

17. Institute for Healthcare Improvement. (n.d.). *Sepsis.* Retrieved from http://www.ihi.org/IHI/Topics/CriticalCare/Sepsis/

18. Stauss, M. P. (2005). A new approach to an old foe: Implementation of an early goal-directed sepsis treatment protocol. *Journal of Emergency Nursing, 31*(1), 34–35.

19. Rubulotta, F., Marshall, J. C., Ramsay, G., Nelson, D., Levy, M., & Williams, M. (2009). Predisposition, insult/infection, response and organ dysfunction: A new model for staging severe sepsis. *Critical Care Medicine, 7*(4), 1329–1335.

20. Howell, M. D., Talmor, D., Schuetz, P., Hunziker, S., Jones, A. E., & Shapiro, N. I. (2011). Proof of principle: The predisposition, infection, response, organ failure sepsis staging system. *Critical Care Medicine, 39*(2), 322–327.

21. Shapiro, N. I., Howell, M. D., Talmor, D., Donnino, M., Ngo, L., & Bates, D. W. (2007). Mortality in Emergency Department Sepsis (MEDS) score predicts 1-year mortality. *Critical Care Medicine, 35*(1), 192–198.

22. Sankoff, J. D., Goyal M., Gaieski, D. F., Deitch, K., Davis, C. B., Sabel, A. L., & Haukoos, J. S. (2008). Validation of the Mortality in Emergency Department Sepsis (MEDS) score in patients with the systemic inflammatory response syndrome (SIRS). *Critical Care Medicine, 36*(2), 421–426.

23. Guven, H., Altintop, L., Baydin, A., Esen, S., Aygun, D., Hokelek, M., … Bek, Y. (2002). Diagnostic value of procalcitonin levels as an early indicator of sepsis. *American Journal of Emergency Medicine, 20*(3), 202–206.

24. Ahrens, T. (2006). Hemodynamics in sepsis. *AACN Advanced Critical Care, 17*(4), 435–445.

25. Finfer, S., Bellomo, R., Boyce, N., French, J., Myburgh, J., & Norton, R. (2004). A comparison of albumin and saline for fluid resuscitation in the intensive care unit. *New England Journal of Medicine, 350*(22), 2247–2256.

26. Vincent, J. L., & Herwig, G. (2004). Fluid resuscitation in severe sepsis and septic shock: An evidence-based review. *Critical Care Medicine, 32*(Suppl. 11), S451–S454.

27. Gaieski, D. F., Mikkelsen, M. E., Band, R. A., Pines, J. M., Massone, R., Furia, F. F., … Goyal, M. (2010). Impact of time to antibiotics on survival in patients with severe sepsis or septic shock in who early goal-directed therapy was initiated in the emergency department. *Critical Care Medicine, 38*(4), 1045–1053

28. Siddiqi, S., & Razzak, J. (2010). Early versus late pre-intensive care unit admission broad spectrum antibiotics for severe sepsis in adults. *Cochrane Database of Systematic Reviews,* (10), CD007081.

29. Bochud, P.-Y., Bonten, M., Marchetti, O., & Calandra, T. (2004). Antimicrobial therapy for patients with severe sepsis and septic shock: An evidence-based review. *Critical Care Medicine, 32*(Suppl. 11), S495–S512.

30. Hayes, M. A., Timmins, A. C., Yau, E. H., Palazzo, M., Hinds, C. J., & Watson, D. (1994). Elevation of systemic oxygen delivery in the treatment of critically ill patients. *New England Journal of Medicine, 330*(24), 1717–1722.

31. Gattinoni, L., Brazzi, L., Pelosi, P., Latini, R., Tognoni, G., Pesenti, A., & Fumagalli, R. (1995). A trial of goal-oriented hemodynamic therapy in critically ill patients. SvO$_2$ Collaborative Group. *New England Journal of Medicine, 333*(16), 1025–1032.

32. Beale, R. J., Hollenberg, S. M., Vincent, J. L., & Parrillo, J. E. (2004). Vasopressor and inotropic support in septic shock: An evidence-based review. *Critical Care Medicine*, *32*(Suppl. 11), S455–S465.

33. Bellomo, R., Chapman, M., Finfer, S., Hickling, K., & Myburgh, J. (2000). Low-dose dopamine in patients with early renal dysfunction: A placebo-controlled randomized trial. Australian and New Zealand Intensive Care Society (ANZICS) Clinical Trials Group. *The Lancet*, *356*(9248), 2139–2143.

34. Goldstein, B., Giroir, B., & Randolph, A. (2005). International pediatric sepsis consensus conference: Definitions for sepsis and organ dysfunction in pediatrics. *Pediatric Critical Care Medicine 6*(1), 2–8.

35. Brierley, J., Carcillo, J. A., Choong, K., Cornell, T., Decaen, A., Deymann, A., … Zuckerberg, A. (2009). Clinical practice parameters for hemodynamic support of pediatric and neonatal septic shock: 2007 update from the American College of Critical Care Medicine. *Critical Care Medicine*, *37*(2), 666–688.

22

Infectious Diseases

William R. Short, Mary Kemper and Jeane Jackson

The emergency department (ED) is one of the most common sites of initial encounter for patients seeking treatment for symptoms caused by an infectious disease. This chapter outlines common infectious diseases categorized according to their mode of transmission. Also addressed are some unusual conditions related to emerging pathogens or potential epidemics. Patients with these illnesses will present for emergency care with signs and symptoms similar to those of common infectious diseases but may pose a grave threat to the hospital and greater community.

ISOLATION PRECAUTIONS

The Centers for Disease Control and Prevention (CDC) has established isolation precautions to prevent the spread of infection in health care institutions. Isolation precautions are divided into two general categories: standard precautions and transmission-based precautions. The three primary routes of disease transmission are contact, droplet, and airborne.[1] Table 22-1 lists examples of common conditions that require isolation.

Standard Precautions

Standard precautions are designed to reduce the risk of transmitting pathogens regardless of a patient's diagnosis or potential risk for an infectious disease. Standard precautions apply to blood, all body fluids, secretions, and excretions (with the exception of sweat), nonintact skin, and mucous membranes.

Transmission-Based Precautions

In addition to using standard precautions, transmission-based precautions should be put in place whenever suspicion of an infectious disease with a specific mode of transmission exists.

Contact Precautions

There are two types of contact precautions:
- Direct—the infectious pathogen is transferred from an infected person directly to another without an intermediate object or person. An example is blood from an infected person that comes in contact with an open wound on the skin.
- Indirect—the infectious pathogen is transferred through an intermediate object or person. An example is the hands of a health care worker transmitting a pathogen to another person.

Droplet Precautions

Droplet transmission, a form of contact transmission, involves contact of the conjunctiva or the mucous membranes of a susceptible person with large droplets (larger than 5 micrometers) containing microbes generated from the respiratory tract of a person who has clinical disease or is a carrier of the organism. Droplets are usually generated when the source person coughs, sneezes, or talks or during procedures such as suctioning, endotracheal intubation, or bronchoscopy.

Airborne Precautions

Airborne transmission involves dissemination of either airborne droplet nuclei (≤5 micrometers) or dust particles containing the infectious agent. Organisms spread in this manner can be dispersed widely by air currents and may become inhaled by or deposited on a susceptible host within the same room or over a longer distance. In this case, special air handling and ventilation are required to prevent airborne transmission.

BLOOD-BORNE INFECTIONS[2]

Blood-borne pathogens cause diseases that spread from person to person through direct contact with infected blood or other bodily fluids.

TABLE 22-1 EXAMPLES OF COMMON CONDITIONS REQUIRING ISOLATION

CONTACT	AIRBORNE	DROPLET
Scabies	Chickenpox (varicella)	Influenza
Impetigo	Tuberculosis	Mumps
Shingles	Herpes zoster (immunocompromised host)	Diphtheria (pharyngeal)
		Neisseria meningitidis
		Pertussis

Human Immunodeficiency Virus

Human immunodeficiency virus (HIV), the virus that causes acquired immune deficiency syndrome (AIDS), is transmitted when there is an exchange of blood, semen, pre-ejaculate, vaginal fluid, or breast milk from an infected individual. Once present in a person's bloodstream, HIV begins to affect the immune system and causes a variety of symptoms and illnesses (known as opportunistic infections) not typically seen in a healthy individual. There is currently no vaccine available to prevent HIV/AIDS. Patients need to be aware of the risk factors involved in HIV transmission and to take precautions against infection.

High-Risk Groups

- Persons who are sexually active: Anyone who is sexually active is at risk for HIV, but this is especially true for men who have sex with men and for those who engage with multiple sex partners without using protection.
- Intravenous (IV) drug users.

Transmission

- Unprotected sexual contact of any kind
- Needle sharing
- Vertical or perinatal transmission—occurs in utero or during birth process from mother to child
- Breastfeeding—an HIV-positive mother can transmit HIV when breastfeeding.

It should be noted that in most developed countries, including the United States, medical technology and the availability of research and resources has significantly lowered the perinatal transmission rate of HIV. Most mothers are educated by their health care providers regarding the risk of breastfeeding and are provided with the necessary resources to reduce the risk of transmission.

Signs and Symptoms (Non-Specific)

- Fever
- Rash
- Malaise
- Myalgia
- Swollen lymph nodes
- Sore throat

Typically these symptoms will be present during the initial stages of infection. Patients may present to an ED without symptoms of HIV and become aware of their diagnosis only if testing is offered and agreed upon. Of course, the reverse is also true, and patients present to the ED with advanced cases of HIV/AIDS seeking treatment because of symptoms associated with an opportunistic infection.

Regardless of presenting symptoms, *all* patients presenting to the ED for *any* form of treatment who report that they are IV drug users or sexually active should be offered an HIV test at that time.

Therapeutic Interventions

Primary Therapeutic Interventions

- Antiretroviral medication
  - Nucleoside reverse transcriptase inhibitors
  - Nonnucleoside reverse transcriptase inhibitors
  - Protease inhibitors
  - Fusion inhibitors
  - Coreceptor antagonists (CCR5)
  - Integrase inhibitors
- Prophylaxis against opportunistic pathogens at certain CD4 criteria
  - CD4 less than 200/mcL—prophylaxis against *Pneumocystis jiroveci* pneumonia (PCP)
  - CD4 less than 100/mcL—prophylaxis against *Toxoplasma gondii*
  - CD4 less than 50/mcL—prophylaxis against *Mycobacterium avium* complex
- Medications and treatment for any current opportunistic infections
- Vaccinations (pneumococcal vaccine polyvalent [Pneumovax], influenza)
- Treatment of patients with latent tuberculosis

Secondary Therapeutic Interventions

- Prophylaxis after patient has completed a course of treatment for certain opportunistic infections (PCP requires a 21-day course of treatment followed by secondary prophylaxis until CD4 is >200 for 6 months)
- Counseling and risk reduction education

Prevention

- Use protective barriers during sexual intercourse.
- Use clean needles during IV drug use.
- Engage in regular HIV testing.

Discharge Instructions

For those who present to the ED and are discharged *with* an HIV diagnosis:

- HIV follow-up care: If possible, schedule an appointment with an HIV care provider prior to discharge from the ED or hospital.
- Provide information on HIV and schedule an appointment for counseling services.
- Provide information regarding HIV transmission prevention.

For those who present to the ED and are discharged *without* an HIV diagnosis:

- Provide information on prevention measures.
- Provide information on community HIV testing sites.

Hepatitis B

Hepatitis B virus (HBV) causes severe infection of the liver and is acquired through contact with blood or body fluids containing blood. HBV can present in two forms: acute and chronic. For those patients presenting with acute HBV infection, treatment needs are minimal. For those with chronic HBV, continuous medical attention is required.

High-Risk Groups

- IV drug users
- Those engaging in unprotected sexual activity
- Undiagnosed pregnant women because of risk of transmission during birth from mother to child

Transmission

- Unprotected sexual contact
- Needle sharing
- Vertical transmission

Signs and Symptoms[3]

- General gastrointestinal symptoms: nausea, vomiting, loss of appetite (31% to 69%)
- Viral symptoms or fever (70% to 94%)
- Pruritus from skin irritation by bile salts
- Body aches
- Dark urine (from bile); clay-colored stool (from lack of bile)
- Jaundice, if bilirubin two to three times the normal value (31% to 69%)

Diagnostic Procedures

- Liver enzymes ALT and AST (also known as SGOT and SGPT) must be at least two times the normal value.
- Hepatitis panel to determine whether patient has HBV, had HBV, or is resistant to the virus.
- If diagnosed with HBV, regular liver function testing will be conducted to measure progression and control side effects (cirrhosis and liver cancer).
- Liver biopsy.

Therapeutic Intervention

Acute HBV infection requires support and monitoring. Chronic HBV infection requires the following:

- Medication—currently, there is no cure available for HBV despite the approval of these seven drugs for treatment:
  - Interferon alpha
  - Pegylated interferon
  - Lamivudine
  - Adefovir dipivoxil (Hepsera)
  - Entecavir
  - Telbivudine
  - Tenofovir
- Medical monitoring—blood work should be drawn on a regular basis.

> Interferon-alpha, one of the medications available for the treatment of hepatitis B, has been known to cause or increase levels of depression. Treatment providers should inquire about baseline levels of depression in a patient and incorporate that information into the treatment decision.[3-5]

Prevention

- Vaccination—HBV vaccination can start at the time of birth. It consists of a series of three injections over the course of 6 months.
- Engage in safe-sex practices.
- Use clean needles or needle exchange programs if an IV drug user.
- Practice universal safety precautions when providing health care.
- Avoid sharing personal items such as razors, toothbrushes, etc.
- If pregnant, participate in prenatal care.

Discharge Instructions

Regardless of HBV type, all patients discharged from the hospital with HBV should be:

- Cautioned against sharing personal items that could spread HBV.

- Made aware of the importance of engaging in safe-sex practices.
- Advised to abstain from illicit drug use, hepatotoxic drug use such as acetaminophen (Tylenol), and alcohol use.
- Given instructions to follow up with their health care providers.
- Educated as to the importance of rest and good nutrition to help the liver regenerate.

Hepatitis D

Hepatitis D virus relies on the presence of HBV to replicate. Hepatitis D and hepatitis B can be transmitted to an individual at the same time or during separate occurrences. Those with hepatitis D will exhibit the same symptoms as those with hepatitis B. While hepatitis D is not common in the United States, it is present in Middle Eastern countries, sub-Saharan Africa, and South America, especially among the IV drug user population. Hepatitis D exacerbates the side effects of hepatitis B and leads to higher incidences of morbidity and mortality, especially among those who go untreated for a significant period of time. The course of treatment and discharge care for hepatitis D are similar to those for hepatitis B.

Hepatitis C

The hepatitis C virus causes inflammation of the liver. Hepatitis C is often thought to be the most dangerous of the hepatitis viruses because patients often live for a long period of time with the virus without exhibiting any signs or symptoms. Like hepatitis B and hepatitis D, hepatitis C is transmitted through contact with infected blood. Diagnosis is commonly made when a patient presents for treatment of symptoms caused by a severe condition that has gone undiagnosed or through routine testing during physical examination with the finding of mildly elevated transaminases. Currently, no vaccination or cure is available for the hepatitis C virus.

Transmission

- IV drug use
- Needlestick in health care setting
- Intranasal cocaine use when straws are shared to snort the drug between multiple individuals
- Unprotected sexual contact

Signs and Symptoms

A patient might not exhibit any signs or symptoms of hepatitis C infection until the disease has progressed to an advanced stage. The following may present throughout the course of illness:

- Tenderness around the area of the liver
- Nausea and loss of appetite
- Increased level of depression
- Fatigue
- Jaundice

Diagnostic Procedures

- Liver function tests
- Hepatitis C antibody test
- Hepatitis C viral load
- Hepatitis C genotype
- Liver biopsy

Therapeutic Intervention

Not all who are infected with hepatitis C require treatment; however, it is important for those infected with hepatitis C to be connected with a health care provider who can monitor liver function over their lifetimes. For those who do require treatment for hepatitis C, the standard regimen is a combination of weekly pegylated interferon in combination with ribavirin. In cases where liver disease has progressed and liver function has deteriorated, there is the possibility of liver transplant when available and appropriate.

Patients with chronic hepatitis C should have serologies ordered to assess their immune status to both hepatitis A and hepatitis B. If there is no evidence of immunity, HAV and HBV vaccination should be administered.

Prevention

- Clean needles (as most hepatitis C infections are acquired through IV drug use)
- Universal precautions
- Health care workers immediately report and obtain treatment after needlestick
- Patient education on risk reduction

AIRBORNE INFECTIONS

Influenza

Viral influenza is a well-established cause of seasonal illness, generally characterized by acute onset of fever, myalgias, and respiratory symptoms. In the United States the peak of flu season occurs between late November and March. In healthy persons the disease usually resolves without sequelae. Unlike the common cold, influenza can cause severe illness and complications in many individuals. Table 22-2 and Table 22-3 list those at risk for complications as well as some of the common complications encountered post influenza.

TABLE 22-2 PATIENTS AT RISK FOR INFLUENZA COMPLICATIONS

- Persons older than 49 years
- Children
- Women who are pregnant or who may become pregnant during flu season
- Adults and children who are immunocompromised
- Adults and children who have a chronic medical condition
- Residents of nursing homes and other long-term care facilities

TABLE 22-3 COMPLICATIONS OF INFLUENZA

- Viral pneumonia
- Secondary bacterial pneumonia
- Exacerbation of underlying cardiac or pulmonary disease
- Myositis
- Rhabdomyolysis
- Reye's syndrome
- Transverse myelitis
- Aseptic meningitis
- Pericarditis
- Myocarditis

Transmission

Influenza viruses are mainly transmitted from person to person in respiratory droplets from coughing and sneezing.

Signs and Symptoms

- Abrupt onset of high fever: 38° C to 40° C (100° F to 104° F)
- Anorexia
- Conjunctivitis, coryza, pharyngitis, nasal discharge
- Dry cough
- General body aches, myalgias
- Headache
- Malaise, lassitude

Diagnostic Procedures

- Diagnosis is usually based on clinical presentation, mostly systemic symptoms.
- Rapid antigen tests from nasal or throat swabs.

Therapeutic Interventions

- Adequate hydration and nutrition.
- Antivirals: zanamivir (Relenza), oseltamivir (Tamiflu), amantadine (Symmetrel), rimantadine (Flumadine).

Prevention

- Annual vaccination is the most effective strategy for preventing influenza.
- Cover nose and mouth with a tissue when coughing or sneezing. Throw the tissue in the trash after use.
- Wash hands often with soap and water. If soap and water are not available, use an alcohol-based hand wash.
- Avoid touching eyes, nose, and mouth.
- Try to avoid close contact with ill people.
- If sick with flulike illness, the CDC recommends staying home for at least 24 hours after the fever is gone, except to get medical care or for other necessities.

Pulmonary Tuberculosis

Tuberculosis is a disease caused by *Mycobacterium tuberculosis*. Infection is transmissible from person to person via aerosolized pulmonary secretions. It is critical to differentiate active (infectious) from latent (inactive) infection:

- Latent—once initial infection occurs, it is contained by the immune system and remains quiescent. Latent tuberculosis is usually asymptomatic and patients are treated with a variety of regimens (isoniazid monotherapy).
- Active—reactivation of the once quiescent disease can take many forms, including active pulmonary disease. These patients require aggressive treatment and respiratory precautions.

Transmission

The major route of transmission is via airborne droplet nuclei produced by coughing, sneezing, and speaking. Droplet nuclei are microscopic (1 to 3 micrometers) and contain hundreds of bacilli. They are capable of remaining suspended in air for prolonged periods of time but are quickly dispersed with air flow, thus special air flow and ventilation are required.

Signs and Symptoms

- Initial infection usually asymptomatic
- Chronic cough (greater than 2 to 3 weeks)
- Night sweats, fevers, chills
- Weight loss, anorexia
- Fatigue

Diagnostic Procedures

- Chest radiograph
- Sputum for acid-fast bacilli
- Routine laboratory work

Therapeutic Intervention

- Standard and airborne precautions
- Adherence to medication regimen
- Avoid close contact with others
- Medication
    - Latent: treatment with isoniazid and pyridoxine for 9 months (most common regimen)
    - Active: usually start with multidrug regimen including isoniazid, rifampin, pyrazinamide, and ethambutol for 2 months (pending drug susceptibility testing); followed by two drugs based on susceptibility testing for an additional 4 months

Chickenpox (Varicella Zoster Virus)

Chickenpox is a highly contagious disease that is caused by varicella zoster virus. Before the advent of routine immunization, chickenpox was a common childhood illness. Most American adults have developed immunity through childhood exposure.

In children, chickenpox is generally a mild illness, although secondary bacterial infections can occur. However, adults who contract the disease can experience complications such as pneumonia or central nervous system disorders. After primary infection, the virus establishes latency in the dorsal root ganglia. As a person gets older or as his or her immune system is compromised, reactivation may occur in the form of shingles.

Transmission

Varicella zoster virus usually is spread through respiratory droplets. It is also possible (although much less common) to acquire the virus through secondary contact with the live virus from skin lesions. Individuals are infectious for 48 hours before the rash appears and remain contagious until all skin lesions have crusted over and no new lesions have formed.[6]

Signs and Symptoms

- Fever
- Headache, anorexia
- Lymphadenopathy
- Malaise
- Pruritus
- Purulent vesicular rash that initially forms on the trunk and face and then becomes generalized
- Urticaria

Diagnostic Procedures

- Routine laboratory work
- Chest radiographs if pulmonary involvement occurs

Therapeutic Interventions

- Respiratory and contact isolation
- Symptomatic care: rest, oral fluid intake
- Medications
    - Antiviral agents: acyclovir (Zovirax), foscarnet (Foscavir) (generally not necessary in uncomplicated cases).
    - Antihistamines: such as diphenhydramine (Benadryl) to control pruritus.
    - Antipyretics and analgesics: acetaminophen (Tylenol), ibuprofen (Motrin).
    - Administration of varicella immunoglobulin for pregnant patients. This drug also can be used for prophylaxis in nonimmune pregnant patients with chickenpox exposure.
    - Systemic antibiotics if a secondary bacterial infection occurs.

Prevention

Administration of varicella vaccine, which contains a live virus, is the primary mode of prevention. One dose is recommended for all children at 12 to 18 months of age. Children and adults who have not been vaccinated and have never had chickenpox should be immunized as well.

> Immunosuppression is a contraindication to immunization.

Measles

Measles, also known as rubeola, is a highly contagious infection of the respiratory system caused by a virus. This once-common childhood illness has largely disappeared from developed nations as a result of aggressive immunization campaigns. The use of vaccination is highly efficacious; however, cases are still seen occasionally in persons who have escaped immunization, such as the elderly, immigrants, and individuals with objections to vaccination.

> The three most common signs and symptoms of measles are the three C's: conjunctivitis, coryza, and cough.

Transmission

Measles is transmitted via nasal secretions, either directly to another individual or via respiratory droplets. The incubation period for the infection is 8 to 12 days. These viruses can be transmitted 5 days after initial exposure and up to 5 days after the rash has appeared.

Signs and Symptoms

- Conjunctivitis, eyelid edema, photophobia
- Dry cough, coryza
- Fever
- Rash
- Koplik spots (diagnostic lesions for measles—small red specks with a blue-white center found on the buccal mucosa, especially near the molars): appear 2 days before the rash and disappear within 48 hours of rash onset
- Malaise, irritability

Diagnostic Procedures

Diagnosis is usually made on the basis of clinical findings. Leukopenia may be present. Viral cultures and antibody testing are possible. Chest radiograph may be necessary for suspected pneumonia.

Therapeutic Interventions

Therapeutic interventions consist of supportive care and symptomatic treatment.

Prevention

Prevention consists of following standard and airborne precautions and immunizations.

Mumps

The mumps virus is a paramyxovirus most frequently seen in the spring months. This virus causes glandular enlargement, primarily involving one of the salivary glands, the parotid gland. Complications include orchitis, in which the testicles become swollen and painful. Twenty to fifty percent of postpubertal males with mumps develop orchitis.[7] Other complications include pancreatitis, aseptic meningitis, and central nervous system involvement.

Transmission

Viral transmission is via respiratory droplets and saliva. Patients are most contagious 1 to 2 days before the appearance of parotitis and remain infectious for up to 5 days after the onset of glandular enlargement.

Signs and Symptoms

- Parotitis: swelling is bilateral in two thirds of cases
- Fever: 37.8° C to 39.4° C (100° F to 103° F)
- Nonspecific symptoms of upper respiratory tract infection: malaise, anorexia, and headache

Diagnostic Procedures

Diagnosis usually is based on clinical findings. Further studies are noncontributory in uncomplicated cases. Other possible studies include the following:

- The virus can be isolated from throat swabs, secretions, cerebrospinal fluid, or urine.
- An immunofluorescence assay indicates viral antigens in oropharyngeal cells.
- An enzyme-linked immunosorbent assay (ELISA) for rapid detection can be performed with unclear cases.
- Leukocytosis with a left shift may be present in severely ill patients.

Therapeutic Interventions

Therapeutic interventions include supportive care, analgesics, and antipyretics. Oral steroids and scrotal support can be used for severe orchitis.

Prevention

Prevention consists of standard and droplet precautions and immunizations.

Pertussis (Whooping Cough)

Pertussis is a highly contagious respiratory disease that is caused by the gram-negative organism *Bordetella pertussis*. These bacteria attach to the respiratory tract's ciliated epithelium and produce a toxin that limits a patient's ability to effectively clear secretions. This may predispose patients to a secondary pneumonia. Pertussis remains a major health issue in countries where vaccination is not standard. Cases have been reported in unimmunized individuals in the United States.

Transmission

B. pertussis is transmitted via respiratory droplets or through contact with airborne respiratory secretions. The incubation period is usually 7 to 10 days but can be variable. Children are infected more frequently than adults and tend to have a more severe disease course. Unimmunized infants are also at risk for acquiring pertussis.

Signs and Symptoms

- Stage I (catarrhal stage; 1 to 2 weeks): Patient presents with coryza, sneezing, low-grade fever, and occasional cough that progressively becomes worse.
- Stage II (paroxysmal stage; 1 to 6 weeks): One to two weeks after onset, the cough worsens. Patients experience unremitting paroxysmal bursts of coughing that end with a high-pitched "whoop." Cyanosis may be

present during the coughing episode. Coughing fits tend to occur more frequently at night.

- Stage III (convalescent stage; weeks to months): Gradual recovery as the cough becomes less severe and frequent. Superinfections can occur at this stage because of trapped secretions.

Diagnostic Procedures

- Diagnosis is usually based on clinical findings.
- Collection of nasopharyngeal cultures for isolation of *B. pertussis.* Use a Dacron® swab and place it directly on the medium. Although the causative organism is difficult to isolate, this procedure may be done during the catarrhal stage of the disease.
- Other diagnostic procedures have been used such as polymerase chain reaction, direct fluorescent antibody, and serological testing.

Therapeutic Interventions

- Respiratory isolation
- Supportive care
- Macrolide antibiotics (azithromycin, clarithromycin, or erythromycin)

Prevention

- Follow standard and droplet precautions.
- Obtain pertussis vaccination.
- Household contacts should be treated with antibiotics regardless of vaccination status.

Diphtheria

Diphtheria is an infection of the mucous membranes caused by the bacteria *Corynebacterium diphtheriae.* This infection is uncommon in the United States largely as a result of vaccination. Diphtheria can still be encountered in unimmunized immigrants, particularly those living in overcrowded situations.

Transmission

Diphtheria is spread by respiratory droplets. The incubation period is 1 to 8 days.

Signs and Symptoms

- Low-grade fever.
- Sore throat.
- A thick, gray, membranous covering forms on the tonsils and pharynx (pseudomembrane). The covering may extend over the larynx, causing airway obstruction.
- Complications include myocarditis, neuritis, and airway obstruction.

Diagnostic Procedures

- Swab the throat for gram stain, culture, and sensitivity.
- Send specimen for toxin analysis.
- Polymerase chain reaction.

Therapeutic Interventions

- Diphtheria antitoxin: dose depends on the extent of the disease
- Erythromycin
- Membrane removal will cause bleeding

Prevention

Prevention consists of standard and droplet precautions and diphtheria vaccination.

WATER-BORNE AND FOOD-BORNE INFECTIONS

Many pathogens are transmitted via contaminated food and water. These infections commonly accompany foreign travel but can also occur in the United States because of inadequate sanitation and poor food preparation or storage practices.

Hepatitis A

The hepatitis A virus (HAV) is a ribonucleic acid (RNA) virus and is prevalent in areas with poor hygiene, poor sanitation, or crowded living conditions. Hepatitis A is a self-limited illness that does not result in chronic liver disease. Infection with HAV provides lifelong immunity. The incubation period is 2 to 6 weeks.

Transmission

HAV is spread via the fecal-oral route from:
- Contaminated food, water, or objects
- High-risk individuals
- Household contact with an infected person
- Persons living in, or traveling to, an area in which HAV is endemic

Signs and Symptoms

- Anorexia, nausea, abdominal pain, diarrhea
- Fatigue
- Jaundice
- Low-grade fever

Diagnostic Procedures

- Serum HAV immunoglobulin M antibody to detect acute infection
- Stool cultures rarely used

Therapeutic Interventions

Therapeutic intervention consists of symptomatic care.

Prevention

- HAV vaccination is recommended for the following individuals[8]:
  - Persons age 1 years or older
  - High-risk individuals
  - Health care workers
  - Travelers to endemic areas
- Immunoglobulin prevents infection if given before, or within 2 weeks, of exposure.
- Wash hands with soap, water, and friction after using the toilet and before eating or food preparation.

Hepatitis E

Hepatitis E virus (HEV), a single-stranded RNA virus, is responsible for most of the non-A, non-B enterically transmitted hepatitis. This organism causes an inflammatory liver disease similar to HAV. The course of the disease is self-limiting. Most patients recover, although mortality rates are higher in pregnant women. HEV does not cause chronic liver disease.

Transmission occurs primarily by the fecal-oral route. The incubation period is 15 to 60 days. Signs and symptoms, diagnostic procedures, therapeutic interventions, and prevention are the same as those for hepatitis A.

Typhoid Fever

Typhoid, or enteric, fever is caused by the organism *Salmonella typhi*. This disease is contracted by ingestion of contaminated food, water, or milk. In the United States typhoid fever is rare but can be found in recent travelers to endemic areas.

Transmission

Transmission is via contaminated food, water, or milk.

Signs and Symptoms

- Altered level of consciousness
- Headache, malaise, anorexia, muscle aches
- High fever and chills for 2 to 3 weeks
- Relative bradycardia (bradycardia in the presence of fever)
- "Rose spots"—erythematous macules usually found on the upper abdomen

Diagnostic Procedures

- Diagnosis generally based on patient history and clinical findings
- Blood cultures (positive in the majority of cases)
- Complete blood count, metabolic panel, urinalysis

Therapeutic Interventions

- Administer antibiotics.
- If the patient has mild disease, typhoid fever can be managed on an outpatient basis.
- For severe disease, the patient is usually admitted to the hospital.

Prevention

- Food and water precautions during travel
- Hygienic food preparation and storage
- Typhoid fever vaccination for those traveling to endemic areas

VECTOR-BORNE INFECTIONS

A vector-borne illness is an illness carried and actively transmitted by an organism, usually an insect, such as a flea or mosquito.

West Nile Virus

West Nile virus, a mosquito-transmitted flavivirus, is a potentially severe illness. Most West Nile virus infections in humans are asymptomatic. Encephalitis may occur in some individuals.

Transmission

The West Nile virus generally is transmitted via the bite of infected mosquitoes. There have been instances of West Nile virus transmission via blood transfusion, organ transplantation, breastfeeding, and percutaneous injury (e.g., laboratory worker needlestick).

Signs and Symptoms

- Anorexia, nausea, vomiting
- Encephalitis or neurologic disorders can develop in severe cases
- Eye pain
- Lymphadenopathy
- Malaise, headache
- Myalgias
- Rash: maculopapular or morbilliform on the neck, trunk, arms, and legs

Diagnostic Procedures

- Lumbar puncture
- West Nile immunoglobulin M antibody in the serum and cerebrospinal fluid

Therapeutic Interventions

- Severe disease requires hospitalization.
- Supportive care includes hydration, respiratory assistance, and prevention and treatment of secondary infections.

Prevention

- Avoid mosquitoes.
  - Use an insect repellant that contains DEET (*N,N*-Diethyl-*m*-toluamide).
  - Wear long sleeves, long pants, and light colors.
  - Avoid outdoor activities at dawn and dusk when mosquitoes are most active.

DERMAL INFECTIONS

Scabies

Scabies is a contagious skin infection caused by the mite *Sarcoptes scabiei*.

Transmission

Scabies is transmitted via direct, close, skin-to-skin contact with an infected person, bedding, or clothing.

Signs and Symptoms

Patients have a red, intensely pruritic rash with burrow channels obvious under the skin. Infestation can occur anywhere on the body but is most common in the webbing between the fingers and toes or in skinfolds over joints. Scratch marks are often present.

> Patients with scabies will have "burrows" of pruritic, white, threadlike patterns with small gray spots at the closed end.

Diagnostic Procedures

Diagnosis usually is made clinically based on patient history and rash characteristics. Skin scrapings can be done to look for mites or eggs.

Therapeutic Interventions

Topical treatment includes lindane 1% lotion (Kwell) or permethrin 5% dermal cream (Lyclear).

Prevention

- Follow standard and contact precautions.
- Wash all linens and clothing in very hot water to prevent insect spread.
- Avoid contact with infected individuals.

Ringworm

Ringworm is a superficial fungal infection of the skin. There are several varieties of tinea (capitis, cruris, pedis), each named for the body region infected. Tinea corporis generally is limited to the arms, legs, and trunk.

Transmission

Ringworm is transmitted through contact with an infected person or animals.

Signs and Symptoms

Patients have sharply marginated anular lesions with raised margins and central clearing.

Diagnostic Procedures

Diagnosis usually is made by clinical examination. Potassium hydroxide–stained skin scrapings are examined under a microscope for hyphae.

Therapeutic Interventions

Antifungal creams generally eradicate the infection. In cases of severe infestation, systemic antifungal agents can be used.

Prevention

- Follow standard and contact precautions.
- Follow good skin hygiene.
- Limit contact with infected pets.

MISCELLANEOUS INFECTIONS

Herpes Zoster (Shingles)

Herpes zoster, commonly known as "shingles," is caused by the reactivation of dormant varicella viruses (see Chickenpox above). Lesions follow along the path of nerve dermatomes, which explains their unilateral distribution (lesions do not cross the midline). Shingles can occur any time after initial varicella infection and may recur repeatedly over the course of a person's lifetime.

Transmission

Vesicles contain live virus and can be contagious to unvaccinated or susceptible hosts.

Signs and Symptoms

- Severe, localized, unilateral pain.
- Within 48 hours of pain onset, vesicular lesions develop along a nerve dermatome.

Diagnostic Procedures

The diagnosis of shingles is usually made clinically. Viral cultures can be obtained, but they rarely contribute to diagnosis or management.

Therapeutic Interventions

- Antiviral medications
- Cover lesions to minimize viral transmission
- Supportive care and comfort measures

Prevention

- Varicella zoster vaccination
- Standard, airborne, and contact precautions around persons with active chickenpox

Meningitis

Meningitis is an acute inflammation of the lining of the brain and spinal cord. It can be either viral or bacterial. Viral (aseptic) meningitis is usually a mild, self-limited condition that resolves spontaneously with basic symptomatic care. Bacterial meningitis is more severe and can cause serious complications if not treated appropriately. Common causative agents for bacterial meningitis are *Streptococcus pneumoniae*, *Haemophilus influenzae*, and *Neisseria meningitidis*.

Transmission

- Bacterial meningitis: via respiratory droplets and secretions
- Viral meningitis: not usually contagious

Signs and Symptoms

- Headache, fever, malaise
- Irritability, restlessness, altered level of consciousness can occur in severe cases
- Nausea, vomiting
- Petechial rash: Characteristic of *N. meningitidis* (meningococcal meningitis)
- Stiff neck, photophobia

Diagnostic Procedures

- Lumbar puncture for cerebrospinal fluid analysis and culture
- Blood cultures

Therapeutic Interventions

- Viral meningitis: supportive care, nutrition, hydration, rest, analgesics, antipyretics.
- Bacterial meningitis: urgent antibiotic therapy targeted at suspected organisms.

- These patients can be extremely ill and progress to septic shock within hours of initial symptoms.
- Place in isolation initially until *N. meningitidis* is ruled out.

Prevention

- Follow standard and droplet precautions.
- Close contacts of patients with *N. meningitidis* should receive antibiotic prophylaxis.
- Vaccines are available for *N. meningitidis* and *H. influenzae* (Hib vaccine).
- Although immunization against *H. influenzae* is effective, *N. meningitidis* vaccination confers immunity only against certain pathogen serotypes.

REFERENCES

1. Siegel, J. D., Rhinehart, E., Jackson, M., & Chiarello, L., Healthcare Infection Control Practices Advisory Committee. (2007). *2007 guideline for isolation precautions: Preventing transmission of infectious agents in healthcare settings.* Atlanta, GA: Centers for Disease Control and Prevention. Retrieved from http://www.cdc.gov/hicpac/pdf/isolation/Isolation2007.pdf
2. Southwick, F. (2007). *Infectious diseases: A clinical short course* (2nd ed.). New York, NY: McGraw-Hill.
3. Chng, Y. M., & Brown, D. F. M. (2006). Jaundice. In S. R. Votey & M. A. Davis (Eds.), *Signs and symptoms in emergency medicine: Literature-based approach to emergent conditions* (2nd ed.). St. Louis, MO: Mosby.
4. Capuron, L., Raison, C. L., Musselman, D. L., Lawson, D. H., Nemeroff, C. B., & Miller, A. H. (2003). Association of exaggerated HPA axis response to the initial injection of interferon-alpha with development of depression during interferon-alpha therapy. *American Journal of Psychiatry, 160,* 1342–1345.
5. Chapman, J., Oser, M., Hockemeyer, J., Weitlauf, J., Jones, S., & Cheung, R. (2011). Changes in depressive symptoms and impact on treatment course among hepatitis C patients undergoing interferon-α ribavirn therapy: A prospective evaluation. *American Journal of Gastroenterology.* doi:10.1038/ajg.2011.252.
6. Panel on Antiretroviral Guidelines for Adults and Adolescents. (2011, January 10). *Guidelines for the use of antiretroviral agents in HIV-1–infected adults and adolescents.* Washington, DC: Department of Health and Human Services. Retrieved from http://www.aidsinfo.nih.gov/ContentFiles/AdultandAdolescentGL.pdf
7. McPhee, S. J., & Papadakis, M. A. (2010). *Current medical diagnosis and treatment 2010* (49th ed.). New York, NY: McGraw-Hill.
8. Centers for Disease Control and Prevention. (2006, March 21). *Hepatitis a vaccine: What you need to know.* Retrieved from http://www.cdc.gov/vaccines/pubs/vis/downloads/vis-hep-a.pdf

Hematologic and Immunologic Emergencies

C.J. Carringer and Belinda B. Hammond

The number of patients presenting to emergency departments (EDs) with hematologic and immunologic emergencies is increasing because of better treatment and enhanced longevity of persons with these conditions. Several pathologic processes directly affect the blood and the organs that produce blood. Three problems commonly encountered by emergency nurses are anemia, sickle cell disease and crisis, and hemophilia. Patients with leukemia and lymphoma experience specific immunologic emergencies related to their disease and its treatment. These complications must be identified and managed. As the result of the dramatic increase in transplant survival, a growing number of organ recipients are being evaluated in EDs for transplant-related complications. Likewise, patients who are human immunodeficiency virus (HIV) positive have an increasing life expectancy and may present with a variety of clinical problems both related and unrelated to their HIV status.

HEMATOLOGIC EMERGENCIES

Anemia

Anemia exists when there is a deficiency in the number of red blood cells (RBCs) and thus a deficiency in the oxygen-carrying ability of the blood. Anemia can be acute or chronic and results from one of three possible mechanisms:

- Excessive blood loss
- Decreased production of RBCs
- Destruction of RBCs

  Management of anemia depends on the acuity of onset and the severity of clinical symptoms. If anemia is suspected, the patient should be assessed for any of the following risk factors:

- Kidney disease
- Diabetes

- Cancer or cancer therapy
- Family history of anemia
- Chronic infection or disease
- Injury
- Anticoagulation therapy
- Gastrointestinal bleeding or malabsorption syndromes
- Abnormal vaginal bleeding
- Medications that suppress bone marrow function

Signs and Symptoms

- Fatigue, decreased energy level
- Dyspnea on exertion
- Chest pain if concurrent coronary artery disease
- Dizziness
- Pallor
- Complaints of "feeling cold"
- Headache

Diagnostic Procedures

- Complete blood count (CBC) with differential and peripheral smear. Anemia is defined as:
  - Hematocrit of less than 39% in men and less than 36% in nonpregnant women
  - Hemoglobin level less than 13.5 g/dL in men and less than 12 g/dL in women
- Coagulation studies if indicated
- Stool sample for occult blood
- Coagulation panel
- Endoscopy or colonoscopy to detect possible gastrointestinal bleeding

---

With acute blood loss, hemoglobin and hematocrit values remain normal until hemodilution occurs. Therefore these are poor early indicators of acute bleeding.

Therapeutic Interventions

- The primary goal of anemia management is to identify the underlying cause.
- If blood loss is acute, measures are aimed at stopping the bleeding. Specific interventions will depend on the source of bleeding.
- Administer supplemental oxygen.
- Anticipate possible need for intravenous volume replacement, type and crossmatching, and blood transfusion.
- Instruct patient to avoid nonsteroidal anti-inflammatory drugs (NSAIDs) and aspirin as these medications may cause or exacerbate gastrointestinal bleeding.
- Arrange outpatient follow up for the patient.

> Anemia in the elderly is common—but it is not normal or harmless. Its causes are multifactorial, with nutritional deficiency accounting for one third of the causes and chronic illness responsible for another third.[1]

Sickle Cell Disease

Sickle cell disease is a congenital hemolytic anemia that occurs primarily, but not exclusively, in those of West African descent. Defective hemoglobin molecules cause RBCs to assume a sickled configuration instead of their usual "jelly doughnut" shape.

An individual with one sickle cell gene possesses the sickle cell trait, but the disease remains clinically inactive. In contrast, a person who inherits two sickle cell genes has sickle cell disease. Early childhood diagnosis and effective treatments have substantially improved the prognosis for individuals with the disease.

Sickled cells carry normal amounts of hemoglobin; however, the cells tend to clump together because of their distinct shape. Clumping increases blood viscosity and can result in capillary obstruction. This is known as a sickle cell crisis (vaso-occlusive crisis). Decreased circulation, edema formation, tissue ischemia, and severe pain ensue. Sickle cell crisis occurs more frequently at night and is associated with a number of precipitants, including:

- Cold ambient temperature
- High altitude
- Infection
- Metabolic or respiratory acidosis
- Stress

If the ischemic state is not corrected, local tissue necrosis soon follows, which can lead to organ dysfunction.

Children generally do not show symptoms of sickle cell anemia until after 4 months of age. Infants and young children may experience hand-foot syndrome (edema secondary to venous stasis). The incidence of ischemic stroke is increasing in children with sickle cell anemia. The disease has a significant psychological influence on patients because of altered body image, frequently missed days of school or work, sexual problems, depression, and fear of a shortened lifespan.

Signs and Symptoms

- Acute, severe pain
  - Acute pain episodes are the single biggest reason for ED visits and hospitalizations in adults with sickle cell disease.[2]
  - Pain described as throbbing, achy, sharp, or dull with sudden onset.[3]
- Weakness due to chronic anemia
- Pallor
- Jaundice resulting from rapid breakdown of RBCs
- Frequent infections resulting from splenic damage

Complications

- Acute chest syndrome
  - Defined as a new pulmonary infiltrate on chest radiograph, fever, cough, worsening anemia, and chest pain
  - Leading cause of morbidity and mortality and a predictor of early death in sickle cell disease[3]
- Chronic hemolytic anemia, transient aplastic crisis
- Frequent infections such as pneumonia, meningitis, and osteomyelitis
- Cholelithiasis and cholecystitis
- Delayed sexual maturation or priapism
- High incidence of spontaneous abortion, perinatal mortality, and maternal mortality
- Renal failure
- Bone disease, particularly infarction leading to avascular necrosis of the femoral head
- High-output cardiac failure
- Autosplenectomy—almost complete disappearance of the spleen because of progressive fibrosis and shrinkage
- Pulmonary embolus
- Cor pulmonale resulting from pulmonary hypertension, a common occurrence in adults
- Chronic skin ulcers
- Jaundice, hepatomegaly, and hepatic infarction
- Blindness resulting from blockage of retinal blood vessels

Diagnostic Procedures

- Elevated reticulocyte count
- Sickled cells on smear
- Leukocytosis
- Thrombocytosis
- Decreased hemoglobin and hematocrit

Therapeutic Interventions

- Pain management is a priority.
  - Many patients report their sickle cell pain management has been inadequate and suboptimal.[2]
  - For mild to moderate pain, use medications such as NSAIDs, acetaminophen (Tylenol), and tramadol (Ultram).
  - For moderately severe to severe pain, use medications such as opioids (codeine, hydrocodone, oxycodone) and ketorolac (Toradol).
- Supplemental oxygen.
- Intravenous rehydration.
- Local application of heat to areas of pain.
- Patients may require blood transfusion if they are significantly anemic.
- Antibiotics if infection is present.
- Maintain warm environment.
- Provide emotional support.

Hemophilia

Hemophilia is a congenital coagulation disorder caused by lack of one of two essential circulating plasma proteins: factor VIII and factor IX. It is an inherited sex-linked (passed from mother to son) disease found primarily in males.

Hemophilia produced by a factor VIII deficiency is referred to as hemophilia A, or classic hemophilia. A majority of patients with hemophilia A produce factor VIII, but it is either entirely nonfunctional or operates below normal capacity. A factor IX deficiency is called hemophilia B, or Christmas disease. Type C, rarely seen in the U.S. population, results from a factor XI deficiency.

Normal clotting is an intricate process that depends on a number of specifically sequenced events:

- Factors VIII, IX, and XI are proteins normally found in the plasma.
- Clotting factors circulate in an inactive form until the clotting cascade, stimulated by a cut or bruise, initiates factor activation.
- Factors in this cascade are activated in a domino-like fashion until fibrinogen becomes fibrin and a clot is formed.
- If any one factor is inactivated or removed from the sequence, proper clot formation will be impeded.

In hemophilia the normal physiological events required for formation of a clot are disrupted by the ineffectiveness of factor VIII, IX, or XI:

- Hemophilia prevents the formation of a firm, fibrin clot; instead, patients with hemophilia have soft, unstable clots. The result is not faster bleeding but rather continuous bleeding.[4]

- Hemophilia severity depends on the extent of factor function in each individual patient.
- Hemophilia is typically diagnosed in infancy but some mild cases go undetected until childhood or adolescence.

Signs and Symptoms

- Bruising with minor injuries
- Prolonged bleeding from cuts, tooth extraction, or surgery
- Bleeding into soft tissues, muscles, or joint capsules
  - Most commonly affected joints are elbow, knee, and ankle
  - Pain and swelling
  - Decreased range of motion
- Paresthesia that progresses to nerve injury following a compressing hematoma
- Epistaxis
- Hematuria (usually not serious)
- Altered mental status, severe headache, and coma if intracranial bleeding is present
- Shock from massive blood loss

Diagnostic Procedures

- In known hemophilia delay diagnostic procedures, including blood work and radiographs, until intravenous factor replacement has been initiated.
- CBC.
- Prothrombin time, platelet count, fibrinogen level—usually normal.[5]
- Decreased levels of factor VIII or factor IX.

> Delay in treatment for the hemophilia patient can result in significant blood loss. Initiate factor VIII replacement immediately, even before obtaining diagnostic procedures.

Therapeutic Interventions

- Replacing the deficient factor with intravenous infusion of factor concentrate is the highest priority.
- Administration of desmopressin acetate (DDAVP) stimulates the release (but not the formation) of factor VIII, making it useful for mild bleeding episodes.
- Immobilize, elevate, and apply ice to affected, painful joints.
- Administer factor replacement before suturing or applying a cast.
- Apply direct pressure for 3 to 5 minutes after venipuncture.
- Consider topical thrombin for nosebleeds.
- Remind patient to avoid NSAIDs and over-the-counter medications that might contain aspirin.

- Listen to the patient and family, most of whom are very knowledgeable concerning their disease and treatment.
- Always consult with the patient's hematologist.

HEMATOLOGIC MALIGNANCIES

Leukemia

Leukemia is a cancer of the blood and blood-forming cells in the bone marrow. It is caused by the malignant proliferation of blasts, the undifferentiated immature white blood cells. Leukemia can be classified according to the type of leukocyte involved and the progression of the disease. See Table 23-1 for a comparison of common types of leukemia.

Risk factors for the development of leukemia have been identified and include the following:
- Previous cancer treatment with either radiation or chemotherapy
- Excessive radiation exposure (occupational or accidental)
- Exposure to certain chemicals such as benzene
- Down syndrome
- Family history of leukemia
- Smoking

Signs and Symptoms

Symptoms are often vague but persistent.
- Fever
- Night sweats
- Fatigue, weakness, and lethargy
- Weight loss
- Bleeding or easy bruising
  - Gum bleeding
  - Epistaxis
  - Petechiae
- Bone or joint pain
- Headache
- Pallor
- Lymphadenopathy
- Hepatomegaly, splenomegaly
- Opportunistic infections

Diagnostic Procedures

- CBC with differential
- Coagulation panel
- Serum chemistries
- Chest computed tomography (CT) or radiograph
- Bone marrow biopsy
- Spinal tap

Therapeutic Interventions

- Definitive diagnosis and initiation of treatment are generally not done in the ED.
- Patient will require care by a hematologist or oncologist; encourage patient to comply with follow-up appointments.
- Definitive therapies may include:
  - Chemotherapy
  - Radiation therapy
  - Stem cell transplant
  - Bone marrow transplant

Lymphoma

Lymphomas are a heterogenous group of malignancies that usually originate in the lymph nodes. They occur more commonly in males and the incidence increases with age.[6] Although the cause of lymphomas is unknown, a viral etiology is possible, particularly with the Epstein-Barr virus and the hepatitis B and C viruses.[6] Lymphomas can be classified

---

TABLE 23-1 FORMS OF LEUKEMIA

TYPE	CELLS AFFECTED	POPULATION AFFECTED
Acute lymphoblastic leukemia (ALL)	Acute leukemia that is aggressive in nature with immature cells multiplying rapidly	• Most common in children • Also called childhood leukemia • Good chance for cure
Acute myelogenous leukemia (AML)	Myeloid cells normally develop into RBCs, WBCs, and platelets	• More common in men • Risk increases with age
Chronic lymphocytic leukemia (CLL)	Certain patients may not require treatment for CLL	• Most common leukemia in adults • Patient generally >55 years of age
Chronic myelogenous leukemia (CML)	Slow-growing cancer that may be found before symptoms are present when the patient has a blood test for other reasons Results from uncontrolled production of immature WBCs called blast cells	• Rare in children • Family history not a risk factor with this cancer

RBC, Red blood cell; *WBC*, white blood cell.

TABLE 23-2	**SIGNS AND SYMPTOMS OF SPECIFIC TRANSPLANTED ORGAN REJECTION**	
KIDNEY	**LIVER**	**HEART**
• Decreased urine output	• Abdominal tenderness	• Shortness of breath
• Shortness of breath	• Jaundice	• Unexplained fatigue, decreased exercise tolerance
• Weight gain or swelling	• Fever	• Fluid retention
• Pain or tenderness over kidney	• Clay-colored stools	• Chest pain
	• Tea-colored urine	• Palpitations

as Hodgkin lymphoma and non-Hodgkin lymphoma (NHL). A patient with a lymphoma may present to the ED with complications related to immunosuppression or obstruction because of enlarged lymph nodes.

Signs and Symptoms

- Painless, swollen lymph nodes (neck, axilla, groin)
- Fatigue, malaise
- Night sweats
- Unexplained weight loss
- Chest pain
- Cough
- Pain in lymph nodes after alcohol consumption and increased sensitivity to alcohol (Hodgkin lymphoma)

Diagnostic Procedures

- CBC, serum electrolytes, platelet count
- Erythrocyte sedimentation rate
- CT and magnetic resonance imaging (MRI) probable
- Positron emission tomography (PET) scan
- Definitive diagnosis by lymph node biopsy and bone marrow aspiration and biopsy

Therapeutic Interventions

- Patient must be referred to oncologist for definitive treatment
- Long-term management may include:
  - Chemotherapy
  - Radiation therapy
  - Bone marrow transplant
  - Stem cell transplant

IMMUNOLOGIC EMERGENCIES

Transplanted Organ Rejection

Organ transplantation is a growing area of treatment for many once-fatal or debilitating clinical conditions. Because of evolving surgical techniques, advanced immunosuppression agents, improved organ preservation, and careful tissue matching, survival after organ transplantation is increasing annually. It is not uncommon for a posttransplant patient

to seek care in the ED because of concerns related to possible infection or drug toxicity resulting from immunosuppression or organ rejection. Because transplant patients are on lifelong immunosuppression drugs, normal inflammatory responses are blunted and symptoms of significant infection may be subtle. Any transplant patient who presents to the ED should be triaged with a minimum priority of "urgent."

Organ rejection may be hyperacute, acute, or chronic. Hyperacute rejection occurs intraoperatively immediately following organ attachment and is not seen in the ED. Acute rejection occurs within the first 6 months following transplant as the body recognizes and responds to foreign tissue. Acute rejection also occurs if the patient stops immunosuppression therapy. A low-grade immunologic response, chronic rejection can occur months to years after the transplant and results in fibrosis and scarring of the transplanted organ.

Signs and Symptoms

- Dysfunction or failure of the transplanted organ
- Pain at the site of transplant
- Flulike symptoms
- Fever
- Pruritus

See Table 23-2 for symptoms related to rejection of specific organs.

Diagnostic Procedures

- CBC, coagulation panel, serum chemistries
- Other blood work specific to the function of the transplanted organ
- Electrocardiogram
- MRI
- Echocardiogram (heart transplant)
- Biopsy of transplanted organ

Therapeutic Interventions

- Consult the patient's transplant center immediately for assistance with patient management.
- Consider infection rather than rejection as a source of the patient's symptoms.

TABLE 23-3 COMMON CLINICAL PROBLEMS IN HIV-POSITIVE PATIENTS

CONDITION SEEN IN ED	CAUSES RELATED TO HIV AND HAART	IMPLICATIONS FOR CARE IN THE ED
Possible adverse effects of antiretroviral medications	Potential complications include: • Hepatotoxicity • Lactic acidosis • Local skin reactions • Pancreatitis	• The incidence of opportunistic infections has decreased in the HIV-positive patient. On the other hand, all antiretroviral medications have the potential for hepatotoxicity.
Cardiovascular disease	• Resulting from increased life expectancy and aging • Protease inhibitors (part of HAART) associated with hyperlipidemia, atherosclerosis, hyperglycemia, and truncal obesity	• Acute coronary syndromes may be present at a younger age. • Management of heart failure is similar to that of patients who are not HIV positive.
Kidney disease	• Kidney disease is now the leading cause of death in HIV-positive patients. • Kidney damage is related to HIV-mediated viral disease or to complications of treatment. • Several protease inhibitors are associated with increased incidence of kidney stones.	• Emergency management of renal failure is similar to that of patients who are not HIV positive.
Neurologic complications	• Incidence of CNS opportunistic infection and CNS lymphoma has decreased in patients on HAART. • Increasing incidence of ischemic and hemorrhagic stroke because of aging of this population and increased atherosclerosis with HAART medications. • HIV itself may be a risk factor for cerebrovascular disease. • Peripheral neuropathies are not uncommon.	• Consider cerebrovascular disease in the HIV-positive patient with altered level of consciousness or focal neurologic changes.
Gastrointestinal and hepatobiliary disease	• Gastrointestinal problems are a common complaint of HIV-positive patients. • Coinfection with hepatitis B and C is a serious complication. • Nearly all medications in HAART are potentially hepatotoxic. • Certain HAART medications are associated with pancreatitis.	• Management of gastrointestinal or hepatobiliary problems is similar to that of patients who are not HIV positive.
Hematologic and oncologic complications	• Anemia, caused by HIV disease and HAART medications, is seen in >50% of HIV-positive patients.* • Incidence of Kaposi sarcoma has decreased because of HAART. • Incidence of Hodgkin lymphoma, anal cancer, and lung cancers has increased.	• Symptomatic anemia may require blood transfusion.
Psychiatric illnesses	• Depression occurs in up to 40% of patients with HIV.* • AIDS dementia complex (ADC) results in a decrease in cognitive functions such as memory, concentration, and reasoning. The patient with ADC may experience personality changes and poor balance.	• Treatment of depression is essential because compliance with HAART is often poor in patients who are depressed. • HAART may delay or prevent ADC and may improve symptoms in those patients already experiencing ADC. • Psychoactive drugs may be needed for acute management.

AIDS, Acquired immune deficiency syndrome; *CNS*, central nervous system; *ED*, emergency department; *HAART*, highly active antiretroviral therapy; *HIV*, human immunodeficiency virus.
*Venkat, A., Plontkowsky, D. M., Cooney, R. R., Srivastava, A. K., Suares, G. A., & Heidelberger, C. P. (2008). Care of the HIV-positive patient in the emergency department in the era of highly active antiretroviral therapy. *Annals of Emergency Medicine, 52*(3), 274–285.

TABLE 23-4 COMMON ONCOLOGIC EMERGENCIES

	OCCURRENCE	PATHOPHYSIOLOGY	CLINICAL FEATURES	THERAPEUTIC INTERVENTIONS
Hypercalcemia of malignancy	• Most common life-threatening metabolic disorder associated with malignancy[a] • Experienced by 10% to 20% of all cancer patients[a,b] • 25% to 35% seen with lung cancer • 30% to 40% seen with breast cancer[a]	• Result of bone destruction by extensive metastatic cells[a,b] • Tumor cells may excrete a parathyroid hormone-like peptide that increases mobilization of bone calcium[a,c] • Factors secreted by the tumor can cause impaired renal clearance and increased tubular resorption of calcium[a]	• Nausea and vomiting leading to dehydration • Thirst and polyuria • Lethargy, confusion • Weakness • Constipation • Elevated serum calcium level	• Fluid replacement • Diuretics may be considered once the patient is rehydrated • Bisphosphonates (pamidronate and zoledronic acid) given intravenously to block bone resorption • Calcitonin, intramuscular or subcutaneous, inhibits bone resorption within a few hours and continues for several weeks • Corticosteroids

Tumor lysis syndrome	• Most commonly occurs with hematologic malignancies such as non-Hodgkin lymphoma[c]	• Acute cell lysis caused by chemotherapy and radiation results in the rapid and massive release of intracellular contents
		• Body's homeostatic mechanisms are overwhelmed and unable to neutralize these products
		• Can lead to multiple organ failure and death
			• Weakness
			• Paralytic ileus
			• Symptoms usually develop 1–5 days after therapy
			• Most life-threatening feature is cardiac arrhythmias
			• Hyperkalemia
			• Hyperuricemia
			• Hyperphosphatemia
			• Hypocalcemia resulting in:
			  • Tetany
			  • Agitation
			  • Acidosis
			• Acute renal failure
				• Hydration or rehydration
				• Treatment of hyperkalemia with glucose, insulin, sodium polystyrene (Kayexalate)
				• Calcium gluconate to treat hypocalcemia
				• Allopurinol to decrease uric acid level
				• Hemodialysis may be required

Spinal cord compression	• Commonly associated with metastasis from breast, lung, prostate, and kidney sites[d]	• Most often because of extradural spread from vertebral metastasis • Compression of vessels or nerves may result in paraplegia and incontinence	• New onset of back pain • Pain may increase in supine position and decrease when upright[b] • Motor weakness • Gait disturbances • Altered bladder and bowel function	• Corticosteroids • Radiation therapy • Possibly emergency chemotherapy • Surgical decompression may be considered

Continued

TABLE 23-4   COMMON ONCOLOGIC EMERGENCIES—cont'd

	OCCURRENCE	PATHOPHYSIOLOGY	CLINICAL FEATURES	THERAPEUTIC INTERVENTIONS
Superior vena cava syndrome	• Lung cancers account for 75% of these cases[a]	• Tumor may compress and obstruct the superior vena cava, resulting in venous congestion of the head, neck, and upper extremities • Increased venous pressure and obstruction decreases blood return to the heart	• Face and neck swelling and discoloration • Edema of upper extremities • Chest pain • Cough, dyspnea • Dysphagia • Jugular venous distension • Conjunctival edema • Altered level of consciousness if cerebral edema is also present	• Radiation therapy • Corticosteroids • Elevate head of bed
Neutropenic fever	• Most common complication of cancer treatment • 50% mortality if untreated[c]	• Chemotherapy destroys neutrophils, leaving the patient vulnerable to infection	• Body temperature greater than 38° C (100.4° F) • Absolute neutrophil count <500/mm^3	• Initiate protective isolation • Obtain blood cultures as needed • Immediate administration of broad-spectrum antibiotics such as ceftazidime and vancomycin[a,b]

[a]Kar, M. (2004). Oncologic emergencies. *Journal, Indian Academy of Clinical Medicine, 4*(1), 32–37.
[b]Krimsky, W. S., Behrens, R. J., & Kerkvliet, G. J. (2002). Oncologic emergencies for the internist. *Cleveland Clinic Journal of Medicine, 69*(3), 209–222.
[c]Higdon, M. L., & Higdon, J. A. (2006). Treatment of oncologic emergencies. *American Family Physician, 74*(11), 1873–1880.
[d]Halfdanarson, T. R., Hogan, W. J., & Moynihan, T. J. (2006). Oncologic emergencies: Diagnosis and treatment. *Mayo Clinic Proceedings, 81*(6), 835–848. doi:10.4065/81.6.835

- Consider reverse isolation to protect the patient.
- Increasing immunosuppressive drugs will be the initial course of treatment for rejection.

Human Immunodeficiency Virus (HIV)

Since the advent of highly active antiretroviral therapy (HAART) in 1995, patients with HIV infection are living longer and presenting to EDs for care of clinical problems unrelated to their HIV status.[7] Prior to the availability of HAART, these patients were generally seen because of infections. Although the possibility of infection should always be considered, HIV-positive patients now commonly seek care for illnesses related to cardiovascular or renal disease, adverse effects of medications, psychiatric problems, or malignancies associated with HIV.[7] Table 23-3 describes common clinical problems in the HIV-positive patient and implications for emergency care. See Chapter 22, Infectious Diseases, for more information.

ONCOLOGIC EMERGENCIES

Cancer patients are at risk for a variety of medical emergencies either as a result of the disease itself or from the effects of the therapeutic modalities used to treat the disease. These emergencies may be metabolic (e.g., hypercalcemia of malignancy, tumor lysis syndrome), neurologic (spinal cord compression), structural (superior vena cava syndrome), or hematologic (neutropenic fever) in nature. As survival from malignancies improves, these emergencies will be encountered more frequently by the emergency nurse. Table 23-4 compares common cancer-associated emergencies.

> New onset of back pain in a cancer patient is a red flag for spinal cord compression.[4]

REFERENCES

1. National Anemia Action Council. (2008, January 7). *Tracking and treating anemia in the elderly patient.* Retrieved from http://www.anemia.org/professionals/feature-articles/content.php?contentid=344
2. Odesina, V., Bellini, S., Leger, R., Bona, R., Delaney, C., Andemariam, B., … Tafas, C. D. (2010). Evidence-based sickle cell pain management in the emergency department. *Advanced Emergency Nursing Journal, 32*(2), 102–111.
3. Pack-Mabien, A., & Haynes, J. (2009). A primary care provider's guide to preventive and acute care management of adults and children with sickle cell disease. *Journal of the American Academy of Nurse Practitioners, 21*(5), 250–257.
4. Laudenbach, L., Jardine, L., & Chin-Yee, I. (2008). *Nursing guidelines for the treatment of hemophilia and other inherited bleeding disorders.* London, ON: London Health Sciences Centre. Retrieved from http://www.lhsc.on.ca/Health_Professionals/Bleeding_Disorders/Nursing_Guidelines.pdf
5. Wulff, K., Zappa, S., & Womack, M. (2003). *Emergency care for patients with hemophilia.* Minneapolis, MN: University of Minnesota. Retrieved from http://www.hemophiliaemergencycare.com/pdf/hp/MinneapolisMN.pdf
6. Lichtman, M. A., Kipps, T. J., Seligsohn, U., Kaushansky, K., & Prchal, J. T. (2010). *Williams hematology* (8th ed.). New York, NY: McGraw-Hill.
7. Venkat, A., Piontkowsky, D. M., Cooney, R. R., Srivastava, A. K., Suares, G. A., & Heidelberger, C. P. (2008). Care of the HIV-positive patient in the emergency department in the era of highly active antiretroviral therapy. *Annals of Emergency Medicine, 52*(3), 274–285.

Stroke

Rita D. Mintmier and Sharon L. Biby

Cerebrovascular disease is the fourth-leading cause of death in the United States and the number one cause of long-term major disability.[1] It is estimated that there are 795,000 stroke incidents in the United States each year, and 1 in 17 deaths is caused by stroke.[1] Of these, 180,000 are recurrent strokes.[1] On average, every 40 seconds someone has a stroke in the United States and every 4 minutes someone dies of a stroke.[1] Because women live longer than men and stroke occurs at older ages, more women than men die of stroke.[2] In addition, stroke is the leading cause of serious, long-term disability and the estimated direct and indirect cost of stroke for 2010 was $73.7 billion.[2]

Strokes are classified as either ischemic or hemorrhagic. Early identification of the type of stroke is critical because appropriate treatment for one classification can be lethal for the other.

Risk factors for stroke include the following:

- Hypertension
- Bacterial endocarditis
- Hyperlipidemia
- Atrial fibrillation
- Prosthetic heart valves
- Diabetes mellitus
- Collagen disorders
- Smoking
- Oral contraceptive use
- Cardiac disease
- Recent neck trauma

INITIAL ASSESSMENT TOOLS

Triage of the patient with a possible stroke must be immediate and accompanied by rapid assessment and intervention. Several prehospital stroke scales are available; the most widely used are the Cincinnati Prehospital Stroke Scale (Table 24-1) and the Los Angeles Prehospital Stroke Screen (Table 24-2). These instruments help identify the patient with a probable stroke and are used by many emergency medical systems (EMS) and emergency departments (EDs) as a quick triage tool. Patients with suspected stroke who present to the ED other than by EMS should be assessed within 10 minutes of arrival. Further assessment should include *immediate* computed tomography (CT).

ISCHEMIC STROKE

Ischemic events account for 80% to 85% of all strokes.[3] These strokes occur when a local thrombus or embolus occludes a cerebral artery. Emboli generally originate in the heart or large arteries following atrial fibrillation, acute myocardial infarction (MI), or surgery. Symptom onset is sudden and, as with acute MI, frequently occurs in the early morning hours.

Signs and Symptoms

- Sudden onset of facial weakness
- Sudden onset of unilateral weakness (involving arm, leg, or both)
- Sudden confusion or trouble speaking (expressive aphasia) or understanding what is being said (receptive aphasia)
- Sudden onset of headache, nausea, and vomiting (most typical of hemorrhagic stroke)
  More subtle deficits may include:
- Dysphagia (difficulty swallowing characterized by a moist voice, drooling, or coughing or frequent throat clearing)
- Sudden visual disturbance (homonymous hemianopsia—loss of vision in the same visual field of both eyes)
- Sudden onset vertigo, ataxia
- Sudden numbness or tingling

TABLE 24-1 CINCINNATI PREHOSPITAL STROKE SCALE

	NORMAL	ABNORMAL*
Facial droop (Have patient smile or show teeth)	Both sides of face move equally	One side of face does not move as well as the other
Arm drift (Ask patient to close eyes and hold both arms straight out for 10 seconds)	Both arms move the same or not at all	One arm does not move or drifts downward
Abnormal speech (Ask patient to say, "You can't teach an old dog new tricks.")	Patient uses correct words without slurring	Patient is unable to speak, uses incorrect words, or slurs words

*Probability of stroke is 72% if any one of these three signs is abnormal.
Data from Jauch, E. C., Cucchiara, B., Adeoye, O., Meurer, W., Brice, J., Chan, Y. Y., … Hazinski, M. F. (2010). Part 11: Adult stroke: 2010 American Heart Association guidelines for cardiopulmonary resuscitation and emergency care. *Circulation, 122,* S818–S828.

TABLE 24-2 LOS ANGELES PREHOSPITAL STROKE SCREEN (LAPSS)

Screening Criteria
Age >45 years
No history of seizure disorder
New onset (past 24 hours) of neurologic symptoms
Patient was ambulatory at baseline (prior to event)
Serum glucose level 60–400

Examination: Look for Obvious Asymmetry

Facial smile or grimace	Normal	Right	Left
Grip	Normal	Right weak	Left weak
		Right no grip	Left no grip
Arm weakness	Normal	Right drifts down	Left drifts down
		Right falls rapidly	Left falls rapidly

Note: Patient may still be experiencing a stroke even if LAPSS criteria are not met.
Data from The Internet Stroke Center. (n.d.). Los Angeles prehospital stroke screen (LAPSS). Retrieved from http://www.strokecenter.org/trials/scales/LAPSS.pdf

Further Assessment and Diagnosis

The emergency department staff must be skilled in recognizing acute stroke to triage and treat patients in a rapid, efficient manner. Communication must be streamlined between EMS and the stroke care team, ensuring that appropriate treatment options based on symptoms and time of symptom onset are available for all patients who present with stroke-like symptoms. To facilitate assessment and diagnosis, five questions need to be explored.

Five basic questions should be answered when a patient presents with stroke-like symptoms:
1. Is this a stroke?
2. When did the symptoms begin?
3. Are airway, breathing, and circulation adequate?
4. Are focal deficits present?
5. What immediate diagnostic procedures are recommended?

Question 1: Is This a Stroke?

Determine whether the following symptoms are the result of a stroke or a stroke mimic:
- Seizures
- Migraine
- Syncope
- Hypoglycemia or hyperglycemia
- Metabolic encephalopathy
- Central nervous system (CNS) tumor
- Other neurologic disease: subdural hematoma, peripheral neuropathy, Bell's palsy, or benign positional vertigo
- Conversion disorder
  Always err on the side of caution and assume that the patient has a true neurologic illness first.

Question 2: When Did the Symptoms Begin?

One of the most challenging parts of the initial assessment is establishing when the symptoms occurred, yet the entire treatment plan hinges on this piece of information. Creative interrogation of the patient, family, EMS personnel, or bystanders is necessary, as is asking the question in several different ways.
- Most witnesses to the event are certain the symptoms occurred when they first were aware of them, so be sure to establish when, *without a doubt*, someone last saw the patient at his or her baseline.

The "last seen normal" time for the patient who woke up with stroke symptoms would not be the time he or she woke up, but rather when he or she was last seen normal before going to bed.

- The Brain Attack Coalition has established goals (Table 24-3) for delivering stroke care for all patients arriving within 6 hours of symptom onset or "last seen normal." If symptoms are present on waking, most likely the patient will be outside the time frame for thrombolytic therapy.

TABLE 24-3	**TIME GOALS FOR STROKE MANAGEMENT**
ED door to physician examination	10 minutes
ED door to CT scan completed	25 minutes
ED door to CT interpretation	45 minutes
ED door to needle (rt-PA started)	60 minutes

CT, Computed tomography; *ED,* emergency department; *rt-PA,* recombinant tissue-type plasminogen activator.
Data from Jauch, E. C., Cucchiara, B., Adeoye, O., Meurer, W., Brice, J., Chan, Y., ... Hazinski, M. F. (2010). 2010 American Heart Association guidelines for cardiopulmonary resuscitation and emergency cardiovascular care science. Part 11: Adult stroke: *Circulation, 122,* S818–S828.

Question 3: Are Airway, Breathing, and Circulation Adequate?

Obtaining a CT scan to determine the type of stroke is a high priority. However, as with all emergency patients, airway, breathing, and circulation (ABC) take top priority. ABC should be rapidly assessed before transporting the patient for CT scan.

- Administer supplemental oxygen for pulse oximetry value less than 94%.
- Measure blood pressure (BP) accurately; make sure the BP cuff is the correct size and check the BP at least twice at 5-minute intervals.
- Obtain a 12-lead electrocardiogram. It is rare to have acute MI concurrently with a stroke, although this can occur. Cardiac enzymes should be part of the initial laboratory studies.

Question 4: Are Focal Deficits Present?

The initial examination is a brief, not full, neurological examination; the Cincinnati Prehospital Stroke Scale is adequate for this brief assessment. If deficits are present and likely associated with stroke, immediately obtain a CT scan of the head.

- For patients who arrive by EMS, this initial neurological examination should be done with the patient still on the EMS stretcher. Do not waste time transferring the patient to a bed, changing monitors, etc.
- For patients presenting to triage, the patient should be placed on a stretcher and have a portable monitor attached, in anticipation of immediate CT scan.
- A mechanism must be in place for having the CT scan read immediately and the results reported to the emergency physician or stroke team as quickly as possible.

Question 5: What Immediate Diagnostic Procedures Are Recommended?

Timing of diagnostic procedures for stroke is controversial. Most stroke centers draw blood for laboratory studies prior

Large left intraparenchymal hematoma

Fig. 24-1 CT scan of intracerebral hemorrhage. (From Moser, D., & Riegel, B. [2007]. *Cardiac nursing: A companion to Brunwald's heart disease* [1st ed.]. Philadelphia, PA: Saunders.)

to the patient going for CT scan since processing the laboratory work is more time consuming than having the CT scan done. Based on the American Heart Association's 2010 guidelines,[2] the following diagnostic procedures should be done:

- Immediate CT scan of the head to rule out hemorrhage and determine course of management
- CT scan completed within 25 minutes and interpreted with 45 minutes of the patient's arrival at the ED.[2] Figure 24-1 shows the CT scan of a patient experiencing a hemorrhagic event.
- Blood glucose
- Serum electrolytes and renal function tests
- 12-lead electrocardiogram
- Cardiac biomarkers
- Complete blood count, including platelet count
- Prothrombin time and international normalized ratio (PT/INR)
- Activated partial thromboplastin time (aPTT)
- Oxygen saturation

Based on the patient's history, other diagnostic procedures that may influence the treatment plan and that may be considered are:

- Hepatic function tests
- Toxicology screen
- Blood alcohol level

TABLE 24-4	COMPONENTS OF THE NATIONAL INSTITUTES OF HEALTH STROKE SCALE (NIHSS)

- Level of consciousness
- Horizontal eye movement
- Visual fields
- Facial palsy
- Arm and leg motor function
- Sensation
- Language and speech
- Neglect and inattention

- Pregnancy test
- Arterial blood gas test (if hypoxia is suspected)
- Chest radiograph
- Lumbar puncture if subarachnoid hemorrhage (SAH) is suspected and CT is negative for blood
- Electroencephalogram (EEG) if seizures are suspected

In-Depth Neurological Examination

The American Stroke Association (ASA) guidelines recommend using a standardized tool for assessing stroke deficits. The most validated tool for determining stroke severity is the National Institutes of Health Stroke Scale (NIHSS). Table 24-4 highlights selected components of the NIHSS. Refer to the ASA website (http://www.strokeassociation.org) or other references to view the complete scale. The ASA website also hosts a free NIHSS tutorial.

Use of the NIHSS ensures a timely examination that is quantifiable, promotes communication with the stroke team, provides information about the probable cause of the neurological deficits, and is essential in determining treatment options for the patient.[1] It is designed to be conducted quickly over 7 minutes. Patients with no deficits and normal mental status will have a score of 0, while scores of 15 to 20 reflect a severe stroke.

Individual institutions may have established protocols for when the NIHSS should be used but most often it is measured at the following times:

- At the time of patient presentation
- Following interventions
- When significant changes in the patient's status occur
- Upon discharge from the ED

Patients with large ischemic and hemorrhagic strokes can decline quickly. The emergency nurse must establish a neurologic baseline and do frequent reassessments for comparison. Close monitoring of vital signs, particularly BP, and neurologic status during imaging studies is also a priority.

Therapeutic Interventions

- The goals of treating the stroke patient are to restore blood flow (arterial recanalization) and to optimize hemodynamics to maintain cerebral perfusion. Minimizing the damage and salvaging the penumbra (area of insulted but viable brain cells around the stroke) are best achieved by maximizing brain perfusion. Establish adequacy of ABCs.
  - Administer supplemental oxygen if oxygen saturation via pulse oximetry is less than 92%.
  - Consider advanced airway as needed.
  - Obtain second intravenous (IV) line with normal saline solution.
- Initiate continuous cardiac monitoring.
- Treat hypoglycemia: do not treat hyperglycemia unless serum glucose is over 185 mg/dL.[4]
- An elevated BP is often noted in the first few hours of a stroke event and is perhaps a stress response. This will often normalize without intervention.
  - If the patient is not eligible for recombinant tissue-type plasminogen activator (rt-PA) administration, do not treat elevated BP unless systolic blood pressure is greater than 220 mm Hg and diastolic blood pressure is greater than 120 mm Hg.
  - See Management of Blood Pressure below.
- Maintain normal body temperature; treat fever greater than 37.5° C (99.5° F).
- Keep patient "nothing by mouth" (NPO) until he or she can be screened for dysphagia.
- Insertion of indwelling urinary catheter is optional but if the patient is a candidate for fibrinolytic therapy, all invasive procedures and tubes (nasogastric, urinary) must be performed or inserted prior to initiating therapy.
- Continuously reassess the patient's neurologic status.
- Initiate venous thromboembolism (VTE) prophylaxis.

> If the patient's neurologic status is spontaneously and rapidly improving to near baseline, fibrinolytic therapy may not be necessary.

Intravenous Thrombolytic Therapy

- Recombinant tissue-type plasminogen activator is the only treatment approved by the U.S. Food and Drug Administration (FDA) for acute ischemic stroke; it is the standard of care and its use does not require written patient consent.
- Once cerebral hemorrhage has been ruled out by CT scan, specific inclusion and exclusion criteria

TABLE 24-5 **INCLUSION AND EXCLUSION CRITERIA FOR TREATING THE PATIENT EXPERIENCING ISCHEMIC STROKE WITH THROMBOLYTIC THERAPY**

INCLUSION CRITERIA	EXCLUSION CRITERIA	RELATIVE EXCLUSION CRITERIA
Stroke resulting from ischemia	Head trauma or previous stroke within previous 3 months	Minor or rapidly improving stroke symptoms
Age ≥18 years	Arterial puncture at noncompressible site in previous 7 days	Major surgery or serious trauma within previous 14 days
Onset of symptoms <3 hours before initiation of treatment	Previous intracranial hemorrhage	Gastrointestinal or urinary tract hemorrhage within previous 21 days
	Current active bleeding	Acute myocardial infarction within previous 3 months
	Presence of bleeding diathesis	Seizure at onset with postictal residual neurological deficits
	• Platelet count <100,000/mm³	
	• INR >1.7	
	• PT >15 seconds	
	Serum glucose <50 mg/dL	
	Elevated blood pressure	
	• Systolic >185 mm Hg	
	• Diastolic >110 mm Hg	

INR, International normalized ratio; *PT,* prothrombin time.
Adapted from Jauch, E. C., Cucchiara, B., Adeoye, O., Meurer, W., Brice, J., Chan, Y. Y., ... Hazinski, M. F. (2010). Part 11: Adult stroke: 2010 American Heart Association guidelines for cardiopulmonary resuscitation and emergency care. *Circulation, 122,* S818–S828.

(Table 24-5) are used to identify the patient as a candidate for thrombolytic therapy.
- Establish a definite time of symptom onset or time "last seen normal." The goal is to begin fibrinolytic reperfusion therapy within 3 hours of onset of symptoms.

> Although it is desirable to know the results of clotting studies prior to giving a thrombolytic, its administration should not be delayed awaiting test results unless one or more of the following is present:
> - There is clinical suspicion of a bleeding abnormality or thrombocytopenia.
> - The patient has received heparin or warfarin.
> - Use of anticoagulants is not known.

- Obtain an accurate patient weight to guide medication dosing.
  - An estimated weight is acceptable as a last resort.
  - Patients weighing over 220 pounds (100 kg) will get the maximum dose; therefore it is not imperative to have an exact weight for these patients.
- Explain the risks and benefits of thrombolytic therapy to the patient and family. The ASA has a reproducible fact sheet available for download at http://www.strokeassociation.org.
- The dose of rt-PA is 0.9 mg/kg.
  - Ten percent of the total dose is given as an IV bolus over 1 minute.
  - The remaining 90% is given as a continuous infusion over 1 hour.

- Following both the bolus and the continuous infusion, the IV line should be cleared with normal saline to ensure that the entire dose has been administered.

> **Caution!**
> - The dosing of recombinant tissue-type plasminogen activator is different for stroke and acute myocardial infarction.
> - Be sure to use the correct dose.
> - Some states require nurses to demonstrate competency prior to administering a thrombolytic.

- Document the following information:
  - Time of onset of stroke symptom or time "last seen normal"
  - NIHSS on admission to the ED
  - If the patient is *not* a candidate for rt-PA, the reason for exclusion
  - Patient's weight
  - Weight-based calculated dose of rt-PA
  - Time rt-PA bolus was started
  - Results of swallow screen if performed in ED
- Provide care for the family of the stroke patient.
  - The flurry of activity surrounding this potentially life-threatening event can be very stressful for the patient and the family. Keep them informed of all procedures and plans.

- Involve a chaplain or other support personnel to communicate with the family.
- Provide a private waiting area if at all possible.
- Assess for complications of thrombolytic therapy:
  - Bleeding
  - Angioedema
  - Anaphylactic reaction
  - Further deterioration in neurologic status
- Though complications are rare, stop the rt-PA infusion should any of these occur and notify the physician.
  - If excessive bleeding or symptomatic intracerebral hemorrhage occur, obtain an immediate type and crossmatch and fibrinogen level.
  - Cryoprecipitate, 10 to 20 units, may be administered. If cryoprecipitate is unavailable, fresh frozen plasma will be used.
- During and following administration of rt-PA:
  - Perform neurologic assessment and obtain vital signs every 15 minutes for the first 2 hours, then every 30 minutes for 4 to 6 hours.
  - The optimal position for the head of the bed has not been determined for stroke patients. Patients with increased intracranial pressure (ICP) or chronic respiratory problems may benefit from elevating the head of the bed to 30 degrees. On the other hand, positioning the head of bed flat can maximize cerebral blood flow in the ischemic stroke.[5]
  - Record an accurate intake and output.
  - For the first 24 hours, do not administer antithrombotics such as aspirin, heparin, clopidogrel, warfarin, or nonsteroidal anti-inflammatory drugs.
- Transfer the patient to the intensive care unit or stroke unit where adequate monitoring can occur. The goal should be to transfer the patient out of the ED within 3 hours of arrival.

Management of Blood Pressure

- Patients with acute ischemic stroke who are not candidates for thrombolytic therapy may require treatment for hypertension.
- Treatment is considered for systolic blood pressure over 220 mm Hg or diastolic blood pressure over 120 mm Hg.[4]
- If treatment for hypertension is indicated, it should be done cautiously, lowering the BP by only 15% to 25% in the first 24 hours.
- Patients who are otherwise eligible for thrombolytic therapy and have a BP over 185/110 mm Hg will require treatment for hypertension to minimize bleeding complications.
  - Labetalol (Trandate) is a first-line agent of choice in stroke because it works quickly, is not too aggressive, and is short acting.

- Administer labetolol, 10 mg intravenously, over 1 to 2 minutes and observe for change in BP.
- Dose may be repeated or increased to 20 mg.
- Nicardipine (Cardene), 2.5 to 5 mg per hour IV infusion, is titrated to desired BP level by increasing the rate by 2.5 mg per hour every 5 minutes to a maximum dose of 15 mg per hour.
  - Once the desired BP is reached, decrease the dose to 3 mg per hour.[4]
  - The response to nicardipine is easily managed and its use does not require an arterial line.
  - The medication should be mixed in normal saline solution.
- Nitroprusside (Nipride) is given as a last resort for BP control in acute stroke.
  - Because nitroprusside causes cerebral vasodilation and increased cerebral blood flow, it should not be used if increased ICP is suspected.
  - Use of nitroprusside requires an arterial line for continuous BP monitoring and administration via a dedicated IV central line.
  - Anticipate rapid drop in BP and monitor closely; reflex tachycardia is a potential side effect.
- To minimize the risk of bleeding, BP must be maintained within approved parameters.
  - Before administration of rt-PA, the goal is a systolic blood pressure less than 185 mm Hg and a diastolic blood pressure less than 110 mm Hg.
  - During and after administration of rt-PA, the target is a systolic blood pressure of 180 mm Hg or less and a diastolic blood pressure of 105 mm Hg or less.

Intra-arterial Thrombolytic Therapy

- Although it is increasing, the use of intra-arterial thrombolysis for ischemic stroke remains controversial.[6]
- Its use may be considered:
  - When the patient misses the 3-hour window for IV thrombolysis
  - As a rescue intervention when IV thrombolysis fails
  - In patients with major stroke resulting from occlusion of the middle cerebral artery[6]

Mechanical Recanalization

The FDA has approved several devices to extract clots from intracranial arteries in acute ischemic stroke. These devices may be used in conjunction with intra-arterial thrombolysis but their efficacy in improving outcomes after stroke is unknown.[7] Patients require transfer to a stroke center with experienced interventional radiologists for this therapy.

TABLE 24-6	HOW TO SCORE THE PATIENT USING ABCD

RISK FACTOR	POINTS
Age ≥60 years	1
Blood pressure	
Systolic BP ≥140 mm Hg *or* Diastolic BP ≥90 mm Hg	1
Clinical features of TIA (choose one)	
Unilateral weakness with or without speech impairment *or*	2
Speech impairment without unilateral weakness	1
Duration of symptoms	
TIA duration ≥60 minutes	2
TIA duration 10–59 minutes	1
Diabetes history	1
Total ABCD^2 score	0–7

BP, Blood pressure; *TIA*, transient ischemic attack.
Data from American Heart Association. (2010). *Heart disease and stroke statistics—2010 update*. Dallas, TX: Author.

TRANSIENT ISCHEMIC ATTACK

In 2009 the definition of transient ischemic attack (TIA) was changed to "brief episodes of neurologic dysfunction resulting from focal cerebral ischemia not associated with permanent cerebral infarction."[8] TIA diagnosis is no longer based on duration or severity of symptoms and imaging is necessary to be certain the patient has not had a stroke.

Transient ischemic attacks are not benign. Numerous studies have demonstrated a high risk of stroke after TIA; 10% to 15% of patients experiencing a TIA have a stroke within 3 months, with half of these occurring within 48 hours.[8] The ABCD^2 assessment tool, illustrated in Table 24-6 and Table 24-7, has been recognized as a means of predicting the patient's risk of having a stroke after a TIA. The score is used to determine which patients should be admitted for a stroke workup and which are safe for follow-up as outpatients.

Many TIA patients will have returned to their baseline by the time they present to the ED. These patients can pose a special challenge for the busy emergency nurse, as they seem to have so few needs.

- It is imperative to know exactly when the patient's symptoms resolved and to "reset" the "last seen normal" clock.
- Neurologic status should be monitored closely since whatever caused the symptoms initially has not yet been identified or treated and the symptoms could reoccur.
- An expedited workup should be the goal and magnetic resonance imaging (MRI) of the brain may be indicated in the ED to rule out stroke.

TABLE 24-7	IMPLICATION OF THE ABCD SCORE

ABCD^2 SCORE	2-DAY STROKE RISK	COMMENT
0–3	1%	Hospital observation may be unnecessary without another indication (e.g., new atrial fibrillation)
4–5	4.1%	Hospital observation justified in most situations
6–7	8.1%	Hospital observation worthwhile

Data from American Heart Association. (2010). *Heart disease and stroke statistics—2010 update*. Dallas, TX: Author.

HEMORRHAGIC STROKE

Stroke symptoms can be the result of intracranial hemorrhage rather than ischemia. The differentiation is important because anticoagulants and fibrinolytic therapy are contraindicated in patients with hemorrhagic stroke.

Classifications of hemorrhagic stroke include the following:

- Intraparenchymal or intracerebral hemorrhage (ICH)
  - Intracerebral hemorrhage accounts for 10% to 15% of first-ever strokes and has a 30-day mortality rate of 35% to 52%; half of the deaths occur in the first 2 days.[9]
  - Infratentorial bleeds carry a higher mortality because of the confined space formed by the tentorium (a fold of the dura mater separating the cerebrum from the cerebellum) and base of the skull. Extra blood in this space often results in herniation.
  - Intracerebral hemorrhage is most often caused by:
    - Hypertension
    - Coagulopathy
    - Anticoagulation
    - Arteriovenous malformation (AVM)
    - Cavernous angioma
    - Illicit drug use
    - Trauma
- Subarachnoid hemorrhage is a cause of stroke, typically as the result of a ruptured cerebral aneurysm.
- Subdural hemorrhage:
  - Trauma is the most common cause of subdural hemorrhage and therefore it is not classified as a stroke.
  - The key piece of history is that symptom onset is gradual as opposed to stroke symptoms, which occur suddenly.

- Epidural hemorrhage is the result of trauma involving the middle meningeal artery between the dura and the skull.
  - Because of higher pressure in the artery, a hematoma can form quickly, causing increased ICP and a high mortality risk.
  - The initial imaging will be definitive in ruling out stroke.

Intracerebral Hemorrhage

Signs and Symptoms

- Patients with ICH can deteriorate quickly; rapid recognition and treatment is essential.
- These patients typically present with sudden onset of focal neurological deficit that progressively worsens.
- Headache.
- Vomiting.
- High blood pressure (often systolic BP >220 mm Hg).
- Decreased level of consciousness, may rapidly progress to coma.
- A standardized tool should be used to assess the patient. The NIHSS has been validated for ischemic stroke only. The Glasgow Coma Scale (GCS) may be more helpful in quantifying neurological deficits in the setting of ICH. See Chapter 36, Head Trauma, for further discussion of the Glasgow Coma Scale.

> Rapid and early deterioration of neurologic status is common in the first few hours following intracerebral hemorrhage.

Diagnostic Procedures

- As with ischemic stroke, after ABCs are assessed and managed, imaging with CT and MRI should be the first priority for a patient with sudden neurological deficits.
- Noncontrast CT is the quickest form of imaging and is very revealing for hemorrhage. It will reveal size and location of the ICH and conditions such as mass effect and obstruction of cerebrospinal fluid with resulting hydrocephalus.

Therapeutic Interventions

- As with ischemic stroke, the ABCs are the first priority.
- Blood pressure management parameters currently are based on incomplete evidence, with clinical trials ongoing. See Table 24-8 for recommended guidelines for treating elevated BP in hemorrhagic stroke.[9]
- Goals for blood pressure management should be to perfuse the brain adequately without increasing the risk for expansion of the hemorrhage.
  - Targets should be adjusted after considering age, ICP, and chronic hypertension.

TABLE 24-8	**RECOMMENDED GUIDELINES FOR TREATING ELEVATED BLOOD PRESSURE IN SPONTANEOUS INTRACEREBRAL HEMORRHAGE**

1. If SBP is >200 mm Hg or MAP is >150 mm Hg, consider aggressive reduction of blood pressure with continuous intravenous infusion, with frequent blood pressure monitoring every 5 minutes.
2. If SBP is >180 mm Hg or MAP is >130 mm Hg and there is evidence or suspicion of elevated ICP, consider monitoring ICP and reducing blood pressure using intermittent or continuous intravenous medications to keep cerebral perfusion pressure >60 to 80 mm Hg.
3. If SBP is >180 mm Hg or MAP is >130 mm Hg and there is no evidence or suspicion of elevated ICP, consider a modest reduction of blood pressure (e.g., MAP of 110 mm Hg or target blood pressure of 160/90 mm Hg) using intermittent or continuous intravenous medications to control blood pressure and clinically reexamine the patient every 15 minutes.

ICP, intracranial pressure; *MAP*, mean arterial pressure; *SBP*, systolic blood pressure.
Data from Morgenstern, L. B., Hemphill, J. C., Anderson, C., Becker, K., Broderick, J. P., Connolly, E. S., ... Tamargo, R. J. (2010). Guidelines for the management of spontaneous intracerebral hemorrhage: A guideline for healthcare professionals from the American Heart Association/American Stroke Association. *Stroke, 41*, 2108–2129.

- Lowering the BP too quickly can result in diminished perfusion and worsening of neurological deficits.
- Antiepileptic therapy is indicated for the treatment of clinical seizures in patients with ICH; prophylactic anticonvulsant medication is not recommended.[9]
- Antipyretics should be used to maintain normothermia.
- Treat increased ICP by raising the head of the bed to 30 degrees and administering analgesia and sedation.
- More aggressive ICP treatment may include osmotic diuretics and hypertonic saline, drainage of cerebrospinal fluid via ventricular drainage system, and neuromuscular blockade. Avoid hyperventilation except in cases when herniation is imminent.
- Keep serum glucose below 140 mm Hg; avoid hypoglycemia.
- Venous thromboembolism prophylaxis should be initiated with intermittent pneumatic compression device and elastic hose.
- As many as 14% of patients with ICH are currently on oral anticoagulants; the patient's international

normalized ratio (INR) needs to be corrected as rapidly as possible using[9]:
- Vitamin K infusion
- Prothrombin complex concentrates
- Fresh frozen plasma
- Monitoring in an intensive care unit is indicated for these patients since deterioration is likely and close monitoring will be required.
- Surgical treatment may be indicated in select patients and will require transfer to a tertiary care facility.

How Aggressive Should Care Be for the ICH Patient?

Determination or prediction of patient outcomes within the first 24 hours after onset of ICH is very difficult and can be inaccurate. Though circumstances may vary and every patient's situation is different, full aggressive care should be provided to the ICH patient in the emergency department. Do Not Resuscitate orders are inappropriate during this time unless they are already in place for other reasons. Most of these deaths are because of removal of life supports.[9]

Subarachnoid Hemorrhage

About 3% of all strokes are spontaneous subarachnoid hemorrhage (SAH) and these account for 5% of stroke deaths.[10] SAH carries a high rate of disability and mortality, with approximately 50% of these patients not surviving the initial injury.[10]

Cerebral aneurysms are the leading cause of nontraumatic SAH. Risk factors for aneurysmal SAH include:
- Family history of SAH
- Hypertension
- Cigarette smoking
- Female gender
- Increasing age
- Alcohol abuse
- Use of stimulants such as cocaine and amphetamines[8]
- Connective tissue disorders such as Marfan syndrome, sickle cell disease, and polycystic kidney disease[10]

Signs and Symptoms
- Sudden intense, unrelenting headache
  - Often described as the "worst headache of my life."
  - In patients with history of headache, this headache is "different" and more severe.
- Altered level of consciousness
  - The NIHSS has not been validated for use with SAH. If a hemorrhagic stroke is identified by CT scan, the GCS is helpful in quantifying level of consciousness.
- Vomiting or nausea
- Photophobia (intolerance to light)

- Nuchal rigidity
- Focal deficits, possibly including hemiparesis
- Prodromal signs may be present 10 to 20 days before rupture[10]
  - Headache
  - Dizziness
  - Diplopia
  - Vision loss

Diagnostic Procedures
- CT without contrast is the first line of imaging
- Lumbar puncture if the CT is negative but SAH is suspected
- Cerebral angiogram to visualize vascular anatomy
- Computed tomography angiogram (CTA) as a noninvasive method to visualize the vasculature

Prognostic Scales for Subarachnoid Hemorrhage

Treatment options are determined by the patient's age and medical condition, size and location of the aneurysm, presence of a clot, and the patient's wishes.[10] In addition, several prognostic scales can be used in making decisions for treating the patient with SAH.
- Hunt and Hess scale uses the patient's presenting symptoms as a predictor of outcomes, with higher scores correlating with higher mortality (Table 24-9).
- The World Federation of Neurological Surgeons classification is based on the Glasgow Coma Scale and findings of aphasia and motor deficits (Table 24-10). Patients with a score of 8 or above have a good chance for recovery; scores of 3 to 5 indicate that the SAH is potentially fatal.

Therapeutic Interventions
- Airway and oxygenation are high priorities because of the patient's decreased level of consciousness and risk of aspiration.
- Initial treatment is focused on preventing rebleeding of the aneurysm.

TABLE 24-9	HUNT AND HESS CLASSIFICATION SCALE
Grade 1	Asymptomatic, mild headache, slight nuchal rigidity
Grade 2	Moderate to severe headache, nuchal rigidity, no neurologic deficit other than cranial nerve palsy
Grade 3	Drowsiness, confusion, mild focal neurologic deficit
Grade 4	Stupor, moderate to severe hemiparesis
Grade 5	Coma, decerebrate posturing

TABLE 24-10	**WORLD FEDERATION OF NEUROLGOICAL SURGEONS SUBARACHNOID HEMORRHAGE GRADING SCALE**	
GRADE	**GLASGOW COMA SCALE SCORE**	**MOTOR DEFICIT**
I	15	Absent
I	14–13	Absent
III	14–13	Present
IV	12–7	Present or Absent
V	6–3	Present or Absent

- Maintain systolic BP of 90 to 140 mm Hg.
- Administer analgesics as needed for pain.
- Short-acting sedatives may be required for agitated patients.
- Perform frequent complete neurologic assessments to detect deterioration.
- Maintain body temperature at less than 37.5° C (99.5° F).
- Keep patient NPO until he or she has passed a bedside swallow test.
- Initiate VTE prophylaxis with elastic stockings or pneumatic compression devices; do not give anticoagulants.
- Admit patient to intensive care unit.
- Patient may require ICP monitoring with a ventricular catheter or subarachnoid screw.

Lowering of an elevated BP should be carefully controlled since a sudden drop may lead to cerebral ischemia.

The patient may be a candidate for surgical clipping or endovascular coiling of the aneurysm; anticipate transfer to a tertiary care center.

REFERENCES

1. Lloyd-Jones, D., Adams, R., Carnethon, M., De Simone, G., Ferguson, T. B., Flegal, K., ... Hong, Y. (2009). Heart disease and stroke statistics—2009 update: A report from the American Heart Association Statistics Committee. *Circulation*, 119(3), e21–e181.
2. American Heart Association. (2010). *Heart disease and stroke statistics—2010 update*. Dallas, TX: Author.
3. Field, J. M. (Ed.). (2008). *ACLS resource text for instructors and experienced providers*. Dallas, TX: American Heart Association.
4. Jauch, E. C., Cucchiara, B., Adeoye, O., Meurer, W., Brice, J., Chan, Y. Y., ... Hazinski, M. F. (2010). Part 11: Adult stroke: 2010 American Heart Association guidelines for cardiopulmonary resuscitation and emergency care. *Circulation*, 122, S818–S828.
5. Summers, D., Leonard, A., Wentworth, D., Saver, J. L., Simpson, J., Spilker, J. A., ... Mitchell, P. H. (2009). Comprehensive overview of nursing and interdisciplinary care of the acute ischemic stroke patient: A scientific statement from the American Heart Association. *Stroke*, 40, 2911–2944.
6. Meyers, P. M., Schumacher, H. C., Higashida, R. T., Barnwell, S. L., Creager, M. A., Gupta, R., ... Wechsler, L. R. (2009). Indications for the performance of intracranial endovascular neurointerventional procedures: A scientific statement from the American Heart Association Council on Cardiovascular Radiology and Intervention; Stroke Council, Council on Cardiovascular Surgery and Anesthesia, Interdisciplinary Council on Peripheral Vascular Disease, and Interdisciplinary Council on Quality of Care and Outcomes Research. *Circulation*, 119, 2235–2249.
7. Molina, C. A. (2010). Reperfusion therapies for ischemic stroke: Current pharmacological and mechanical approaches. *Stroke*, 42(1), 2108–2129.
8. Easton, J. D., Saver, J. L., Albers, G. W., Alberts, M. J., Chaturvedi, S., Feldmann, E., ... Sacco, R. L. (2009). Definition and evaluation of transient ischemic attack: A scientific statement for healthcare professionals from the American Heart Association/ American Stroke Council; Council on Cardiovascular Surgery and Anesthesia; Council of Cardiovascular Radiology and Intervention; Council on Cardiovascular Nursing; and the Interdisciplinary Council on Peripheral Vascular Disease. *Stroke*, 40(6), 2276–2293.
9. Morgenstern, L. B., Hemphill, J. C., Anderson, C., Becker, K., Broderick, J. P., Connolly, E. S., ... Tamargo, R. J. (2010). Guidelines for the management of spontaneous intracerebral hemorrhage: A guideline for healthcare professionals from the American Heart Association/American Stroke Association. *Stroke*, 41, 2108–2129.
10. Alexander, S., Gallek, M., Presciutti, M., & Zrelak, P. (2009). *Care of the patient with aneurysmal subarachnoid hemorrhage*. Glenview, IL: American Association of Neuroscience Nurses. Retrieved from http://www.aann.org/pdf/cpg/aannaneurysmalsah.pdf

Neurologic Emergencies

Robin Walsh

The function of the nervous system is to control all motor, sensory, autonomic, cognitive, and behavioral activities. A wide variety of neurologic disorders can bring a patient to the emergency department (ED). Neurologic disorders involve some portion of the nervous system, which includes the central nervous system, the peripheral nervous system, and the autonomic nervous system. These disorders may result from infections, physiologic derangements, or trauma. Severity ranges from minor discomfort to life-threatening conditions requiring emergent medical or surgical intervention. Regardless, the normal function of the nervous system has been altered. As with any focused assessment, airway, breathing, and circulation should be assessed and appropriate interventions implemented prior to the focused neurologic assessment.

NEUROLOGIC ASSESSMENT

For the emergency nurse, a comprehensive neurologic assessment may include but is not limited to the following:
- General appearance and affect
- Level of consciousness
- Responsiveness
- Pupil assessment
- Mental status exam
- Cranial nerve assessment

Some of these are discussed in more detail below.

Level of Consciousness

Level of consciousness is the earliest and most reliable indicator of a change in a patient's neurologic status and exists on a continuum from lethargy to violent and mild confusion to coma.

Level of consciousness has two components: arousal (wakefulness) and awareness.
- Arousal is controlled by the brainstem and is the most fundamental part of level of consciousness.
- Awareness is assessed by orientation, memory, calculation, and foundation of knowledge.

Level of consciousness is affected by structural abnormalities, metabolic imbalances, medications, and injury. A thorough assessment is required to intervene in potentially lethal situations. Use the AEIOU–TIPS mnemonic for a list of common conditions that can lead to an alteration in a patient's level of consciousness.

Frequent causes of altered mental status include:
- Hypoglycemia: Perform a bedside glucose test and administer glucose, if needed.
- Hypoxia: Check pulse oximetry and administer oxygen, if needed.

AEIOU-TIPS for Assessment of the Patient with Altered Level of Consciousness:
- A—Alcohol (acute intoxication, withdrawal)
- E—Epilepsy (or any seizure), environmental conditions (hypothermia, heatstroke)
- I—Insulin (too much or too little)
- O—Oxygen (underdose or overdose)
- U—Uremia (or other metabolic disorders)
- T—Trauma, toxicity, tumors, thermoregulation
- I—Infection, ischemia
- P—Psychiatric, poisoning
- S—Stroke, syncope (or other neurologic or cardiovascular cause)

TABLE 25-1 GLASGOW COMA SCALE

CATEGORY	SCORE	RESPONSE
Eye opening	4	Spontaneous: eyes open spontaneously without stimulation
	3	To speech: eyes open with verbal stimulation but not necessarily to command
	2	To pain: eyes open with noxious stimuli
	1	None: no eye opening regardless of stimulation
Verbal response	5	Oriented: accurate information about person, place, time, reason for hospitalization, and personal data
	4	Confused: answers not appropriate to question but use of language is correct
	3	Inappropriate words: disorganized, random speech, no sustained conversation
	2	Incomprehensible sounds: moans, groans, and incomprehensible mumbles
	1	None: no verbalization despite stimulation
Best motor response	6	Obeys commands: performs simple tasks on command; able to repeat performance
	5	Localizes to pain: organized attempt to localize to remove painful stimuli
	4	Withdraws from pain: withdraws extremity from source of painful stimuli
	3	Abnormal flexion: decorticate posturing spontaneously or in response to noxious stimuli
	2	Extension: decerebrate posturing spontaneously or in response to noxious stimuli
	1	None: no response to noxious stimuli; flaccid

Data from Urden, L. D., Stacy, K. M., & Lough, M. E. (2010). *Critical care nursing: Diagnosis and management* (6th ed.). St. Louis, MO: Mosby.

Responsiveness

There are tools to help provide objectiveness in assessing a patient's level of consciousness. A tool familiar to most health care providers is the Glasgow Coma Scale (GCS) (Table 25-1). Possible GCS scores range from 15 (best) to 3 (worst). A patient with a GCS score of 8 or less is considered severely altered (comatose). A score of 9 to 12 indicates moderate abnormality; those who score 13 to 15 are considered only mildly altered.[1]

Another tool in assessing level of consciousness is the Full Outline of UnResponsiveness (FOUR) score of neurologic assessment.[2,3] FOUR score (Table 25-2) was developed by neurologists at the Mayo Clinic as an alternative to the GCS in assessing and monitoring patients. Some practitioners believe that it is easier to use and provides more detailed information about the patient's level of consciousness. FOUR score assesses eye, motor, brainstem, and respiratory function and assigns a score of 0 to 4 in each category. The lower the score, the more serious the patient's condition. FOUR score does not assess a patient's verbal abilities.

> Neurologic assessments should be trended to monitor for deterioration and for response to interventions.

Mental Status Exam

The most commonly used tool to assess cognitive function is the Mini-Mental State Examination (MMSE). Cognitive testing is focused on evaluating memory, ability to calculate, language, visuospatial skills, and degrees of alertness. It does not assess mood or thought processes and patients with mild dementia may be able to compensate.

> **Components of the Mini-Mental State Examination**
> - Orientation (order in which orientation is lost: time, then place, and finally person).
> - Registration and memory: Name three unrelated items to the patient and ask him or her to state them back.
> - Foundation of knowledge: Ask the patient what is on the national news.
> - Attention span and calculation: For example, have the patient subtract backwards by 7 from 100.
> - Naming: Show the patient an object and have him or her name it.
> - Repetition: Have the patient repeat a statement.
> - Comprehension: Give the patient simple directions to follow and see if he or she is able to follow the directions.
> - Reading: Tell the patient to read a directive statement and then do what the statement says. For example, "Raise your hand."
> - Writing.
> - Drawing.

Cranial Nerve Assessment

Table 25-3 lists the cranial nerves and their functions. See Chapter 36, Head Trauma, for more information.

TABLE 25-2 FULL OUTLINE OF UNRESPONSIVENESS SCORE

EYE RESPONSE	MOTOR RESPONSE	BRAINSTEM REFLEXES	RESPIRATION
4 = eyelids open or opened, tracking, or blinking to command	4 = thumbs-up, fist, or peace sign	4 = pupil and corneal reflexes present	4 = not intubated, regular breathing pattern
3 = eyelids open but not tracking	3 = localizing to pain	3 = one pupil wide and fixed	3 = not intubated, Cheynes-Stokes breathing pattern
2 = eyelids closed but open to loud voice	2 = flexion response to pain	2 = pupil or corneal reflexes absent	2 = not intubated, irregular breathing
1 = eyelids closed but open to pain	1 = extension response to pain	1 = pupil and corneal reflexes absent	1 = breathes above ventilator rate
0 = eyelids remain closed with pain	0 = no response to pain or generalized myoclonus status	0 = absent pupil, corneal, and cough reflex	0 = breathes at ventilator rate or apnea

Data from Wijdicks, E. F., Bamlet, W. R., Maramattom, B. V., Manno, E. M., & McClelland, R. L. (2006). Validation of a new coma scale: The FOUR score. *Annals of Neurology, 58*(4), 585–593.

TABLE 25-3 CRANIAL NERVES AND THEIR FUNCTION

NUMBER	NAME	FUNCTION
I	Olfactory	Smell
II	Optic	Vision
III	Oculomotor	Elevate upper lid, papillary constriction, most extraocular movements
IV	Trochlear	Downward, inward movement of the eye
V	Trigeminal	Chewing, clenching of the jaw, lateral jaw movement, corneal reflexes, face sensation
VI	Abducens	Lateral eye deviation
VII	Facial	Facial motor, taste, lacrimation, salivation
VIII	Vestibulocochlear	Equilibrium, hearing
IX	Glossopharyngeal	Swallowing, gag reflex, taste on posterior tongue
X	Vagus	Swallowing, gag reflex, abdominal viscera, phonation
XI	Spinal accessory	Head and shoulder movement
XII	Hypoglossal	Tongue movement

TABLE 25-4 DIFFERENTIAL DIAGNOSIS FOR COMA

CATEGORY	DIFFERENTIAL DIAGNOSIS
Structural	Abscess, aneurysm, hematoma, hemorrhage, inflammation (i.e., meningitis, encephalitis), subarachnoid hemorrhage, stroke, trauma, tumor
Metabolic	Cardiopulmonary arrest, decreased cardiac output, elevated serum ammonia, fluid or electrolyte imbalance, hepatitis, hepatic dysfunction, hypoglycemia, hypothermia, hypothyroidism, seizure, vitamin deficiencies
Toxicity	Alcohol, anticholinergics, benzodiazepines, carbon monoxide, cyanide, opiates, salicylates, sedatives, tricyclic antidepressants, gamma hydroxybutyrate (GHB)
Psychiatric	Hysteria, malignant catatonia, psychogenic unresponsiveness

SELECTED EMERGENCIES

Unconsciousness

Unconsciousness is defined as a lack of awareness of self or of anything surrounding oneself, despite application of various stimuli. Assessment of the patient who is unconscious or who has an altered level of consciousness must be done concurrently with emergent interventions for airway, breathing, and circulation. Causes of unconsciousness can be categorized as structural, metabolic, toxic, or psychiatric (Table 25-4).

Therapeutic Interventions

Therapeutic interventions for altered level of consciousness include the following:

- Support the patient's airway, breathing, and circulation.
  - Administer supplemental oxygen and titrate to oxygen saturation levels. Anticipate endotracheal

intubation if the patient is unable to maintain adequate oxygenation or ventilation.
- Patients with a GCS score of 8 or less generally require endotracheal intubation for airway protection regardless of their ability to oxygenate and ventilate.
- Protect the patient from further deterioration.
- Identify and treat the underlying cause.
  - Evaluate serial vital signs for indications of shock or hypothermia.
  - Measure blood glucose to identify hypoglycemia.
    - Administer 25 to 50 mL of dextrose 50% (D_{50}) intravenously if the adult patient is hypoglycemic.
    - Give thiamine 50 to 100 mg intravenously before D_{50} infusion if alcohol abuse is suspected to prevent the development of Wernicke-Korsakoff syndrome.
  - Obtain serum electrolyte levels, a complete blood count, a 12-lead electrocardiogram, toxicology screens, a urinalysis, and chest radiographs, as indicated by the patient's history and condition.
  - Administer naloxone (Narcan) 0.4 to 2 mg intravenously to patients with suspected opiate toxicity.
  - Consider flumazenil (Romazicon) administration 0.1 to 0.2 mg intravenously for patients with suspected benzodiazepine toxicity.
  - Immobilize the spine and obtain spinal radiographs if trauma is suspected.
  - Facilitate a computed tomography scan of the head if focal neurologic findings or signs of trauma are present.
- Perform and document serial neurologic examination score and pupillary evaluations.

Wernicke-Korsakoff Syndrome[4]

Wernicke encephalopathy and Korsakoff syndrome are different conditions that both result from brain damage caused by a lack of vitamin B_1, which is common in people with alcoholism. It is also common in persons whose bodies do not absorb food properly, as sometimes occurs following bariatric surgery. Korsakoff syndrome, or Korsakoff psychosis, tends to develop as Wernicke symptoms go away. Wernicke encephalopathy causes brain damage in lower parts of the brain called the thalamus and hypothalamus. Korsakoff psychosis results from damage to areas of the brain involved in memory.

Seizures

A seizure is an episode of abnormal electrical activity in the brain. Like a headache, a seizure is a symptom rather than a disease. The three most common seizure categories are generalized, focal, and status epilepticus. Seizure frequency is slightly higher in males than in females, with a peak incidence in those over the age of 65 years.[5] Seizures may result in physiologic abnormalities including hypoxia and apnea, transient hyperthermia, hypoglycemia, and acidosis.

Critical information related to seizure assessment includes the following:
- Events immediately before the seizure
- History of recent or past head trauma
- Drugs or other substances the patient has consumed—including over-the-counter, recreational, and herbal agents—or failed to take (e.g., missed prescribed medications)

Seizure Types

Generalized Tonic-Clonic. Tonic-clonic seizures, formerly referred to as grand mal seizures, involve a sudden loss of consciousness and organized muscle tone, accompanied by extensor muscle spasms, apnea or irregular respirations, and bilateral clonic movements. Once the seizure ends, the patient fades into a postictal state characterized by muscle relaxation, deep breathing, and depressed level of consciousness.

Febrile Seizures. Febrile seizures are a type of tonic-clonic seizure. They occur as a single seizure, without focal features. Febrile seizures, triggered by a rapid rise in body temperature, typically last less than 15 minutes. Treatment is directed at protecting the patient from injury, lowering the fever, and managing any underlying infectious conditions.

Partial Seizures. Clinical manifestations of a partial (focal) seizure may be sensory, motor, or autonomic. Obsolete names for this type of seizure include Jacksonian, psychomotor, and minor motor. Focal brain lesions such as tumors, abscesses, infarctions, or scars cause partial seizures. Seizure activity is usually unilateral, does not produce loss of consciousness, and is not considered life threatening. Single seizures, lasting less than 5 minutes, rarely require pharmacologic therapy. Medications for long-term control of partial seizures include carbamazepine (Tegretol), phenytoin (Dilantin), gabapentin (Neurontin), and sodium valproate (Depakene). Lamotrigine (Lamictal) and levetiracetam (Keppra) may also be considered.

Seizure Management

Emergency department management of the patient who is having a seizure (or presents following a recent seizure) focuses on:
- Assessment of airway, breathing, and circulatory status
- Immediate control of any current seizure activity
- Investigation of possible causes

Therapeutic Interventions

Therapeutic interventions for seizures (beyond altered level of consciousness measures) include the following:

- Administer oxygen as needed to maintain saturation.
- Maintain airway, breathing, and circulation.
- Safeguard the patient from injury.[6]
  - Turn patient on side and suction oropharynx as needed
  - Protect the head
  - Side rails up at all times
  - Pad side rails with blankets
- Most seizures spontaneously resolve. Administer benzodiazepines (e.g., diazepam [Valium], lorazepam [Ativan]) intravenously to control unresolved seizure activity, as ordered. Intravenously administer anticonvulsants, such as phenytoin (Dilantin) or phenobarbital, once seizures have been controlled, as ordered.
- Obtain and send therapeutic drug level samples for any anticonvulsant agents that may have been prescribed for the patient.
- Consider administering intravenous fosphenytoin (Cerebyx) for short-term control of generalized convulsive status epilepticus.
  - Monitor the patient's electrocardiogram, blood pressure, and respirations continually during infusion and for 10 to 20 minutes after the infusion is complete.

> Never force any object into the patient's mouth while he or she is actively seizing.

Documentation

Document the details of seizure activity, including but not limited to:

- Body parts involved
- Progression
- Duration
- Continent or incontinent of bowel and bladder
- Patient injury during seizure

Monitor the patient's postictal period and continue to document the patient's condition, including vital signs, level of consciousness, and response to interventions. If possible, discuss with the patient or family the patient's typical seizure activity, presence of an aura, and postictal recovery.

> The COLD mnemonic can be used.[7]
> - C—Character (What type of seizure activity occurred?)
> - O—Onset (When did it start? What was the patient doing?)
> - L—Location (Where did the activity start?)
> - D—Duration (How long did it last?)

Discharge Instructions

- Take seizure medications as directed.
- Try to avoid triggers, which include stress, fatigue, hypoglycemia, alcohol, excessive caffeine, and illegal drugs.
- Make sure the home is safe to prevent injuries.
- Wear a medical alert or identification bracelet.
- Do not drive until cleared by the primary care provider and check with the state Department of Motor Vehicles regarding driving restrictions.
- Include family and friends in learning more about seizures and what to do during a seizure.

Status Epilepticus

The patient in status epilepticus experiences a series of consecutive seizures (without normal mentation between) or one continuous seizure lasting more than 5 minutes that does not resolve spontaneously and is unresponsive to traditional treatment. This situation is a medical emergency that requires immediate intervention. The resulting acidosis, hypoglycemia, hypercalcemia, muscle damage, and autonomic dysfunction are associated with significant morbidity and mortality.

Therapeutic Interventions. Therapeutic interventions for status epilepticus (beyond altered level of consciousness interventions) include the following:

- Open and clear the airway.
  - Administer oxygen as needed to maintain saturation. Consider endotracheal intubation if the seizure is prolonged. Rapid sequence intubation (RSI) should be considered. If using RSI, short-acting paralytics should be used to ensure that ongoing seizure activity is not masked.
- Establish intravenous (IV) or intraosseous (IO) access.
- Identify and treat the cause as soon as possible.
  - Administer IV naloxone (Narcan) 0.4 to 2 mg if narcotic toxicity is a potential cause.
  - Infuse D_{50}, 25 to 50 mL if the patient is hypoglycemic. First give thiamine 50 to 100 mg intravenously to alcoholic patients.
- Initiate anticonvulsant therapy.
  - Benzodiazepines (i.e., diazepam [Valium], lorazepam [Ativan], midazolam [Versed]) either intravenously, IO, or per rectum until seizures are controlled.
  - Fosphenytoin sodium (Cerebyx) 20 mg phenytoin equivalents (PE)/kg intravenously infused at 100 to 150 mg PE/min. Unlike phenytoin, fosphenytoin may be diluted in 5% dextrose in water or normal saline. Orders for fosphenytoin must always be written in PE units. Cardiac monitoring and observation for hypotension are essential. Fosphenytoin may be given intramuscularly.

TABLE 25-5	CHARACTERISTICS OF VARIOUS TYPES OF PRIMARY HEADACHES			
HEADACHE	**PATIENT POPULATION**	**FAMILY HISTORY**	**AURA**	**QUALITY (PAIN) LOCATION**
Migraine without aura	Onset age: 6–25 years Female-to-male 3:1, but 1:1 at extremes of age	Positive	No	Begins as unilateral or bilateral dull penetrating pain that progresses to moderate or severe throbbing pain
Migraine with aura	Onset age: 6–25 years Female-to-male 3:1, but 1:1 at extremes of age	Positive	Yes	Throbbing unilateral pain
Migraine	Any age or gender	Positive	No	Dull, diffuse bilateral squeezing, nonthrobbing and not exacerbated by routine activity
Cluster	Age 20–40 Male-to-female 9:1	Occasionally positive	Uncommon	Boring unilateral, especially orbit, severe boring tearing like a "hot poker in the eye"
Subarachnoid hemorrhage	80% of patients are aged 40–65 years	Positive	No	Throbbing variable, severe; patient says it is "the worst headache of my life"
Chronic paroxysmal hemicranias	Average age of onset: 33 years Female-to-male 2:1	Absent	No	Severe, sharp, boring, throbbing, unilateral orbital, supraorbital, or temporal pain always the same side

Data from Martin, C. O. (2001). Neurology. In M. A. Graber & M. L. Laternier (Eds.), *University of Iowa family practice handbook* (4th ed.). Iowa City, IA: University of Iowa. Retrieved from http://web.archive.org/web/20040402145750/www.vh.org/adult/provider/familymedicine/FPHandbook/09.html

- Phenytoin (Dilantin) 18 to 20 mg/kg intravenously. Do not inject intramuscularly. Always mix and infuse phenytoin with normal saline, *not* a dextrose-containing solution. Place the patient on a cardiac monitor and give the drug slowly; do not exceed an infusion rate of 50 mg/min.
- Phenobarbital 130 mg intravenously every 10 to 15 minutes up to 1 gram, as needed (adult dose).
- Consider general anesthesia if status epilepticus does not respond to any of these medications.
- Paralytic agents may be given but will only stop muscle activity; they do nothing to control brain activity, so seizures will continue despite the lack of external evidence.

> Dilantin for elderly patients should be infused at a rate of 25 mg/min or less.

Headache

Among the United States population, 70% report having had a headache and 5% have seen a physician for one.[8] Even 35% of children have reported infrequent headaches by age 7.[8] Headache is not a diagnosis per se but rather a symptom of some underlying disorder. The most common are tension and vascular etiologies. Table 25-5 summaries the characteristics of various headache types.[6]

Tension Headache

Tension headaches usually occur in times of physical or emotional stress. Tension headache pain is described as dull, tight, or constricting. Pain is typically nonpulsating and bilateral and is located in the frontal or occipital regions. Interventions focus on identifying and treating the casual factors. Tension headaches usually respond to mild analgesics such as nonsteroidal anti-inflammatory agents. Severe tension headaches may be indistinguishable from migraines and stronger drugs are necessary.

> Tension headaches tend to get worse as the day progresses.

Traumatic Headache

Traumatic headaches are a sequela of minor and severe head injuries. Local tissue damage from trauma can lead to muscle contraction and tension on the extracranial vasculature. Concussions and contusion may be followed by intermittent headaches that persist for months. Intracerebral bleeds generally are accompanied by a severe headache of sudden onset. Refer to Chapter 36, Head Trauma, for further discussion of intracerebral hemorrhage.

Temporal Arteritis

Temporal arteritis is a systemic arterial vasculitis. It produces severe, unilateral, throbbing frontotemporal pain. Palpation of the temporal area causes great discomfort or a cordlike artery can be felt. Pain may involve the neck or jaw, and jaw claudication (if present) is strongly suggestive of the disorder. Loss of vision can occur because of ischemic optic neuritis. Steroids should be given immediately to prevent vision loss. Patients with temporal arteritis are usually over 50 years of age and have a history of polymyalgia rheumatica.[6] A biopsy is required for definitive diagnosis.

Vascular Headaches

Cluster headaches and migraines are two types of vascular headaches.

Cluster Headaches. Fortunately, cluster headaches are rare and short lived. Cluster headaches are more common in men and are typically not familial. Believed to be caused by dysfunction of the trigeminal nerve, these headaches are characterized by intense unilateral pain in the orbital or temporal region and last 15 to 180 minutes. The headaches tend to occur in clusters—that is, daily on the same side of the face for several weeks before going into remission. Associated findings include ipsilateral conjunctival injection, lacrimation, nasal congestion, rhinorrhea, and facial swelling.[9] Oxygen relieves 90% of cluster headaches within 15 minutes.[6]

Migraine Headaches. Migraine presentation can vary considerably between patients but a patient's migraine constellation of symptoms tends to be similar with each attack. Migraines affect women twice as frequently as men and are familial. Most migraines are not spontaneous but instead occur in response to a variety of environmental, emotional, hormonal, food, and medication triggers. Table 25-6 lists common headache triggers. Migraine headaches tend to

start before age 30 years; always be reluctant to assume it is the patient's first time ever migraine.[6] Helping patients to identify their triggers is key to preventing or minimizing future attacks. In a meta-analysis, combination treatment of dihydroergotamine (DHE-45, Migranal) and an antiemetic (e.g., metoclopramide [Reglan]) outperformed treatment with meperidine (Demerol), valproate (Depakote), or ketorolac (Toradol).[10]

A migraine presentation varies between patients but an individual patient's migraine headache tends to be similar on each occurrence. Be suspicious if this "migraine" is different.

Headache Assessment

Emergency department management of the patient with headache focuses on the assessment and initial treatment of symptoms. Most headaches are benign and tend to recur and be similar from one episode to the next. However, headaches can be an indication of a serious underlying disorder. A response to analgesic does not exclude life-threatening causes of headaches. A more thorough evaluation is required. Complaints of headaches that would be considered "red flag" situations include the following:

- Never experienced a headache, this is the patient's first
- First headache after age of 55 years
- Atypical headache pain for the patient
- Headaches increasing in frequency and severity
- Elderly patient
- New onset or at risk for cancer, human immunodeficiency virus (HIV), or immunosuppression
- Focal, abnormal neurologic findings
- The patient states, "This is the worst headache of my life"

If an entire family wakes up with headaches (and especially if the family pet is sick), consider carbon monoxide poisoning as the cause of the headaches.

The PQRST mnemonic (Provokes/Palliates, Quality, Radiates, Severity, Time) can be used to guide the patient interview. The following are other subjective and objective considerations:

- Is this the first headache (or the first of this type) ever experienced?
- If similar headaches before, why did the patient come to the ED this time?
- When and how did the headache start?
- Is there a history of trauma (long ago or recent)?
- Is the headache associated with nausea or vomiting?
- Activity at the onset of the headache.
- Are there signs of meningeal irritation (e.g., stiff neck, photophobia, fever)?

TABLE 25-6	**MIGRAINE HEADACHE TRIGGERS**
CATEGORY	**EXAMPLES**
Environmental	Changes in weather, season, or barometric pressure; bright or unusual colors; sun glare; flickering lights; television; tobacco, including secondhand smoke
Emotional or hormonal	Stress; anxiety; fatigue; altered sleep cycles; menstruation; pregnancy; hypoglycemia; intense physical exertion, including sexual activity
Food	Alcohol, especially red wine; aged cheeses; chocolate; monosodium glutamate; caffeine; aspartame
Medications	Cimetidine (Tagamet), nifedipine (Procardia), theophylline

- Have there been personality changes or unusual behaviors since the onset of the headache?
- Is there memory loss or confusion related to the headache?
- Has the patient had any recent infections?
- Are there visual changes? Blurring? Diplopia? Hemianopia?
- Have there been any new neurologic deficits?
- Has blood pressure been elevated? For how long?
- Does the patient have a history of emotional or psychiatric problems?
- What medications (i.e., prescription, over-the-counter, herbals) is the patient currently taking? Not taking? This includes drugs for the treatment of this headache.
- Has the patient ever had a seizure? When? What kind?

> Do a visual acuity assessment when a patient reports visual changes, even if the patient indicates the changes are a result of the migraine.

Therapeutic Interventions

Therapeutic interventions for headaches include the following:
- Nonsteroidal anti-inflammatory drugs can be given orally (e.g., ibuprofen) or parenterally (i.e., ketorolac).
- Provide relief of nausea and vomiting with antiemetics such as metoclopramide (Reglan), ondansetron (Zofran), chlorpromazine (Thorazine), and prochlorperazine (Compazine). These agents are highly effective. When these agents are given intravenously some patients also obtain headache relief.
- Manage vascular headache pain with dihydroergotamine or serotonin inhibitors such as sumatriptan (Imitrex).
- Cluster headaches may be treated with calcium channel blockers (e.g., verapamil) and with antiseizure medications such as divalproex (Depakote), topiramate (Topamax), and gabapentin (Neurontin).
- Use narcotic analgesics if headache-specific agents are ineffective.
- Consider a computed tomography scan to rule out life-threatening causes (e.g., subarachnoid hemorrhage).

Discharge Instructions

- Understand headache triggers; using a headache diary can be helpful.
- Learn and practice stress management.
- Get plenty of sleep, eat a healthy diet, exercise regularly, and use proper posture.
- Have routine eye exams.

- Contact the health care provider if experiencing:
  - The "worst headache of your life"
  - Change in headache patterns or pain
  - Speech, vision, balance, or motion difficulties
  - Medication side effects

Neuromuscular Disorders

Guillain-Barré Syndrome

Guillain-Barré syndrome is an acute paralytic disease that decreases myelin in the nerve roots and peripheral nerves. About half of all patients with Guillain-Barré syndrome experience a mild febrile illness several weeks before the onset of symptoms. Risk factors for this ascending paralytic condition include infection with HIV, cytomegalovirus, or hepatitis B; pregnancy; and Hodgkin lymphoma.[5]

Signs and Symptoms

- A tingling sensation in the hands and feet that may be present for hours or weeks before diagnosis
- Severely diminished superficial and deep tendon reflexes (particularly in the lower extremities)
- Symmetrical paralysis, usually beginning in the lower extremities, that gradually ascends to the respiratory muscles
- Urinary retention
- Ileus
- Postural hypotension
- Respiratory insufficiency

Therapeutic Interventions

- Support the patient's airway, breathing, and circulatory status.
- Assess for alternative causes of neuropathy such as heavy metal poisoning, diabetes, vitamin B_{12} deficiency, myasthenia gravis, multiple sclerosis, amyotrophic lateral sclerosis, and botulism.
- Provide general supportive care until the condition spontaneously resolves, generally weeks after onset.

> Because of the potential for hypoventilation due to respiratory muscle weakness, monitor the depth and adequacy of respirations in a patient with Guillain-Barré syndrome.

Myasthenia Gravis

Myasthenia gravis is a defect of neuromuscular transmission. The original translation of its name meant grave weakness. Onset generally occurs around 20 to 30 years of age.[11] This condition occurs more frequently in females than in males and may have a familial connection.[11] Many commonly prescribed drugs such as antibiotics and psychotropic and antidysrhythmic drugs can precipitate a myasthenic crisis. The hallmark of myasthenia gravis is weakness, particularly of the ocular, facial, and neck muscles or in the upper extremities. Patients in myasthenic crisis can experience fatal respiratory paralysis.

Signs and Symptoms
- Increasing fatigue
- Delayed recovery of muscle strength after exercise
- Weak eye muscles, visual changes, and diplopia (but *not* pupillary changes)
- An abnormal smile because of weak facial and jaw muscles
- Dysphagia, weak pharyngeal muscles
- Inability to handle oral secretions

Therapeutic Interventions
- Support the patient's airway, breathing, and circulatory status.
- Anticholinesterase medications, particularly pyridostigmine bromide (Mestinon) and neostigmine bromide (Prostigmin), are used for ongoing management of myasthenia gravis.
- Symptoms of myasthenic crisis and cholinergic crisis are similar. To differentiate between the two, administer edrophonium chloride (Tensilon), an anticholinesterase inhibitor, in a Tensilon challenge. If symptoms improve, the test is considered positive, indicating that the patient is in myasthenic crisis. Treat myasthenic crisis with neostigmine (Prostigmin) 1 mg intravenously. If symptoms worsen, it is a cholinergic crisis and reverses with atropine intravenously.

Other Neurologic Emergencies

Neurogenic Shock

Although neurogenic shock is most often the result of spinal cord injury, it may also occur with certain neurologic disorders, cord compression from oncology emergencies, regional anesthesia, and some medications (e.g., nitrates, opioids, adrenergic blockers). In neurogenic shock there is a disruption in sympathetic nervous system function. It is characterized by the triad of hypotension, bradycardia, and massive vasodilation. Impairment of the descending sympathetic pathways in the spinal cord results in ineffective circulating volume and inadequate organ and tissue perfusion. As the blood vessels dilate, blood pools away from the heart. Inadequate blood returns to the heart so the heart is unable to effectively pump blood throughout the body. Neurogenic shock differs from hypovolemic shock in that there is no compensatory increase in cardiac output (tachycardia) because of the decrease in sympathetic tone. Treatment focuses on airway management, intravenous fluids, and medications that increase peripheral vascular resistance (i.e., norepinephrine, dopamine).[1]

> Patients with neurogenic shock are more likely to be warm and dry than cool and clammy as compared with patients in hypovolemic shock.

Shunt Problems

Ventricular shunts decrease intracranial pressure by diverting cerebrospinal fluid from the lateral ventricles to the torso. Complications related to shunts are infection and shunt malfunction. Malfunction occurs when the shunt becomes obstructed by debris, blood clots, or brain tissue. Obstruction also results if the shunt ends become disconnected or malpositioned. Regardless of the underlying problem, the patient usually has an altered level of consciousness because of increased intracranial pressure. If the problem develops rapidly, the patient experiences acute changes; if the problem develops over time, changes in level of consciousness occur gradually. Infection generally is associated with fever; shunt malfunction is not.

Therapeutic Interventions
- Determine the patient's neurologic status at the time of emergency department presentation.
- Elicit a history of acute or gradual changes in level of consciousness.
- In addition to changes in level of consciousness, signs of increased intracranial pressure include headache and nausea progressing to projectile vomiting, lethargy, and coma.
- Identify other neurologic findings such as ataxia, incontinence, and pupillary changes.
- Assess for signs of infection, including fever and meningeal irritation.
- Treatment includes lumbar puncture or shunt tapping to aspirate cerebrospinal fluid. If infection is suspected, send cultures and institute antibiotic therapy.
- Surgical intervention is required for obstructed, fractured, or malpositioned catheters.

> **Internet Neuroscience Nursing Resources:**
> - American Association of Neuroscience Nurses, http://www.aann.org
>   - Offers certification as neuroscience registered nurse (CNRN)
>   - Certification effective for 5 years
> - American Academy of Neurology, http://www.aan.com
> - National Institute of Neurological Disorders and Stroke (NINDS), http://www.ninds.nih.gov
> - National Headache Foundation, http://www.headaches.org
> - American Headache Society Committee for Headache Education, http://www.achenet.org
> - Epilepsy Foundation, http://www.epilepsyfoundation.org

REFERENCES

1. Dennison, R. D. (2007). *Pass CCRN* (3rd ed.). St. Louis, MO: Mosby.

2. Wijdicks, E. F., Bamlet, W. R., Maramattom, B. V., Manno, E. M., & McClelland, R. L. (2006). Validation of a new coma scale: The FOUR score. *Annals of Neurology, 58*(4), 585–593.

3. Stead, L. G., Wijdicks, E. F., Bhagra, A., Kashyap, R., Bellolio, M. F., Nash, D. L., ... William, B. (2009). Validation of a new coma scale, the FOUR score, in the emergency department. *Neurocritical Care, 10*(1), 50–54.

4. Dugdale, D. C. (2010, February 6). *Wernicke-Korsakoff syndrome.* Retrieved from http://www.nlm.nih.gov/medlineplus/ency/article/000771.htm

5. Ferri, F. (2010). *Ferri's clinical advisor: Instant diagnosis and treatment.* St. Louis, MO: Mosby.

6. Jordan, K. S. (Ed.), (2007). *Emergency nursing core curriculum* (6th ed.). Philadelphia, PA: Saunders.

7. Hall, K. N. (2006). Seizures. In V. J. Markovchick & P. T. Pons (Eds.), *Emergency medicine secrets* (4th ed., pp. 101–107). St. Louis, MO.

8. Decker, W. W., & Haro, L. H. (2006). Headache. In V. J. Markovchick & P. T. Pons (Eds.), *Emergency medicine secrets* (4th ed., pp. 91–95). St. Louis, MO.

9. Denny, C. J., & Schull, M. J. (2004). Headache and facial pain. In J. E. Tintinalli, G. D. Kelen, & J. S. Stapczynski (Eds.), *Emergency medicine: A comprehensive study guide* (6th ed., pp. 1375–1381). New York, NY: McGraw-Hill.

10. Colman, I., Brown, M. D., Innes, G. D., Grafstein, E., Roberts, T. E., & Rowe, B. H. (2005). Parenteral dihydroergotamine for acute migraine headache: A systematic review of the literature. *Annals of Emergency Medicine, 45*, 393–401.

11. Goldenberg, W. D. (2011, July 15). *Emergency management of myasthenia gravis.* Retrieved from http://emedicine.medscape.com/article/793136-overview.

Facial, ENT, and Dental Emergencies

Darcy Egging

Medical problems of the face, ears, nose, throat, and mouth involve multiple conditions including infections, foreign bodies, and thrombotic or embolic events. Regardless of the patient's chief complaint, the first priority for these patients is assessment and management of airway, breathing, and circulation. The focus of this chapter is medical emergencies related to the face; see also Chapter 41, Facial, Ocular, ENT, and Dental Trauma.

FACIAL EMERGENCIES

Bell's Palsy

Bell's palsy is a unilateral facial paralysis caused by damage to the facial nerve (cranial nerve VII), often the result of the herpes simplex virus. Symptoms can take weeks or months to resolve and some individuals will have permanent sequelae. Bell's palsy is a diagnosis of exclusion. Patients must be fully evaluated to rule out stroke, meningitis, or a tumor affecting the facial nerve.[1]

Signs and Symptoms

- Unilateral facial paralysis with facial drooping (Fig. 26-1)
- Inability to blink or close the affected eye
- Postauricular pain
- Increased or decreased unilateral tear production
- Drooling
- Ipsilateral loss of taste (one side of the tongue)
- A perception that sound is louder in the ear on the affected side (hyperacusis)
- Headache

Diagnostic Procedures

- Clinical examination is the hallmark for diagnosing this problem.
- There is no specific diagnostic study to confirm the diagnosis.

- Specific imaging studies are not recommended. Testing to rule out other diagnoses, such as stroke, may be indicated.

Therapeutic Interventions

- Antiviral medications and corticosteroids may shorten the disease course
- Analgesics for pain
- Eye care: artificial tears during the day, lubricants for nighttime eye protection
- Consider facial massage to prevent contracture or paralyzed muscles

Trigeminal Neuralgia (Tic Douloureux)

Trigeminal neuralgia, also known as tic douloureux, is defined by the International Association for the Study of Pain as "a sudden, usually unilateral, severe, brief, stabbing, recurrent pain in the distribution of one or more branches of the fifth cranial nerve."[2] The trigeminal nerve (cranial nerve V) divides into three branches: ophthalmic nerve (V1), maxillary nerve (V2), and mandibular nerve (V3). The two branches most often affected are V2 and V3. Trigeminal neuralgia is often accompanied by facial spasm called a tic and occurs most often in females over the age of 60 years. The pain may be precipitated by normal daily activities such as brushing one's teeth or chewing.[3]

Signs and Symptoms

- Excruciating, stabbing, electric shock–like pain lasting seconds to several minutes
- Generally unilateral, rarely bilateral
- Usually involves the lips, cheeks, jaw, eyes, forehead, scalp, and nose (Fig. 26-2)

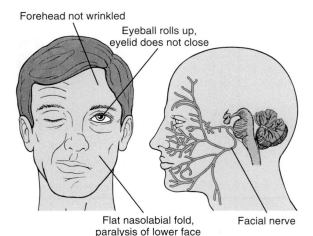

Forehead not wrinkled

Eyeball rolls up, eyelid does not close

Flat nasolabial fold, paralysis of lower face

Facial nerve

Fig. 26-1 Bell's palsy: facial characteristics. (From Lewis, S. M., Heitkemper, M. M., & Dirksen, S. R. [2004]. *Medical-surgical nursing: Assessment and management of clinical problems* [6th ed.]. St. Louis, MO: Mosby.)

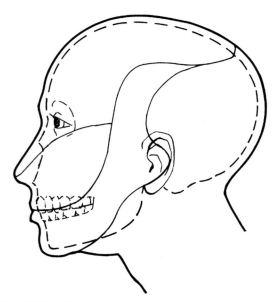

Fig. 26-2 Distribution of trigeminal nerve. (Reprinted with permission from Thompson, J. M., McFarland, G. K., Hirsch, J. E., & Tucker, S. M. [2005]. *Mosby's clinical nursing* [5th ed.]. St. Louis, MO: Mosby.)

Therapeutic Interventions

- A trial of carbamazepine (Tegretol) can be therapeutic as well as diagnostic. If this drug does not ease the pain, it suggests that trigeminal neuralgia is not the cause of the pain.
- Other medications include:
  - Phenytoin (Dilantin)
  - Oxcarbazepine (Trileptal)
  - Clonazepam (Klonopin)
  - Lamotrigine (Lamictal)
  - Valproic acid (Depakene)
  - Gabapentin (Neurontin)
- Carbamazepine and baclofen have been suggested as a synergistic combination to decrease pain.[4,5]
- Inform the patient that exacerbations generally occur in fall and spring months.

Periorbital (Preseptal) and Orbital Cellulitis

Periorbital and orbital cellulitis are infections caused by common respiratory pathogens such as *Streptococcus pneumoniae* (most common organism), *Staphylococcus aureus*, *Streptococcus pyogenes*, and *Haemophilus influenzae*. Diagnosis is based on clinical examination; computed tomography (CT) scan and magnetic resonance imaging (MRI) may be obtained nonetheless. One of the greatest concerns with periorbital or orbital cellulitis is the potential for it to lead to meningitis. Table 26-1 compares periorbital and orbital cellulitis.

Cavernous Sinus Thrombosis

Cavernous sinus thrombosis (CST) (Fig. 26-3) is a rare but potentially life-threatening infection of a blood clot in one or both of the cavernous sinuses. The cavernous sinuses are located at the base of the skull and receive venous blood from the facial veins. As a result, infections of the face, tonsils, and orbits can spread to the cavernous sinuses. CST usually follows midfacial cellulitis or paranasal sinus infection. *S. aureus* (70%) and *Streptococcus* are the most frequent causative pathogens.[6] The mortality rate for CST is 30% in all patients; in those with underlying sphenoid sinusitis, mortality is up to 50%.[6] Death occurs from overwhelming sepsis or neurologic infection.

Signs and Symptoms

- History of sinusitis or midfacial infection
- Symptoms of CST are similar to those of periorbital and orbital cellulitis
- Headache is the most common symptom
- Chemosis—edema of the conjunctiva and mucous membrane of the eyelid

TABLE 26-1   PERIORBITAL (PRESEPTAL) AND ORBITAL CELLULITIS

	DEFINITION	CAUSES	SIGNS AND SYMPTOMS	THERAPEUTIC INTERVENTIONS
Periorbital (preseptal) cellulitis	Inflammation of tissues anterior to the nasal septum More common	Spread of a local infection from facial or eyelid trauma Insect bite Conjunctivitis Chalazion Sinusitis	Tenderness, swelling, warmth, redness of the eyelid Visual acuity and EOM not affected	Broad-spectrum antibiotics on an outpatient basis with close follow-up Consider MRSA
Orbital cellulitis	Inflammation of tissues within the orbit posterior to the orbital septum More severe clinical situation and more severe complications	Spread of a sinus infection	Tenderness, swelling, warmth, redness of the eyelid Pain with EOM Decreased visual acuity Exophthalmos Fever, malaise, headache	Hospitalization for IV antibiotics Ophthalmology consult Surgery may be necessary to decompress the abscess

EOM, Extraocular eye movement; *IV*, intravenous; *MRSA*, methicillin-resistant *Staphylococcus aureus*.
Nolan, E. G. (2010) Dental, ear, throat, and facial emergencies. In P. K. Howard & R. A. Steinmann (Eds.), *Sheehy's emergency nursing: Principles and practice* (6th ed., pp. 590–601). St. Louis, MO: Mosby; Lowery, R. S. (2009, July 30). Blepharitis, adult. Retrieved from http://emedicine.medscape.com/article/1211763-overview.

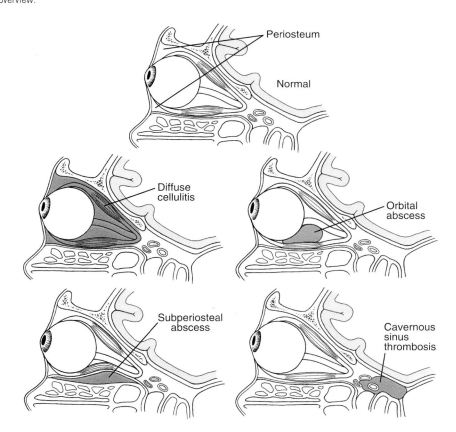

Fig. 26-3   Location of orbital cellulitis and cavernous sinus thrombosis. (Reprinted with permission of Garrity, J. (2008, September). Preseptal and orbital cellulitis. *The Merck manuals online.* Retrieved from http://www.merckmanuals.com/professional/eye_disorders/orbital_diseases/preseptal_and_orbital_cellulitis.html?qt=prespetal%20and%20orbital%20cellulitis&alt=sh.)

- Decreased visual acuity resulting from increased intra-ocular pressure
- Ptosis and impaired eye movement resulting from dysfunction of cranial nerves III, IV, V, and VI
- Exophthalmos
- Facial pain
- Fever, tachycardia, sepsis
- Meningeal signs such as nuchal rigidity and Kernig and Brudzinski signs

Diagnostic Procedures

- This is a clinical diagnosis and laboratory tests are not specific. Blood cultures and complete blood count (CBC) are usually obtained.
- CT scan or MRI with contrast to confirm diagnosis.
- Magnetic resonance venogram shows absence of venous flow in the affected sinus.[6]

Therapeutic Interventions

- Immediate intravenous administration of broad-spectrum antibiotics.
- Administration of anticoagulants and steroids is questionable.[6] Steroids may be considered to prevent adrenal crisis if the course of CST leads to pituitary insufficiency.
- Infectious disease and surgical consults are recommended.
- Possible admission to intensive care unit if sinus drainage is indicated.

EAR, NOSE, AND THROAT EMERGENCIES

Infections of the Ear

Infections of the ear and their possible complications are compared in Table 26-2.

Cerumen Impaction

Cerumen is produced in the outer ear to repel moisture and trap debris and microorganisms. Cerumen normally moves to the opening of the ear canal, where it can be washed away. Overproduction of cerumen or anatomical narrowing of the external canal may cause an impaction of the cerumen. Impaction may also occur if cotton-tipped swabs push the cerumen deep into the inner ear canal, where it can obstruct the tympanic membrane.[7]

Signs and Symptoms

- Itching or pain of ear
- Feeling of fullness in the ear
- Loss of hearing
- Tinnitus
- Dizziness

Therapeutic Interventions

- Instill cerumenolytics such as triethanolamine polypeptide oleate-condensate (Cerumenex) or liquid docusate sodium (Colace) to soften and loosen the wax.
- Irrigate ear with warm water if ruptured tympanic membrane is *not* suspected.
- Curettage may be necessary to remove impacted cerumen.
- Instruct patients to avoid placing any object into ear; emphasize that high-energy instrumentation, such as a water pick, should never be used in the ear.

Foreign Body in the Ear

Foreign bodies, such as beads, beans, small toys, and live bugs, are seen most commonly in the ears of pediatric patients. Bleeding and rupture of the tympanic membrane can occur if the patient attempts to remove the foreign object. Live insects trapped in the ear cause the patient great distress as they move and buzz inside the ear canal. This movement may also rupture the tympanic membrane.

Signs and Symptoms

- Adult patients are usually able to identify what is in their ear.
- Pediatric patients may complain of ear pain, discharge, and foul odor from the ear.
- Hearing loss on the affected side.
- Movement of live insect may cause dizziness, nausea, or vomiting.

Therapeutic Interventions

- Live insects should be killed prior to removal by instilling lidocaine or mineral oil into the ear canal.
- Suction or use of alligator forceps may be necessary to grasp and remove the foreign object.
- Irrigating the ear should be avoided if the foreign body is organic in nature, as it will absorb liquid and become more difficult to remove.
- Avoid pushing the object further into the ear canal.
- Procedural sedation may be required for patient cooperation and successful removal.

How to Perform Ear Irrigation

1. Consider instilling a ceruminolytic in the affected ear canals before the procedure.
2. Use a large syringe (e.g., 30 mL) with a soft intravenous catheter attached (e.g., an 18-gauge butterfly catheter with the needle cut off). Trim the catheter to avoid perforation of the tympanic membrane. Do not irrigate with a Waterpik; the stream is too forceful.

Box continued on page 280.

TABLE 26-2 EAR INFECTIONS AND POSSIBLE COMPLICATIONS

	DESCRIPTION	SIGNS AND SYMPTOMS	THERAPEUTIC INTERVENTIONS
Otitis externa	Infection of the external auditory canal Also known as "swimmer's ear" Usually bacterial infection Excessive moisture and trauma are common predisposing factors[a]	Pain with movement of the tragus and auricle Swelling and erythema of the ear canal Discharge from the ear (often purulent) Hearing loss Possible periauricular cellulitis	Topical or systemic analgesics Topical or otic antibiotics Warm otic drops by rotating bottle between hands prior to administration to avoid dizziness Apply heat with heating pad or warm compresses Keep ear dry; may require an ear wick Instruct patient not to insert cotton-tipped swabs or other objects into ear canal Swimmers should wear ear plugs
Otitis media	Infection of the inner ear Blockage of the eustachian tube causes a buildup of fluid behind the tympanic membrane Often seen in children ages 6 months to 3 years following a UTI Most infections are viral but may be bacterial Common pathogens are *Streptococcus pneumoniae*, *Haemophilus influenzae*, and *Moraxella catarrhalis*[b]	Sharp middle ear pain Sensation of fullness in ear Hearing loss Fever Bulging tympanic membrane History of UTI Infants and children may be irritable and pull at ear Possible nausea and vomiting	Systemic antibiotics Analgesics Treat fever as necessary with acetaminophen or ibuprofen Instruct parents or family of importance of completing antibiotic course
Mastoiditis	Rare complication of otitis media Decreased incidence since advent of antibiotic therapy for otitis media Infection may erode mastoid and invade surrounding structures, leading to intracranial infection[c]	Recent or recurrent otitis media Pain and swelling in mastoid area Otalgia Hearing loss Fever Headache Possible rupture of tympanic membrane	Hospital admission with infectious disease consult Intravenous antibiotics Analgesics Possible surgery: mastoidectomy or myringotomy
Labyrinthitis	Inflammation of the inner ear or labyrinth Often follows acute otitis media, UTI, or allergies Causes include bacterial or viral infections, ototoxic medications, or autoimmune disorders Rarely seen in children[d,e]	Symptoms may last for weeks but condition is usually self-limiting History of recent infective process Vertigo associated with movement Hearing loss Tinnitus Nausea and vomiting Otalgia Fever Nystagmus	CT or MRI is needed to rule out neurological cause of vertigo Bed rest and adequate hydration Possible medications include: • Antiemetics • Benzodiazepines • Oral corticosteroids • Antibiotics Instruct patient in the following: • Avoid sudden changes in head or body position • Use assistive devices if unsteady gait • Do not drive or operate machinery while taking medications or while symptoms are present

CT, computed tomography; *MRI*, magnetic resonance imaging; *UTI*, urinary tract infection.

[a]Morrissey, T. (2008). Ear emergencies. In J. G. Adams (Ed.), *Emergency medicine*. Philadelphia, PA: Saunders Elsevier.

[b]Guest, J. F., Greener, M. J., Robinson, A. C., & Smith A. F. (2004). Impacted cerumen: Composition, production, epidemiology and management. *QJM, 97*(8), 477–488.

[c]Chase, K. S., & Doty, C. I. (2009, September 28). *Mastoiditis in emergency medicine*. Retrieved from http://emedicine.medscape.com/article/784176-overview.

[d]Nolan, E. G. (2010) Dental, ear, throat, and facial emergencies. In P. K. Howard & R. A. Steinmann (Eds.), *Sheehy's emergency nursing: Principles and practice* (6th ed., pp. 590–601). St. Louis, MO: Mosby.

[e]Baloh, R. W. (2003). Clinical practice: Vestibular neuritis. *New England Journal of Medicine, 348*(11), 1027–1032.

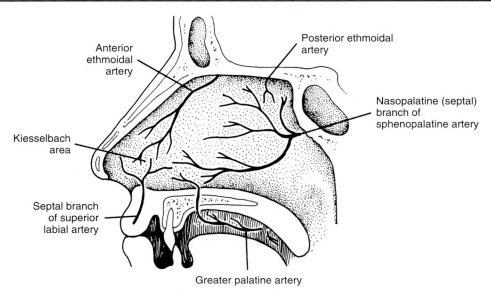

Fig. 26-4 Arterial supply to nasal septum. (From Rosen, P., & Barkin, R. [Eds.]. [1998]. *Emergency medicine: Concepts and clinical practice* [4th ed.]. St. Louis, MO: Mosby.)

3. Use water at body temperature. (The water may be mixed with hydrogen peroxide.) Water that is too hot or too cold causes dizziness when it contacts the tympanic membrane.
4. With the patient sitting upright, straighten the ear canal by pulling it up and back for adults or down and back for young children.
5. Fill the syringe with water, insert it into the outer portion of the ear canal, and direct the stream at the *side* of the canal. Be careful not to scratch the ear canal with the catheter.
6. If the patient feels water in the mouth or throat, *stop immediately*. This indicates perforation of the tympanic membrane.
7. Collect the irrigation water in a basin held under the patient's ear.
8. Repeat the procedure until all cerumen has been removed from the ear canal.

Epistaxis

Epistaxis, or nasal hemorrhage, can occur from either anterior or posterior vessels. Anterior bleeding is the most common source and is usually from the area of the Kiesselbach plexus (Fig. 26-4). Posterior bleeding is usually seen in older adults and is often more profuse. Common causes of epistaxis include:
- Nose-picking
- Nasal trauma
- Inhalant use
- Hypertension
- Dry nasal mucosa
- Infections
- Tumors
- Septal perforation
- Intranasal drug administration (cocaine)
- Anticoagulation
- Coagulopathies

Signs and Symptoms
- Bleeding from one or both nares
- Dizziness from severe blood loss
- Nausea and vomiting from swallowed blood

Therapeutic Interventions
- Caregivers should observe universal precautions, including goggles, mask, and gown as needed.
- Ensure patent airway; have suction available.
- Elevate the head of the bed.
- Have the patient sit upright, lean forward, and pinch nostrils for at least 10 minutes.
- If bleeding is severe, obtain intravenous (IV) access and administer fluids.
- Anticipate chemical cautery with silver nitrate sticks.
- Prepare for nasal packing with:
  - Vaseline gauze
  - Pledget soaked with:

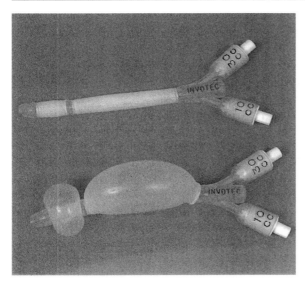

Fig. 26-5 Epistaxis balloon. (Courtesy of Invotec International, Jacksonville, FL.)

- 4% cocaine
- Neo-Synephrine
- Lidocaine with epinephrine
- Merocel nasal sponge
- Epistaxis balloon (Fig. 26-5)
- Patients with posterior bleeds may require more extensive treatment and hospitalization.
- Arrange for follow-up with ear, nose, and throat (ENT) physician within 48 to 72 hours.

Nasal Foreign Bodies

Foreign bodies in the nose occur most often in the pediatric population. The chief concern with nasal foreign bodies is the potential for aspiration.

Signs and Symptoms
- Nasal and sinus pain
- Purulent nasal discharge
- Recurrent epistaxis
- Fever

Therapeutic Interventions
- Determine the type of nasal foreign body; a magnet, button battery, or organic matter requires prompt removal.
- Have the patient block the unaffected nares and blow his or her nose; this creates positive pressure and is a noninvasive technique.
- More invasive methods for removal include:

- Direct instrumentation using an alligator forceps or right angle hook
- Balloon catheter such as a small urinary catheter
- Suction
- Decongestants may be used prior to treatment to facilitate foreign body removal.
- ENT physician consultation may be necessary.
- Educate the caregivers concerning the dangers of small play objects for young children.

Pharyngitis and Tonsillitis

Acute pharyngitis and tonsillitis are common viral or bacterial illnesses that cause inflammation of the oropharynx. The bacteria usually causing these illnesses are group A beta-hemolytic *Streptococcus* (GABHS), *Mycoplasma*, and *Chlamydia*. Viral causes include the Epstein-Barr virus, which is also the main cause of mononucleosis.[8,9]

Signs and Symptoms
- Sore throat
- Fever and myalgias
- Dysphagia
- Halitosis
- Headache
- Ear pain

Therapeutic Interventions
- Obtain "quick strep" or throat culture.
- Antibiotics for positive strep tests; instruct the patient to take the full prescription.
- Antipyretics for fever as well as for pain; advise the patient to avoid aspirin and products that contain aspirin.
- Instruct the patient of need to increase fluid intake.
- Patients may receive some relief from gargling with warm salt water.

Peritonsillar Abscess

A peritonsillar abscess is a collection of purulent material around the tonsils that may lead to a deep tissue infection. Often following an episode of pharyngitis or tonsillitis, this infection must be diagnosed early and quickly to avoid complications, particularly those related to airway patency.

Signs and Symptoms
- Deviation of uvula toward the unaffected side
- Drooling and dysphagia
- Fever
- Halitosis
- Muffled voice ("hot potato voice")
- Pain in throat, radiating to ear
- Swollen soft palate on affected side

- Cervical lymphadenitis
- Erythematic tonsils with exudates
- Trismus from pain and inflammation

Diagnostic Procedures

- Laboratory studies depend on the severity of the patient's symptoms and may include the following:
  - CBC and electrolytes
  - Monospot
  - Culture and sensitivity of throat exudate
- Soft tissue neck radiograph
- CT scan may be necessary

Therapeutic Interventions

- First priority is to ensure patent airway and adequate breathing.
- Establish IV access for hydration or rehydration.
- Administer IV antibiotic.
- Administer IV steroids, such as dexamethasone (Decadron), to decrease edema.
- Administer systemic analgesics.
- Consult an ENT specialist.
- Prepare for needle aspiration or incision and drainage.

DENTAL EMERGENCIES

Ludwig's Angina

Ludwig's angina is a fast-moving, potentially lethal, bacterial cellulitis involving the floor of the mouth and neck. The infection can spread rapidly to the mediastinum, pericardium, and pleural cavity.[10,11] Causes include:

- Untreated dental abscess
- An abscess unresponsive to antibiotic therapy
- Trauma to the mouth

Signs and Symptoms

- Respiratory distress with stridor, tachypnea, and dyspnea
- Swelling of submandibular and sublingual spaces
- Pain and tenderness
- Dysphagia, drooling, and muffled voice
- Fever
- Trismus
- Patient anxiety resulting from respiratory distress

Therapeutic Interventions

- Airway patency is the priority.
  - Maintain elevated head of bed.
  - Administer supplemental oxygen.
  - Prepare for possible emergency airway intervention, including intubation or cricothyrotomy.
- Obtain blood for CBC, blood chemistries, and cultures.

- If airway patency is assured, CT or soft tissue films may be obtained.
- Obtain IV access for fluid and antibiotic administration.
- Systemic analgesia.
- Consult an ENT specialist and prepare for possible surgical intervention and admission to the intensive care unit.

Odontalgia (Dental Pain)

The initial considerations for patients with dental pain are ensuring a patent airway and being prepared for definitive airway management.[10,11] Odontalgia has numerous causes, including:

- Poor oral hygiene
- Oral infection
- Recent dental procedures
- Trauma

Table 26-3 and Table 26-4 describe common dental problems seen in the emergency department.

BODY PIERCING OF THE FACE, EARS, AND TONGUE

All forms of body piercing have the potential to cause serious local or systemic infections. Potential issues related to unsafe piercing practices include tetanus, hepatitis, and human immunodeficiency virus (HIV).[12-14] Other complications related to facial piercing are listed below. Figure 26-6 illustrates different types of body jewelry and their removal.

Ear

- Perichondrial hematoma ("cauliflower ear")
- Keloid formation
- Embedded earring
- Perichondritis
- Deformed earlobe

Mouth

- Airway compromise
- Tooth fracture or chipping
- Speech impediment
- Various infections
- Gingival infection or trauma
- Ludwig's angina
- Perforation of lingual vessels causing bleeding or hematoma formation

Nose

- Infection
- Aspiration or swallowing of jewelry
- Perichondritis and necrosis of the cartilage of the nasal wall

TABLE 26-3 **PERIODONTAL EMERGENCIES REQUIRING DENTAL REFERRAL**

TYPE	DESCRIPTION
Gingivitis	Inflammation of the gums characterized by redness, swelling, and bleeding caused by plaque buildup. Usually painless. Good dental hygiene can prevent or reverse this condition.
Periodontitis (pyorrhea)	Occurs when gingivitis extends into the surrounding structures and bone is destroyed. The patient has symptoms of severe gingivitis. Radiographs are used to determine the amount of bone loss. Eventually teeth will loosen and fall out. Antibiotics and surgery may be required.
Vincent's angina (necrotizing ulcerative gingivitis or trench mouth)	Painful bleeding, halitosis, lymphadenopathy, chills, fever, dysphagia, and malaise are present. The tops of the gums (between the teeth) erode and become covered with a layer of gray-colored, dead tissue that must be debrided by a dentist.
Pericoronitis	A flap of gum overlying an erupting tooth, often a wisdom tooth, under which bits of food and bacteria accumulate. Accompanied by swelling, lymphadenopathy, and trismus. Treatment involves removing the tissue over the tooth. Rinse with warm saline, take antibiotics, and follow up with a dentist for possible tooth extraction.

TABLE 26-4 **COMPARISON OF DENTAL ABSCESS, BLEEDING, AND ALVEOLAR OSTEITIS**

	CAUSES	SIGNS AND SYMPTOMS	THERAPEUTIC INTERVENTIONS
Dental and periodontal abscesses	Extension of pulpal necrosis from oral cavities or a traumatic injury Abscess may involve supporting structures of the teeth	Pain Facial swelling; neck swelling if severe infection Fever Halitosis Difficulty swallowing Possible airway compromise	Systemic analgesics Possible antibiotics Ensure adequate hydration
Bleeding after dental procedure	If severe enough, bleeding may interfere with airway patency	Bleeding Pain Difficulty breathing	Direct pressure to bleeding site Pack socket with hemostatic dressing (Gelfoam) Topical thrombin Low-temperature cautery Instruct patient not to eat or drink for 2–3 hours after procedure; only cold drinks and soft food until seen by dentist or oral surgeon
Alveolar osteitis (dry socket)	Localized osteomyelitis occurring when a clot becomes dislodged following tooth extraction Commonly occurs 3–4 days after extraction[10]	Exposed bone over the site of extraction Increasing pain radiating to ear Halitosis	Prepare for nerve block and socket irrigation Assist with packing socket using material containing lidocaine and antiseptic Possible antibiotics Instruct patient: • Follow up with dentist or oral surgeon • No smoking for 72 hours (supply patient with nicotine patch if needed) • Do not drink from a straw • Cool beverages and soft foods only • If sinus cavity is involved, do not fly or scuba dive for 2 weeks

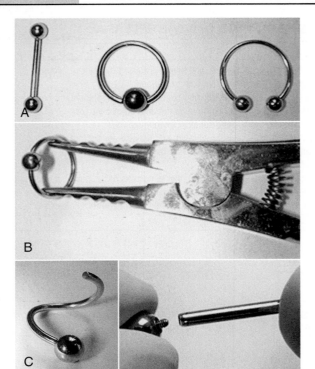

Fig. 26-6 Removal of body jewelry. **A,** Barbell, bead ring, circular band. **B,** Ring-expanding pliers with bead ring. **C,** Bead ring removed with hemostats; removal of internal threaded barbell. (Courtesy of Association of Professional Piercers, Chamblee, GA.)

REFERENCES

1. Taylor, D. C., Bessman, E., Dorion, D., Hedges, T. R., Huff, J. S., Khoromi, S., ... Zalvan, C. H. (2011, March 29). *Bell palsy.* Retrieved from http://emedicine.medscape.com/article/791311-overview
2. IASP Task Force on Taxonomy. (1994). Part III: pain terms, a current list with definitions and notes on usage. In H. Merskey & N. Bogduck (Eds.), *Classification of chronic pain* (2nd ed., pp. 209–214). Seattle, WA: IASP Press.
3. Huff, J. S. (2010, March 24). *Trigeminal neuralgia in emergency medicine.* Retrieved from http://emedicine.medscape.com/article/794402-overview
4. Gronseth, G., Cruccu, G., Alksne, J., Argoff, C., Brainin, M., Burchiel, K., ... Zakrzewska, J. M. (2008) Practice parameter: The diagnostic evaluation and treatment of trigeminal neuralgia (an evidence-based review): Report of the Quality Standard Subcommittee of the American Academy of Neurology and the European Federation of Neurological Societies. *Neurology, 71*(15), 1183–1190.
5. Jeffery, S. (2008, August 21). *New guideline on diagnosis and treatment of trigeminal neuralgia.* Retrieved from http://www.medscape.com/viewarticle/579404
6. Sharma, R., & Bessman, E. (2010, February 26). *Cavernous sinus thrombosis.* Retrieved from http://emedicine.medscape.com/article/791704-overview
7. Guest, J. F., Greener, M. J., Robinson, A. C., & Smith A. F. (2004). Impacted cerumen: Composition, production, epidemiology and management. *QJM, 97*(8), 477–488.
8. Hern, H. G. (2008). Pharynx and throat emergencies. In J. G. Adams (Ed.), *Emergency medicine.* Philadelphia, PA: Saunders Elsevier.
9. Benko, K. (2008). Dental emergencies. In J. G. Adams (Ed.), *Emergency medicine.* Philadelphia, PA: Saunders Elsevier.
10. Murchison, D. F. (2009, March). Overview of dental emergencies. *The Merck manuals online.* Retrieved from http://www.merckmanuals.com/professional/dental_disorders/dental_emergencies/overview_of_dental_emergencies.html?qt=dental%20emergencies&alt=sh
11. DeBoer, S., McNeil, M., & Amundson, T. (2008). Body piercing and airway management: Photo guide to tongue jewelry removal techniques. *AANA Journal, 76*(1), 19–23.
12. Theodossy, T. (2003). A complication of tongue piercing: A case report and review of literature. *British Dental Journal, 194*(10), 551–552.
13. Meltzer, D. I. (2005). Complications of body piercing. *American Family Physician, 72*(10), 2029–2034.
14. Garrity, J. (2008, September). Preseptal and orbital cellulitis. *The Merck manuals online.* Retrieved from http://www.merckmanuals.com/professional/eye_disorders/orbital_diseases/preseptal_and_orbital_cellulitis.html?qt=preseptal%20and%20orbital%20cellulitis&alt=sh

Ocular Emergencies

Darcy Egging

As in all other emergency situations, potentially life-threatening conditions must be addressed prior to the assessment and management of ocular problems. However, ocular problems are high priority because of the potential effect on vision.

> Do *not* instill topical ocular agents if ruptured globe is suspected.

> Contact lenses should be removed prior to eye examination other than for visual acuity.

DETERMINING VISUAL ACUITY

Visual acuity is considered a "vital sign" for patients with ocular problems and should be obtained on all patients presenting with a visual complaint. The exception to this rule is the patient with a chemical burn to the eye; this is a true medical emergency and the nurse should immediately initiate treatment in the form of eye irrigation prior to measuring visual acuity.

- Determine visual acuity before manual eye examination because manipulation increases blurring and decreases visual acuity.
- Consider instilling a topical anesthetic agent before examination to facilitate obtaining visual acuity.
- Measure visual acuity with and without corrective lenses.
  - Use the Snellen chart, placed at a distance of 20 feet, to test the affected eye first, then the unaffected eye, and finally both eyes.
  - Use the "E Chart" with patients who are illiterate or non-English speaking.
- If the patient is unable to see the Snellen chart, assess visual acuity by walking toward the patient holding up several fingers. Stop walking when the patient is able to tell how many fingers are being held up. Document the number of fingers and the distance from the patient (e.g., "three fingers at 15 feet"). Near-vision cards are also available for nonambulatory patients.
  - If the patient is unable to see fingers, assess for the patient's perception of light and dark.

CONJUNCTIVITIS (PINK EYE)

Acute conjunctivitis is an infection of the conjunctiva, the membrane that lines the eyelid and sclera. Causes of conjunctivitis include bacterial, viral, and fungal infections and allergic and chemical irritation.[1]

Signs and Symptoms

- Eyelids "crusted" shut upon awakening in the morning
- Sensation of foreign body in the eye
- Conjunctival erythema
- Purulent drainage (bacterial infection)
- Serous discharge (allergic or viral cause)
- Pruritus (allergic conjunctivitis)

Diagnostic Procedures

- Diagnosis based on clinical examination
- Culture discharge only if conjunctivitis is severe ("waterfall" discharge of gonorrhea), chronic, or unresponsive to treatment.

Therapeutic Interventions

- Antibiotic ophthalmic drops or ointment for bacterial infections.
- Cool compresses and decongestants for allergic conjunctivitis.
- If conjunctivitis is gonococcal, consider that the patient may also have chlamydial conjunctivitis; systemic therapy and appropriate referrals will also be needed.

- Treat chemical conjunctivitis as a chemical burn with immediate eye irrigation.

Patient Education

- Bacterial and viral conjunctivitis are highly contagious; teach the following infection control measures:
  - Practice frequent hand washing using good technique.
  - Keep children home from school until infection has cleared.
  - Do not share objects such as towels, washcloths, and pillows that may come in contact with discharge.
  - Stay out of swimming pools until symptoms have resolved.
  - Do not handle food while infection is present.
  - Discard eye make-up.
- Warm soaks may help to gently remove crusted exudates from eyelids and lashes after sleep.
- Cool compresses can be applied to eyelids for comfort and to decrease swelling.
- Wear sunglasses to decrease photophobia.
- Do not wear contact lenses or eye makeup until symptoms have resolved.
- Follow up with health care provider or ophthalmologist in 2 to 3 days.

How to Instill Ophthalmic Medications

Ophthalmic Drops
1. Explain the procedure to the patient.
2. Pull the lower eyelid down.
3. Have the patient look up.
4. Instill one or two drops of solution into the cul-de-sac (the center of the lower lid).
5. Have the patient blink gently to distribute the solution.
6. Instruct the patient not to squeeze the eyelids shut tightly; this will cause the solution to leak out.

Ophthalmic Ointment
1. Explain the procedure to the patient.
2. Pull the lower eyelid down.
3. Have the patient look up.
4. Apply ointment in a 1-cm line into the inner aspect of the lower lid.
5. Have the patient blink to distribute the ointment.
6. Instruct the patient not to squeeze the eyelids shut tightly; this will expel the ointment.

INFECTIONS OF THE EYELIDS AND CORNEA

Infections of the eyelids (i.e., blepharitis, hordeolum, chalazion) or the cornea (keratitis) are not uncommon complaints of patients presenting to the emergency department.

The most likely causative pathogen for these infections is *Staphylococcus aureus*. Table 27-1 summarizes the signs and symptoms and therapeutic interventions for these ocular infections.

CORNEAL ABRASION AND CORNEAL ULCER

Corneal abrasions are the most commonly seen eye injury in the emergency department. On the other hand, corneal ulcers are a true medical emergency; left untreated, they can cause blindness in 24 to 48 hours.[2] Visual acuity determinations should be attempted on these patients but may be difficult due to pain and photophobia. Fluorescein staining and slit lamp examination are also indicated. Table 27-2 compares corneal abrasions and corneal ulcers.

UVEITIS

Uveitis refers to inflammation of the middle layer of the eye. The uvea, or middle layer, consists of the iris, the ciliary body, and the choroid. Inflammation may involve the *anterior* uvea affecting the iris (iritis) or both the iris and the ciliary body (iridocyclitis). *Posterior* uveitis includes inflammation of the choroid (choroiditis) or the choroid and the retina (chorioretinitis); panuveitis indicates involvement of structures of both the anterior and the posterior uvea.[3]

Acute uveitis most frequently has an idiopathic cause.[3] Other causes include trauma, infections, and autoimmune diseases such as systemic lupus erythematosus (SLE) and rheumatoid arthritis.

Signs and Symptoms

- Unilateral painful red eye
- Blurred vision
- Photophobia
- Tearing
- Floaters more common with posterior uveitis

Diagnostic Procedures

- Visual acuity may be decreased in the affected eye.

Therapeutic Interventions

- Main goal is to reduce pain and inflammation
- Cycloplegics to decrease pain and photophobia
- Ophthalmology consultation must be obtained
- Topical or oral steroids only as directed by ophthalmologist

TABLE 27-1   EYELID AND CORNEAL INFECTIONS

	DESCRIPTION	SIGNS AND SYMPTOMS	THERAPEUTIC INTERVENTIONS
Blepharitis	• Acute or chronic inflammation of the lid margins • Usually allergic or chemical reaction • May also result from rosacea, herpes simplex, varicella zoster, seborrhea, or staphylococcus dermatitis[a,b]	• Burning and tearing of the eyes • Sensation of foreign body in the eye • Crusting of the lashes • Reddened lids and sclera • Pain and photophobia • Decreased vision	• Antibiotic ophthalmic ointment • Instruct patient to keep lids clean, gently remove crust, apply warm compresses, and then wash area thoroughly but gently with baby shampoo and water
Hordeolum	• Also known as a "sty" • Infection of an eyelid oil gland • May occur with blepharitis and is usually self-limiting	• Small external abscess • Pain • Redness • Swelling	• Warm compresses 3–4 times per day • Ophthalmic antibiotic ointment • Will usually rupture spontaneously but may require incision and drainage • Instruct patient in the importance of *not* trying to express purulent discharge
Chalazion	• Internal hordeolum caused by inflammation of the meibomian gland on the inner surface of the eyelid[a]	• Painless localized swelling beneath the eyelid	• Topical antibiotic ointment • Apply warm compresses 3–4 times per day • Consult ophthalmologist if chalazion does not resolve in 3–4 weeks • Incision and drainage may be required if chalazion affects vision
Keratitis	• Generic term for inflammation of the cornea • Causes may be viral (herpes simplex or zoster), bacterial, fungal, or amoebic • Use of contact lenses and ultraviolet light exposure are risk factors for keratitis • Untreated it can cause permanent corneal damage and blindness[a]	• Pain and photophobia • Mucopurulent drainage (usually bacterial) • Pus in the anterior chamber (hypopyon) • Decreased vision • Reddened sclera	• Oral or topical antibacterial, antiviral, or antifungal agent, depending on causative organism • Topical cycloplegic to decrease pain • Systemic analgesics to help control pain • Do *not* patch eye

[a]Egging, D. (2010). Ocular emergencies. In P. K. Howard & R. A. Steinmann (Eds.), *Sheehy's emergency nursing: Principles and practice* (6th ed., pp. 602–618). St. Louis, MO: Mosby.
[b]Vision Partners. (n.d.). *Blepharitis*. Retrieved from http://www.vp2020.com/common_education.php?p_id=26

TABLE 27-2   CORNEAL ABRASIONS AND CORNEAL ULCERS

	CAUSES	SIGNS AND SYMPTOMS	THERAPEUTIC INTERVENTIONS
Corneal abrasions	• Foreign body scratches the corneal epithelium	• Pain • Photophobia • Tearing • Sensation of foreign body • Eyelid spasms	• Topical anesthetic ocular drops prior to examination • Ophthalmic antibiotic drops • Topical ophthalmic nonsteroidal agents • Systemic analgesics

Corneal ulcers	• Usually caused by an infectious process
	• Risk factors include:
	  • Contact lenses
	  • Eye trauma
	  • Immunosuppression
		• Pain and photophobia
		• Sensation of foreign body
		• Tearing and blurry vision
		• Eyelid swelling
		• Possible purulent discharge
		• Appearance of "white spots" on cornea
			• Treatment depends on cause
			• Parenteral, oral, or topical antibiotics depending on severity of clinical presentation
			• Cycloplegic agents to decrease pain
			• Follow-up with ophthalmologist within 24 hours

OCULAR FOREIGN BODY

Ocular foreign bodies are generally superficial (conjunctiva or cornea) but can create long-term problems if not removed promptly. It is important to ascertain the identity of the foreign body:

- Organic foreign bodies have a higher rate of infection.
- Metallic objects leave a rust ring unless removed promptly.
- A foreign body as a result of high-speed velocity increases the index of suspicion for intraocular penetration.[2]

Signs and Symptoms

- Sensation of "something in the eye"
- Excessive tearing, pain, and photophobia

Diagnostic Procedures

- Visual acuity generally decreased
- Identification of foreign body on slit lamp examination

Therapeutic Interventions

- Instill ophthalmic anesthetic agents before examination.
- Invert upper eyelid, irrigate eye with normal saline, and gently remove the foreign body with a *moistened* cotton-tipped applicator.
- If the foreign body is adhered to the cornea, use a 25- or 27-gauge needle or an ophthalmic burr to remove it.
- After removal of foreign body, examine the cornea for other objects or rust ring.[2] Use the burr to remove a rust ring.
- Treat the resulting corneal abrasion.

OCULAR BURNS

Ocular burns are a true medical emergency and pose an immediate threat to the patient's vision. Burns to the eye may result from chemicals, thermal heat, or radiation. Thermal burns usually involve the eyelids, not the cornea, and are treated in the same way as thermal burns to other parts of the body. Chemical burns result from acids, alkalis, or petroleum-based substances.[4] Acid burns precipitate tissue proteins and limit, to some extent, penetration. Alkali burns are particularly devastating; alkali substances such as concrete and drain cleaners containing lye continue to penetrate until completely removed.

Signs and Symptoms

- Severe pain (radiation burns are particularly painful)
- Decreased visual acuity
- Excessive tearing and photophobia
- Blepharospasm
- Foreign body sensation

Diagnostic Procedures

- Decreased visual acuity
  - Do not delay eye irrigation to determine visual acuity

Therapeutic Interventions

- Begin eye irrigation with normal saline or Lactated Ringer solution *immediately*.
  - Check pH of eye prior to beginning irrigation.
  - Instill topical anesthetic drops.
  - Irrigate until eye pH is 7.0 to 7.5.
  - Irrigation may take up to 60 minutes if alkaline burn is present.
- Update tetanus immunization if needed.
- Ocular radiation burn treatment includes cycloplegics, topical antibiotics, and avoiding light.
- Severe ocular burns require ophthalmology consultation and possible patching for comfort and protection.

> Accidental application of cyanoacrylate (also known as Krazy Glue or Super Glue) to the eye may result in the eyelid being glued shut. Do not try to pry the lid open; some suggest trimming the eyelashes while others advocate waiting until the glue naturally flakes off (which may take a week). If the eye remains open, irrigate it immediately with copious amounts of water; treat as subsequent corneal abrasion.

CENTRAL RETINAL ARTERY OCCLUSION

Central retinal artery occlusion produces sudden, painless, unilateral blindness and is a medical emergency. Circulation to the retina must be restored within 60 to 90 minutes to prevent permanent loss of vision. Occasionally patients experience transient episodes of blindness (called amaurosis fugax) before total occlusion occurs.[4] Causes of central retinal artery occlusion include the following:

- Emboli (possibly from atrial fibrillation)
- Thrombosis
- Hypertension
- Giant cell arteritis
- Angiospasm

Signs and Symptoms

- Sudden, painless, unilateral blindness
- Often described as "curtain or shade coming down over eye"

Diagnostic Procedures

- Elevated intraocular pressure: normal intraocular pressure as measured by tonometer is 10 to 21 mm Hg.
- Electrocardiogram may demonstrate atrial fibrillation.
- Laboratory blood tests may indicate coagulopathies.

Therapeutic Interventions

- Place patient in supine position to optimize circulation to head.
- Having the patient breathe into a paper bag may increase arterial pCO_2 and cause vasodilation.
- Physician may attempt intermittent eye massage to reestablish blood flow.
- Acetazolamide (Diamox), 500 mg intravenously, and a topical beta-blocker such as timolol (Timoptic) may decrease intraocular pressure.
- Sublingual nitroglycerin may be used to dilate retinal vessels.
- Fibrinolytic therapy may be considered.

ACUTE RETINAL DETACHMENT

Acute retinal detachment is an ocular emergency. A tear in the retina allows vitreous humor to leak between the retina and the choroid, diminishing blood supply to the retina; permanent vision loss may ensue. Detachment may result from trauma or from an unknown cause. Spontaneous retinal detachment is more frequent in nearsighted individuals because the retina is thinner with myopia.[4]

Signs and Symptoms

- Flashes of light
- Shower of "floaters" or "cobwebs" in visual field
- Sudden decrease or loss of vision
- "Veil" or "curtain" effect in visual field

Diagnostic Procedures

- Visual acuity determination
- Dilated fundus and slit lamp examination
- Ophthalmic ultrasonography

Therapeutic Interventions

- Immediate referral to ophthalmologist
- Prepare patient for surgical intervention

ACUTE ANGLE CLOSURE GLAUCOMA

Acute angle closure glaucoma occurs when aqueous humor cannot escape the anterior chamber. Intraocular pressure increases and eventually the optic nerve becomes compressed. Acute angle closure glaucoma is a medical emergency that progresses quickly and, if left untreated, causes blindness within hours.

Signs and Symptoms

- Acute eye pain
- Decreased peripheral vision
- Halo around lights
- Nausea and vomiting
- Severe headache
- Reddened eye
- Fixed or slightly dilated pupil
- Cornea with foggy appearance
- Globe may feel very firm

Diagnostic Procedures

- Elevated intraocular pressure

Therapeutic Interventions

- Therapy focuses on facilitating drainage of aqueous humor and decreasing intraocular pressure.
- Topical miotic eye drops such as pilocarpine (Isopto Carpine) increase outflow of aqueous humor.
- Topical beta-blockers such as timolol maleate (Timoptic) decrease aqueous humor production.
- Carbonic anhydrase inhibitors such as acetazolamide (Diamox) also decrease aqueous humor production.
- Antiemetic to control nausea and vomiting.
- Narcotics for pain control.
- Instruct patient in ways to avoid increasing intraocular pressure:
  - Do not have head lower than waist.
  - Avoid coughing and straining.
  - Do not lift more than 5 pounds.
- Stress the need for ophthalmic follow-up.
- If medical management is unsuccessful in lowering intraocular pressure within the first few hours, laser surgery will need to be performed to penetrate the anterior chamber and drain aqueous humor.

REFERENCES

1. Bhatia, K., & Sharma, R. (2008). Eye emergencies. In J. G. Adams (Ed.), *Emergency medicine*. Philadelphia, PA: Saunders Elsevier.
2. Egging, D. (2010). Ocular emergencies. In P. K. Howard & R. A. Steinmann (Eds.), *Sheehy's emergency nursing: Principles and practice* (6th ed., pp. 602–618). St. Louis, MO: Mosby Elsevier.
3. Tsang, K., & Sinert, R. H. (2011, May 4). *Iritis and uveitis.* Retrieved from http://emedicine.medscape.com/article/798323-overview
4. Kaufman, D. V., Galbraith, J. K., & Wallane, M. J. (2009). Ocular emergencies. In P. Cameron, G. Jelinek, A. Kelly, L. Murray & A. F. T. Brown (Eds.), *Textbook of adult emergency medicine* (3rd ed., pp. 568–575). Edinburgh, United Kingdom: Churchill Livingstone.

Abdominal Pain and Emergencies

Lisa Wolf and Polly Gerber Zimmermann

Abdominal pain is present in about 6% of approximately 100 million emergency department visits and is one of the most common chief complaints.[1] Although most abdominal pain is benign, as many as 10% of patients in the emergency department setting have a severe or life-threatening cause of abdominal pain or require surgery.[2]

Abdominal pain is categorized as visceral, parietal, or referred. The gastrointestinal (GI) tract contains both visceral and parietal pain receptors. The visceral receptors are located throughout the abdomen, while the parietal pain receptors are located in the peritoneum. Irritation of the somatic or parietal receptors causes more localized, sharper pain.

> Visceral pain replaced by somatic pain often signals need for a surgical intervention.[3]

Pain can further be reduced to intra-abdominal or extra-abdominal; causes of abdominal pain can be classified as GI, genitourinary, cardiac, pulmonary, or neurogenic (Table 28-1). Because initial determination of pain etiology is frequently not possible, the patient presenting with abdominal complaints should be treated as urgent or emergent until proven otherwise. Initial treatment should be directed toward identifying and treating the cause of the pain.

INITIAL EVALUATION

History
- Focus on the patient's pain history. The location of pain should drive the evaluation; also ask about pain radiation and the effect of movement or change in body position on the pain.[2] Pain preceding vomiting (as compared to vomiting before pain) and severe pain lasting 6 or more hours are more likely associated with a surgical condition.

Other considerations[3]:
- Anorexia, nausea, and vomiting are directly proportional to the severity and extent of peritoneal irritation.
- Colic—sharp localized abdominal pain that increases, peaks, and subsides—may indicate a class of diseases of hollow viscera contracting related to a calculi, obstruction, etc.
- Determine the date of last bowel movement especially in the elderly and post-operative patient.
- Determine positive past medical history of abdominal surgery and infectious illnesses.

> In the patient with abdominal pain, hypovolemia should always be considered if the patient's heart rate is greater than 130 beats per minute, especially in the presence of anorexia, nausea, or vomiting.

Physical Assessment
Vital Signs
Out-of-range vital signs may be indicators of pain but, more importantly, can give insight into possible processes such as the following:
- Tachycardia and relative hypotension can be indicators of volume depletion or sepsis. These responses can be blunted in the elderly and in those on beta-blockers.
- Tachypnea and decreased oxygen saturation can indicate an acute infectious process.
- Fever suggests infection but its absence does not rule it out, especially in the elderly and in the immunosuppressed.

Respiratory and Cardiac Assessment
- This assessment should be noted particularly in patients with upper abdominal pain because they could suggest pneumonia or cardiac ischemia.

TABLE 28-1	ABDOMINAL PAIN PATTERNS AND POSSIBLE ETIOLOGIES	
Diffuse Pain • Acute gastroenteritis • Sickle cell crisis • DKA • Peritonitis • IBS • Intestinal obstruction • Constipation	**Epigastric Pain** • Acute gastroenteritis • PUD • GERD • AAA • Early perforated viscus • Acute pancreatitis • Acute MI	**Left Upper Quadrant** • Gastritis or PUD • Left lower lobe pneumonia • Splenic infarct or rupture • Splenic enlargement: mononucleosis or leukemia • Left renal colic or pyelonephritis • Herpes zoster
Left Lower Quadrant • Ovarian torsion or cyst rupture • PID or salpingitis • Inguinal hernia • Diverticulitis • Ruptured ectopic or mittelschmerz	**Right Upper Quadrant** • Hepatitis or biliary tract disease or abscess • Right lower lobe pneumonia • Right pyelonephritis or colic • Herpes zoster • Hepatomegaly	**Right Lower Quadrant** • Inguinal hernia • Acute appendix • Ovarian torsion, cyst, or mittelschmerz • Ruptured ectopic • PID, tubo-ovarian abscess, or salpingitis • Mesenteric adenitis or Meckel's diverticulitis

AAA, Abdominal aortic aneurysm; *DKA,* diabetic ketoacidosis; *GERD,* gastroesophageal reflux disease; *IBS,* irritable bowel syndrome; *MI,* myocardial infarction; *PID,* pelvic inflammatory disease; *PUD,* peptic ulcer disease.

Abdominal Assessment[4,5]

- Inspection: Consider the patient's facial expression, use of abdominal muscles, position of comfort, and body movement during the examination for cues as to location, intensity, and possible etiology of pain.
- Auscultation: Auscultate the abdomen in all four quadrants for the presence, frequency, and character of bowel sounds. Normal bowel sounds are 5 to 35 clicks or gurgles per minute. Listen for bruits over the abdominal aorta and the renal, iliac, and inguinal arteries. The best indicator of peristalsis is the ability to pass flatus.
- Percussion: Percuss for liver and splenic borders. The liver edge should be soft, distinct, and even with the right costal margin. Assess for normal tympany over hollow organs and normal dullness over solid organs.
- Palpation: Palpate for rigidity, guarding, pain, rebound, masses, and hernias.

Position[4]

- A patient comfortably moving in the bed is less likely to have a serious etiology.
- A patient laying rigidly still or in the fetal position is classic of peritonitis; these positions are assumed by the patient to avoid peritoneal irritation.

Diagnostic Procedures

- Basic laboratory procedures, including complete blood count (CBC) and complete metabolic panel, are routinely ordered. Simultaneous amylase and lipase measurements are recommended in patients with epigastric pain.[2]

- The American College of Radiology recommends ultrasonography to assess right upper quadrant pain[6] and computed tomography (CT) to assess right and left lower quadrant pain.[7,8] These should also be considered in special populations, such as the elderly, who may present with atypical symptoms ("the atypical is typical in the elderly").

Symptoms with abdominal pain that are suggestive of surgical or emergent conditions include[2]:
- Fever
- Protracted vomiting
- Syncope or presyncope
- Evidence of GI blood loss

SPECIFIC ABDOMINAL EMERGENCIES

Peritonitis[4,5]

Primary peritonitis occurs when blood-borne organisms enter the peritoneal cavity. Secondary peritonitis, a much more common occurrence, results when abdominal organs perforate and release their contents (bile, enzymes, bacteria) into the peritoneal cavity. An initial chemical peritonitis is followed by bacterial peritonitis a few hours later. Possible causes include the following:
- Ruptured appendix
- Pancreatitis
- Trauma from a gunshot or knife wound
- Peritoneal dialysis

Signs and Symptoms

- Evidence of hypovolemic shock because of a massive fluid shift into the peritoneum.
- Tenderness over the involved area. However, if perforation exists, the patient can feel temporary relief from the release of the pressure, followed by a return of significant, generalized pain.
- "Guarding," or protection of the area by positioning, or refusing to allow examination of the area.
- Rigid, "boardlike" abdomen (muscles spasm from the irritation).

Diagnostic Procedures

For all conditions, a history, physical assessment, and general laboratory work (CBC, electrolytes) are routinely prescribed. In addition to the routine diagnostic procedures, physical assessments include the following:

- Positive rebound tenderness: Apply deep palpation pressure. Pain is worse when released because of the irritation of the perineum.
- Heel drop (Markle test): Patient stands, rises on tiptoes with knees straight, and forcibly drops down on both heels to test for generalized peritoneal irritation. An alternative is to have the patient hop on one leg. When the patient is in severe discomfort, the same assessment can be made by firmly striking the supine patient's heel to cause jarring in the peritoneum.

Therapeutic Interventions

Acute abdominal conditions require standard treatment:

- Keep patient nothing by mouth (NPO), insert nasogastric tube (NGT), and initiate bowel rest
- Obtain intravenous (IV) access and replace fluid and electrolytes as indicated
- Administer analgesics, antiemetics, and antibiotics as prescribed
- Anticipate surgical intervention

Acute Gastroenteritis[7,8]

Acute gastroenteritis can be bacterial, viral, or chemical in origin. The patient may present with dehydration; the very young or the elderly may experience hypovolemia.

Signs and Symptoms

- Diarrhea with nausea and vomiting.
- Pain is usually characterized as diffuse, sometimes crampy, lower abdominal pain.
- Fever.
- Signs of dehydration such as tachycardia and warm, dry skin.

- Splenomegaly may be noted, indicating gastroenteritis of bacterial origin.
- Ask about similar symptoms in family members or others who ate the same food to rule out food poisoning. Inquire about recent travel to an underdeveloped country where the patient might have contracted an intestinal parasite.

Diagnostic Procedures

- Ova and parasite testing for stool as appropriate.
- Electrocardiogram is recommended for women, patients with diabetes, and the elderly as nausea and vomiting can be indicative of a cardiac event.
- Digoxin (Lanoxin) levels in the elderly population on this drug. Digoxin is excreted by the kidney, which decreases function by 1% every year of life after age 30 years. Early signs of toxicity are nausea and vomiting.
- Rule out appendicitis, as the conditions can imitate each other. See "Appendicitis" below.
- Differentiate from gastritis (left upper quadrant or epigastric pain or tenderness), which is a gastric mucosa irritation most commonly caused by smoking, alcohol, or medications.

Therapeutic Interventions

- Establish IV access to replace fluid and electrolytes as indicated.
- Administer antiemetics.
- Facilitate pain control if needed.
- Most gastroenteritis is self-limiting. The patient should be NPO until vomiting has ceased. As soon as tolerated, encourage oral intake of fluids with glucose and electrolytes (e.g., Pedialyte).

Appendicitis[1,2,9,10]

Appendicitis occurs when an obstruction of the appendiceal lumen results in a decrease in blood supply which, if left untreated, may progress to necrosis, perforation, and peritonitis.

Appendicitis is the most common surgical cause of abdominal pain. Overall, 7% of the population will be affected over their lifetime. One to three percent of emergency department visits for abdominal pain are appendicitis.[1] It is most commonly found in males between the ages of 10 and 30 years. The elderly and children are more likely to have atypical presentations.

Signs and Symptoms

- The classic presentation of appendicitis is a mild fever with dull steady periumbilical pain, anorexia, and nausea.
  - Over the course of 12 to 48 hours, the pain typically moves to the right lower quadrant at McBurney's

point, the point on the lower abdomen that lies between the umbilicus and the right superior iliac spine.

- Anorexia; nausea and vomiting.
- Psoas sign may be present 6% to 30% of the time.
  - To assess for the psoas sign, the nurse passively extends the right thigh of a patient lying on his or her side with knees extended or asks the patient to actively flex his or her right thigh at the hip. If right lower quadrant abdominal pain results, it is a "positive" psoas sign.
  - Pain results because the psoas muscle borders the peritoneal cavity and moving it causes friction against the nearby inflamed tissues.
- Rebound tenderness.
- Abdominal rigidity.

Diagnostic Procedures[2,5]

Appendicitis can be difficult to diagnose, as the patient presents at various points in the protracted course or can be an atypical presentation. Misdiagnosis occurs with a frequency of 20% to 40% in some populations.[1]

- CBC to detect leukocytosis ("shift to the left")[11]: One study of patients 15 to 83 years of age with suspected appendicitis found that a white blood cell count greater than 10,000/mm^3 was 77% sensitive and 63% specific for the diagnosis. The white blood cell count is normal in 10% to 30% of patients with appendicitis.[1]
- Urinalysis and a pregnancy test are routine.
- Imaging: CT with contrast is recommended by the current literature (70% to 94%) over ultrasonography for diagnosing appendicitis and can detect extracolonic causes of abdominal pain. It has a sensitivity of 92% to 98% and is specifically recommended for men with atypical presentation and for women in whom pelvic pathology may mimic appendicitis.

Therapeutic Interventions

- Keep patient NPO
- Perform frequent abdominal reassessment
- Obtain IV access and initiate fluid volume replacement
- Administer parenteral analgesics and antiemetics as needed
- Administer broad spectrum IV antibiotics
- Prepare patient for probable surgical intervention

In appendicitis, vomiting generally does not precede the abdominal pain. This is an important due to delineate appendicitis pain from gastroenteritis or some other etiology.[3]

Gastroesophageal Reflux Disease and Esophagitis[5,12]

Gastroesophageal reflux disease (GERD) occurs when the reflux of gastric secretions back into the esophagus causes symptoms; there may be associated esophageal mucosal injury or esophagitis.[13] Esophagitis also may result from infections, radiation, or the ingestion of a caustic substance such as a strong acid or alkali.

Signs and Symptoms

- Steady, substernal pain that increases with swallowing, may be positional, worsening when the patient is supine
  - Discomfort of "heartburn" often mimics that of myocardial ischemia both in radiation and intensity
- Occasional vomiting
- Weight loss
- Sore throat, raspy voice
- Episodes of upper GI bleeding

Diagnostic Procedures

- Diagnosis is made mainly by history and physical assessment.

Therapeutic Interventions

- Assess airway and breathing (inflammatory response to an insult can cause compromise and can be a trigger for asthma or sleep apnea).
- Lifestyle modifications such as weight loss, avoiding foods that relax the lower esophageal sphincter, such as alcohol, chocolate, coffee, fatty foods, and eliminating smoking.[13]
- Home measures to minimize reflux include elevating the head of the bed (e.g., 4 to 6 inches) and avoiding large volumes of food or drink, especially before bedtime.
- The "GI cocktail" (a mixture of a liquid antacid, viscous lidocaine, and an anticholinergic such as Donnatal elixir), 30 mL orally, may be the initial intervention.
- Medications including antacids, proton pump inhibitors (PPI), or histamine (H$_2$) blockers.
  - PPIs include:
    - Omeprazole (Prilosec)
    - Lansoprazole (Prevacid)
    - Esomeprazole (Nexium)
  - H$_2$ blockers include:
    - Ranitidine (Zantac)
    - Cimetidine (Tagamet)
    - Famotidine (Pepcid)

Upper Gastrointestinal Bleeding

Upper GI bleeding is a potentially life-threatening condition. The most common causes of nonvariceal upper GI bleeding are duodenal and gastric ulcers (50%), gastric erosions (30%), Mallory-Weiss syndrome (10%), and esophagitis.[14] The frequent use of non-steroidal anti-inflammatory drugs puts patients at risk for upper GI bleeding as does the presence of esophageal varices.

Comorbid illnesses are present in 98.3% of the patients who die with upper GI bleeding; it is these comorbid conditions that are the primary cause of death rather than the bleeding.[15]

Signs and Symptoms[14]

- Hematemesis or melena (31% to 69%) may be the only symptom.
  - "Coffee-ground" emesis is a specific finding for the patient with upper GI bleeding
- Weakness, dizziness, syncope
- Postural hypotension
- Possible signs of hypovolemic shock (tachycardia, hypotension, prolonged capillary refill time)

Diagnostic Procedures

- CBC and serial hemoglobin levels.
- Basic metabolic panel (BMP).
- Coagulation panel including PT, aPTT, INR, and platelet count.
- Type and crossmatch in anticipation of transfusion with packed red blood cells.
- CT or GI bleeding scan if necessary.
- Endoscopy to identify site of bleeding.

Therapeutic Interventions

- Airway management may require endotracheal intubation in the actively hemorrhaging patient
- Obtain IV access with large-bore catheter and begin volume replacement. See Chapter 20, Shock, for further discussion of the management of a patient with hemorrhagic hypovolemic shock.
- Place NGT to empty and decompress the stomach, and to identify characteristics of the aspirate (bright red blood or "coffee ground" material)
- Lavage with iced or room temperature saline is no longer recommended as it may lyse clots and contribute to further bleeding.[11]
- Blood transfusion may be initiated in a patient whose hemoglobin level is less than 7 g/dL.[16]
- H_2 blockers, somatostatin and octreotide are not routinely used for actively bleeding patients.[16]
- Anticipate endoscopic therapy to control bleeding site.

Peptic Ulcer Disease[2,9]

Peptic ulcer disease (PUD) is characterized by a circumscribed area of mucosal inflammation and ulceration. There are three types of ulcers related to PUD: duodenal, gastric, and stress ulcers. Peptic ulcers are generally the result of a disruption of protective mucosal barriers and increased acid secretion. Common contributing factors include the use of nonsteroidal anti-inflammatory drugs (NSAIDs) or infection with *Helicobacter pylori* (present in 75% to 95% of duodenal ulcers and 65% to 95% of gastric ulcers).

Duodenal ulcers, the most common type of PUD, are characterized by increased parietal cells, which results in increased acid and gastrin production. The patient has a rapid gastric emptying time and pain occurs when the stomach is empty. The pain is typically relieved with food or antacids; therefore it is critical to ask the patient if he or she has pain before or after eating to differentiate duodenal ulcers from other types. Duodenal ulcers heal spontaneously and recur frequently, so asking the patient about similar episodes can yield a probable etiology more quickly.

Gastric ulcers usually occur in the antrum near parietal cells and tend to become chronic. The hallmark of this problem is complaints of pain after eating, and patients may present with some weight loss. The patient with a history of gastric ulcers may be at higher risk for gastric cancer.

Stress ulcers generally result from ischemic stress and tend to develop after a prolonged period of physical stress, such as a severe illness, trauma, or neural injury. The stress response shunts blood away from the gastric mucosa, causing ischemia and mucosal damage that result in ulceration of the gastric mucosa. This type of ulcer is most often seen in the intensive care unit rather than in the emergency department, but a patient with a recent history of severe illness or stress may present with this type of ulcer.

Signs and Symptoms

- Concurrent, episodic gnawing or burning pain
- Pain relieved or exacerbated by food
- Pain often accompanied by feelings of fullness or bloating
- Pain may awaken patient during the night
- History of frequent NSAID or low-dose aspirin use
- Upper GI bleeding may be the initial manifestation of PUP

Diagnostic Procedures

- Routine laboratory tests are not helpful
- Non-invasive tests for *H. pylori* infection include fecal antigen and urea breath testing

Therapeutic Interventions

Most stable patients with PUD are treated on an outpatient basis with a combination of acid-inhibiting drugs and antibiotics.

- Standard dose H_2 blockers or proton pump inhibitors to promote healing of the ulcer.
- If patient is positive for *H. pylori*, a course of antibiotics such as clarithromycin and amoxicillin is recommended.
- NSAID use must be discontinued.

Mallory-Weiss Syndrome[12,14]

Mallory-Weiss syndrome is the result of violent retching and vomiting that is not synchronized with gastric regurgitation. Persistent retching causes a longitudinal mucosal tear at the gastroesophageal junction (the gastric cardia).[17]

Signs and Symptoms

- History of retching or vomiting of normal stomach contents (31% to 69%), followed by hematemesis (70% to 94%).
- May also have a history of alcohol consumption (6% to 30%), aspirin use, heavy lifting, coughing, bulimia, or pregnancy.
- Red or "coffee-ground" hematemesis (with or without melena). The volume of hematemesis is a poor guide for estimating volume loss.
- Hematochezia (maroon-colored stool) may be present.

Diagnostic Procedures

- An NGT for aspirate may be used to assess for occult blood.
- Upper GI endoscopy is often used for diagnosis if bleeding is active.
- Additional laboratory studies as indicated in "Upper Gastrointestinal Bleeding" section

Therapeutic Interventions

- Obtain IV access and administer antiemetic drugs as needed.
- Prepare patient for endoscopy to cauterize or repair bleeding vessels.
- Balloon tamponade should be avoided unless other efforts have failed or are not available.
- Refer to "Therapeutic Interventions" for patient experiencing upper GI bleeding.

Bleeding Esophageal Varices[3,5]

The portal vein drains approximately 1500 mL/min of blood from the intestines, spleen, and stomach to the liver. Obstruction to this venous flow (often from liver disease or cirrhosis) increases portal venous pressure and causes collateral vessels to form between the stomach and the systemic veins of the lower esophagus. These extremely dilated sub-mucosal veins (esophageal varices) can rupture and are a leading cause of death in more than one third of cirrhotic patients.

Signs and Symptoms

- The patient may have a history of liver disease (cirrhosis), portal hypertension, or chronic alcohol intake.
- Signs of upper GI bleeding and hypovolemic shock. (See "Upper Gastrointestinal Bleeding.")

Diagnostic Procedures

Laboratory tests include the following:
- Coagulation panel
- Hepatic function studies

Imaging studies include the following:
- Upper GI endoscopy
- Abdominal ultrasound or CT scan

Therapeutic Interventions

Therapeutic treatment focuses on the management of bleeding and hemorrhagic hypovolemic shock, including airway management, oxygen administration, and initiation of large-bore IV access and fluid replacement.

- NGT insertion has a risk of inadvertent esophageal rupture and hemorrhage and must be undertaken cautiously.
- Pharmacological therapy using somatostatin or octreotide (to decrease portal pressure by relaxing mesenteric vascular smooth muscle) *or* a combination of IV vasopressin and sublingual or transdermal nitroglycerin intravenously.
- Endoscopic injection sclerotherapy.
- Direct pressure through balloon tamponade is used only after pharmacological therapy or endoscopic have failed. Options include a Sengstaken-Blakemore tube (triple lumen, double balloon), Minnesota tube (quadruple lumen), or Linton-Nachlas tube (greater gastric balloon and a port to drain the esophagus).

Cholecystitis[5,9]

Cholecystitis is an acute or chronic inflammation of the gallbladder, usually resulting from an impacted stone in the neck of the gallbladder or in the cystic duct (90% to 95%). Symptoms are usually secondary to obstruction of the flow of bile.

The classical example of a patient at risk for cholecystitis is referred to as the "6 F's":
- Fat
- Female
- Forties
- Fertile
- Fair (higher frequency in Caucasians)
- Flatulent

Pregnant woman are also at a greater risk for developing cholecystitis.

Signs and Symptoms[2,9,18]

- Right upper quadrant pain (70% to 94%) that can radiate to the back, or right shoulder or scapula, particularly after consuming a meal with high fat content.
  - Pain may initially be colicky but will become constant.
- Positive Murphy sign (62%): pause of inspiration (gasp) during palpation beneath right costal arch below hepatic margin, which occurs because the fingertips have touched an enlarged gallbladder.[3]
- Signs of infection or inflammation (37%), including a low-grade fever and tachycardia.
- Jaundice (25%) if obstruction is significant.
- GI upset: nausea and vomiting (31% to 69%), anorexia, eructation, flatulence, or fat intolerance.

Diagnostic Procedures[9]

- Routine laboratory studies which may reveal the following:
  - Leukocytosis
  - Elevated bilirubin level
  - Increased ALT and AST
- Pregnancy test should be performed in women of childbearing age
- Ultrasound is sensitive in identifying stones (70% to 94%). It is quick, noninvasive, and readily available.
- Radionuclide cholescintigraphy (also known as a hepatobiliary iminodiacetic acid, or HIDA, scan) is the most sensitive and specific diagnostic procedure available to rule out cholecystitis and common bile duct obstruction.
- Other imaging studies include abdominal CT scan, cholangiogram, cholecystogram, endoscopic retrograde cholangiopancreatography (ERCP), and flat and upright radiographs.

Therapeutic Interventions

- Keep patient NPO. Some patients may require insertion of a NG tube with suction because of vomiting and pain.

- Obtain IV access for rehydration and correction of electrolyte imbalances.
- Administer antiemetics and analgesics as needed.
- Administer broad-spectrum antibiotics because of the potential for gangrene and perforation.
- Anticipate possible surgical or endoscopic intervention.

Pancreatitis[5,8,9]

Pancreatitis results from release of digestive pancreatic enzymes into the tissue of the pancreas, with autodigestion, inflammation, tissue destruction, and injury to adjacent structures and organs. Acute pancreatitis usually is caused by excessive ethanol ingestion or by a gallstone that blocks the pancreatic duct, trapping digestive enzymes in the pancreas. Other etiologies include recent surgery or ERCP, viral illness, trauma, or hypertriglyceridemia. Approximately 15% are idiopathic.

Acute pancreatitis can resolve spontaneously or progress to a severe, life-threatening condition. Of the approximately 80,000 cases of pancreatitis that occur in the United States each year, about 20% are considered severe.

Chronic pancreatitis occurs when digestive enzymes slowly destroy the pancreas and surrounding tissues, generally following years of alcohol abuse. This results in an inability to digest fats, proteins, and carbohydrates properly. Insulin production also is affected, causing hyperglycemia. Hemorrhagic pancreatitis is an emergent condition in which digestive enzymes have eroded through a major abdominal vessel.

Signs and Symptoms[9]

- Sudden onset of pain that gradually increases in severity
  - Pain described as dull and steady.
  - Located in left upper abdomen or epigastum.
  - Because of the pancreas's retroperitoneal location, pain may radiate through abdomen to back.
  - Pain may lessen when patient is in sitting or fetal position.
- Abdominal tenderness and guarding
- Nausea, vomiting, anorexia
- Fever and tachycardia
- In severe cases, hypovolemia (up to 6 L can be third-spaced; up to 30% can have renal failure) and sepsis may result

Diagnostic Procedures

- Serum amylase and lipase follow a classic pattern. Amylase rises quickly but returns to normal 24 to 72 hours later. Serum lipase rises more slowly but is detected in the bloodstream up to 2 weeks later. (Urine amylase is detected for up to 2 weeks.) Lipase is an important diagnostic procedure, as other disorders can cause a rise in amylase.

- Other laboratory tests include electrolytes (including calcium and magnesium), CBC, hepatic profile, and blood glucose.
- A contrast-enhanced CT abdominal scan is considered the best imaging study, but usually is not ordered in the emergency department.
- Ultrasound can view the biliary tract but is often unable to visualize the pancreas.
- Abdominal series may be used to check for free air and perforation.

Therapeutic Interventions

- Obtain IV access for fluid resuscitation and medication administration.
- Pain management with IV meperidine (Demerol) as morphine can cause spasms in the sphincter of Oddi.
- Administer antiemetics as needed.
- Replace serum calcium with IV infusion as indicated.
- Frequent patient reassessment is needed to detect complications related to breathing, blood glucose levels, hypocalcemia, and sepsis.
- IV antibiotics may be administered if patient develops pancreatic abscess or sepsis.

Intestinal Obstruction

Intestinal obstructions are caused by a variety of conditions, including the following[10]:
- Physical obstructions, such as fecal impaction, hernias, tumors, intussusceptions, volvulus, and incarcerated hernias. In developed countries, approximately 50% to 70% of all small bowel obstructions are caused by post-operative adhesions.
- Nervous system disorder (paralytic ileus).
- Inflammatory conditions (abscess, pancreatitis causing an ileus, inflammatory bowel disease).

Following intestinal obstruction, the accumulation of GI secretions and swallowed air lead to intestinal distention, increased intraluminal pressure, and massive third spacing of fluid.

Signs and Symptoms[2,9]

- History of previous abdominal surgery (47%), particularly appendectomy.
- Abdominal pain (95% to 100%), often colic in nature (48%). The pain may be crampy and "wavelike."
- Nausea and vomiting (70% to 94%): Patients with small bowel obstructions usually vomit stomach contents, then bile, then copious feculent material. Pain usually decreases after vomiting (60%).

- Tachycardia and hypotension
- Abdomen distension and tenderness (70% to 94%).
- No flatus (obstipation) or stool passage (75%), despite feeling the need.
- Bowel sounds can have high-pitched, hyperactive sounds immediately proximal to the obstruction, with hypoactive or absent bowel sounds distal to the obstruction.

Diagnostic Procedures[9]

- Routine serum chemistries.
  - Elevated white blood cells
  - An elevated blood urea nitrogen may be result of dehydration
- Abdominal radiography, supine or flat and upright views, to detect air/fluid levels and dilated small bowel loops. However, early in the process of the condition the results can be negative.
- CT has a high sensitivity and specificity in complete small bowel obstruction.

Therapeutic Interventions

- The immediate complication of intestinal obstruction is dehydration from third-spacing. Other potential complications include bowel infarction and possible perforation, and infection, particularly sepsis.[6]
- Aggressive fluid resuscitation is necessary to prevent hypovolemic shock.
- Bowel decompression with NGT suction.
- Administer analgesics, antiemetics, and possibly IV antibiotics.
- Surgical consultation.

Incarcerated Hernia

A hernia is the protrusion of a bowel loop (or other abdominal contents) through the abdominal musculature, but not through the skin. Hernias most commonly are found in the inguinal, femoral, and umbilical regions. If the blood supply to the hernia is good, no urgent care is required. If the hernia becomes incarcerated or trapped, blood supply is compromised; this is a medical emergency.

Inguinal hernias occur in 1% to 4% of children; approximately 10% of these become incarcerated hernias. The male to female ratio of hernia occurrence is 4:1 but the incarceration rate is higher in girls.[19]

Signs and Symptoms

- Pain and swelling at the site of herniation.
- Inguinal hernias are typically noted as firm, tender masses in the inguinal canal and superior scrotum, typically ipsilateral.

- Nausea and vomiting.
- Possible signs of intestinal obstruction.

Diagnostic Procedures

- Diagnosis is usually based on physical examination.
- CBC should be obtained but results are usually nonspecific.
- Abdominal radiographs can be used to rule out intestinal obstruction.
- Ultrasonography to help detect strangulation.

Therapeutic Interventions

- Anticipate manual reduction of hernia.
  - Provide adequate sedation and analgesia prior to attempt at reduction.
  - Ice packs to hernia and Trendelenburg positioning may be used 20 to 30 minutes prior to reduction.
- Surgical consultation may be necessary.

Lower Gastrointestinal Bleeding[5,9,14]

Lower GI bleeding refers to blood loss originating distal to the ligament of Treitz. It occurs less frequently and generally has a less severe course than upper GI bleeding; many lower GI bleeds stop spontaneously. Bleeding from the large bowel or rectum usually is caused by inflammatory bowel disease, bleeding polyps or ulcers, cancer, hemorrhoids, perirectal abscess, or diverticulosis.

Signs and Symptoms

- Bleeding is usually modest, but may be severe and life-threatening.
- Rectal bleeding is usually bright red (hematochezia) and may contain clots; darker blood indicates the source of bleeding is higher up in the bowel.
- Bleeding is usually painless.
- Pallor, fatigue, postural changes, syncope, tachycardia.
- With extensive blood loss, the patient may exhibit signs of hemodynamic instability.
- Hypotension is a late sign (typically after 1500 mL blood loss); tachycardia can be an earlier sign.

Diagnostic Procedures

- History of anticoagulant use
- CBC, coagulation panel
- Stool specimen for occult blood
- Colonoscopic examination can be both diagnostic and therapeutic.

> Occult GI bleeding from GI cancer should be considered in a patient age 50 years or older with anemia.

Therapeutic Interventions

- The hemodynamically unstable patient will require aggressive resuscitation for hypovolemic shock (see Chapter 20, Shock).
- Reverse any coagulopathies.
- Colonoscopy may involve thermal coagulation or vasoconstrictor or sclerosing agents.

Irritable Bowel Syndrome[4,5]

Irritable bowel syndrome (IBS) is characterized by abdominal pain and altered bowel function without structural or biochemical abnormalities; it may be a diagnosis of exclusion. IBS has three components: altered GI motility, visceral hyperanalgesia, and psychopatholgy.[20]

Recent theories suggest that IBS may be undiagnosed celiac disease (gluten-sensitive enteropathy, celiac sprue), a sensitivity to the gluten in grain (barley, rye, oats, wheat), or related to enteric infections.

Signs and Symptoms

- Abdominal pain in association with changes in bowel habits (constipation, diarrhea, or both)
  - Pain is usually in the lower abdomen (although location and intensity vary)
  - Pain may be described as crampy or as a generalized ache with superimposed periods of abdominal cramps
  - Pain and abdominal discomfort may be relieved with a bowel movement
- Anxiety or psychological stress may be a factor
- Weight loss if diarrhea is a predominant symptom

Diagnostic Procedures

- CBC to detect anemia, erythrocyte sedimentation rate (ESR), complete metabolic panel.
- Stool for occult blood, ova and parasites, and enteric pathogens including *Clostridium difficile*.
- Abdominal CT scan to rule out other problems such as tumors or intestinal obstruction.
- Colonoscopy often prescribed to rule out more serious etiologies.

Therapeutic Interventions

Therapeutic treatments include the following:
- Symptom-targeted medications such as analgesics, antidiarrheals, anticholinergics, prokinetics, and antidepressants.
- Psychiatric or psychological referral.
- Peppermint is a "natural" aid, as it works like a calcium channel blocker to relax smooth muscles.

- Dietary modifications include:
  - Adding more bulk to aid regular peristalsis.
  - Avoid fluids with meals, as this tends to cause abdominal distension.
  - Limit or avoid lactose, fructose, or gluten if these are problematic for the patient.
  - If constipation is a predominant symptom, increase daily fluid intake.

Inflammatory Bowel Disease

Inflammatory bowel disease refers to disorders in which the intestines become inflamed probably as a result of an autoimmune reaction. The two major types of inflammatory bowel disease are ulcerative colitis and Crohn's disease; both disorders are characterized by exacerbations and remissions and are chronic conditions with significant emotional and social impact.[5,8] Ulcerative colitis involves the large colon while Crohn's disease can affect any part of the GI tract from the mouth to the anus.

Signs and Symptoms[21]

The signs and symptoms of ulcerative colitis and Crohn's disease are compared in Table 28-2.

Diagnostic Procedures

- Routine laboratory tests including CBC and complete metabolic panel to rule out other diagnoses.
- Serum albumin as an indicator of nutritional status.

TABLE 28-2	**SIGNS AND SYMPTOMS OF ULCERATIVE COLITIS AND CROHN'S DISEASE**
ULCERATIVE COLITIS	**CROHN'S DISEASE**

• Bloody stool
• Severe diarrhea, cramps, and dehydration in severe disease
• Left lower quadrant tenderness
• Abdominal distention
• Fever and tachycardia
• Weight loss
	• Abdominal pain
	  • Crampy or steady
	  • Periumbilical or right lower quadrant
	• Intermittent low grade fever
	• Weight loss
	• Signs of intestinal obstruction
	• Associated anal fissures, perianal fistulae, or abscesses

Data from Basson, M. D. (2011, May 25). *Ulcerative colitis.* Retrieved from http://emedicine.medscape.com/article/183084-overview; Rangasamy, P. (2011, June 16). *Crohn disease.* Retrieved from http://emedicine.medscape.com/article/172940-overview/

- Definitive diagnosis is made by endoscopic examination.
- Abdominal radiographs may demonstrate colonic dilatation, evidence of perforation, or obstruction.

Therapeutic Interventions

- Initial management includes bowel rest with IV rehydration.
- Corticosteroids and anti-inflammatory and anti-diarrheal agents are mainstays of medical management.
- Crohn's disease is also managed with immunosuppression or infliximab (Remicade), a drug to block the body's inflammatory response.
- Surgery may be considered if medical management fails
  - Because ulcerative colitis is confined to the colon, surgery can be curative.
  - Surgery for Crohn's disease is most commonly required for complications such as strictures, fistulae, or bleeding; surgery is non-curative in Crohn's disease.

Diverticulitis[9]

Diverticula are small outpouchings anywhere in the GI tract, most commonly in the sigmoid colon. *Diverticulosis* refers to the presence of un-inflamed diverticula and is thought to be associated with a low-fiber diet, constipation, and obesity. *Diverticulitis* is defined as inflammation of one or more diverticula. This inflammation, and subsequent focal necrosis and perforation, may be the result of obstruction of the diverticula by fecal material or undigested food.[22]

Diverticulosis occurs in 50% of people over 70 years of age and in up to 80% of those over 80 years old.[22] Approximately 25% of persons with diverticulosis will have an episode of acute diverticulitis.

Signs and Symptoms

- Left lower quadrant abdominal pain and tenderness (70% to 94%), often referred to as "left-sided appendicitis"
- Anorexia, nausea, vomiting
- Possible change in bowel habits (constipation or diarrhea)
- Fever and signs of peritonitis if perforation

Diagnostic Procedures

- Diagnosis is based on history and clinical presentation.
- CBC with differential may indicate leukocytosis if infection is present.
- BMP to determine electrolyte imbalances.
- CT scan or abdominal radiographs may indicated.

Therapeutic Interventions

- Mild symptoms can be managed on an out-patient basis with clear liquid diet and broad spectrum antibiotics.
- IV fluids for rehydration as needed.
- Hospitalization and aggressive management will be necessary if infection or peritonitis is present. See "Peritonitis."

Esophageal Obstruction

The most common cause of esophageal obstruction in children is an ingested foreign body. Obstruction in adults is usually because of a bone or food bolus.

Signs and Symptoms

- Patient complains of "something stuck" in the throat
- History of foreign body ingestion, especially if the patient is a child, may not exist
- Difficulty swallowing
- Drooling
- Subcutaneous emphysema of the neck may be present if esophageal perforation has occurred

Diagnostic Procedures

- Chest and neck radiographs may be performed.

Therapeutic Interventions

Airway compromise is a major concern
- IV administration of glucagon to relax the smooth muscle and allow for passage of the object.
- Appropriate upright positioning of the patient to facilitate passage of the object.
- Esophagoscopy to remove the object.
- If the object does not have sharp edges and can pass into the stomach, it usually proceeds through the intestines without difficulty.

REFERENCES

1. Adams, J. G. (2003, June). Missed appendicitis. *Web M&M: Morbidity & Mortality Rounds on the Web*. Retrieved from http://www.webmm.ahrq.gov/case.aspx?caseID=17
2. Cartwright, S. L., & Knudson, M. P. (2008). Evaluation of acute abdominal pain in adults. *American Family Physician, 77*(7), 971–978.
3. McPheeters, R. A., & Purcell, T. B. (2006). Abdominal pain. In V. J. Markovchick & P. T. Pons (Eds.), *Emergency medicine secrets* (4th ed.). St. Louis, MO: Mosby.
4. Zimmermann, P. G., & Herr, R. D. (2006). *Triage nursing secrets*. St. Louis, MO: Mosby.
5. Schmeltzer, M. (2011). Nursing management: Lower gastrointestinal problems. In S. L. Lewis, S. R. Dirksen, M. M. Heitkemper, L. Bucher, & I. A. Camera (Eds.), *Medical-surgical nursing: Assessment and management of clinical problems* (8th ed., pp. 1006–1057). St. Louis, MO: Mosby.
6. American College of Radiology. (2010). *ACR appropriateness criteria: Right upper quadrant pain*. Retrieved from http://www.acr.org/SecondaryMainMenuCategories/quality_safety/app_criteria/pdf/ExpertPanelonGastrointestinalImaging/RightUpperQuadrantPainDoc13.aspx
7. American College of Radiology. (2010). *ACR appropriateness criteria: Right lower quadrant pain*. Retrieved from http://www.acr.org/SecondaryMainMenuCategories/quality_safety/app_criteria/pdf/ExpertPanelonGastrointestinalImaging/RightLowerQuadrantPainDoc12.aspx
8. American College of Radiology. (2008). *ACR appropriateness criteria: Left lower quadrant pain*. Retrieved from http://www.acr.org/SecondaryMainMenuCategories/quality_safety/app_criteria/pdf/ExpertPanelonGastrointestinalImaging/LeftLowerQuadrantPainDoc8.aspx
9. Char, E. A., & Haing, E. F. (2006). Abdominal pain. In M. A. Davis & S. R. Votey (Eds.), *Signs and symptoms in emergency medicine* (2nd ed.). St. Louis, MO: Mosby.
10. Zimmermann, P. G. (2008). Is it appendicitis? *American Journal of Nursing, 108*(9), 27–31.
11. Kessler, N., Cyteval, C., Gallix, B., Lesnik, A., Blayac, P.M., Pujol, J., … Taourel, P. (2004). Appendicitis: Evaluation of sensitivity, specificity, and predictive values of US, Doppler US, and laboratory findings. *Radiology, 230*(2), 472–478.
12. Smeltzer, S. C., & Bare, B. G. (2003). *Brunner and Suddarth's textbook of medical-surgical nursing* (10th ed.). Philadelphia, PA: Lippincott Williams & Wilkins.
13. Patti, M. G. (2011, August 19). *Gastroesophageal reflux disease*. Retrieved from http://emedicine.medscape.com/article/176595
14. McCullough, L., & Sachs, C. J. (2006). Bleeding. In M. A. Davis & S. R. Votey (Eds.), *Signs and symptoms in emergency medicine* (2nd ed.). St. Louis, MO: Mosby.
15. Geibel, J. (2011, June 13). *Upper gastrointestinal bleeding*. Retrieved from http://emedicine.medscape.com/article/187857
16. Barkun, A. N., Bardou, M., Kuipers, E. J., Sung, J., Hunt, R. H., Martel, M., & Sinclair, P. (2010). International consensus recommendations on the management of patients with nonvariceal upper gastrointestinal bleeding. *Annals of Internal Medicine, 152*(2), 101–113.
17. Wong Kee Song, L-M. (2011, March 29). *Mallory-Weiss tear*. Retrieved from http://emedicine.medscape.com/article/187134
18. Trowbridge, R. L., Rutkowski, N. K., & Shojania, K. G. (2003). Does this patient have acute cholecystitis? *Journal of the American Medical Association, 189*(1), 80–86.
19. McQueen, A., McCabe, F., & Peeples, N. (2006). Vomiting, pediatric. In S. R. Votey & M. A. Davis (Eds.), *Signs and symptoms in emergency medicine* (2nd ed.). St. Louis, MO: Mosby.
20. Lehrer, J. K. (2011, June 16). *Irritable bowel syndrome*. Retrieved from http://emedicine.medscape.com/article/180389
21. Devuni, D., Rossi, L. M., Wu, G. Y., Liu, J. H., & Ko, C. Y. (2009, April 14). *Megacolon, toxic*. Retrieved from http://emedicine.medscape.com/article/181054-overview
22. Nguyen, M. C. T. (2011, July 6). *Diverticulitis*. Retrieved from http://emedicine.medscape.com/article/173388-overview

Metabolic Emergencies

Benjamin E. Marett

The endocrine system is instrumental in regulating metabolism, tissue function, growth, development, moods, and emotions. Additionally, it works to maintain homeostasis in response to physiological stress.[1] Dysfunction of one endocrine gland can affect the physiology of the entire body.[2] Disruption in the production, supply, or use of hormones or electrolytes can result in a medical emergency that requires prompt assessment, diagnosis, correction, and identification of the precipitating cause. Figure 29-1 shows the location of the major endocrine glands.

DIABETIC EMERGENCIES[1–4]

Diabetes mellitus is a chronic condition in which the body is unable to metabolize glucose because of a lack of effective insulin. There are two major types of diabetes mellitus:
- Type 1, formerly called insulin-dependent diabetes or juvenile-onset diabetes, results from an absolute insulin deficiency.
- Type 2, previously referred to as non–insulin-dependent diabetes or adult-onset diabetes, is characterized by insulin resistance, increased hepatic glucose release, impaired glucose storage, and eventual insulin deficiency. Type 2 is the more prevalent form and tends to be progressive, eventually requiring a second oral drug or insulin.

The short-term goals of diabetes management are to balance food intake with energy expenditure and ensure a sufficient amount of insulin (endogenous or exogenous) to maintain blood glucose levels at or near normal. When these goals are not achieved, a diabetic crisis can occur.

Hypoglycemic Emergencies[2,3]
Etiology
Hypoglycemia is the most common acute complication of diabetes. Normal blood glucose levels range from 80 to 120 mg/dL (4.4 to 6.6 mmol/L). Sources vary, but hypoglycemia is defined as a blood glucose level less than 60 to 70 mg/dL and severe hypoglycemia is defined as a blood glucose level less than 40 mg/dL. How quickly the serum glucose decreases can influence the patient's symptoms; if glucose levels drop too quickly in relation to the body's compensatory ability, the patient may become symptomatic at levels of 60 to 80 mg/dL.[2]

Patients at risk for hypoglycemia may be taking[4]:
- Sulfonylureas (first generation: tolbutamide; second generation: glipizide, glyburide; third generation: glimepiride)
- Meglitinides including repaglinide (Prandin) and nateglinide (Starlix)
- Intensive insulin therapy regimens due to type 1 diabetes
- Long-acting oral hypoglycemic agents, such as chlorpropamide (Diabenese), due to type 2 diabetes[4]

Other causes of hypoglycemia include the following:
- Insufficient food intake including inadequate caloric intake or missed meals (most common cause)
- Too much insulin (includes unintentional and intentional overdoses of insulin or oral hypoglycemic agents)
- Sulfonylurea potentiation of insulin action in the liver
- Increased exercise or activity
- Alcohol consumption

Oral hypoglycemic agents that do *not* cause hypoglycemia[3,4]:
- Biguanides (metformin [Glucophage]): Decreases hepatic production of glucose and increases insulin sensitivity. Risk: Lactic acidosis.
- Thiazolidinediones (rosiglitazone [Avandia], pioglitazone [Actos]): Increases sensitivity to insulin in peripheral tissue. Risk: Hepatotoxicity.
- Alpha-glucosidase inhibitors (acarbose [Precose], miglitol [Glyset]): Decreases gastrointestinal glucose absorption. Risk: Diarrhea.

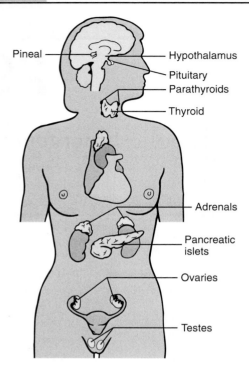

Pineal

Hypothalamus

Pituitary

Parathyroids

Thyroid

Adrenals

Pancreatic islets

Ovaries

Testes

Fig. 29-1 Location of major endocrine glands. (From Lewis, S. L., Heitkemper, M. M., & Dirksen, S. R. (2007). *Medical-surgical nursing: Assessment and management of clinical problems* (7th ed.). St. Louis, MO: Mosby.)

Presentation

Mild. In mild hypoglycemia, adrenergic symptoms are the predominant findings:

- Shaking
- Sweating
- Tachycardia
- Hunger
- Pallor
- Tingling of the lips
- Anxiety
- Palpitations
- Restlessness

However, these symptoms are masked ("hypoglycemic unawareness") in patients:

- With long-standing diabetes (because diabetes neuropathy affects the autonomic system)
- Who have had recent severe episodes of hypoglycemia (because of diabetic autonomic neuropathy, there is loss of the typical autonomic response)
- Who are taking beta-blocker medications (these drugs block the typical epinephrine response).

- Who are alcoholics (inhibition of gluconeogenesis by alcohol)

Moderate. Moderate hypoglycemia is characterized by neuroglycopenic symptoms as a result of insufficient glucose to the brain.[3,5]

- Behavioral changes, irritability
- Confusion[3]
- Headache
- Drowsiness
- Slurred speech
- Weakness, staggering gait
- Blurred vision

Severe. Severe hypoglycemia is a medical emergency. If left untreated, it can result in seizures, coma, or permanent neurological damage.

> Hypoglycemia is the most common cause of altered mental status in persons with diabetes.

Treatment

If unsure whether hypoglycemia or hyperglycemia is being experienced and unable to obtain a glucose level, treat as if hypoglycemia is the problem. Giving a small amount of additional glucose is not harmful to patients with hyperglycemia, but its lack is harmful to patients with hypoglycemia.

> Identify possible causes for a hypoglycemic incident to prevent future attacks. Frequent or prolonged bouts of hypoglycemia contribute to permanent neurologic damage.

Treatment of Hypoglycemia in the Conscious Patient

- Measure the serum glucose level. A fingerstick blood glucose test is adequate to begin treatment.
- Obtain a laboratory analysis of serum glucose for confirmation of the meter reading. However, do not delay treatment while awaiting laboratory results if the patient is symptomatic.
- Administer 15 to 20 g of a rapid-acting oral glucose preparation (Table 29-1).
- If the serum glucose level does not improve within 15 minutes, administer a second dose of carbohydrates orally. (Sympathetic nervous system symptoms should resolve quickly but neurogenic symptoms may continue for 1 hour or longer even if blood glucose levels are greater than 100 mg/dL.)
- After an increase in serum glucose, follow with oral complex carbohydrate administration (usually lasting less than 2 hours). A complex carbohydrate snack or meal eaten soon after blood glucose begins to rise will decrease the risk of recurrent hypoglycemia.

TABLE 29-1 TREATMENT OF HYPOGLYCEMIA

Each of the following contains 15 g of carbohydrates:
- 1 cup of milk
- 1 small tube of glucose gel
- 10 jelly beans
- 3 glucose tablets
- 8 small sugar cubes or 4 tsp of sugar
- ½ cup regular soda (avoid in patients with renal failure)
- ½ cup orange juice (avoid in patients with renal failure)
- ⅓ cup apple juice
- ½ oz box of raisins
- 3 tsp of honey or syrup
- 8 Life Savers candies
- 1 small tube of cake frosting

Treatment of Hypoglycemia in the Semiconscious or Unconscious Patient

- Measure the blood glucose level (as previously discussed).
- Administer 50% dextrose, 25 to 50 mL intravenously for adult patients. In children, administer 25% dextrose; administer 10% to 12.5% dextrose to neonates and infants.
- Consider continuous infusion of 5% dextrose in water (D_5W) or 10% dextrose in water ($D_{10}W$) to maintain serum glucose within the normal range as prescribed. Cerebral edema is a rare but possible complication, especially in children.
- Initiate seizure precautions.

When Intravenous Access Is Not Readily Available

- Administer glucagon 1 mg intramuscularly (0.5 mg in children ages 3 to 5 years; 0.25 mg in children less than 3 years).
- Glucagon should be prescribed for all individuals at significant risk of severe hypoglycemia and caregivers or family members of these individuals should be instructed in its administration. Glucagon administration is not limited to health care professionals.
  - If there is no improvement in 20 minutes, repeat the same glucagon dose.
  - Once the patient can swallow, give 20 g of carbohydrates by mouth to restock depleted glycogen stores and to prevent recurrence of hypoglycemia.
  - Glucagon may not be effective if liver glycogen stores have been depleted—for instance, in hypoglycemia caused by alcoholism.

Vomiting is common following the administration of glucagon; position the patient to avoid aspiration.

Hyperglycemic Emergencies
Diabetic Ketoacidosis[2,3,5–7]

Diabetic ketoacidosis (DKA) accounts for most hyperglycemic emergencies. This acute diabetic complication in some cases may be the initial presentation of new-onset diabetes, particularly type 1.

Etiology. DKA results from an inadequate amount of available insulin and is characterized by profound dehydration, electrolyte losses, ketonuria, and acidosis. When insulin is unavailable to transport glucose into the cells, the liver metabolizes fatty acids into ketone bodies. This accumulation of ketones produces metabolic acidosis.

The classic findings include:
- Blood glucose over 250 mg/dL
- pH less than 7.3 (metabolic acidosis)
- Serum HCO_3 less than 15 to 20 mmol/L
- Ketonemia

DKA usually is limited to type 1 diabetic patients, but under conditions of extreme stress, it may occur in those with type 2 diabetes.[2]

Causes[3]
- New-onset diabetes
- Inadequate insulin dosing or omission of insulin doses
- Illness or infection in a known diabetic patient (most common cause of DKA)
- Alcohol or drug abuse
- Myocardial infarction
- Pancreatitis and abdominal disorders

Signs and Symptoms[3]
- Tachycardia, hypotension
- Volume depletion: dry skin and poor skin turgor, dry mucous membranes
- Fatigue
- Acute mental status changes from drowsiness to coma
- Acetone on the breath (fruity-smelling breath)
- Kussmaul respirations (rapid, deep breathing): the body is attempting to compensate for the metabolic acidosis by blowing off carbon dioxide
- Abdominal pain without rebound tenderness, diminished bowel sounds

Diagnostic Procedures
- Measure the serum glucose level. A fingerstick blood glucose test is adequate to begin treatment. (Obtain serum glucose to validate.)
- Test for glucose and ketones in urine.
- Obtain urinalysis (infection is a frequent precipitant of DKA).
- Obtain a complete blood count with differential, electrolytes, blood urea nitrogen (BUN), creatinine, phosphate, and amylase.
- Obtain arterial blood gas.

- Obtain a chest radiograph, 12-lead electrocardiogram (ECG), and blood cultures as indicated.

Therapeutic Interventions. Although the condition requires emergent intervention, correction that occurs too rapidly may result in cerebral edema, hypoglycemia, or hypokalemia.[2]

Fluid Replacement

- Restore intravascular volume and renal perfusion. Volume losses in DKA can be extensive. Total body fluid deficits average 6 L (adults) or 100 mL/kg of body mass. The exact rate will depend on the patient's condition and response. Begin fluid replacement before initiating insulin therapy or electrolyte replacement.
- Administer normal saline at 1 to 2 L per hour over the first 1 to 2 hours and then at 100 to 500 mL per hour for adults. For pediatric patients, replace 20 mL/kg of body mass in the first hour. More aggressive fluid replacement is indicated if the patient is in hypovolemic shock.
- Change intravenous (IV) solution to 0.45% saline if hypovolemia has been reversed and the serum sodium level is still high or normal.

Reverse Ketonemia and Hyperglycemia and Administer Insulin

> Ketogenesis is considered reversed when:
> - Serum glucose is less than 200 mg/dL
> - Anion gap is 12 mEq/L or less
> - Venous pH is greater than 7.3
> - Serum bicarbonate level is 18 mEq/L or higher

- Administration of IV insulin is recommended; injected insulin is absorbed erratically in the presence of hypovolemia. The treatment of choice for moderate to severe DKA is regular insulin by continuous IV infusion.
- Give an IV bolus of 0.1 units of regular insulin per kilogram of body mass and then start a continuous IV infusion at 0.1 unit/kg per hour.[8] Prime the tubing and discard the first 30 to 50 mL of the insulin–normal saline solution because insulin binds to plastic.
- Measure serum glucose hourly. Too rapid a decrease in serum glucose will increase the risk of cerebral edema. Many institutions have implemented insulin protocols to guide the titration of the insulin infusion according to glucose levels. When serum glucose falls to 250 mg/dL, consider changing the IV fluid to a dextrose-containing solution (e.g., D_5W/0.45% saline) and decreasing the insulin according to physician order to maintain a serum glucose level of 150 to 200 mg/dL. Depending on the insulin type, subcutaneous insulin therapy must be initiated 1 to 4 hours before discontinuation of the IV insulin infusion to avoid recurrence of hyperglycemia and ketogenesis.

> An anion gap measures the amount of negatively charged ions in the serum that are not bicarbonate or chloride. An elevated anion gap means some unmeasured anion, toxic, or organic acid is in the blood and is an alert to a potentially serious disease or overdose.
>
> To calculate an anion gap, add the serum bicarbonate and serum chloride levels and then subtract this number from the serum sodium level [Anion gap = $Na^+ - (HCO_3 + Cl^-)$]. A normal anion gap is 12 ± 2 mEq/L.
>
> Another formula used for anion gap is $(Na^+ + K^+) - (Cl^- + HCO_3)$ with a normal range of 5 to 15.[17]

Replace Electrolytes

- Measure serum electrolytes at the time of patient arrival and every 2 to 4 hours thereafter. In most cases the serum potassium level initially will be elevated. Fluid resuscitation, insulin therapy, and acidosis correction reduce extracellular potassium levels.
- Once serum potassium is less than 5 mEq/L, begin IV potassium replacement to keep blood levels between 4 and 5 mEq/L. If the initial serum potassium is less than 3.3 mEq/L, delay insulin therapy and start potassium replacement immediately.
- Begin potassium replacement only after it has been established that the patient has adequate urine output and is not in renal failure.
- Phosphate replacement also may be necessary.
- Sodium bicarbonate can be given intravenously if the arterial pH is 7 or less.

Hyperosmolar Hyperglycemic Syndrome or State[2,3,5,7]

Formerly known as hyperosmolar hyperglycemic non-ketotic coma, hyperosmolar hyperglycemic syndrome (HHS) accounts for 10% to 20% of hyperglycemic emergencies and is associated with a 10% to 60% mortality, depending on the severity of the precipitating illness[2] (Table 29-2).

The higher mortality is related to an insidious onset, delay in treatment, and more elderly population. A higher serum osmolarity and higher serum sodium correlate with a poor outcome. *Osmolality* is a measure of the osmoles of solute per kilogram of solvent (osmol/kg or Osm/kg).

Etiology. HHS is frequently associated with type 2 diabetes, although as many as half of patients with HHS are not diabetic. Many have a precipitant medical or surgical condition such as infection, acute myocardial infarction, or stroke. Medications, such as thiazide diuretics, steroids, phenytoin (Dilantin), propranolol (Inderal), and cimetidine

TABLE 29-2	COMPARISON OF DIABETIC KETOACIDOSIS AND HYPEROSMOLAR HYPERGLYCEMIC SYNDROME PATIENT PRESENTATIONS	

FEATURE	DIABETIC KETOACIDOSIS	HYPEROSMOLAR HYPERGLYCEMIC SYNDROME
Patient's age	Usually <40 years	Usually >60 years
Duration of symptoms	Usually <2 days	Usually >5 days
Glucose level	Usually <600 mg/dL	Usually >600 mg/dL
Sodium level	Likely to be low or normal	Likely to be normal or high
Potassium level	High, normal, or low	High, normal, or low
Bicarbonate level	Low	Normal
Ketone bodies	At least 4+ in a 1:1 dilution	<2+ in a 1:1 dilution
pH	Low, usually <7.3	Normal
Serum osmolality	Usually <350 mOsm/kg	Usually >350 mOsm/kg
Cerebral edema	Often subclinical, occasionally clinical	Rapid glucose decline increases the risk
Prognosis	3% to 10% mortality	20% to 60% mortality
Subsequent course	Ongoing insulin therapy usually required	Insulin therapy often not required
Diabetes mellitus	Most commonly seen with type 1	Most commonly seen with type 2

(Tagamet) can be a cause. Other causes include total parenteral nutrition (TPN), tube feeding without sufficient free water, and renal disorders.

Signs and Symptoms.[2,3] Clinical findings include dehydration, extreme hyperglycemia, electrolyte imbalances, hyperosmolarity, and altered mental status.

- Weakness.
- Polyuria, polydipsia.
- Significant volume depletion with dry mucosa, dry skin, orthostatic hypotension, and tachycardia in severe cases.
- Anorexia and nausea and vomiting.
- Acute mental status changes, lethargy, or coma. Mental status correlates with serum osmolarity.
- Seizures.

Diagnostic Procedures. The main difference between HHS and DKA is that HHS is indicated by a more severely elevated serum glucose and an absence of ketoacidosis. In order to make a diagnosis, obtain a basic metabolic panel, arterial blood gas, and urinalysis. HHS is defined by the following laboratory findings:

- Hyperglycemia greater than 600 mg/dL
- Elevated plasma osmolality greater than 315 mOsm/kg
  - Plasma osmolality is determined by the following formula: 2(serum sodium) + (serum glucose/18 + BUN/2.8)
- Serum bicarbonate greater than 15 mEq/L
- Arterial pH within normal limits
- Negative serum ketones
- Urine positive for glucose but no ketones

Hyperglycemia and hyperosmolarity should be corrected gradually to prevent hypokalemia and cerebral edema.

Therapeutic Interventions.[2,3] Treatment is similar to DKA (see above), though less insulin is needed.

Replace Fluids

- The average fluid deficit is 9 to 12 L. Begin fluid resuscitation with 1 L of normal saline over the first hour to restore blood pressure and urine output. Change to 0.45% saline at 5 to 15 mL/kg per hour if the serum sodium level is normal or high.
- Insert an indwelling urinary catheter to strictly monitor intake and output. Incorporate urinary losses into fluid replacement calculations.

Hydration with IV normal saline is the cornerstone therapy for HHS.

Serum Glucose Reduction

- Administer insulin: The goal of insulin therapy in patients with HHS is to reduce serum glucose levels by around 50 to 70 mg/dL per hour.
- When the blood glucose drops to 300 mg/dL, change to a dextrose-containing IV solution such as D_5W/0.45% saline. Adding dextrose to IV fluids reduces the risk of cerebral edema associated with rapid decreases in serum glucose levels.
- Monitor serum glucose levels hourly.

Replace Electrolytes

- Check serum chemistries every 2 to 4 hours until the patient is stable.
- Replace potassium at 20 to 30 mEq/L in IV fluid if adequate urine output. If potassium is less than 3.3 mEq/L, delay insulin therapy until hypokalemia has been corrected.

PITUITARY EMERGENCIES

Diabetes Insipidus[6]

Etiology

Diabetes insipidus (DI) may be a temporary or a permanent condition, depending on the amount of hypothalamic secretory tissue remaining and the extent of renal impairment. It should be considered in patients who have experienced head trauma, recently undergone intracranial surgery or have a history of oat cell carcinoma. Although the names are similar, DI has no association with diabetes mellitus. There are two types of DI: neurogenic and nephrogenic.

Neurogenic Diabetes Insipidus. The antidiuretic hormone (ADH) is produced in insufficient quantities by the hypothalamus or is not released by the posterior pituitary gland.

Some causes of neurogenic DI include the following:
- Tumors of the hypothalamus or pituitary region
- Head injury
- Surgical brain trauma
- Ischemia or infection of the hypothalamus or pituitary
- Meningitis or encephalitis
- Cerebral aneurysm
- Drugs: phenytoin, lithium

Nephrogenic Diabetes Insipidus. Adequate amounts of ADH are produced and released, but the renal tubules are unresponsive to the hormone. This renders the kidneys unable to concentrate urine appropriately, and excessive amounts of dilute urine are excreted. Causes of nephrogenic DI include the following:
- Polycystic kidney disease
- Pyelonephritis
- Sickle cell disease
- Sarcoidosis
- Familial genetic disorders

Signs and Symptoms

- Polydipsia, polyuria (5 to 20 L/day)
- Urine specific gravity less than 1.005
- Urine osmolality less than 300 mOsm/kg
- Serum osmolality greater than 295 mOsm/kg
- Serum sodium greater than 145 mEq/L
- Weight loss, fatigue

Therapeutic Interventions

- Fluid replacement.
  - Rehydrate orally if the patient is asymptomatic and the total body water deficit is not extreme.
  - Sometimes, in an emergency, patients with DI cannot drink enough fluid to replace their urine losses. Replace the losses with dextrose and water or

IV fluid that is hypo-osmolar to the patient's serum. Avoid hyperglycemia, volume overload, and overly rapid correction of hypernatremia. A good rule of thumb is to reduce serum sodium by 0.5 mEq/L per hour.
- Neurogenic DI: Replace ADH with the following:
  - Aqueous pitressin (IV or subcutaneous)
  - Lysine vasopressin spray (nasal)
  - Desmopressin acetate (DDAVP)
- Nephrogenic DI: Does not respond to ADH replacement therapy.
  - Dietary sodium and protein restrictions
  - Thiazide diuretics
  - Nonsteroidal anti-inflammatory drugs (NSAIDs)

Syndrome of Inappropriate Antidiuretic Hormone Secretion[2,3]

Etiology

The syndrome of inappropriate antidiuretic hormone (SIADH) secretion results when abnormal amounts of ADH are released from the pituitary, producing water intoxication.

Possible causes of SIADH include the following:
- Head trauma
- Infections: Brain abscesses, meningitis, human immunodeficiency virus, pneumonia
- Stroke, cerebral aneurysm, other central nervous system disorders
- Malignancies
- Adrenal insufficiency
- Pain, stress
- Drugs: oral hypoglycemic agents, psychotropics, antineoplastic agents, general anesthetics, narcotics

---

Hyponatremia and hypo-osmolality characterize SIADH.

Signs and Symptoms

- Headache
- Fatigue
- Confusion, decreased level of consciousness
- Seizures
- Nausea, vomiting
- Diminished deep tendon reflexes
- Weight gain without edema

Diagnostic Procedures

- Draw a basic metabolic panel, which will show dilutional hyponatremia and decreased plasma osmolality
- Obtain a urinalysis, which will show increased urine osmolality, sodium, and specific gravity

Therapeutic Interventions

Treatment is determined by symptom severity and the extent of hyponatremia.

- If the patient is asymptomatic, water intake simply may be restricted to 500 to 1000 mL per day.
- Symptomatic patients who have severe hyponatremia require IV hypertonic saline (3% to 5%) and furosemide (Lasix) until symptoms improve. Follow institutional policies on administration of hypertonic saline. A hypertonic solution is one that has greater tonicity than the fluid within the body's cells. When this type of fluid is injected, it causes the cells to lose fluid into the surrounding spaces. If too much hypertonic solution is injected, the cells will shrink and shrivel. The cells become irritated, and this will probably cause pain at the site of administration. As a result, some patients will require infusion through a central line and critical care–level monitoring.
- Monitor serum sodium levels every 1 to 2 hours

THYROID EMERGENCIES

Thyroid emergencies are rare but can be life threatening. The thyroid gland regulates the body's metabolic rate through the hypothalamic-pituitary-thyroid counter-regulatory system.[2]

Severe thyroid dysfunction, both hypothyroid and hyperthyroid states, is a medical emergency.

Thyroiditis and Thyroid Storm (Hyperthyroid Crisis)[2,9]

Thyroiditis is an inflammation of the thyroid gland characterized by anterior neck pain that may appear following an upper respiratory infection (usually viral) There are several types of thyroiditis and, depending on the phase of the condition, may be associated with either hypo- or hyperthyroidism.

Thyrotoxicosis, and the more severe form thyroid storm, is a hyper metabolic state associated with hyperthyroidism. Approximately 60% to 80% of thyrotoxicosis are due to Graves disease, an autoimmune disorder causing continuous stimulation of the thyroid gland.[10]

Etiology

- Stress
- Manipulation of the thyroid gland
- Severe drug reactions
- Surgery
- Trauma
- Myocardial infarction
- Infection

- DKA
- Embolism

Signs and Symptoms[11]

The differentiation between hyperthyroidism and thyroid storm is clinical judgment.

- Elevated temperature of 38.7°C (101.7°F) but may be as high as 41°C (105.8°F)
- Central nervous system dysfunction: Patients may be restless, with a shortened attention span, anxiety, emotional lability, agitation, and tremors
- Cardiovascular dysfunction
  - Sinus tachycardia is almost always present (indicates the severity of catecholamine excess)
  - Atrial fibrillation
  - Angina from unmasked previously existing coronary artery disease
- Gastrointestinal dysfunction (nausea and vomiting, diarrhea, pseudodiarrhea [hyperdefecation], e.g., increased frequency [more than 3 times a day])

Diagnostic Procedures

A serum thyroid panel should be drawn. Expect patients to have elevated levels of triiodothyronine (T_3), thyroxine (T_4), and free thyroxine (free T_4), with decreased thyroid-stimulating hormone (TSH) levels.[2,10]

Therapeutic Interventions

If not promptly identified and treated, this condition progresses to exhaustion, cardiac failure, and death in as little as 2 hours. Untreated, hyperthyroid crisis carries a high mortality of 90%.[11]

Care of the patient with thyroid storm involves identification and treatment of the underlying cause, thyroid hormone level reduction, and emergent management of systemic manifestations, such as hyperthermia and cardiac dysrhythmias.

- Give acetaminophen (not aspirin) to reduce hyperthermia.
  - Acetaminophen is preferable to aspirin, which can increase serum free T_4 and T_3 concentrations by interfering with protein binding.
- Administer a beta-blocking agent to counteract sympathetic hyperstimulation. Use with extreme caution in patients with asthma or heart failure. Propranolol (Inderal) intravenously, followed by oral administration, is frequently used, but esmolol can be used. Propranolol inhibits both the tachycardia and the T_4 from changing to T_3.
- Antithyroid drugs.
  - Propylthiouracil (PTU) or 6-n-Propylthiourical (PROP): prevents thyroid hormone synthesis. As the

result of a 2003 U.S. Food and Drug Administration alert related to the risk of serious liver disease, PTU is no longer recommended as the frontline drug for nonpregnant adults and children.[12]

- Methimazole (Tapazole, Thiamazole): inhibits the synthesis of T_3 and T_4.
- Iodine (sodium iodide, potassium iodide, or Lugol iodine): inhibits thyroid hormone release. Iodine needs to be administered one hour after either PTU or methimazole, as iodine can increase thyroid production.
- Reserpine.
- Guanethidine.
- Glucocorticoids (dexamethasone): inhibits peripheral conversion of T_4 to T_3. Glucocorticoids also help replace the use of the cortisol in a stressed situation.
- Ensure that fluid and calorie intake are adequate for the increased metabolic demands.

Myxedema Coma (Hypothyroid Coma)[3]

Myxedema coma is a rare but serious hypothyroid emergency. Generally, myxedema coma results from a new stress in patients with preexisting hypothyroidism. This disorder occurs most often in older patients (older than 60 years of age), in women, and during winter months. Approximately one third of patients have a history of hypothyroidism; coexistence of a precipitating factor often delays diagnosis.

Etiology
- Infection
- Heart failure
- Drugs: amiodarone, interferon, general anesthesia, sedatives, antidepressants, narcotics (there is an increased sensitivity to opioids in this population), beta-blockers, several anticonvulsants, lithium
- Trauma, surgery
- Exposure to cold temperatures
- Stress

Signs and Symptoms[3,11]
- Signs of decreased metabolism. Hypothermia (T <35.5°C [95.9°F]) without shivering; bradycardia; systolic blood pressure less than 100; hypoventilation.
- Signs of long-standing hypothyroidism: periorbital edema, macroglossia (tongue swelling), hoarse voice, dry skin, nonpitting edema of the lower extremities, fatigue, lethargy.
- Coma; seizures in patients with coma.
- Myxedema madness: 5% to 15% of myxedema patients exhibit some form of psychosis.[12] Most commonly this includes manifestations of thought disorders, such as delusions and hallucinations.[13]

Diagnostic Procedures
- Thyroid panel: expect thyroxine (T_4) level to be decreased and TSH to be elevated.
- Basic metabolic panel: expect hyponatremia and hypochloremia.
- ECG.

Therapeutic Interventions
- Advanced airway management as needed
- Gentle rehydration and sodium replacement
- Passive warming to correct hypothermia
- Intravenous thyroid hormone replacement (levothyroxine, thyroxine)
- Glucocorticoids (to treat possible coexisting adrenal insufficiency)

ADRENAL EMERGENCIES

The adrenal cortex (outer portion of the adrenal gland) produces glucocorticoids (cortisol), which largely control metabolism. The cortex also produces mineralocorticoids (aldosterone), which contribute to fluid and electrolyte balance. The adrenal medulla (inner core of the adrenal gland) secretes epinephrine and norepinephrine, which are autonomic nervous system stimulants.

Cushing Syndrome

Excessive steroids, usually from systemic exogenous administration, result in temporary hypernatremia (fluid retention), hypokalemia, hyperglycemia, and hypocalcemia. Immunosuppression and appropriate precautions are required. If a patient does not wean down the dose, an Addisonian crisis from insufficient glucosteroids can result.

Acute Adrenal Insufficiency[2,14]

Acute adrenal insufficiency (adrenal crisis, Addisonian crisis) results from a sudden decrease in cortisol and aldosterone levels.

Primary adrenal insufficiency occurs in individuals with preexisting chronic adrenal insufficiency (Addison disease). A common trigger is an acute illness or stressor.

Secondary adrenal insufficiency (suppression of adrenal hormone release) is much more common. Long-term glucocorticoid use (hydrocortisone, prednisone) causes adrenal gland suppression, primarily reducing cortisol production. Consequently, abrupt discontinuation of supplemental steroids may precipitate acute adrenal crisis.

Etiology

- Stress, infection, burns, or trauma in individuals with preexisting chronic adrenal insufficiency or in patients who have adequate adrenal function in the absence of stressors
- Damage of the adrenal or pituitary glands
- Abrupt withdrawal of glucocorticoid therapy
- Head injury with pituitary or hypothalamic injury

Signs and Symptoms[14]

- Weakness, fatigue
- Hypotension
- Anorexia, weight loss if chronic
- Nausea and vomiting, abdominal pain, diarrhea or constipation
- Hyperpigmentation, particularly of the knuckles, axillae, gums, and the creases of the hands in chronic primary adrenal insufficiency

Diagnostic Procedures

- Obtain a complete metabolic panel. Typical findings include the following:
    - Hyponatremia, hypochloremia, and hyperkalemia (in patients with primary adrenal insufficiency)
    - Hypoglycemia
- Obtain a creatinine level
- Draw cortisol and adrenocorticotropic hormone levels

Therapeutic Interventions

- Stabilization related to fluids and electrolytes.
- Hydrocortisone intravenously. Patients who are receiving chronic steroid treatment and the acutely ill or injured may be treated with additional steroids for the current physiologic stress in addition to therapies for the primary medical condition.
- Dexamethasone.

Catecholamine Excess and Pheochromocytoma

Etiology

Catecholamine excess has many causes, including sympathomimetic overdose (e.g., cocaine, amphetamines, diet pills), withdrawal from alcohol or sedative-hypnotics, monoamine oxidase inhibitor interactions with certain foods (e.g., foods high in the amino acid tyramine, such as alcohol, aged cheese, sauerkraut, and processed meats such as salami), and pheochromocytoma. Pheochromocytoma is a tumor (usually benign) of the chromaffin cells in the adrenal medulla. These tumors stimulate excessive catecholamine secretion (especially norepinephrine) and produce active peptides.

Signs and Symptoms

- Hypertension
- Headache, visual disturbances
- Anxiety
- Diaphoresis
- Palpitations, tachyarrhythmias
- Abdominal discomfort

Diagnostic Procedures

- 24-hour urine for catecholamines and metanephrines

Therapeutic Interventions

- Control the hypertensive crisis with an intravenous alpha-blocking agent (phentolamine), nitroprusside (Nipride), or labetalol (Normodyne). Beta-blockade without alpha-blockade is contraindicated as it may worsen the hypertension.
- Maintain a normal volume status.
- Observe for cardiac dysrhythmias and treat as indicated.

ELECTROLYTE DISORDERS[7,9,15]

Electrolytes, ions that conduct electrical current, are essential for proper cellular functioning and maintenance of fluid and acid-base balance. An excess or deficit of any vital electrolyte can result in a life-threatening crisis. Table 29-3 summarizes cardiac rhythm changes associated with major electrolyte disturbances.

Calcium Disturbances[7,9]

About 45% of calcium in the blood is physiologically available for cellular needs. This portion is referred to as "active," "free," or "ionized" calcium. Another 40% is bound to serum protein (primarily albumin) and is not physiologically active. The remaining calcium (about 15%) is combined with other electrolytes. Changes in blood pH alter the amount of ionized calcium. As blood pH rises, more calcium binds with serum proteins thus decreasing ionized calcium levels. As pH decreases, less calcium is protein-bound and ionized calcium levels rise. Likewise, when serum protein drops, total serum calcium also decreases. Understanding these relationships allows clinicians to identify signs and symptoms of calcium disorders.

Hypocalcemia

Hypocalcemia is defined as ionized calcium less than 2 mEq/L.

Etiology[3,6,7,9]

- Impaired absorption: small bowel resection, Crohn's disease, malnutrition

- Increased renal loss: renal failure, diuretics
- Alkalosis (usually hyperventilation syndrome)
- Pancreatitis
- Multiple rapid blood transfusions of banked blood (citrate toxicity results when the preservative citrate in the transfused blood begins to bind calcium in the patient)
- Parathyroid disorder (parathyroid affects calcium excretion); thyroid or parathyroid surgery
- Gram-negative bacterial sepsis (20% may have hypocalcemia)[11]

Signs and Symptoms. Clinical findings in patients with hypocalcemia depend on actual calcium levels and the severity of ionized calcium loss.

- Numbness and tingling (mouth, hands, feet)
- Nausea and vomiting
- Muscle and nerve effects: tremor, twitching
- Chvostek's sign: tetany of the facial muscles when the facial nerve is tapped against the bone, anterior to the ear
- Trousseau's sign: occlusion of the brachial artery (with an inflated blood pressure cuff) for 3 minutes results in carpal spasm
- Hyperactive reflexes
- Seizures
- Prolonged QT interval

Therapeutic Interventions

Acute

- Ten milliliters of 10% calcium gluconate solution intravenously over 10 to 15 minutes (rapid administration can cause hypotension). Calcium chloride may be substituted but infiltration of this drug causes local tissue

---

TABLE 29-3   COMMON CARDIOVASCULAR RHYTHM CHANGES FROM MAJOR ELECTROLYTE DISTURBANCES

ELECTROLYTE	RHYTHM CHANGES
Calcium: Normal—total serum Ca^{++}, 8.5–10.5 mg/dL; Ionized serum Ca^{++}, 4–5 mg/dL	
Hypocalcemia	Prolonged ST segment and QT interval
	Inverted T waves
	Not usually associated with life-threatening dysrhythmias
Hypercalcemia	Shortened ST segment and QT interval
	Flatteneing of T wave
	Severe bradycardia
	Heart blocks
	Paroxysmal atrial fibrillation
	Cardiac standstill or arrest
Magnesium: Normal—1.3–2.1 mEq/L	
Hypomagnesemia	Prolonged QT interval
	Torsades de pointes
	Supraventricular tachycardia
	Ventricular ectopy including ventricular fibrillation
Hypermagnesemia	Prolonged PR interval
	Widened QRS complex
	Heart blocks progressing to cardiopulmonary arrest
Phosphorus: Normal—2.5–4.5 mg/dL	
Hypophosphatemia	Changes similar to hypercalcemia
Hyperphosphatemia	Changes similar to hypocalcemia
	Tachycardias
Potassium: Normal—3.5–5 mEq/L	
Hypokalemia	Prolonged PR interval
	Flattened or inverted T waves
	ST segment depression
	Development of "u" waves
	Ventricular ectopy
	Torsades de pointes
	Potentiates digitalis toxicity

TABLE 29-3 **COMMON CARDIOVASCULAR RHYTHM CHANGES FROM MAJOR ELECTROLYTE DISTURBANCES—cont'd**

ELECTROLYTE	RHYTHM CHANGES
Hyperkalemia	Tall, peaked, tented T waves
	Widened QRS
	Shortened QT interval
	Increased PR interval and QRS complex duration
	P wave prolongation with decreased amplitude
	P waves disappear as potassium level rises
	T waves and QRS complexes merge
	Bradycardia or AV block
	Progression to VF or asystole
Sodium: Normal—135–145 mEq/L	Not typically a *direct* cause of rhythm changes, but abnormal levels involve fluid shifts and signs of hypovolemia or hypervolemia with tachycardia or bradycardia

AV, Atrioventricular; *PAC,* premature atrial contraction; *PVC,* premature ventricular contraction; *SVT,* supraventricular tachycardia; *VF,* ventricular fibrillation; *VT,* ventricular tachycardia.

Data from Futterman, L. G. (2008). Electro cardiography: Abnormal electrocardiogram. In D. K. Moser & B. Riegel, *Cardiac nursing: A companion to Brunwald's heart disease* (pp. 620–621). St. Louis, MO: Saunders Elsevier; Felver, L. (2010). Fluid and electrolyte and acid-base balance. In S. L. Woods, E. S. S. Froelicher, S. U. Motzer, & E. J. Bridges, *Cardiac nursing* (6th ed., pp. 157–165). Baltimore, MD: Wolters Kluwer. Gibbs, M., Wolfson, A., & Tayal, V. (2002). Electrolyte disturbances. In J. Marx, R. Hockenberger, & R. Walls (Eds.), *Rosen's emergency medicine: Concepts and clinical practice* (5th ed.). St. Louis, MO: Mosby; Irwin, R., & Rippe, J. (Eds.). (2003). *Intensive care medicine* (5th ed.). Philadelphia, PA: Lippincott, Williams & Wilkins; Kee, J., & Paulanka, B. (2000). *Handbook of fluid, electrolyte, and acid-base imbalances.* New York, NY: Delmar; Kruse, J., Fink, M., & Carlson, R. (Eds.). (2003). *Saunders' manual of critical care.* Philadelphia, PA: Saunders; Achinger, S. G., & Ayus, J. C. (2009). Fluids and electrolytes in the critically ill. In J. Civetta, R. Taylor, & R. Kirby (Eds.), *Critical care* (4th ed., pp. 609–630). Philadelphia, PA: Lippincott, Williams & Wilkins; Marino, P. (2000). *The ICU book* (2nd ed.). Philadelphia, PA: Lippincott, Williams & Wilkins; Rice, V. (1983). Home study program. Magnesium, calcium, and phosphate imbalances: Their clinical significance. *Critical Care Nursing, 3*(3), 88–112; Foster, C., Mistry, N. F., Peddi, P. F., & Sharma, S. (Eds.). (2010). *The Washington manual of therapeutics* (33rd ed.). Philadelphia, PA: Lippincott, Williams & Wilkins; Alspach, J. G. (2005). *Core curriculum for critical care nursing* (6th ed.). Philadelphia, PA: Saunders.

necrosis. Patient should be on a cardiac monitor while calcium is infused.

- Institute seizure precautions.
- Calcifediol (a secondary hormone that is converted to vitamin D).

Chronic

- Vitamin D orally (ergocalciferol [D_2] therapy): vitamin D must be present for calcium to be absorbed from the gastrointestinal tract.
- Increase dietary calcium intake.
- Provide oral calcium supplementation.

Hypercalcemia[3,6,7,9]

Etiology. Hypercalcemia is usually a complication of a malignancy, most commonly in the presence of primary bone disease or bony metastasis. The malignancies that commonly present initially with signs of hypercalcemia are adult T-cell lymphoma and multiple myeloma.

Other possible causes include hyperparathyroidism, thiazide diuretics, hypervitaminosis D, hyperthyroidism, Addison disease, renal failure, and overingestion of calcium. Hypercalcemic crisis is defined as a total calcium concentration usually greater than 14 mg/dL with acute signs and symptoms.

Signs and Symptoms

- Polyuria and polydipsia[3]
- Signs and symptoms of dehydration: dry mucous membranes, tachycardia, orthostatic hypotension
- Weakness, fatigue
- Lethargy, confusion, coma

Therapeutic Interventions

- The goal of hypercalcemia treatment is to identify the underlying cause and reduce serum levels. Calcium level reduction usually can be accomplished by rehydration.
- Furosemide (Lasix) may be given to prevent fluid overload and promote renal elimination of calcium. Furosemide diuretic can worsen hypercalcemia unless adequate amounts of saline are administered. Avoid thiazide diuretics because they increase the absorption of calcium.
- Calcitonin, a normal peptide hormone, lowers plasma calcium and phosphate levels without augmenting calcium accretion.

Magnesium Disturbances[2,3,7,9]

Hypomagnesemia

Dietary magnesium is consumed primarily in green vegetables. Magnesium is absorbed in the small bowel and is excreted by the kidneys. The enzyme systems that control cell membrane permeability, muscle contraction, oxidative phosphorylation, and fat and nucleic acid synthesis are activated by magnesium.

Etiology[4,7,9]

- Decreased intake, especially when needs increase (pregnancy, growth spurts)
- Chronic alcohol abuse
- Nasogastric suctioning, vomiting, and diarrhea
- Malabsorption syndromes
- Excess renal loss, diuretic abuse
- DKA treatment (correction of acidosis may deplete magnesium levels)
- Massive transfusions of citrated blood
- Cisplatin, nephrotoxic agents (aminoglycosides, amphotericin B)
- Concurrent with acid-base abnormalities

Signs and Symptoms

- Similar to hypocalcemia (see above)
- Anorexia, nausea, and vomiting
- Tremors, leg cramps, muscle fibrillation, hyperreflexia, ataxia, tetany
- Positive Chvostek and Trousseau signs
- Seizures (if serum levels less than 1.5 mEq/L)
- Cardiac irritability and dysrhythmias, especially torsades de pointes

Therapeutic Interventions

- Administer magnesium orally if levels are mildly depleted.
- Administer magnesium replacement intravenously (or by deep intramuscular injection) to symptomatic patients and those with greatly reduced levels.
- Supplemental magnesium is excreted readily in the urine, necessitating repeated doses. Long-term replacement therapy often is required.
- Initiate seizure precautions.

Hypermagnesemia

Hypermagnesemia is an uncommon but life-threatening condition associated with severe fluid loss or renal failure.

Etiology. The cause of this condition is usually iatrogenic, resulting from excessive administration of magnesium-containing products such as antacids, enemas, and dialysate solution or from lithium overdose. Hypermagnesemia also may be seen in patients with DKA, Addison disease, viral hepatitis, hypothermia, and renal failure without dialysis and in those receiving magnesium therapy for pregnancy-induced hypertension.[2,7]

Signs and Symptoms

- Mild (3 to 5 mEq/L)
  - Bradycardia
  - Hypotension
  - Nausea, vomiting
  - Muscular weakness, decreased deep tendon reflexes (DTRs)
- Moderate (5 to 10 mEq/L)
  - Prolonged PR interval, QT interval, and QRS complex duration
  - Loss of DTRs
  - Decreased level of consciousness
- Severe (greater than 10 mEq/L)
  - Third-degree heart block, asystole
  - Respiratory muscle paralysis

Therapeutic Interventions

- Administer fluids and diuretics intravenously to enhance excretion (if renal function is normal).
- Administer IV calcium gluconate 10 mL of 10% solution. This treatment antagonizes the neuromuscular effects of magnesium.[16]

> If hypomagnesemia is present, evaluate the patient's calcium and potassium levels, as they are often low.

Phosphorus Disturbances

Hypophosphatemia

In humans, 80% to 85% of the phosphate in the body is contained in the bones and teeth and 15% to 20% is intracellular. Food products are the main source of phosphate, which is excreted by the kidneys. This ion plays an essential role in cellular structure and function, glycolysis, oxygen delivery, and maintenance of serum calcium levels.

Etiology. Hypophosphatemia may be seen in patients with chronic alcohol abuse, diabetes, chronic bowel disease, or severe burns. Phosphorus levels drop when the electrolyte is lost through the intestines or kidneys or when sepsis, respiratory alkalosis, epinephrine administration, or hepatic failure cause intracellular phosphate shifts. In patients with chronic obstructive pulmonary disease or asthma, hypophosphatemia can be a reversible cause of respiratory muscle hypocontractility and impaired tissue oxygenation.

Signs and Symptoms

- Moderate decrease
  - Weakness, tremors, and muscle pain
  - Tingling of the fingers and circumoral area
  - Joint stiffness, pain in the bones, fractures

- Anorexia
- Confusion
- Chest pain
- Severe decrease
  - Hemolytic anemia
  - Impaired oxygen delivery
  - Paralysis
  - Seizures, coma, death

Therapeutic Interventions

- Decrease the intake of substances such as phosphorus-binding antacids.
- In cases of mild to moderate hypophosphatemia, replace phosphorus orally with 1 to 3 grams per day by giving skim milk or Neutra-Phos.
- If the condition is severe or the patient is symptomatic, IV phosphorus replacement is required.

> Intravenous phosphorus replacement can lead to a rapid decrease in serum calcium levels.

Hyperphosphatemia

Hyperphosphatemia is defined as a serum phosphorus level greater than 4.5 mg/dL.

Etiology. This electrolyte abnormality is most commonly the result of poor renal phosphorus excretion but occasionally is caused by phosphorus moving from the intracellular to the extracellular space as a result of cellular tissue destruction (e.g., rhabdomyolysis).

Signs and Symptoms

- Anorexia, nausea, vomiting
- Pruritus
- Muscle weakness, tetany
- Tachycardia
- Calcium phosphate deposition in the joints, muscles, kidneys, and blood vessels

Therapeutic Interventions

- Administer a phosphate-binding agent such as magnesium or a calcium-containing antacid.
- Decrease dietary intake of phosphorus.

Potassium Disturbances

As the primary intracellular ion, potassium is responsible for muscle depolarization and neurologic function.

Hypokalemia

Hypokalemia is defined as a serum potassium level less than 3.5 mEq/L.

Etiology

- Excess potassium excretion in the urine (diuresis) or feces (diarrhea or malabsorption).
- Metabolic alkalosis.

- Insulin therapy.
- High-dose steroids.
- Inadequate potassium intake.
- Trauma patients may experience short-term hypokalemia because of elevated serum epinephrine levels.

Signs and Symptoms

- Fatigue, muscle weakness (mostly noted in the legs), leg cramps
- Nausea, vomiting, anorexia, paralytic ileus
- Polydipsia
- Decreased reflexes, central nervous system irritability, paresthesias, paralysis
- Ventricular dysrhythmias
- Flattened or inverted T waves, ST segment depression

Therapeutic Interventions

- Monitor closely for dysrhythmias; treat as indicated.
- Correct mild hypokalemia with increased dietary potassium or oral supplements.
- Never give potassium intramuscularly.
- Intravenous replacements must be diluted and given slowly; never give a potassium bolus to patients.
- Typically, IV replacement therapy involves 40 mEq of potassium chloride infused over 4 hours (adjusted to actual replacement needs). In emergent situations as much as 15 mEq/h can be administered.
- Potassium IV infusion is irritating to the veins. Check peripheral sites frequently and consider infusions containing lidocaine. Administration through a large vein or a central line improves patient comfort.
- Monitor serum potassium levels and other pertinent electrolytes.
- Hold supplemental potassium in oliguric patients.

> A coexisting magnesium deficiency makes it more difficult to correct hypokalemia.

Hyperkalemia[7,9,15]

Etiology. Hyperkalemia is defined as a serum potassium level greater than 5 mEq/L. Its most common causes are:

- Chronic renal failure
- Acidosis (potassium moves out of the cell as the pH falls)
- Drugs (NSAIDs, potassium-sparing diuretics, digoxin [Lanoxin], angiotensin-converting enzyme inhibitors)
- Cell death (potassium comes out of an injured muscle or red blood cell)—for example, burns, crush injuries, rhabdomyolysis, tumor lysis syndrome

Signs and Symptoms

- Muscle weakness (early sign) progressing to paralysis starting in the legs
- Abdominal cramping, hyperactive bowel sounds, diarrhea

- ECG changes: tall, tented T waves progressing to a widened QRS complex, a prolonged PR interval, ventricular fibrillation, or asystole

Therapeutic Interventions. Treatment depends on serum levels, the presence (or absence) of ECG changes, and underlying renal function. If life-threatening ECG changes exist:

- Slowly administer 10 mL of a 10% calcium chloride solution (or 20 mL of 10% calcium gluconate) intravenously. This helps protect cardiac cells from potassium-induced irritability but does not actually decrease potassium levels. Calcium chloride has a rapid onset of action that lasts for 30 to 60 minutes and is especially useful in hyperkalemic dialysis patients, particularly those in cardiac arrest situations.
- Administer IV insulin and glucose to drive the potassium back into the cell. Guidelines include giving 1 ampule of $D_{50}W$ (50 mL) and 10 units of regular insulin. Monitor serum glucose levels and observe the patient closely for hypoglycemia. This is a temporary measure to decrease the serum potassium; more definitive measures, such as Kayexalate and hemodialysis, must follow.
- Administer nebulized albuterol (Proventil, Ventolin) 10 to 20 mg over 15 minutes. (Catecholamines activate the sodium-potassium ATPase pump through beta-2 receptor stimulation in a manner that is additive to the effects of insulin.)
- Consider sodium bicarbonate slow IV, 1 to 3 ampules (44 mEq/ampule), over 20 to 30 minutes. The onset of action is immediate and lasts 1 to 2 hours. Sodium bicarbonate infusion can shift potassium from the extracellular to intracellular space by increasing blood pH. Venous or arterial pH should be monitored.
- If the patient has adequate renal function, administer furosemide (Lasix) 40 to 80 mg and normal saline intravenously (100 mL/h) to promote diuresis and potassium loss.
- Administer sodium polystyrene sulfonate (Kayexalate), a cation exchange resin, orally or by rectal enema. Onset of action is slow, making this drug a poor choice for the initial treatment of life-threatening hyperkalemia.
- Hemodialysis if potassium levels are life-threatening, especially in patients with renal failure who are unable to excrete excess potassium.[9]

Verify that the blood specimen is not hemolyzed as a cause of false hyperkalemia.

Sodium Disturbances[15]

Hyponatremia

A serum sodium level less than 135 mEq/L is considered hyponatremia. This condition occurs with an actual decrease in the amount of extracellular sodium or an increase in the extracellular fluid volume, resulting in dilutional hyponatremia.

Etiology. Mild hyponatremia (>125 to 130 mEq/L) is usually related to sodium loss from diuretic use (most common in the elderly) or some degree of fluid overload. The fluid overload is seen from heart failure, renal failure, or liver disease related to developing a secondary hyperaldosteronism (aldosterone is released because of renal hypoperfusion). Infants may develop hyponatremia if given only water as fluid replacement when they have gastroenteritis or from having their formula diluted too much.

Moderate to severe hyponatremia (less than 125 mEq/L) most commonly results from SIADH and psychogenic polydipsia.

Signs and Symptoms. The severity of clinical findings depends on the serum sodium level and the rapidity with which the reduction of sodium occurred. Signs and symptoms of severe hyponatremia include neurologic effects (cerebral edema leading to headache, dizziness, confusion, coma, and seizures) because of its effects on osmolality.

Therapeutic Interventions

- Identify and treat the underlying cause.
- In conscious patients, begin with conservative therapies such as water restriction and oral sodium replacement.
- For severe hyponatremia (serum Na^+ <109 mEq/L), consider slow IV sodium replacement with a 3% to 5% saline solution followed by diuretics to promote water excretion. Defined formulas are available as suggested guidelines for hypertonic saline administration. Hypertonic solutions pose inherent dangers and are given only until symptoms subside. Be sure to follow institutional policies regarding hypertonic saline administration.

Treat hyponatremia cautiously. Aggressive correction is dangerous and associated with pituitary damage (from cells shrinking) and osmotic demyelinating syndrome (demyelinization from rapid sodium replacement).

Hypernatremia

Hypernatremia is defined as a serum sodium level greater than 145 mEq/L. This condition can result from an increase in total sodium or a decrease in body water. It is relatively rare, as people with normal mentation and intact thirst mechanisms have a thirst response to even a slight increase in the serum sodium level (3 mEq/L) above baseline that triggers water intake.

Etiology. Volume depletion may occur as a result of urinary losses, fever, hyperventilation, water deprivation, diarrhea, or excessive perspiration.

An increased serum sodium level causes water to move from the intracellular to extracellular space in an attempt to achieve osmotic equilibrium. The resulting cellular dehydration produces central nervous system depression and (occasionally) intracerebral hemorrhage.[7]

Signs and Symptoms

- Thirst
- Fatigue, lethargy, confusion, coma

Therapeutic Interventions

- To avoid cerebral edema, treat the underlying condition and slowly restore serum sodium levels to normal.
- If water loss is the cause, begin gradual hypotonic fluid replacement with oral water ingestion, D_5W, or a D_5W and 0.45% saline solution intravenously.

REFERENCES

1. Collier, J., & Longmore, M. (Eds.). (2006). *Oxford handbook of clinical specialties* (7th ed.). Oxford, United Kingdom: Oxford University Press.
2. Emergency Nurses Association. (2010). *Sheehy's emergency nursing: Principles and practice* (6th ed.). St. Louis, MO: Mosby.
3. Lis, J. G. (2006). Mental status change and coma. In S. R. Votey & M. A. Davis (Eds.), *Signs and symptoms in emergency medicine* (2nd ed.). St. Louis, MO: Mosby.
4. Skidmore-Roth, L. (2010). *Mosby's nursing drug reference* (23rd ed.). St. Louis, MO: Mosby.
5. Buchanan, J. A. (2006). Diabetes mellitus. In V. J. Markovchick & P. T. Pons (Eds.), *Emergency medicine secrets* (4th ed.). St. Louis, MO: Mosby.
6. Chulay, M., & Burns, S. (2006). *AACN Essentials of critical care nursing.* New York, NY: McGraw-Hill.
7. American Heart Association. (2008). *ACLS resource text for instructors and experienced providers.* Dallas, TX: Author.
8. Trachtenbarg, D. E. (2005). Diabetic ketoacidosis. *American Family Physician, 71*(9), 1705–1714.
9. Kronenberg, H., Melmed, S., Polonsky, M. D., & Larson, P. R. (2007). *Williams textbook of endocrinology* (11th ed.). Philadelphia, PA: Saunders.
10. Lee, S. L. (2011, July 29). *Hyperthyroidism.* Retrieved from http://emedicine.medscape.com/article/121865
11. Herbert, M. E., & Lanctot-Herbert, M. L. (2006). Palpitations and tachycardia. In S. R. Votey & M. A. Davis (Eds.), *Signs and symptoms in emergency medicine* (2nd ed.). St. Louis, MO: Mosby.
12. Bahn, R. S., Burch, H. S., Cooper, D. S., Garber, J. R., Greenlee, C. M., Kline, I. L., ... Stan, M. N. (2009). The role of propyl-thiouracil in the management of Graves' disease in adults: Report of a meeting jointly sponsored by the American Thyroid Association and the Food and Drug Administration. *Thyroid, 19*(7), 673–674.
13. Heinrich, T. W., & Grahm, G. (2003). Hypothyroidism presenting as psychois: Myxedema madness revisited. *Primary Care Companion to the Journal of Clinical Psychiatry, 5,* 260–266.
14. Griffey, R. T., & Ilgen, J. S. (2006). Weakness and fatigue. In S. R. Votey & M. A. Davis (Eds.), *Signs and symptoms in emergency medicine* (2nd ed.). St. Louis, MO: Mosby.
15. Slovis, C. M. (2006). Fluids and electrolytes. In V. J. Markovchick & P. T. Pons (Eds.), *Emergency medicine secrets* (4th ed.). St. Louis, MO: Mosby.
16. Kuiper, B. L. (2007). Fluid and electrolyte abnormalities. In Emergency Nurses Association, *Emergency nursing core curriculum* (6th ed., pp. 361–386). St. Louis, MO: Saunders.
17. Dennison, R. (2007). *Pass CCRN* (3rd ed.). St. Louis, MO: Mosby.

Toxicologic Emergencies

Scott Schaeffer, Randal Bryan Badillo, and Kimberly Hovseth

According to the *2009 Annual Report of the American Association of Poison Control Centers' National Poison Data System*, approximately 2.5 million cases of human exposure to poisons were reported in that year.[1] The five substances most frequently involved in all human exposures were analgesics; cosmetics/personal care products; household cleaning substances; sedatives/hypnotics/antipsychotics; and foreign bodies/toys/miscellaneous. The five most common exposures in children ages 5 years and under were cosmetics/personal care products; analgesics; household cleaning substances; foreign bodies/toys/miscellaneous; and topical preparations.[1]

Exposures can be occupational, environmental, recreational, or therapeutic. Toxic exposures occur through inhalation, ingestion, injection, or contact with skin and mucous membranes. Most poisonings are unintentional, relatively mild, and do not require emergency services. Treatment in a health care facility is required for about 24% of those who contact a poison control center, approximately half of whom are treated and released.[1] Only about 16% of these patients are admitted to a critical care unit.[1]

The field of toxicology, the science of poisons and their effects on living organisms, is evolving rapidly, and practices routinely change as better interventions are identified. Because it is difficult for individual practitioners to keep current, poison control centers located throughout the United States have assumed a vital role in the identification and management of toxic emergencies. Poison control center experts help clinicians to assess patients and can suggest current management practices. These centers have access to POISINDEX and other toxicology databases that are updated regularly. Poison center contact should be made by an emergency department clinician for each poisoned patient. This not only allows poison control centers to be of assistance to emergency departments, but also helps them to track patients

and gather demographic and statistical information on poisonings.

> Nationwide Poison Control Center phone number: 1-800-222-1222

Because most patients with a poison exposure will have no significant problems, it is important to be able to recognize those at greatest risk for serious complications and death. Consider persons in the following categories as "red flag" patients:

- Age: The older the patient, the more likely the patient is to die from ingestion.
- Pharmaceuticals: Pharmaceutical agents are generally more toxic than plants, household chemicals, and recreational drugs.
- Polypharmacy: Patients exposed to multiple substances are at increased risk for death.
- Intentional poisonings: Persons who intentionally expose themselves to toxic substances are considerably more likely to sustain adverse events than are those with unintentional exposures.
- Altered mental status or other severe symptoms on presentation: Patients who are significantly compromised upon arrival to the emergency department are more likely to have a poor outcome.

GENERAL PRIORITIES FOR POISONED PATIENTS

Give basic and advanced supportive care (physiological and psychological) as needed. Support the patient's airway, breathing, and circulation; airway protection is critical in patients with an altered mental status. Specifically:

- Administer supplemental oxygen as needed.
- Establish intravenous access and infuse lactated Ringer solution or normal saline solution.

TABLE 30-1 TOXIDROMES

	HEART RATE	PUPIL SIZE	BLOOD PRESSURE	BODY TEMPERATURE	BOWEL SOUNDS	RESPIRATIONS	DIAPHORESIS
Anticholinergic	↑	↑	↑	↑	↓	↔	↓
Cholinergic	↕	↓	↕	↔	↑	↕	↑
Sedatives	↓	↔	↓	↓	↓	↓	↔
Opioid	↓	↓	↓	↓	↓	↓	↔
Sympathomimetic	↑	↑	↑	↑	↔	↑	↑

Note: ↓, decreased; ↑, increased; ↕, may increase or decrease; ↔, no change.

- Give naloxone (Narcan) 0.4 to 2 mg intravenously, endotracheally, intramuscularly, subcutaneously, intraosseously, or sublingually if the patient has a potential opioid exposure.
- Check blood glucose level and infuse dextrose 50% at 50 mL (25 g) intravenously as needed to maintain normoglycemia.
- Administer 50 to 100 mg thiamine intravenously to adult patients with suspected chronic alcohol abuse.
- Initiate continuous cardiac monitoring and obtain 12-lead electrocardiograms as indicated.
- Monitor urinary output.
- Draw arterial blood gases as indicated.
- Perform serial monitoring of electrolyte levels, vital signs, and respiratory, cardiac, and neurologic status.
- Obtain an exposure history:
  - To what substance or substances was the patient exposed?
  - When did the exposure occur? Is this an acute or chronic exposure?
  - What was the route of exposure?
  - Are there currently any signs or symptoms of poisoning?
  - How much of the substance is involved?
  - Was the exposure intentional or unintentional?
  - Does the patient have a history of previous toxic exposures?
  - What treatment was rendered before arrival of emergency medical services?
  - How old is the patient?
  - What is the patient's medical history (especially cardiac, hepatic, psychiatric, and renal disorders)?
  - Are any psychological, social, or environmental risk factors involved?
- Administer the appropriate antidote (if one is available).
- Provide education to patients, families, and significant others to prevent future incidents.

IDENTIFYING THE POISON

Toxidromes

A toxidrome is a set of toxic symptoms caused by a particular class of medication or type of poison. In the patient with an unknown poisoning, early recognition of a toxidrome will enable emergency personnel to rapidly initiate appropriate treatment. Table 30-1 summarizes common toxidromes that can aid in identification of the poison. Table 30-2 lists some other diagnostic clues for identifying unknown toxins.

Anticholinergic Toxidrome

- Includes antihistamines, tricyclic antidepressants, cyclobenzaprine, Parkinson's disease medications, antispasmodics, mydriatics, and certain plants (e.g., jimsonweed)
- Signs and symptoms include the following:
  - Increased blood pressure, heart rate, and temperature
  - Mydriasis, decreased bowel sounds, dry mucous membranes, flushing, urinary retention, agitation, delirium, and hallucinations
  - A helpful memory aid is HOT as a hare (hyperthermia), RED as a beet (flushing), DRY as a bone, BLIND as a bat (mydriasis), MAD as a hatter (delirium, hallucinations)

Cholinergic Toxidrome

- Includes organophosphates and carbamate insecticides, physostigmine, pilocarpine, and nicotine
- Combination of muscarinic and nicotinic effects (Table 30-3)

Sedative Toxidrome

- Includes ethanol and benzodiazepines
- Signs and symptoms include the following:
  - Decreased blood pressure, heart rate, and respirations

TABLE 30-2 DIAGNOSTIC CLUES IN UNKNOWN EXPOSURES

CLUE OR SYMPTOM	POSSIBLE AGENT OR CAUSE
Metabolic acidosis	MUDPILES mnemonic: **M**ethanol, **U**remia, **D**iabetic ketoacidosis, **P**araldehyde, **I**soniazid/Iron, **L**actic acidosis, **E**thanol/Ethylene glycol, **S**alicylates/**S**ympathomimetics
Radiopaque medications	CHIPE mnemonic: **C**hloral hydrate, **H**eavy metals, **I**ron, **P**henothiazines, **E**nteric-coated tablets
Breath Odors	
Alcohol	Ethanol, chloral hydrate, phenols
Acetone	Acetone, salicylates, isopropyl alcohol, diabetic ketoacidosis
Bitter almond	Cyanide
Coal gas	Carbon monoxide
Garlic	Arsenic, phosphorus, organophosphates
Nonspecific	Consider inhalant abuse
Oil of wintergreen	Methylsalicylates
Urine Color	
Red	Hematuria, hemoglobinuria, myoglobinuria, pyrvinium, phenytoin, phenothiazines, mercury, lead, anthocyanin (food pigment found in beets and blackberries)
Brown-black	Hemoglobin pigments, melanin, methyldopa, cascara, rhubarb, methocarbamol
Blue or blue-green	Amitriptyline, methylene blue, triamterene, Clorets gum, *Pseudomonas*
Brown or red-brown	Porphyria, urobilinogen, nitrofurantoin, furazolidone, metronidazole, aloe, seaweed
Orange	Rifampin, phenazopyridine, sulfasalazine

Data from Dart, R. D. (Ed.). (2000). *The 5-minute toxicology consult.* Philadelphia, PA: Lippincott Williams & Wilkins.

TABLE 30-3 MUSCARINIC AND NICOTINIC EFFECTS OF CHOLINERGIC TOXIDROMES

MUSCARINIC EFFECTS (DUMBELS MNEMONIC)	NICOTINIC EFFECTS
Diarrhea, diaphoresis	Tachycardia
Urination	Hypertension
Miosis	Fasciculations
Bradycardia, bronchorrhea	Paralysis
Emesis	Mydriasis
Lacrimation	
Salivation	

- Normothermic to hypothermic
- Central nervous system (CNS) depression, decreased bowel sounds, hyporeflexia, and ataxia

Opioid Toxidrome

- Includes opiates and narcotics
- Signs and symptoms include the following:
  - Decreased blood pressure, heart rate, respiratory rate, and temperature
  - CNS depression, miosis, hyporeflexia.
- Rapid response to naloxone

Sympathomimetic Toxidrome

- Includes cocaine, amphetamines, and other stimulants
- Signs and symptoms include the following:
  - Increased blood pressure, heart rate, respiratory rate, and temperature
  - CNS excitation, tremors, seizures, hyperreflexia, mydriasis, and diaphoresis

THERAPEUTIC INTERVENTIONS FOR POISONINGS AND OVERDOSES

Gastrointestinal Decontamination

Decontamination of the digestive system can be done in several ways, including by induced emesis, administration of activated charcoal or multiple-dose activated charcoal, gastric lavage, cathartics, and whole-bowel irrigation (WBI). Hemodialysis and charcoal hemoperfusion are also used in some severe poisonings.

Induced Emesis

Although once a mainstay of care, the role of syrup of ipecac in the management of the poisoned patient has significantly decreased in recent years. Routine use of syrup of ipecac is no longer recommended.[2] Some of the serious side effects of ipecac include:

- Risk of aspiration
- Inducing vomiting may lead to increased intracranial pressure
- Increases risk for hemorrhagic bleeding and profound fluid and electrolyte disorders

Syrup of ipecac is only marginally effective at emptying the stomach, and its use is associated with numerous contraindications and complications. Emesis can delay charcoal administration significantly. However, there are rare circumstances under which ipecac *may* be considered appropriate,[2] and as a result, the drug is still available over the counter and at hospitals throughout the United States.

Activated Charcoal

Recently, some research has indicated that the use of activated charcoal alone is equivalent or even superior to other poisoning treatment modalities and combinations. However, no well-controlled studies have documented significant improvement in patient outcome.[3]

Given by mouth or gastric tube, activated charcoal has the advantage of being minimally invasive, relatively easy to administer, and safe for both children and adults. Activated charcoal absorbs and binds most commonly ingested substances. Specific contraindications to use of activated charcoal include the following:[4]

- Ingestion of a corrosive agent or hydrocarbons.
- Decreased or absent bowel sounds (relative contraindication).
- Toxins not bound by charcoal, such as iron, lead, and lithium.

Substances _Not_ Absorbed by Activated Charcoal
• Caustics
• Heavy metals (lead, zinc, mercury)
• Hydrocarbons
• Iron preparations
• Lithium
• Toxic alcohols

Recommendations for the administration of activated charcoal are as follows:

- In rare cases where syrup of ipecac has been administered, activated charcoal should not be administered until induced emesis has subsided (usually 60 to 90 minutes after the patient last vomited).
- Alert, cooperative patients can drink activated charcoal through a straw.
- Activated charcoal is gritty but not particularly unpleasant tasting. Flavoring (e.g., cherry or chocolate syrup) makes the charcoal more palatable and does not decrease its effectiveness.
- Small, intermittent doses may reduce vomiting.

- Shake the activated charcoal mixture (slurry) thoroughly to eliminate clumping.
- More dilute slurries are easier to drink or pass through a gastric tube, particularly tiny pediatric tubes.
- In patients with an altered mental status, aggressively protect the airway (endotracheal intubation) before administration of activated charcoal. Visualization of the epiglottis is difficult *after* activated charcoal has been vomited. Aggressive suctioning of aspirated charcoal appears to improve patient outcome.
- A standard-sized Salem sump tube is adequate for activated charcoal instillation.
- Securely anchor gastric tubes to prevent retraction from the stomach to the esophagus.
- Reconfirm appropriate gastric tube placement immediately before administration of activated charcoal.

Multiple-Dose Activated Charcoal

Multiple-dose ("multidose" or "repeated dose") activated charcoal may be considered for poisonings involving extended-release medications, carbamazepine, dapsone, quinine, theophylline, and medications that may form bezoars or concretions (e.g., enteric-coated tablets). Multiple-dose activated charcoal commonly is used for other substances as well.

Indications for Multiple-Dose Activated Charcoal[5]	
Evidence-Based	**Frequently Used**
• Carbamazepine	• Digoxin
• Dapsone	• Phenytoin
• Phenobarbital	• Salicylates
• Quinine	• Sustained-release preparations
• Theophylline	• Tricyclic antidepressants

Dosing for Multiple-Dose Activated Charcoal

- Administer 0.5 g/kg (25 to 50 g in adults) every 4 to 6 hours for up to 12 to 24 hours.[5]
- Seek consultation with the poison center for pediatric patients.
- Use aqueous formulation, without sorbitol, to prevent fluid loss and electrolyte disturbances.

Gastric Lavage

Gastric lavage may be considered for potentially life-threatening poisonings. Routine use is not recommended, and it should never be performed punitively.[6] Gastric lavage may be of benefit in the following situations:

- Symptomatic patients who present within 1 hour of ingestion.
- Symptomatic patients who have ingested an agent that slows gastrointestinal motility.

- Patients who have ingested a sustained-release medication.
- Patients who have taken massive or life-threatening amounts of a substance.

Like induced emesis, to be of any benefit gastric lavage should be initiated within 1 hour of ingestion. Complications of this procedure include unintentional endotracheal intubation, aspiration, decreased oxygenation during the procedure, and stomach or esophageal perforation.

Cathartics

Cathartics—such as magnesium sulfate, magnesium citrate, or sorbitol—have long been added to activated charcoal to enhance gastrointestinal elimination of poisons. However, overuse of cathartics causes diarrhea, nausea and vomiting, abdominal pain, increased magnesium levels, electrolyte imbalances, and hypovolemia.[7] Cathartics should not be given if bowel sounds are absent. Never administer cathartics to children under 1 year of age; cases of fatal diarrhea have been reported in this population.[4]

Whole-Bowel Irrigation

Whole-bowel irrigation involves the use of an electrolyte solution (GoLYTELY, CoLyte) administered orally or by gastric tube. Caution must be taken in the pediatric population, and WBI for pediatric patients should be guided by a poison center clinician. WBI produces a rapid catharsis, eliminating most matter from the gastrointestinal tract within a few hours. It most commonly is given following ingestion of an agent that is not well adsorbed by activated charcoal, such as enteric- or sustained-release products, iron, lead, lithium, or zinc. Adverse effects of WBI include nausea, vomiting, and severe cramping as well as increased risk of electrolyte imbalance. It is contraindicated in cases of preexisting gastrointestinal pathology or in patients with increased risk of ileus or obstruction. Swallowed button batteries and cocaine-filled condoms or other packets of illicit drugs can also be removed by WBI.[4]

Hemodialysis and Charcoal Hemoperfusion

Hemodialysis is indicated for certain serious poisonings associated with severe metabolic acidosis, electrolyte abnormalities, or renal failure. Peritoneal dialysis also can be used for short-term treatment. Early consultation with the local poison center can help determine when hemodialysis or charcoal hemoperfusion may be appropriate.

Dialysis is not indicated for the following:
- Ingestion of substances that are highly protein bound
- Agents that are rarely lethal or for which an effective antidote exists
- In patients who are too hemodynamically unstable
- In patients with bleeding disorders

Poisons That Respond to Hemodialysis[4,7]	
• Acetaminophen	• Paraldehyde
• Alcohols	• Phenacetin
• Amphetamine	• Phenytoin
• Antibiotics	• Potassium
• Arsenic	• Quinidine
• Chloral hydrate	• Quinine
• Ergotamine	• Salicylate
• Ethylene glycol	• Strychnine
• Isoniazid	• Sulfonamide
• Meprobamate	• Theophylline
• Methanol	• Valproic acid

- In patients with poor vascular access
- In small children

Similar to hemodialysis, charcoal hemoperfusion is an extracorporeal technique that involves filtering blood through a cartridge containing activated charcoal. However, charcoal hemoperfusion is performed infrequently and there are only a handful of substances for which hemoperfusion is indicated. Extracorporeal membrane oxygenation and liver dialysis are two other highly invasive interventions occasionally used to manage serious poisonings.

Poisons That Respond to Charcoal Hemoperfusion
• Digitalis
• Paraquat
• Phenobarbital
• Tegretol
• Theophylline

SPECIFIC TOXICOLOGIC EMERGENCIES

Analgesics

Poisonings related to nonprescription analgesics such as acetaminophen (Tylenol), salicylates (aspirin), and nonsteroidal anti-inflammatory drugs (NSAIDs) have increased rapidly since 1999. These medications come in a variety of strengths, colors, sizes, and combinations, making dosing errors common even by persons with the best intentions. Complacency and easy availability add to the high incidence of exposures.

Acetaminophen

According to the U.S. Food and Drug Administration, acetaminophen (Tylenol), a metabolite of phenacetin, and unintentional acetaminophen overdose are consistently the leading cause of acute liver failure in the United States.[8] This drug is found in varying quantities in more than 200 miscellaneous remedies for pain, sleep, coughs, and colds.

The toxic metabolites of acetaminophen destroy hepatocytes, resulting in hepatic necrosis and massive liver damage. Hepatotoxicity is seen following ingestion of more than 140 mg/kg. Patients with a history of alcohol abuse or other liver disease are at increased risk for acetaminophen toxicity.

Signs and Symptoms of Toxicity[9]

- Initial stage (0 to 24 hours after ingestion)
  - Symptoms may be mild or absent in the early phase, even in significantly toxic individuals.
  - Gastrointestinal irritation (nausea, vomiting, anorexia)
  - In rare cases of massive poisoning (4-hour blood level >800 mg/L), metabolic acidosis and coma can develop within the first 24 hours.
- Dormant stage (24 to 48 hours after ingestion)
  - This is a relatively symptom-free stage of toxicity. Gastrointestinal distress tends to subside, and hepatic failure is not yet significant enough to produce overt findings.
  - Even though the patient is asymptomatic, liver failure has begun.
  - Laboratory studies show elevations of serum transaminases (AST, ALT) and elevated coagulation studies (international normalized ratio, prothrombin/partial thromboplastin time).
  - Right upper quadrant pain may be present.
- Hepatic stage (48 to 96 hours after ingestion)
  - Progressive hepatic encephalopathy develops, characterized by confusion, lethargy, and coma.
  - Vomiting.
  - Jaundice.
  - Significant right upper quadrant pain.
  - Bleeding disorders.
  - Hypoglycemia.
  - Transient elevation of liver enzymes.
  - Renal damage.

Therapeutic Interventions

- Provide basic and advanced supportive care as indicated.
- Obtain baseline liver enzymes, prothrombin time, blood urea nitrogen, and blood glucose levels.
- Consider gastric lavage if the ingestion was recent and the dose was more than 7.5 g (>140 mg/kg in a pediatric patient).
- Administer activated charcoal.
- Consult your regional poison control center.
- Draw a quantitative acetaminophen level 4 hours from the time of (acute) ingestion and plot the results on a Rumack-Matthew nomogram. Serum levels drawn before 4 hours have no clinical value.
  - The nomogram is applicable only to single, acute ingestions and is valid only for levels drawn between 4 and 24 hours after ingestion. For chronic ingestions and those in which more than 24 hours have elapsed, contact a poison center clinician about antidotal therapy.
- If the patient's plasma level falls within the toxic range of the nomogram, administer the antidote, N-acetylcysteine (Mucomyst).
- For best results, initiate therapy within 8 hours of acetaminophen ingestion. However, N-acetylcysteine may still be effective when started up to 24 hours after poisoning.
- N-acetylcysteine dosing:
  - Oral[10]
    - Loading dose: 140 mg/kg.
    - Maintenance dose: 70 mg/kg every 4 hours for 17 additional doses.
    - If the patient is vomiting, administer antiemetics. They may be administered via gastric tube; instill N-acetylcysteine slowly.
  - Intravenous[11]
    - Loading dose: 150 mg/kg in 200 mL D_5W over 60 minutes
    - First maintenance dose: 50 mg/kg in 500 mL D_5W over 4 hours
    - Second maintenance dose: 100 mg/kg in 1000 mL D_5W over 16 hours
- In pediatric patients, the volume of diluents must be decreased to prevent fluid overload resulting in seizures because of hyponatremia.
- Liver dialysis and liver transplant have been used in the management of severe acetaminophen toxicity.

Salicylates

With the emergence of other over-the-counter analgesics, the number of salicylate poisonings has decreased over the past 20 years. Aspirin and other salicylates interfere with a variety of organ systems, including central nervous, hematologic, cardiovascular, and gastrointestinal systems. Salicylates also affect both acid-base and electrolyte status. Management of overdose is complex and consultation with a medical toxicologist or poison center clinician is recommended.

Signs and Symptoms of Toxicity

- Tachypnea and tachycardia
- Nausea, vomiting, and abdominal pain
- Diaphoresis, fever, and dehydration
- Tinnitus
- Hypoglycemia and electrolyte imbalances
- Altered mental status or seizures
- Hemorrhagic gastritis
- Coagulation abnormalities

Therapeutic Interventions

- Provide basic and advanced supportive care as indicated.
- Maintain fluid balance and urine output through administration of intravenous fluids.
  - Correct fluid and electrolyte imbalances (these may be profound).
  - Use caution in patients with pulmonary edema.
- Endotracheal intubation may be necessary.
- Consider WBI. Gastric emptying still can be effective several hours following ingestion if the patient consumed enteric-coated pills.
- Activated charcoal has a high affinity for aspirin. Multiple-dose activated charcoal may be effective.
- Repeat salicylate level measurements every 6 to 12 hours.
- Cautious alkalinization with sodium bicarbonate will both help acidosis and enhance salicylate excretion.
- Provide conventional treatment for hypoglycemia, seizures, and pulmonary edema.
- Hyperthermia usually subsides with rehydration and external cooling.
- Hemodialysis may be indicated in cases of severe poisoning and in patients with renal failure. Hemodialysis can correct fluid and electrolyte disturbances and remove salicylates from the blood.
- Hemodialysis may be indicated in the following situations:
  - Salicylate level greater than 75 mg/dL
  - Decreased renal function
  - Significant acidosis
  - Severe fluid or electrolyte disturbances[9]

Nonsteroidal Anti-inflammatory Drugs

Since the introduction of NSAIDs for nonprescription use in 1984, their use has skyrocketed. Ibuprofen (Motrin, Advil), the most popular NSAID, has a short half-life and is absorbed and eliminated rapidly. Fortunately, the toxicity of these agents is low. In 2009 there were 88,850 poisonings related to NSAIDs. Of 11,350 treated in a health care facility, there was only one death.[1] Acute ingestion of less than 100 mg/kg is regarded as nontoxic. Ingestions of more than 300 mg/kg are considered severe. Ibuprofen has a high safety profile compared with the incidence of death associated with acetaminophen and aspirin.

Signs and Symptoms of Toxicity

- Drowsiness, lethargy, seizures (particularly in children who ingest more than 400 mg/kg)
- Gastrointestinal irritation
- Hypotension, bradycardia
- Renal failure, hepatotoxicity
- Apnea
- Metabolic acidosis

Therapeutic Interventions

- Provide basic and advanced supportive care as indicated.
- Monitor the cardiac rhythm continuously in patients with significant overdoses.
- Serum NSAID levels are not clinically useful.
- Consider gastric lavage if the ingestion was recent and involved a large dose.
- Administer activated charcoal.
- Institute seizure precautions.

Common Prescription Medications

Beta-Blockers and Calcium Channel Blockers

Patients with toxic levels of calcium channel blockers or beta-blockers present unique and problematic profiles. Because of the sustained-release nature of many of these agents, onset of toxicity may be late, characterized by waxing and waning deterioration. Medications in these classes produce a variety of negative chronotropic, dromotropic, and inotropic effects. They may cause severe toxicity with as little as one tablet or capsule in pediatric patients. Death frequently occurs more than 24 hours after the overdose.[1] Symptoms may be rapid in their progression and may be resistant to conventional therapies.

Signs and Symptoms of Toxicity

- Hypotension
- Cardiac disturbances, especially conduction abnormalities, atrioventricular blocks, and bradycardia
- Confusion, altered mental status, syncope, seizures, and coma
- Nausea and vomiting
- Hyperglycemia with calcium channel blockers *or* hypoglycemia with beta-blockers

Therapeutic Interventions

- Provide basic and advanced supportive care as indicated.
- Administer crystalloids such as normal saline (0.9%) or lactated Ringer solution.
- Monitor cardiac rhythm continuously. Obtain a 12-lead electrocardiogram.
- Quantitative drug levels are of little value in the management of acute toxicity.
- Consider gastric lavage if ingestion was recent.
- Administer activated charcoal.
- WBI can be used for significant ingestion of sustained-release products.
- Institute cardiac pacing as needed for atrioventricular blocks and bradycardia.
- Several drugs may be used to manage calcium channel blocker or beta-blocker overdose. Treat patients symptomatically.[12–14]

- *Calcium:* Effective in small or therapeutic overdoses but is relatively ineffective in massive overdoses.
  - Administer 1 g of calcium chloride over 5 minutes; may repeat every 15 to 20 minutes for an additional three to four doses.[12]
  - Calcium gluconate should *not* be used, as it has a reduced bioavailability of calcium.
- *Atropine:* May be useful for the treatment of symptomatic sinoatrial node bradycardia but will not reverse bradycardia caused by atrioventricular blocks. Transcutaneous pacing is preferred.
- *Glucagon:* Glucagon has both positive inotropic and positive chronotropic effects. It is an antidote for drugs that reduce intracellular calcium. Administration may reverse myocardial depression in cases of intractable bradycardia.
  - The optimum dose is not well established.
  - A suggested glucagon regimen is 5 to 10 mg slow intravenous push followed by an infusion of 1 to 5 mg/h.[15]
- *Vasopressors:* Treat hypotension with fluids, dopamine, or norepinephrine.
- *Hyperinsulinemia and euglycemic therapy*[14]: Some research suggests that insulin and glucose administration increases myocardial carbohydrate metabolism and contractility in calcium channel blocker overdose. Before beginning treatment, consider the patient's baseline glucose level.
  - Bolus dose of insulin 1 IU/kg
  - 25 g of dextrose (50 mL of $D_{50}W$) in adults
  - Pediatric dose: 0.25 g dextrose per kilogram (as in $D_{25}W$)
  - Insulin infusion of 0.5 to 1 IU/kg per hour
  - Dextrose infusion of 0.5 g/kg per hour for both pediatric and adult patients

Tricyclic Antidepressants

Tricyclic antidepressants are highly protein bound and lipid soluble. This results in falsely low serum levels, inability to remove this chemical through dialysis, and a long elimination half-life. The patient may also be too unstable to undergo dialysis, if needed. Onset of action is rapid and symptoms may peak as soon as 60 minutes after ingestion. The three pharmacological features responsible for the toxic manifestations most commonly observed in tricyclic antidepressant overdose are the following:
- Cardiotoxicity: Decreased cardiac conduction results.
- Adrenergic compromise: Alpha-adrenergic stimulation is blocked, and catecholamines are depleted.
- Anticholinergic activity: Although prominent, anticholinergic symptoms have little impact on morbidity and mortality.

TABLE 30-4	THE ANTICHOLINERGIC TOXIDROME: COMMON SIGNS AND SYMPTOMS
PERIPHERAL ANTICHOLINERGIC EFFECTS	**CENTRAL NERVOUS SYSTEM EFFECTS**
• Blurred vision	• Anxiety
• Decreased bowel motility	• Confusion
• Dilated pupils	• Delirium
• Dry mouth	• Disorientation
• Dry skin	• Hallucinations
• Fever	• Impaired recent memory
• Flushed skin	• Incoherent speech
• Increased heart rate	• Paranoia
• Reduced secretions	• Purposeless movements
• Urinary retention	

Signs and Symptoms of Toxicity
- Anticholinergic effects
- Nausea and vomiting
- Tachydysrhythmias, prolonged PR interval, widened QRS complex, prolonged QT, heart blocks, and asystole
- Hypotension
- Syncope, seizures, and coma
  See Table 30-4 for more information.

Therapeutic Interventions
- Provide basic and advanced supportive care as indicated.
- Serum tricyclic antidepressant levels are not clinically useful in overdose situations.[16]
- Institute gastric lavage. Endotracheal intubation is usually advisable before lavage because of the rapid onset of toxic symptoms.
- Consider giving multiple doses of activated charcoal (first check for the presence of an ileus).
- Consider cathartic agents to counteract drug-induced decreased bowel motility.
- Monitor continuously for cardiac dysrhythmias; these can be severe and lethal.
- Give sodium bicarbonate intravenously. Mild alkalosis reduces the incidence of dysrhythmias. Keep serum pH between 7.45 and 7.55.[16]
- Manage hypotension with isotonic fluids and dopamine or norepinephrine as needed.
- Administer benzodiazepines for seizures.

Digoxin

Digoxin is prescribed for the treatment of heart failure. Digoxin also is given to reduce ventricular response rates in certain supraventricular tachycardias. Digitalis works by

TABLE 30-5	**SIGNS AND SYMPTOMS OF DIGITALIS TOXICITY**
MILD TOXICITY	**SEVERE TOXICITY**
• Anorexia	• Blurred vision
• Bradycardia	• Delirium
• Confusion	• Diarrhea
• Headache	• Disorientation
• Malaise	• Hallucinations
• Nausea and vomiting	• Sinoatrial or atrioventricular block
• Premature ventricular contractions	• Ventricular fibrillation
• Visual disturbances	• Ventricular tachycardia

slowing atrioventricular nodal conduction and augmenting contractility (positive inotropic effect). The concurrent use of other cardiac drugs and diuretics or the presence of hypokalemia can increase the incidence of mild toxicity in patients receiving therapeutic doses. Following acute ingestion, symptoms can peak in as little as 30 minutes or up to 12 hours later.[17]

Signs and Symptoms of Toxicity
- Dysrhythmias, especially bradycardia
- Hyperkalemia
- Anorexia, nausea, and vomiting
- Mental status changes or vision disturbances
  See Table 30-5 for more information.

Therapeutic Interventions
- Provide basic and advanced supportive care as indicated.
- Obtain a quantitative serum digoxin level immediately and 6 hours after acute ingestion. Further digoxin levels are of no value.
- Administer activated charcoal.
- Correct electrolyte imbalances, hypoglycemia, and hypovolemia.
- Give atropine or use cardiac pacing for bradycardia.
- Administer Digoxin Immune Fab (Digibind), the digitalis antidote.[17]
- Indications for Digoxin Immune Fab
  - Large ingestions in previously healthy individuals (adult patients, 10 mg; pediatric patients, 4 mg)
  - Bradycardia unresponsive to atropine
  - Ventricular dysrhythmias
  - Digoxin levels in excess of 10 ng/mL
  - Hyperkalemia (>5.5 mEq/L)
- Dosage
  - Each vial binds 0.5 mg of digoxin.
  - Number of vials = (Digoxin level [ng/mL] × Patient weight in kg) ÷ 100

- Administer over 30 minutes. If situation is life-threatening, Digoxin Immune Fab may be administered as an intravenous bolus. Seek advice from the poison center clinician.
- Precautions
  - Digoxin Immune Fab has an excellent safety profile but allergic reactions are possible.
- Check for precipitous drops in potassium levels.
- Monitor for new-onset dysrhythmias and symptoms of congestive heart failure in patients who have been taking digoxin therapeutically.

Benzodiazepines

Benzodiazepines are administered for anxiety, sedation, seizures, and muscle relaxation. Designed to depress the CNS, these drugs also can cause hypotension and respiratory suppression in overdose quantities. Fortunately, mortality related to these substances is low. Death usually involves coingestion of another CNS depressant such as ethanol.

Signs and Symptoms of Toxicity
- Intoxicated behavior without the odor of alcohol, slurred speech, impaired memory, or coma
- Respiratory depression
- Dilated pupils
- Weak and rapid pulse

Therapeutic Interventions
- Provide basic and advanced supportive care as indicated.
- Monitor closely for respiratory and CNS depression.
- Do not induce emesis because of CNS depression.
- Consider gastric lavage if the amount ingested was large or was combined with other medicines.
- Consider activated charcoal.
- With supportive care (possibly including mechanical ventilation), benzodiazepine overdoses generally self-resolve.
- Administer flumazenil (Romazicon), a specific antidote for benzodiazepine reversal.[18]

Precautions
- Do not give flumazenil to patients who have also ingested a tricyclic antidepressant, cocaine, or other seizure-inducing agent.
- Do not give flumazenil to chronic benzodiazepine users. This can precipitate seizures due to withdrawal.
- Monitor respiratory status and watch for resedation 30 to 60 minutes after flumazenil administration.

Oral Diabetic Medications

There are three groups of diabetic medications, each with a different toxic profile: sulfonylureas, meglitinides, and biguanide. Sulfonylureas include glipizide, glyburide, glimepiride, chlorpropamide, acetohexamide, tolazamide, and tolbutamide. Meglitinides include nateglinide and repaglinide. These two groups of medications are highly toxic in pediatric patients even at low doses. Biguanide (metformin) may produce significant lactic acidosis; hypoglycemia is not the primary toxic effect.

Signs and Symptoms of Toxicity
- Sulfonylureas and meglitinides
  - Hypoglycemia
  - CNS depression, including coma
  - Seizures
- Biguanide (metformin)
  - Lactic acidosis

Therapeutic Interventions
- Supportive care as indicated, including intravenous fluids and airway management.
- Consider administration of activated charcoal.
- Food or juice if the patient is alert.
- Dextrose infusion or boluses for hypoglycemia.
- Octreotide may be used for hypoglycemia unresponsive to food or dextrose.
  - Octreotide antagonizes insulin release.
  - Adult dose: 50 mcg subcutaneously or intravenously; repeat every 6 hours as needed.
  - Pediatric dose: 1 mcg/kg subcutaneously or intravenously; repeat every 6 hours as needed.
- Dialysis may be considered for elevated lactate levels because of metformin toxicity.
- Lactic acidosis may be treated with sodium bicarbonate. Consult with a poison center clinician.

Environmental Poisons

Iron

Toxic levels of iron are most commonly a result of iron supplement ingestion. Treatment is complicated by the fact that there is no physiologic mechanism for iron excretion. It is important to identify the type of iron ingested and the amount in the compound, as 40 to 60 mg/kg of elemental iron may lead to severe symptoms.[4]

Signs and Symptoms of Toxicity
- Initial stage (0 to 2 hours after ingestion)
  - Nausea, vomiting, and abdominal pain
  - Hematemesis, bloody stools
  - Hypotension
- Second stage (2 to 48 hours after ingestion)
  - Resolution of gastrointestinal disturbances
  - Dehydration may be the only symptom present
- Third stage (48 to 96 hours after ingestion)
  - Metabolic acidosis
  - Coagulopathy
  - Hemorrhage and shock
  - Hepatic and renal failure

Therapeutic Interventions
- Provide basic and advanced supportive care as indicated.
- Induced emesis may be preferred over gastric lavage in pediatric patients because most adult-strength pills (e.g., prenatal vitamins) are large and will not fit through a pediatric lavage tube. Seek advice from a poison center clinician.
- Activated charcoal does *not* bind well with iron.
- Obtain abdominal radiographs. Some types of iron tablets are radiopaque on abdominal films. Chewable vitamins containing iron are usually not visible.
- Initiate WBI if there is radiographic evidence of iron tablets past the pylorus or if iron remains in the stomach after other attempts at decontamination.
- Draw and send a serum iron level 4 to 6 hours after ingestion.
- Consider chelation therapy with deferoxamine (Desferal) with a maximum dose of 15 mg/kg per hour by continuous infusion. Continuation of deferoxamine therapy beyond 24 hours greatly increases the risk of severe side effects.[19]
- Indications for deferoxamine
  - Symptomatic patients when an iron level is not readily available.
  - Ingestion of more than 20 mg/kg of elemental iron.
  - Significant signs of iron toxicity such as metabolic acidosis, hypotension, and altered mental status.
  - Serum iron levels greater than 500 mcg/dL.
  - Deferoxamine administration turns the urine a pink "vin rosé" color.
  - Continue deferoxamine infusion until urine color normalizes.
- Emergency surgery may be performed for the removal of iron bezoars from the gastrointestinal tract. Bezoars can cause necrosis, gut perforation, and massive intra-abdominal hemorrhage. Although rarely indicated, some patients have required exchange transfusions for massively toxic levels.

Pesticides

Organophosphates and carbamates are two related classes of insecticides that are commonly available, and both can cause serious poisonings. Patients with a toxic exposure to either of these agents have similar clinical presentations, but the duration of carbamate symptoms is usually shorter. Organophosphates and carbamates bind acetylcholinesterase, allowing accumulation of acetylcholine at the neuroreceptor sites. This produces a cholinergic crisis. Pesticides are readily absorbed by oral, dermal, and inhalation routes of exposure. Geriatric and pediatric patients may be more at

TABLE 30-6	CLINICAL EFFECTS OF PESTICIDE POISONING (ACETYLCHOLINE EXCESS)

TISSUE OR ORGAN	EFFECT
Muscarinic Effects	
Sweat glands	Sweating
Pupils	Pupillary constriction
Lacrimal glands	Lacrimation
Salivary glands	Excessive salivation
Bronchial tree	Wheezing
Gastrointestinal	Cramps, vomiting, diarrhea, tenesmus
Cardiovascular	Bradycardia, fall in blood pressure
Ciliary bodies	Blurred vision
Bladder	Urinary incontinence
Nicotinic Effects	
Striated muscle	Fasciculations, cramps, weakness, twitching, paralysis, respiratory embarrassment, cyanosis, respiratory arrest
Sympathetic ganglia	Tachycardia, elevated blood pressure
Central nervous system	Anxiety, restlessness, ataxia, convulsions, insomnia, coma, absent reflexes, Cheyne-Stokes respirations, respiratory and circulatory depression

risk for serious side effects from organophosphate exposures because of their lower cholinesterase levels.[4]

Signs and Symptoms of Toxicity. Table 30-6 summarizes the signs of pesticide toxicity.

Therapeutic Interventions

- Decontaminate the patient to reduce further absorption and prevent secondary exposure of health care providers.
- Provide basic and advanced supportive care as indicated.
- Treat hypotension with fluids and vasopressors. (Resolving bradycardia will improve blood pressure.)
- Administer antidotes.
  - *Atropine:* This drug may need to be given for up to 24 hours. Massive quantities may be required. Continue to give atropine until secretions are minimal and bradycardia has resolved.
  - *Pralidoxime chloride (Protopam):* This antidote is administered as a loading dose followed by a continuous intravenous infusion in cases of severe organophosphate poisoning; effects are often dramatic.

Cyanide

Cyanide is used in many industrial processes and has been linked with terrorism attacks. Exposure may occur through inhalation, dermal contact, ingestion, or parenteral (extended nitroprusside infusion) routes. Ingestion of apricot seeds, cassava, or other plant sources may liberate cyanide. Cyanide exposure secondary to smoke from fires is an occupational hazard for firefighters. Because cyanide levels generally are not readily available, consider the diagnosis of cyanide poisoning in a patient with an elevated lactate level and minimal difference between arterial and venous oxygen saturation levels.

Signs and Symptoms of Toxicity

- Hypoxia
- Seizures
- Metabolic acidosis
- Hypotension
- Dysrhythmias
- Respiratory arrest

Therapeutic Interventions. As soon as cyanide poisoning is suspected, rapid intervention must be performed because of the potential for severe decline in patient status.[20]

- Provide basic and advanced supportive care as indicated.
- Oxygen via nonrebreather mask
  - Endotracheal intubation and mechanical ventilation as needed
- Administer antidote medications from a commercial cyanide antidote kit. These kits usually include amyl nitrite ampoules, sodium nitrite, and sodium thiosulfate. Hydroxocobalamin may also be available. The patient must be closely monitored, as hypotension and headache may occur with administration of nitrites.
  - Amyl nitrite: Crush the ampoule and hold under the patient's nose. Have the patient inhale deeply for 15 seconds, if able. Remove for 15 seconds and repeat. Change the ampule every 3 minutes. Discontinue when sodium nitrite has been administered.
    - Amyl nitrite may be delivered via bag-mask.
    - Health care team members should avoid inhalation of amyl nitrite.
  - When intravenous access is established, administer sodium nitrite.
    - Adult dose: 300 mg (10 mL of 3% solution) over 2 to 4 minutes
    - Pediatric dose: 0.2 mL/kg of 3% solution (maximum 10 mL) over 5 minutes[11]
  - Once sodium nitrite has been administered, give sodium thiosulfate.

○ Adult dose: 12.5 g (50 mL of 25% solution) over 30 minutes
○ Pediatric dose: 7 g/m^2 (maximum 12.5 g)[20]

If adequate response is not obtained within 30 minutes, sodium nitrite and sodium thiosulfate may be repeated at half the initial dose for both adult and pediatric patients.

Petroleum Distillates

Kerosene, lighter fluid, mineral oil, furniture polish, turpentine, gasoline, and many insecticides contain petroleum distillates. Complications usually occur as a result of aspiration or other pulmonary problems. Hydrocarbon aspiration produces transient CNS depression or excitation. As with pesticides, the skin, gut, and lungs readily absorb petroleum products.

Signs and Symptoms of Toxicity

- Respiratory difficulty (aspiration of petroleum distillates can initiate a massive pulmonary inflammatory response)
- Infiltrates on chest radiographs
- Abnormal arterial blood gases
- Dysrhythmias

Therapeutic Interventions

- Decontaminate the patient to reduce further absorption and prevent secondary exposure of health care personnel.
- Provide basic and advanced supportive care as indicated.

- Administer oxygen. Endotracheal intubation may be required.
- Gastric emptying is not indicated unless the patient has a history of a large ingestion of hydrocarbons known to produce renal, liver, or CNS toxicity (e.g., halogenated hydrocarbons, petroleum, or petroleum distillates with additives).
- Monitor arterial blood gases in patients with respiratory symptoms (coughing, choking, dyspnea).
- Obtain a chest radiograph. (Changes should be diagnostic within 6 hours of exposure.)

CURRENTLY AVAILABLE ANTIDOTES

An antidote is a physiological antagonist that reverses the signs or symptoms of poisoning. Table 30-7 provides a brief guide to poisons and their antidotes.[4,7] New drugs are added to and old drugs are deleted from this list regularly. For current information and help with patient management, contact the experts at your regional poison control center.

PREVENTION AND EDUCATION

Since its passage in 1970, the Poison Prevention Packaging Act has succeeded in reducing the number of pediatric exposures and poison-related deaths. This legislation mandated child-resistant caps on toxic substances. Nonetheless, child-resistant containers are not a substitute for prevention

TABLE 30-7 ANTIDOTES

EXPOSURE OR CONDITION	ANTIDOTE	COMMENTS
Carbamates	Atropine, pralidoxime	Very large quantities of atropine may be required.
Organophosphates		Give a pralidoxime loading dose followed by continuous infusion.
Neuroleptic drugs (haloperidol, phenothiazines, thioxanthenes) and metoclopramide	Benztropine (Cogentin)	Reverses drug-induced dystonias through competitive inhibition of muscarinic receptors and blockade of dopamine reuptake.
Calcium channel blockers	Calcium chloride (drug of choice unless the patient is acidotic)	Large amounts may be required. Keep serum Ca^{++} <11 mg/dL.
Hydrofluoric acid burns	Calcium gluconate	2.5% calcium gluconate gel for dermal exposure. 10% calcium gluconate infiltrated locally around hydrofluoric acid burns (or can be given as an intra-arterial infusion into the affected limb).
Hyperkalemia and hypermagnesemia	Calcium gluconate intravenously	Administer slowly.
Cyanide and hydrogen sulfide	Cyanide kit	Follow the instructions in the kit. Oxygen and methemoglobin levels need to be monitored closely. Do not use methylene blue if excessive methemoglobinemia occurs. For hydrogen sulfide poisoning, do *not* use sodium thiosulfate. Use the nitrites only.

TABLE 30-7 ANTIDOTES—cont'd

EXPOSURE OR CONDITION	ANTIDOTE	COMMENTS
Iron	Deferoxamine mesylate (Desferal)	Deferoxamine forms ferrioxamine complexes that are excreted. This red complex is water-soluble and is excreted readily by the kidneys. Vin rosé–colored urine indicates the presence of iron in the urine.
Digitalis	Digoxin Immune Fab (Digibind)	Antigen-binding fragments bind with digoxin.
Arsenic, lead encephalopathy, gold, and mercury	Dimercaprol (BAL, British anti-Lewisite)	Heavy metals inhibit sulfhydryl-containing enzymes; the resulting chelated mercaptide product is less toxic and more easily excreted from the body than the heavy metals.
Phenothiazines	Diphenhydramine (Benadryl)	Diphenhydramine reverses drug-induced extrapyramidal effects.
Benzodiazepines	Flumazenil	Use cautiously in persons with unknown drug ingestions. Seizures can occur with reversal of benzodiazepine effects in chronic users, especially with tricyclic antidepressant or cocaine coingestions.
Beta-blockers	Glucagon	Bypasses beta-adrenergic blockade by activating nonbeta receptors; increases cardiac contractility.
Nitrites and local anesthetics	Methylene blue	Methylene blue is a reducing agent that converts methemoglobin to hemoglobin.
Sulfonylureas (oral hypoglycemic agents)	Octreotide	Stimulates release of insulin from the beta islet cells of the pancreas. Use for overdoses refractory to glucose administration.
Acetaminophen	*N*-acetylcysteine (Mucomyst)	*N*-acetylcysteine is a glutathione substitute that prevents the formation of toxic intermediary metabolites. Best when given within 8 hours of ingestion but can be given up to 24 hours after ingestion.
Opioids	Naloxone (Narcan), Nalmefene (Revex)	Opioid antagonists used to reverse central nervous system and respiratory depressant effects.
Anticholinergics *(rarely)* and tricyclic antidepressants *(last resort only)*	Physostigmine	Inhibits the destructive action of acetylcholinesterase. Should *not* be used routinely because of its potential for serious adverse effects.
Warfarin and long-acting anticoagulants	Phytonadione (vitamin K)	Reverses the inhibitory action of warfarin on blood clotting factors II, VII, IX, and X.
Tricyclic antidepressants	Sodium bicarbonate	Aside from gastric decontamination, sodium bicarbonate is the most useful single intervention for the management of overdose.

education or aggressive poison-proofing of homes frequented by young children. Recently, denatonium benzoate (Bitrex), a taste-aversive agent, has been added to many household products to dissuade children from drinking toxic quantities. Expanding the use of this product to an even greater number of poisonous agents could decrease pediatric morbidity and mortality even further.

Emergency nurses are in an excellent position to teach patients and communities about proper medication use, safe storage of toxins, and the risks associated with recreational substance abuse.

REFERENCES

1. Bronstein, A. C., Spyker, D., Cantilena, L. R., Green, J. L., Rumack, B. H., & Giffin, S. L. (2010). 2009 annual report of the American Association of Poison Control Centers' National Poison Data system (NPDS): 27th annual report. *Clinical Toxicology, 48*(10), 979–1178.
2. Manoguerra, A. S., & Cobaugh, D. J.; Guidelines for the Management of Poisoning Panel. (2005). Guideline on the use of ipecac syrup in the out-of-hospital management of ingested poisons. *Clinical Toxicology, 43*(1), 1–10.

3. Chyka, P. A., Seger, D., Krenzelok, E. P., & Vale, J. A.; American Academy of Clinical Toxicology; European Association of Poisons Centres and Clinical Toxicologists. (2005). Position paper: Single-dose activated charcoal. *Clinical Toxicology*, *43*(2), 61–87.

4. Phillips, M. (2007). Toxicologic emergencies. In Emergency Nurses Association (Ed.), *Emergency nursing core curriculum* (6th ed., pp. 604–658). St. Louis, MO: Saunders.

5. Howland, M. A. (2006). Activated charcoal. In N. Flomenbaum, L. Goldfrank, R. Hoffman, M. A. Howland, N. Lewin, & L. Nelson (Eds.), *Goldfrank's toxicologic emergencies* (8th ed, pp. 128–134). New York, NY: McGraw-Hill.

6. Vale, J. A., & Kulig, K. (2005). Position paper: Gastric lavage. *Clinical Toxicology*, *43*(2), 61–87.

7. Sturt, P. (2010). Toxicologic emergencies. In P. K. Howard & R. A. Steinmann (Eds.), *Sheehy's emergency nursing: Principles and practice* (6th ed., pp. 564–577), St. Louis, MO: Mosby.

8. U.S. Food and Drug Administration. (2011, January 13). *FDA drug safety communication: Prescription acetaminophen products to be limited to 325 mg per dosage unit; Boxed warning will highlight potential for severe liver failure.* Retrieved from http://www.fda.gov/Drugs/DrugSafety/ucm239821.htm

9. Goldfrank, L. R., & Flomenbaum, N. (Eds.). (2006). *Goldfrank's toxicologic emergencies* (8th ed.). New York, NY: McGraw Hill.

10. Rowden, A. K., Norvell, J., Eldridge, D. L., & Kirk, M. A. (2005). Updates on acetaminophen toxicity. *Medical Clinics of North America*, *89*(6), 1145–1159.

11. Acetadote [package insert]. (2008). Nashville, TN: Cumberland Pharmaceuticals.

12. DeRoos, F. (2006). Calcium channel blockers. In L. R. Goldfrank & N. Flomenbaum (Eds.), *Goldfrank's toxicology emergencies* (8th ed., pp. 911–923). New York, NY: McGraw Hill.

13. Lheureux, P. E., Zahir, S., Gris, M., Derrey, A. S., & Penaloza, A. (2006). Bench-to-bedside review: Hyperinsulinaemia/euglycaemia therapy in the management of overdose of calcium-channel blockers. *Critical Care*, *10*(3), 212.

14. Kerns, W. (2007). Management of beta-adrenergic blocker and calcium channel antagonist toxicity [abstract viii]. *Emergency Medicine Clinics of North America*, *25*(2), 309–331.

15. Bailey, B. (2003). Glucagon in beta-blocker and calcium channel blocker overdoses: A systematic review. *Journal of Toxicology Clinical Toxicology*, *41*(5), 595–602.

16. Liebelt, E. L. (2006). Cyclic antidepressants. In L. R. Goldfrank & N. Flomenbaum (Eds.), *Goldfrank's toxicologic emergencies* (8th ed., pp. 1083–1097). New York, NY: McGraw Hill.

17. Schaider, J., Hayden, S. R., Wolfe, R., Barkin, R. M., & Rosen, P. (Eds.). (2003). *Rosen and Barkin's 5-minute emergency medicine consult* (2nd ed.). Philadelphia, PA: Lippincott Williams & Wilkins.

18. Fullwood, D., Sargent, S., & Fernandes, T. (2010). An overview of sedation for adult patients in hospital. *Nursing Standard*, *24*(39), 48–56.

19. Howland, M. A. (2006). Deferoxamine. In L. R. Goldfrank & N. Flomenbaum (Eds.), *Goldfrank's toxicologic emergencies* (8th ed., pp. 638–642). New York, NY: McGraw Hill.

20. Hamel, J. (2011). A review of acute cyanide poisoning with a treatment update. *Critical Care Nurse*, *31*(1), 72–81.

Environmental Emergencies

S. Kay Sedlak

This chapter discusses specific emergencies that occur because of the body's exposure to changes in or extremes of environmental conditions. The most common environmental emergencies involve the body's inability to thermoregulate due to exposure to cold or heat.

Thermoregulation, or the maintenance of a fairly constant body temperature, is important because the human body functions optimally within a specific temperature range. The body attempts to maintain a temperature of 37°C (98.6°F) and the hypothalamus reacts to changes in blood temperature of as little as 0.5°C (roughly 1°F). There can be negative consequences to both too little heat and too much heat.

COLD-INDUCED INJURIES

Cold-induced injuries include both tissue injuries (chilblains, immersion foot, and frostbite) and a decrease in core body temperature. Table 31-1 lists factors that increase susceptibility to cold.

Chilblains[1]

Chilblains, also known as pernio, are localized areas of itching, painful redness, and recurrent edema on exposed areas such as the earlobes, fingers, and toes. Chilblains are a mild form of frostbite that develop in cool, damp climates when temperatures are above freezing. Symptoms (usually numbness and tingling) are generally self-limiting and resolve with symptomatic treatment.

Immersion Foot

Immersion foot, or "trench foot," occurs when the feet are wet and subjected to cold temperatures for prolonged periods inside a nonbreathing boot or shoe. This condition is typically seen in foot soldiers, hunters, and the homeless. Initially the foot appears pale and wrinkled. Tissue sloughing can develop if the condition is allowed to persist. Dry shoes and socks are necessary to prevent this condition.

Frostbite[2–6]

Frostbite is a traumatic condition that results when ice crystals form in the cells and extracellular spaces, causing direct cellular damage. In addition, there is indirect damage secondary to vasospasm and arterial thromboses. Once the cells are frozen, damage is irreversible. Further exposure or trauma worsens the injury. Protecting the tissues surrounding frostbitten areas helps prevent additional tissue loss. The full extent of injury will not be apparent for several days. Frostbite can be accompanied by hypothermia. Depending on the extent of hypothermia, treatment of this condition may take precedence over frostbite interventions.

Superficial Frostbite

Superficial frostbite usually involves the fingertips, ears, nose, cheeks, or toes. The skin will retain some resistance when pressed down upon.

Signs and Symptoms
- Local burning, numbness, tingling
- Whitish, waxy skin color
- Stinging, hot feeling after the skin thaws
- Large blisters, depending on length of exposure

Deep Frostbite

Deep frostbite produces local vascular and tissue changes resulting in cellular injury and death. Deep frostbite can involve muscle, fat, bones, and tendons as well as skin. Factors that influence the probability of sustaining frostbite include the following:
- Ambient temperature
- Windchill factor
- Duration of exposure
- Contact with moisture or metal objects
- Type and number of layers of clothing

TABLE 31-1 FACTORS THAT INCREASE SUSCEPTIBILITY TO COLD

GENERAL	DRUG USE	ENDOCRINE SYSTEM	CARDIOVASCULAR SYSTEM	NEUROLOGIC SYSTEM	TRAUMA	INFECTION
Infancy Advanced age Malnutrition Exhaustion	Alcohol Sedatives Clonidine	Hypoglycemia Hypothyroidism Adrenal insufficiency Diabetes	Peripheral vascular disease Nicotine use	Peripheral neuropathy Spinal cord damage Autonomic neuropathy Hypothalamic disease	Falls (head or spinal injury) Fracture causing immobility	Sepsis (diaphoresis and hypothalamic dysfunction)

Data from Patel, N. N., & Patel, D. N. (2008). Frostbite. *American Journal of Medicine*, *121*(9), 765–766.

Signs and Symptoms

- Slight burning pain followed by a feeling of warmth and then numbness as the area freezes
- Whitish or yellow-white discoloration of the skin followed by a waxy appearance
- Swelling and intense burning accompanying thawing
- Blisters (usually appear in 1 to 7 days)
- Edema of the entire extremity that may persist for months
- Severe discoloration and gangrene are late findings

Therapeutic Interventions

Escharotomy is indicated for treatment of severe vascular compromise in deep frostbite.

Amputation of body parts affected by frostbite is not an emergency procedure. As edema resolves, early necrosis becomes apparent. Final demarcation often is delayed for more than 60 to 90 days. Hence the aphorism "frostbite in January, amputate in July."

General guidelines for the management of cold-related tissue injury are listed in Table 31-2.

Prevention

- Dress properly for the climate; wear layers of loose-fitting clothing.
- When outdoors in cold areas, eat a diet high in carbohydrates and fats.
- Do not smoke or drink alcoholic or caffeinated beverages in extreme weather.
- Prevent bare skin contact with metal objects.
- Keep skin and clothing dry.
- Avoid exhaustion.
- Protect previously frostbitten parts from re-exposure.

Hypothermia

Hypothermia is defined as a core body temperature of less than 35°C (95°F). Severe hypothermia occurs at a core body temperature of 32.2°C (90°F). Below this temperature, profound physiologic derangements take place. Death usually

TABLE 31-2 GENERAL MANAGEMENT PRINCIPLES FOR COLD-RELATED TISSUE INJURY

- Do not thaw areas if they are likely to be refrozen before definitive care. Repeated freeze-thaw cycles cause additional tissue necrosis.
- Protect the injured part from further damage.
- Do not use ice or snow and friction to massage the frozen extremity. This outmoded intervention promotes further tissue damage.
- Immerse the injured part in circulating water that is temperature controlled at 37°C–40°C (98.6–104°F).
- Encourage gentle motion of the injured part in water, but do *not* rub injured tissues.
- Once thawed, protect and immobilize the extremity with splints and bulky sterile dressings (avoid pressure).
- Administer nonsteroidal anti-inflammatory medication and additional analgesics if necessary.
- Provide topical care for areas of open wounds.
- Ensure tetanus prophylaxis.
- Rehydrate patient and address other medical and surgical conditions.

results when core body temperature falls below 25.6°C (78°F). The following populations are especially prone to hypothermia:

- Neonates, because of limited body fat and an inability to shiver or seek warmth
- Elderly persons, because of medications, loss of body fat, and cardiovascular changes associated with aging
- Alcoholics and the homeless, because of poor nutrition and environmental exposure

Pathophysiology

Body heat loss occurs by four different means, which alone or in combination can result in losses that overwhelm the body's ability to compensate: convection, conduction, radiation, and evaporation (Table 31-3).

> Normal body heat lost by conduction is only 2% but it may increase 5 times with wet clothes or 25 times with cold water immersion.[7]

Most of the metabolic and enzymatic processes of the body are temperature dependent and changes evolve with decreasing temperatures. At core body temperatures less than 32°C (90°F), defined as profound or severe hypothermia, pathologic changes are noted as the cold directly affects various body functions. Table 31-4 summarizes potential changes in various body systems.

Rewarming

Rewarming measures can be classified into three categories: passive or spontaneous rewarming, active external or surface rewarming, and active internal or core rewarming. Methodologies for each as well as their advantages and disadvantages are summarized in Table 31-5.

Some additional principles to consider when rewarming severely hypothermic patients include the following:

- Ventricular fibrillation will not respond to conventional advanced cardiac life support interventions unless the

TABLE 31-3 MECHANISMS OF HEAT LOSS

CONVECTION	CONDUCTION	RADIATION	EVAPORATION
• Caused by movement of air in proximity to body when air flows across exposed skin • Normally the major mode of heat loss • Varies according to wind velocity and amount of protective clothing worn	• Caused by direct contact between the skin and a colder substance (e.g., ground or water) • Normally only 2% of losses, but may increase by 5 times with wet clothes or 25 times with cold water immersion	• Results when skin is exposed to the environment • Losses are determined by the difference between body and ambient temperatures, as well as position (which influences amount of body surface exposed)	• Occurs as water is converted from its liquid to its gaseous state • Normally accounts for 20% of heat loss • Losses are accelerated with presence of wet clothing, diaphoresis, and breathing dry air

TABLE 31-4 POTENTIAL PATHOLOGICAL CHANGES IN VARIOUS BODY SYSTEMS

BODY SYSTEM	POTENTIAL PATHOLOGICAL CHANGE
Central nervous system	Progressive decline in level of consciousness as temperature decreases Sluggish pupillary response Decrease in cerebral metabolism, causing impaired judgment and disorientation Consciousness may be lost between 32°C (89.6°F) and 30°C (86°F)
Cardiovascular system	Initially, increased blood pressure, heart rate, and cardiac output; later, bradycardia Atrial fibrillation commonly occurs and spontaneously resolves with rewarming Prolonged QT interval Asystole almost universal at temperatures ≤18°C (64.4°F) Death most commonly from asystole Dysrhythmias refractory to defibrillation, medications, and artificial pacing until heart rewarmed to >28°C (82.4°F) Osborn or J wave (extra deflection at QRS-ST junction) may be seen
Respiratory system	Depressed cough reflex, bronchodilation, and bronchorrhea lead to aspiration pneumonia Decreased ciliary motility Increased viscosity and amount of secretions Noncardiogenic pulmonary edema

Continued

TABLE 31-4 POTENTIAL PATHOLOGICAL CHANGES IN VARIOUS BODY SYSTEMS—cont'd

BODY SYSTEM	POTENTIAL PATHOLOGICAL CHANGE
Renal system	"Cold diuresis" caused by peripheral vasoconstriction leading to central hypervolemia
	Large quantities of urine with low specific gravity
	Renal hypoperfusion
	Myoglobinuria
	Acute tubular necrosis
Hematologic system	Hemoconcentration results from diuresis, fluid shifts, and decreased intake
	Hemoconcentration, low temperature, and low flow state cause increased blood viscosity
	Coagulopathies and DIC may develop
	Platelets sequester in liver and spleen
Digestive system	Bowel peristalsis is slowed at temperatures <34°C (93.2°F)
	Paralytic ileus develops when core temperature drops to 28°C (82.4°F)
	Hepatic function slows with cooling
	Insulin is ineffective at core temperature <30°C (86°F)
	The most uniform finding at autopsy in hypothermia is pancreatic necrosis

DIC, Disseminated intravascular coagulation.

TABLE 31-5 REWARMING MEASURES

	PASSIVE OR SPONTANEOUS REWARMING	ACTIVE EXTERNAL OR SURFACE REWARMING	ACTIVE INTERNAL OR CORE REWARMING
Underlying principle	Minimize heat loss	• Exogenous heat is applied to patient externally	• The core is actively rewarmed by convection
Treatment	• Remove victim from cold • Provide insulation • Maximize basal heat production • Remove wet clothing and linens • Dry patient's skin • Cover with warm, dry blankets • Protect from air flow • Radiant lights (ambient air at >21°C [69.8°F]) • Cover head	• Heating blankets • Bair Hugger • Warm water immersion	• Heated, humidified gas (up to 44°C [111.2°F]) • Warm IV solutions (up to 37°C [98.6°F]) • Peritoneal lavage with heated dialysate (up to 45°C [113°F]) • Irrigation of stomach, colon, bladder, pleural cavity (limited value) • Extracorporeal circulation via cardiac bypass, rapid fluid infuser (e.g., Level I) or hemodialysis
Advantages	• Easily accomplished • Inexpensive • Slow resolution of fluid shifts	• Rapid and noninvasive	• The most rapid means of rewarming
Disadvantages	• Patient must be capable of generating heat by thermogenesis • Humans are poikilothermic at <30°C (86°F) • Shivering ceases at 32°C (89.6°F)	• Increased mortality from development of aftershock and afterdrop • Nonphysiologic: increases needs of periphery before heart is rewarmed • May inhibit shivering • Potential skin burns	• Invasive • May require advanced skills • Expensive

IV, Intravenous.

patient is rewarmed. Limit defibrillation to three shocks (along with intravenously administered medications) until the core body temperature reaches 28°C (86°F).

• Replace volume. Rewarming causes peripheral vasodilation, and hypotension can occur as a result of this relative hypovolemia.

• Core rewarming of the severely hypothermic patient is essential to prevent rewarming shock. Rewarming shock occurs when the periphery is warmed faster than the core. This causes the lactic acid accumulated in cold extremities to be shunted rapidly to the heart, where it can induce fibrillation.

• Give medications judiciously. Hypothermic patients metabolize drugs poorly and may receive a large bolus once rewarmed.

• No one is dead until he or she is warm and dead!

> Give medication judiciously when rewarming patients. Hypothermic patients metabolize drugs poorly and may receive a large bolus once rewarmed.

HEAT-INDUCED ILLNESSES[8-13]

A variety of heat-induced illnesses can occur and range in severity from mildly annoying to life-threatening. Nursing care relating to the most common conditions is listed in Table 31-6.

> No pharmacologic agents have been proven to be beneficial in managing heatstroke. This includes dantrolene sodium, which has been postulated to accelerate cooling.

LIGHTNING INJURIES[14-21]

Each year in the United States, 150 to 300 lightning-related fatalities and 1000 to 1500 serious injuries occur, making this the third most common cause of death from isolated environmental injuries. Five different mechanisms by which these injuries can occur are described in Table 31-7.

Signs and Symptoms

Lightning strikes can potentially cause injury to any body system. There is extreme variability in the injuries resulting from lightning strikes between individuals, however,

TABLE 31-6 HEAT-INDUCED ILLNESSES

	HEAT CRAMPS	HEAT EXHAUSTION	HEATSTROKE
Causes	• Sweat-induced electrolyte depletion during intense physical activity in hot weather • Patients generally in good health but have not replaced lost fluids and electrolytes adequately	• A combination of prolonged periods of fluid loss (from perspiration, diarrhea, or diuretic use) and exposure to warm ambient temperatures without adequate fluid *and* electrolyte replacement • Symptoms generally have a rapid onset • Condition is common in the very young and the very old • Untreated, may progress to heatstroke	• Exercise-induced heatstroke results from strenuous physical activity in a hot environment when a person is unable to dissipate body heat effectively • Non–exercise-induced heatstroke occurs in individuals who are vulnerable to high environmental temperatures, particularly young children and the elderly • Heatstroke also can be precipitated by medications that affect heat production (thyroid preparations, sympathomimetics), decrease thirst (haloperidol), or limit diaphoresis (antihistamines, anticholinergics, phenothiazines, and propranolol) • As the body temperature rises to 41°C (105.8°F), central nervous system, cardiac, and cellular functions are affected. For every 1°C (33.8°F) rise in temperature, the metabolic rate increases by approximately 13%. Such tremendous metabolic demands cannot be sustained indefinitely and death follows if body temperature is not lowered

Continued

TABLE 31-6 HEAT-INDUCED ILLNESSES—cont'd

	HEAT CRAMPS	HEAT EXHAUSTION	HEATSTROKE

Signs and symptoms	• Cramps, especially in shoulders, lower extremities, and abdominal wall muscles
	• Weakness
	• Thirst
	• Nausea
	• Tachycardia
	• Profuse diaphoresis
	• Pale, cool, moist skin
		• Symptoms of heat cramps *and*
		  • Anorexia, vomiting
		  • Anxiety, general malaise
		  • Core body temperature normal or elevated (37–44°C/98.6–111.2°F)
		  • Headache
		  • Dehydration, orthostatic hypotension
		  • Muscle incoordination
		  • Syncope
			• Rapid symptom onset
			• Hyperthermia: core temperature greater than 41°C (105.8°F)
			• Nausea, vomiting, diarrhea
			• Classically, the skin is hot and dry but perspiration is often present in the early stages, particularly in young, healthy individuals (e.g., athletes)
			• Tachycardia, tachypnea
			• Decreased level of consciousness, abnormal posturing, seizures
			• Dilated, unresponsive pupils
			• Hypotension, decreased urinary output
			• Coagulopathies

Therapeutic interventions	• Replace sodium chloride orally or intravenously, depending on the patient's clinical status
	• Commercially prepared balanced electrolyte drinks (e.g., Gatorade, Powerade) work well for oral electrolyte replacement
	• Move the patient to a cool location
	• Encourage rest. Following an episode of heat cramps, patients should not return to the hot environment for 1–2 days
		• Basic and supportive care as indicated
		• Encourage rest
		• Place patient in cool environment
		• Administer fluids and electrolytes intravenously
			Heatstroke is a true medical emergency. Provide the following interventions:
			• Provide basic and advanced supportive care as indicated
			• Cool the patient as rapidly as possible:
			  • Remove clothing
			  • Spray and fan the patient. This involves repeatedly spraying patients with a fine mist and blowing a fan over the skin. This technique minimizes shivering and promotes evaporative cooling
			  • Place ice packs in the groin and axilla
			  • Iced peritoneal lavage and cardiopulmonary bypass have been used in refractory cases
			• Rehydrate patients with room temperature intravenous fluids
			• Monitor electrolytes and clotting factors
			• Check urine for the presence of myoglobin (indicates rhabdomyolysis)
			• Other supportive measures include the following:
			  • Control shivering with chlorpromazine (Thorazine). Shivering causes the body temperature to rise
			  • Prepare for inpatient admission

TABLE 31-7 TYPES OF LIGHTNING STRIKE

DIRECT STRIKE	SIDE FLASH OR SPLASH	CONTACT INJURY	GROUND CURRENT EFFECTS	INJURIES CAUSED BY BLUNT TRAUMA
Passage of current directly through person between head or upper body and feet	Individual is close to (but not in contact with) an object through which the direct current discharges	A person touches an object that is part of a lightning current circuit	Current spreads through the ground from site of the strike	Both from current-induced muscular contractions and from superheating of air causing concussive effect to organs

because of the varying resistance of body tissues (Table 31-8), ranges in body size, position, and use of protective gear. The cardiac and neurologic systems are most seriously affected (Table 31-9).

Therapeutic Interventions[22]

Therapeutic interventions for injury from lightning include the following:
* Provide basic and advanced supportive care as indicated.

* Institute continuous cardiac monitoring and obtain a 12-lead electrocardiogram.
* Collect and send laboratory studies based on symptom severity: complete blood count, electrolytes, troponin I, creatinine phosphokinase, urinalysis, blood urea nitrogen, and creatinine.
* Watch for evidence of rhabdomyolysis (dark urine, elevated creatinine phosphokinase).
* Perform radiographic studies of injured areas.
* Observe for the development of compartment syndrome. See Chapter 40, Musculoskeletal Trauma.
* Clean and dress burn wounds.

Prevention

The optimal way to reduce morbidity and mortality associated with lightning injuries is prevention. During a lightning storm, one should seek shelter in a large structure. Ideally, individuals should stay indoors during lightning storms and stay clear of windows. A fully enclosed metal vehicle is also relatively safe. Baths and water immersion should be avoided. Telephones (landlines) should not be used, as they serve as a conduit for the lightning charge to enter a building. Cell phones, however, may be used without increased risk. Interestingly, a single case report indicates that an implantable cardioverter-defibrillator restored a

TABLE 31-8	**RESISTANCE OF BODY TISSUES**	
LEAST	**INTERMEDIATE**	**MOST**
• Nerves	• Dry skin	• Tendon
• Blood		• Fat
• Mucous membranes		• Bone
• Muscle		

Data from Price, T. G., & Cooper, M. A. (2006). Electrical and lightning injuries. In J. S. Marx (Ed.), *Rosen's emergency medicine: Concepts and clinical practice* (6th ed., pp. 2267–2278). St. Louis, MO: Mosby.

TABLE 31-9 SIGNS AND SYMPTOMS ASSOCIATED WITH LIGHTNING INJURIES

CARDIAC	NEUROLOGIC	RENAL	INTEGUMENTARY AND MUSCULOSKELETAL	OTHER
• Alterations in conduction system • Cardiac dysrhythmias (including ventricular fibrillation, asystole) • Release of cardiac biomarkers • ECG changes (T wave inversion, current of injury, ST segment elevation, prolonged QT interval) • Motion abnormalities; hypokinesia • Cold, pulseless extremities (indicates vasomotor instability)	• Altered level of consciousness (confusion, amnesia, loss of consciousness) • Fixed and dilated pupils: generally transient • Autonomic nervous system impairment (hypertension, vasovagal syncope, complex regional pain syndrome) • Cognitive impairment • Long-term peripheral neuropathy • Keraunoparalysis (muscular stunning: temporary paralysis)	• Acute renal failure • Myoglobinuria	• Burn wounds (superficial to deep tissue): look for entrance and exit sites • Spiderlike cutaneous burns (from path of lightning over surface of body; see Fig. 31-1) known as Lichtenberg flowers • Traumatic injury to muscles	• Cardiopulmonary arrest (primary cause of death after strike) • Apnea • Temporary hearing loss, possible tympanic membrane rupture • Hypotension: may be related to intra-abdominal hemorrhage, pelvis fracture, or extremity fracture

ECG, Electrocardiogram.

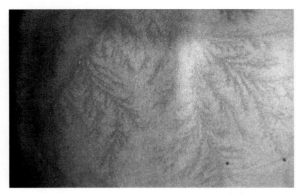

Fig. 31-1 Spiderlike cutaneous burns from path of lightning over surface of body. (Courtesy Mary Ann Cooper, MD. From Marx, J. A., Hockberger, R. S., & Walls, R. M. [2009]. *Rosen's emergency medicine* [7th ed.]. Philadelphia, PA: Mosby.)

normal cardiac rhythm in an individual who experienced ventricular fibrillation after a lightning strike.[23]

30-30 Rule for Lightning Safety
- Seek shelter if lightning is seen and thunder is heard before counting to 30.
- Do not resume outdoor activities until at least 30 minutes after the last flash of lightning is seen or thunder is heard.

Lightning rule of thumb: "If you see it, flee it; if you hear it, clear it."

DIVING EMERGENCIES[24-28]

Dive Depth and Gas Volumes

Scuba divers are exposed to atmospheric pressures far greater than those on land. Such hyperbaric conditions produce an array of medical problems unique to the underwater diving environment. At sea level the pressure exerted on the body is 1 atmosphere. At a water depth of 33 feet, pressure on the body is 2 atmospheres. With increasing depth, the pressures continue to increase proportionately. According to Boyle's law, gas volume is related inversely to pressure at a constant temperature. In other words, as pressure increases (i.e., descent), gas volume decreases, and vice versa (Table 31-10).

When a diver inhales air from the tank, the amount inspired remains the same regardless of submersion depth. However, with ascent, gas in the pulmonary system expands.

TABLE 31-10	THE EFFECT OF WATER DEPTH ON GAS VOLUME	
DEPTH	**GAS VOLUME (mL)**
Sea level: 0 feet (0 meters)	2000
1–33 feet (0.3–10 meters)	1000
34–100 feet (10.4–30.5 meters)	500
101–233 feet (30.8–71 meters)	250

If the diver fails to exhale on the way up, the volume of air in the lungs will increase as atmospheric pressure decreases. As this gas expands, it stretches the lungs and rupture can occur, resulting in pneumothorax and air embolism. Consequences of the pressure changes to which a diver is subjected can be summarized in four categories, as described in Table 31-11.

Martini law for nitrogen narcosis: For every 50 feet of descent, the effect is equivalent to roughly one martini.

Recompression Therapy

Arterial gas embolism, decompression illness, and breathing possibly contaminated air (carbon monoxide poisoning) may necessitate recompression therapy. If the patient must be flown to a hyperbaric chamber, pressurize the aircraft cabin to 1 atmosphere. Transport in nonpressurized aircraft (e.g., helicopters) should be done at an altitude of no more than 500 feet (152 meters) above the departure point, if at all possible.

Resources for Diving Emergencies
- The Divers Alert Network is based out of Duke University Medical Center. Experts are available 24 hours a day for telephone consultation related to any diving emergency. These specialists can help facilitate transfer to a hyperbaric oxygen recompression chamber. Call 919-684-8111.
- U.S. Navy Experimental Diving Unit in Washington, DC. Hotline (202-433-2790): The line is open 24 hours a day, 7 days a week. The duty officer can provide the name, location, and telephone number of the nearest recompression chamber.
- *Directory of Worldwide Decompression Chambers* is available from the Superintendent of Diving, U.S. Navy, Naval Ships Systems Command, National Center Building #3, Washington, DC 20360.

TABLE 31-11 POSSIBLE CONSEQUENCES OF UNDERWATER DIVING

	BAROTRAUMA (MIDDLE EAR BAROTRAUMAS, "EAR SQUEEZE")	NITROGEN NARCOSIS	ARTERIAL GAS EMBOLISM	DECOMPRESSION ILLNESS (GAS BUBBLE DISEASE, THE BENDS, DYSBARISM, DIVER'S PARALYSIS)
Description and etiology	With increasing depths, pressure increases against intact TM.	When air is breathed under pressure (e.g., when scuba diving), nitrogen is dissolved slowly in the blood, producing neurodepressant symptoms.	High-pressure air is forced into the circulatory system, causing an air embolism.	Results from the presence of gas bubbles in the blood and tissue.
Prevention	Perform maneuvers to force passage of additional air into the middle ear through the Eustachian tubes.	Avoid extreme depths: the deeper one dives, the greater the degree of nitrogen narcosis.	Exhaling during a slow, controlled ascent.	Avoid air travel after diving. Awareness of issues that may increase severity: extreme water temperatures, heavy exercise, poor conditioning, increasing age, alcohol ingestion, obesity, preexisting peripheral vascular disease, fatigue.
Signs and symptoms	Pain increases as there is a negative differential pressure in the middle ear. Increasing pressure can cause the TM to rupture.	"Martini law": for every 50 feet of descent, the effect is equivalent to roughly one martini. Progression from drowsiness and decreased muscle strength to decreased strength and impaired coordination to further deterioration and finally to unconsciousness and death.	Respiratory: Chest tightness; shortness of breath; pink, frothy sputum; pneumothorax symptoms. Neurologic: Vertigo (loss of visual point of reference), unilateral or bilateral limb paresthesias, sensory loss or paralysis, confusion, loss of consciousness, seizures.	Clinical manifestations are related to nitrogen bubbles in the joints, pulmonary system, central nervous system, and skin: shortness of breath, crepitus, cough; petechial rash, itching; headache; visual loss, diplopia; fatigue, dizziness, unconsciousness, seizures; paresthesias, paralysis; joint soreness, progressive pain.
Therapeutic interventions	Treat presenting signs and symptoms.	Gradual ascent to shallow water with decompression stops along the way to allow nitrogen reabsorption.	Prompt therapy is crucial: basic and advanced supportive care, oxygen, needle decompression if indicated. *Avoid* head-down Trendelenburg position. Arrange urgent recompression in hyperbaric chamber.	Prompt therapy is crucial: basic and advanced supportive care, oxygen, fluid resuscitation to maintain urinary output of 1–2 mL/h, analgesia (avoid narcotics). Arrange urgent recompression in hyperbaric chamber. Consider antiplatelet or antithrombin medications. Consider helium-oxygen to increase bubble shrinkage.

TM, Tympanic membrane.

HIGH ALTITUDE PULMONARY EDEMA[29]

High altitude pulmonary edema (HAPE) is the most common cause of death related to altitude. Early recognition and treatment significantly improve outcome. HAPE typically occurs 2 to 4 days after rapid ascent to an altitude above 8000 feet (2438 meters). It is also seen in patients who normally live at high altitudes, go to sea level for 2 weeks or more, and then return home. Symptoms are usually worse at night. HAPE is a form of noncardiogenic pulmonary edema. The exact etiology remains unclear but appears to be related to increased pulmonary artery pressures that occur in response to significant elevation.

Signs and Symptoms

- Dyspnea at rest
- Cough, may be productive of pink, frothy sputum
- Weakness, fatigue, exercise intolerance
- Chest tightness or congestion
- Tachypnea
- Tachycardia
- Crackles, wheezing
- Confusion
- Central cyanosis

Therapeutic Interventions

- The most effective treatment is descent to a lower altitude. This usually reverses the disease process.
- Administer high-flow oxygen to maintain normal saturation levels.
- Keep the patient warm.
- Provide bed rest.
- Pressurize the patient in a hyperbaric chamber; a portable, inflatable, hyperbaric chamber commonly used in wilderness situations (e.g., Gamow bag) can be used.
- Consider medication administration.
  - Nifedipine may be effective in dilating the pulmonary vasculature; may improve SaO_2 in a few minutes.
  - Acetazolamide is often used in the prevention of HAPE (there are no documented studies that confirm the effectiveness of this treatment once HAPE is diagnosed).
  - Other medications may be prescribed as clinically indicated.

REFERENCES

1. Prakash, S., & Weisman, M. H. (2009). Idiopathic chilblains. *American Journal of Medicine, 122*(12), 1152–1155.
2. Danzl, D. F. (2010). Frostbite. In J. A. Marx, R. S. Hockberger, & R. M. Walls, *Rosen's emergency medicine* (7 ed., pp. 1861–1867). St. Louis, MO: Elsevier.
3. Danzl, D. F. (2006). Hypothermia and frostbite. In V. J. Markovchick & P. T. Pons (Eds.), *Emergency medicine secrets* (4th ed., p. 390). St. Louis, MO: Mosby.
4. Golant, A., Nord, R. M., Paksima, N., & Posner, M. A. (2008). Cold exposure injuries to the extremities. *Journal of the American Academy of Orthopaedic Surgeons, 16*(12), 704–715.
5. McGillion, R. (2005). Frostbite: Case report, practical summary of ED treatment. *Journal of Emergency Nursing, 31*(5), 500–502.
6. Patel, N. N., & Patel, D. N. (2008). Frostbite. *American Journal of Medicine, 121*(9), 765–766.
7. Minnesota Sea Grant. (2011). *Hypothermia preventions: Survival in cold water*, Retrieved from http://www.seagrant.umn.edu/coastal_communities/hypothermia
8. Anderson, B. H., & Vukich, D. J. (2006). Heat illness. In V. J. Markovchick & P. T. Pons (Eds.), *Emergency medicine secrets* (4th ed., pp. 392–395). St. Louis, MO: Mosby.
9. Hadal, E., Cohen-Sivan, Y., Heled, Y., & Epstein, Y. (2005). Clinical review: Treatment of heat stroke: Should dantrolene be considered? *Critical Care, 9*(1), 86–91.
10. Lewis, A. M., (2010). Emergency: Heatstroke in older adults: In this population it's a short step from heat exhaustion. *American Journal of Nursing, 107*(6), 52–56.
11. McDermott, B. P., Casa, D. J., Ganio, M. S., Lopez, R. M., Yeargin, S. W., Armstrong, L. E., & Maresh, C. M. (2009). Acute whole-body cooling for exercise-induced hyperthermia: A systematic review. *Journal of Athletic Training, 44*(1), 84–93.
12. Platt, M., & Vicario, S. (2010). Heat Illness. In J. A. Marx, R. S. Hockberger, & R. M. Walls, *Rosen's emergency medicine* (7 ed., pp. 1882–1892). St. Louis, MO: Elsevier.
13. Wagner, C., & Boyd, K. (2008). Pediatric heatstroke. *Air Medical Journal, 27*(3), 118–122.
14. Adekoya, N., & Nolte, K. B. (2005). Struck-by-lightning deaths in the United States. *Journal of Environmental Health, 67*(9), 45–50.
15. Alyan, O., Ozdemir, O., Tufekcioglu, O., Geyik, B., Aras, D., & Demirkan, D. (2006). Myocardial injury due to lightning strike: A case report. *Angiology, 57*, 219–223.
16. Bier, M., Chen, W., Bodnar, E., & Lee, R. C. (2005). Biophysical injury mechanisms associated with lightning injury. *NeuroRehabilitation, 20*, 53–62.
17. Cherington, M. (2005). Spectrum of neurologic complications of lightning injuries. *NeuroRehabilitation, 20*, 3–8.
18. Price, T. G., & Cooper, M. A. (2010). Electrical and lightning injuries. In J. A. Marx, R. S. Hockberger, & R. M. Walls, *Rosen's emergency medicine* (7 ed., pp. 1893–1902). St Louis, MO: Elsevier.
19. Grubb, B. P., & Karabin, B. (2007). New onset postural tachycardia syndrome following lightning injury. *Pacing and Clinical Electrophysiology, 30*(8), 1036–1038.
20. Jost, W. H., Schonrock, L. M., & Cherington, M. (2005). Autonomic nervous system dysfunction in lightning and electrical injuries. *NeuroRehabilitation, 20*, 19–23.
21. Shockley, L. W. (2006). Lightning and electrical injuries. In V. J. Markovchick & P. T. Pons (Eds.), *Emergency medicine secrets* (4th ed., pp. 369–373). St. Louis, MO: Mosby.

22. Okafor, U. V. (2005). Lightning injuries and acute renal failure: A review. *Renal Failure, 27*, 129–134.

23. Kondur, A. K., Afonso, L. C., Berenbom, L. D., & Lakkireddy, D. R. (2008). Implantable cardioverter defibrillators save lives from lightning-related electrocution too! *Pacing and Clinical Electrophysiology, 31*, 256–257.

24. MacDonald, R. D., O'Donnell, C., Allan, M., Breeck, K., Chow, Y., DeMajo, W., ... Wax, R. (2006). Interfacility transport of patients with decompression illness: Literature review and consensus statement. *Prehospital Emergency Care, 10*, 482–487.

25. Shockley, L. W. (2006). Scuba diving and dysbarism. In J. S. Marx (Ed.), *Rosen's emergency medicine: Concepts and clinical practice* (6th ed., pp. 2279–2295). St. Louis, MO: Mosby.

26. Smerz, R. W. (2006). Age associated risks of recreational scuba diving. *Hawaii Medical Journal, 66*, 140, 141, 153.

27. Tetzlaff, K., Shank, E. S., & Muth, C. M. (2003). Evaluation and management of decompression illness—an intensivist's perspective. *Intensive Care Medicine, 29*, 2128–2136.

28. Flarity, K. (2010). Environmental emergencies. In P. K. Howard & R. A. Steinmann (Ed.), *Sheehy's emergency nursing: Principles and practice* (6th ed., pp. 535–553). St. Louis, MO: Mosby.

29. Bärtsch, P., Maggiorini, M., Ritter, M., Noti, C., Vock, P., Oelz, O. (1991). Prevention of high-altitude pulmonary edema by nifedipine. *New England Journal of Medicine, 325*(18), 1284–1289.

Bite and Sting Emergencies

S. Kay Sedlack

Between 2001 and 2005 approximately 94,552 instances of animal bites and stings were reported in the United States.[1] Most are successfully managed medically, but death can and does occur. More than half (52%) of these deaths are from insect bites and stings, followed by 30% from snakebites and 13% from spider bites.[2] Other considerations are potential infection and systemic complications.

RABIES

Rabies, one of the world's oldest diseases, is most commonly transmitted through the saliva of an infected mammal but is also known to spread via the airborne route. There are an estimated 55,000 deaths worldwide each year from rabies.[3] In the United States, however, prevention measures have resulted in only one or two actual cases developing in the 16,000 to 39,000 individuals exposed to potentially rabid carnivores and bats.[4] The Centers for Disease Control and Prevention (CDC) reported in 2007 that the canine strain of rabies has been eliminated in the United States, and most human incidents of rabies are now the result of exposure to wildlife such as bats, raccoons, skunks, and foxes.[4]

Signs and Symptoms

- *Initial stage* rabies includes paresthesias, pain, or itching at the bite site. This is thought to be related to viral replication and may progress over several days to a week. The incubation period is usually 1 to 3 months but can vary from days to years.[3]
- *Prodrome stage* rabies includes nonspecific findings such as headache, fever, runny nose, sore throat, myalgias, and gastrointestinal symptoms. The virus progresses along the peripheral nervous system toward its ultimate destination: the central nervous system.

- *Acute, progressive encephalitis* includes:
  - Hydrophobia, an overwhelming fear of seeing or feeling water, is considered pathognomonic for rabies.
  - Aerophobia, a fear elicited by the movement of air.

Prevention

Once the virus becomes established in a human, the disease is almost 100% fatal. However, early aggressive wound management is suggested to prevent viral replication. This includes the following interventions:
- Scrub (do not irrigate) with a virucidal agent such as povidone-iodine (Betadine).
- Soap is preferred over plain water if povidone-iodine is not available.
- Sunlight and drying also kills the rabies virus.

Postexposure Prophylaxis

Postexposure prophylaxis is imperative (Table 32-1). For those who have not previously been exposed, the rabies vaccine human rabies immunoglobulin provides rapid, passive immunity. When the rabies vaccine is administered properly, detectable rabies virus neutralizing antibodies have been shown to develop in approximately 7 to 10 days.[4] These antibodies persist for several years. Reactions to prophylactic therapies are rarely severe.[4]

TICK-BORNE ILLNESSES

Ticks are responsible for a number of illnesses in humans and are second only to mosquitoes as a vector for disease transmission. With strong jaws and a cementlike adhesive, ticks attach to humans, other mammals, birds, and reptiles. Ticks engorge themselves on blood and transmit disease through their saliva. Because their digestive tract has no exit (anus), when they are well fed they burst, spreading potential pathogens.

TABLE 32-1	RABIES POSTEXPOSURE PROPHYLAXIS
THOSE *NOT* PREVIOUSLY VACCINATED FOR RABIES (i.e., GENERAL PUBLIC)	**THOSE PREVIOUSLY VACCINATED FOR RABIES (i.e., VETERINARIANS)**
Immediate aggressive cleaning and scrubbing of wound with virucidal agent (rinse with water or saline and dry after).	Immediate aggressive cleaning and scrubbing of wound with virucidal agent (rinse with water or saline and dry after).
Administer human rabies immunoglobulin (20 IU/kg or 0.133 mL/kg). If anatomically feasible, inject as much as possible directly into proximal area of wound (virus will travel along nerve tracts toward the central nervous system). Any remaining volume is administered intramuscularly at a site distal to the vaccine site.	Do *not* administer rabies immunoglobulin.
Administer human diploid cell vaccine or purified chick embryo 1 mL dose on days 0, 3, 7, and 14.[a]	Administer human diploid cell vaccine or purified chick embryo 1 mL dose on days 0 and 3.[a]

Data from Centers for Disease Control and Prevention. (2010). Use of a reduced (4-dose) vaccine schedule for postexposure prophylaxis to prevent human rabies: Recommendations of the Advisory Committee on Immunization Practices. *MMWR Recommendations and Reports, 59*(RR-2), 1–9.

[a]Mitka, M. (2010). CDC advisors suggest streamlining postexposure prophylaxis for rabies. *Journal of the American Medical Association, 303*(16), 1586.

Note: More detailed information is available from Centers for Disease Control and Prevention.

Unfortunately, because of the tick's small size many people are unaware that they have been bitten. Initial symptoms are often nonspecific but a history of travel or a characteristic rash can provide clues. Search for the tick if it is suspected. It is most often in the scalp but may also reside in the axilla, pubic or perianal area, popliteal fossa, or ear canal.

Table 32-2 lists a sampling of common tick-borne illnesses that occur in the United States. In addition to spreading infection, certain ticks contain a neurotoxin that can induce tick paralysis. This disease is characterized by a

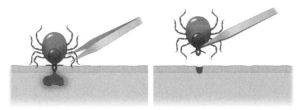

Fig. 32-1 Tick removal technique. (From Raoult, D. [2008]. Rickettsioses. In L. Goldman & D. Ausiello [Eds.], *Cecil medicine* [23rd ed.]. Philadelphia, PA: Saunders.)

descending paralysis that resembles Guillain-Barré syndrome. Paralysis quickly resolves when the tick is removed.

Tick Removal[5,6]

Ticks should be removed as soon as possible to decrease the amount of time for microorganisms to be transferred to the host. Guidelines for safe tick removal are included in Table 32-3 and depicted in Figure 32-1. Avoid squeezing or crushing the tick, as this may cause the inadvertent release of the tick's internal contents. Avoid handling the tick. Occasionally, the tick may be sent to a local laboratory or health department for analysis and evaluation.

Prevention

Avoidance of tick habitats is the best prevention measure. Table 32-4 lists ways to avoid tick exposure that can be included in patient discharge instructions.

> Always report removal of a tick to a health care provider.

SNAKEBITES

Only about 5 to 10 individuals die annually in the United States as a consequence of a snakebite.[2] The actual incidence of snakebites is estimated at 45,000, with 7000 to 8000 from venomous snakes.[2] Most bites occur when handling, teasing, or playing with snakes and 40% of persons bitten have a blood alcohol level greater than 0.1%.[7] Around 85% of bites are on the fingers or hand and 15% involve the foot or ankle.[7]

Of the 120 species of snakes indigenous to the United States, only 20 (from four different species) are venomous. Three of the species of poisonous snakes are from the family known as pit vipers (*Crotalidae*): rattlesnakes, copperheads, and cottonmouths (also known as water moccasins). The fourth species of poisonous snake is the coral snake, which looks similar to the nonvenomous king snake.

TABLE 32-2 COMMON TICK-BORNE ILLNESSES

TICK-BORNE DISEASE	CAUSATIVE VECTOR	EARLY SIGNS AND SYMPTOMS	LATER SIGNS AND SYMPTOMS	TREATMENT	SPECIAL CONSIDERATIONS[a]
Rocky Mountain spotted fever	*Rickettsia rickettsii*	Fever, headache, rash (small, flat, pink, nonpruritic spots [macules] on the palms, wrists, forearms, soles, and ankles during the first 10 days. Initially, the spots blanch when pressure is applied. They eventually become raised bumps.), nausea, vomiting, tenderness in large muscle groups.	Maculopapular rash: characteristic red, spotted (petechial) rash of Rocky Mountain spotted fever seen 2–5 days after symptoms onset. The rash typically spreads in a centripetal fashion to cover most of the body, including the palms, soles, and face. Patient can develop circulatory collapse, coma, renal failure, and electrolyte imbalances.	Doxycycline 100 mg bid for 10–14 days or chloramphenicol 50 mg/kg/day.	Consider with unexplained febrile illness, even in absence of rash or known tick bite. Delayed treatment may result in fatal outcome.
Lyme disease (most common; peaks between April and September)	*Borrelia burgdorferi*	Target, bull's-eye rash formation (erythema migrans)—this annular lesion, with bright red borders and a fading center, is present in only 25% of cases. "Viral syndrome," lymphadenopathy, malaise, headache.	Bell's palsy (common); chronic arthritic and neurologic abnormalities (meningoencephalitis), fatigue.	Doxycycline 100 mg orally twice a day for 21 days.	A significant attachment time (48 hours) is required to transmit the bacteria. Consider with viral illness, monoarticular arthritis, meningitis, multiple neurologic abnormalities, or heart block.
Tularemia	*Francisella tularensis*	Most common skin lesion at site of inoculation which ulcerates in 2–3 days; regional adenopathy.	If untreated may progress to pulmonary tularemia.	Streptomycin 30–40 mg/kg/day in two divided doses IM for 3 days, then half dose for next 4–11 days.	Suspect with slow-healing extremity ulcers and regional adenopathy.
Colorado tick fever	*Orbivirus*	Severe flulike illness—fever, chills, headache, myalgia, lethargy, anorexia, nausea.	Biphasic course in 50% of patients—symptoms resolve after 2–3 days, patient improves, followed by a second and possibly third febrile period.	Self-limiting disease; essentially all patients recover without sequelae.	Supportive treatment is indicated. Some clinicians suggest the use of Ribivirin.
Relapsing fever	*Borrelia hermsii*	Fever, chills, headache, arthralgias, nausea, vomiting.	Relapsing cycles of fever and illness, repeating 3–5 times, each less severe.	Tetracycline or erythromycin 500 mg for 5–10 days.	Suspect with recurrent viral-like illness and high fever. Confirm with presence of spirochetes on blood smear during period of rising temperature.

bid, Twice daily; *IM,* intramuscularly.

[a]Bolgiano, E. B., & Sexton, J. (2006). Tick-borne illnesses. In J. S. Marx (Ed.), *Rosen's emergency medicine: Concepts and clinical practice* (6th ed., pp. 2116–2145). St. Louis, MO: Mosby.

To tell the difference between a poisonous coral snake and a nonvenomous king snake, remember this rhyme[7]:
- Red on yellow, kill a fellow (coral snake)
- Red on black, venom lack (king snake)

Table 32-5 describes the differences between most venomous and nonvenomous snakes in the United States.[8]

Signs and Symptoms

Snake venoms contain varying combinations of neurotoxic, cardiotoxic, and hemolytic proteins designed to immobilize the prey, stop the heart, and begin the digestive process. A summary of the range of consequences appears in Table 32-6.

The amount of venom a snake injects varies according to the following:
- Size of its prey (food source)
- If the bite was the result of a defensive attack
- Age of the snake; baby snakes are not as capable of controlling the amount of venom they release

TABLE 32-3 TICK REMOVAL

Do
- Wear gloves to avoid contact with the tick.
- Using narrow-tipped tweezers, grasp the tick as close to the skin as possible.
- Pull upward slowly and steadily.
- If tick is to be sent for analysis, place it in a sterile specimen container and label.
- Thoroughly disinfect the bite site.
- Wash hands.

Do Not
- Squeeze or crush the tick.
- Handle the tick.

TABLE 32-4 AVOIDING TICK-BORNE ILLNESS

Awareness
- Ticks live in moist, wooded, bushy, or grassy areas. Avoid thick underbrush and stay near the center of trails.
- Perform a "tick drag" to determine whether ticks exist in a specific area. Drag a 3-foot stick with white flannel on each end across an area of concern several times. Examine the stick and flannel to identify any ticks that have latched on.

Clothing
- Wear light-colored clothing. This makes it easier to see ticks.
- Wear long-sleeved shirts tucked into pants and pants tucked into socks or boot tops. Wear a hat.

Insect Repellent
- Use a 35% DEET (N,N-Diethyl-m-toluamide) product on exposed skin (not under clothes).
- Use permethrin-containing products on clothing, footwear, and camping gear.

Inspection
- After spending time outdoors, check your entire body for ticks. Shower afterward.
- Check clothes for ticks. Launder immediately. A hot dryer will kill ticks.
- Check pets for ticks. Use a tick collar.

Early Removal
- If a tick is identified, remove it in a timely manner. Save it for a health care provider in a baggie or sealed container.
- Wash area. Observe area over time for development of rash or other symptoms.

Notify a Health Care Provider
- Always advise your health care provider if you have removed a tick or have been in a tick-prone area and develop signs or symptoms of illness.

TABLE 32-5 VENOMOUS VERSUS NONVENOMOUS SNAKES IN THE UNITED STATES

SNAKE CHARACTERISTICS	VENOMOUS	NONVENOMOUS
Pupils	Elliptical (except coral snake)	Round
Bite	Fangs (two, unless one is broken), which produce punctures	Several rows of small teeth, which produce scratches
Head shape	Triangular (from venom glands)	Rounded
Presence of pit between eye and nostril	Yes, in pit vipers	No
Tail: row of subcaudal plates	Single row	Double row

TABLE 32-6	CONSEQUENCES OF ENVENOMATION

TYPE OF VENOM	CLINICAL FINDINGS (FROM MINOR TO LIFE-THREATENING)
Hemotoxic	• Capillary fragility • Petechiae • Bullae • Anemia • Hemolysis • Coagulopathy • Disseminated intravascular coagulation
Neurotoxic	• Periorbital paresthesias • Pain or numbness at site of injury • Constricted pupils (unilateral or bilateral), ptosis, diplopia • Muscle twitching: mouth, face, and affected extremity • Difficulty speaking, confusion • Weakness, paresthesia • Seizures • Paralysis
Cardiotoxic	• Tachycardia • Hypotension • Shock • Cardiopulmonary arrest

Up to 45% of bites by venomous snakes are "dry," meaning that no poison is injected. This is secondary to an indirect hit, a failure of the gland-fang mechanism, or an insufficient amount of venom being injected.

The severity of response to envenomation is extremely variable and depends on the following:
- Species and size of the snake
- Location and depth of the bite—muscle absorbs venom faster than fat
- Number of bites
- Amount of venom injected
- Age of the snake
- Age, size, and health of the patient
- Individual sensitivity to venom and the number of previous venom exposures
- Concentration of microorganisms in the mouth of the snake
  Some specific symptoms include:
- Pit vipers: pain at the site that is out of proportion to the puncture, metallic or rubber taste in the mouth, oral or facial numbness, rapid onset of slow spreading edema (80%)
- Rattlesnakes: fang marks oozing nonclotted blood with surrounding ecchymosis and severe burning pain, microhematuria

- Coral snake: nonspecific early signs, systemic signs 12 hours later

Therapeutic Interventions

Therapeutic interventions for snakebites include the following:
- Provide basic and advanced supportive care as indicated.
- Remove potentially constricting clothing or jewelry.
- Immobilize the involved area at or below the level of the heart.
- Send blood for a complete blood count, type and cross-match, electrolytes, and coagulation studies (prothrombin time and international normalized ratio, activated partial thromboplastin time, fibrinogen, D-dimer).
- Do not use ice, tourniquets, constricting bands, electrotherapy, or wound suction. Clinical trials do not support the use of these traditional interventions. In fact, these measures may worsen outcomes.
- Cleanse the wound and provide tetanus prophylaxis as indicated.
- Give analgesics for pain.
- Monitor patient for at least 6 hours to determine need for antivenin. Antivenin is not used for mild or resolving symptoms. Generally, antivenin is indicated in the presence of any progressive pain, swelling, or ecchymosis.
- Antivenins are specific to the type of snake involved. Most U.S. emergency departments have access to crotalid (pit viper) antivenin. Contact the poison control center as needed.
- Ideally, antivenin administration should be initiated within 4 hours of exposure but may be effective up to 24 hours after exposure.
- Because antivenin is made from animal serum, its use is associated with potentially life-threatening allergic reactions. However, with the newer formulations, pretesting for allergy is no longer recommended.[9] Watch for signs of an antigen-antibody response.

SPIDER (ARACHNID) BITES

Most spider bites involve local reactions such as itching, swelling, redness, and stinging pain. The two spiders of clinical importance in the United States are the black widow and brown recluse. See Table 32-7 for a comparison of black widow and brown recluse spider bites. Suspect a spider bite if there are two tiny red fang marks at the point of venom entry surrounded by a papule.

The presence of multiple bite marks usually excludes spider envenomation; arachnids rarely bite more than once. A common phenomenon is "Mustov's disease," or blaming any lesion on a spider (e.g., "I have this spot. I *must*

TABLE 32-7 COMPARISON OF BLACK WIDOW AND BROWN RECLUSE SPIDER BITES

	LATRODECTUS (BLACK WIDOW)	*LOXOSCELES* (BROWN RECLUSE)[a]
Location	All United States Dark, secluded, damp, cool places (woodpile)	Mainly southwest, south central, southeast United States Dark, undisturbed places (attics, boxes) Active at night
Markings	Red hourglass on ventral abdomen (female)	Dark violin-shaped spot anterodorsally
Symptoms	Neurotoxic Pain at site with halo around bite into large muscle cramping (e.g., abdomen) Differentiate from peritonitis because no local tenderness	Cytotoxic, hemolytic, local necrosis Minor pain into bluish ring with irregular borders, local edema into local errhythema, edema (8 hours) into necrotic site 2–4 days. Eschar, may require surgery Potential systemic reaction Fever, nausea, vomiting, myalgias
Length of signs and symptoms	Peak in 2–3 hours Last for 2–3 days	Local: 8 hours Necrosis: 2–4 days Eschar: weeks or months
Specific treatment	Control muscle spasms Antihistamines for systemic edema[b] Antivenin cautiously	No specific antidote is available in the United States (Brazil produces an antivenom)

[a]Nunnelee, J. D. (2006). Brown recluse spider bites: A case report. *Journal of Perianesthesia Nursing, 21*(1), 12–15.
[b]Frundle, T. C. (2004). Management of spider bites. *Air Medical Journal, 23*(4), 24–26.

have been bitten by a spider."). It is said of all bites that are blamed on spiders, 80% of these diagnoses are erroneous.[10]

> The presence of multiple bite marks usually excludes spiders, as most arachnids bite only once.

Therapeutic Interventions

For all spider bites:
- Apply ice to the area to decrease venom absorption.[11]
- Elevate the extremity.
- Check the patient's tetanus immunization status and vaccinate as needed.
- Treat symptomatically.

For black widow spider bites:
- Some sources recommend benzodiazepines for associated muscle spasms.[9] Calcium gluconate, traditionally used for muscle spasms, has been shown to be of no benefit.
- *Latrodectus* antivenin administration can shorten the course of the illness significantly. However, its use is reserved for more severe cases because of the potential for acute hypersensitivity and delayed serum sickness. Indications for antivenin administration include worsening pain or muscle spasms, rigidity to abdomen or head, development of hypertension, or increasing

diaphoresis.[9] A skin sensitivity test is recommended before administration.

For brown recluse spider bites:
- Over the years many therapies—including antihistamines, antibiotics, steroids, hyperbaric oxygen, electrical shock, and surgical excision—have been advocated. None of these has been demonstrated to be effective.
- Dapsone (Avlosulfon) inhibits the progression of crater lesions but must be used cautiously because of the risk of blood dyscrasias. The dose is 50 mg twice daily for 10 days.

> **Rules of Thumb**
> - Black widow: neurotoxic
> - Brown recluse: necrotic

SCORPION STINGS

Scorpions are found throughout the world, particularly in warm climates, but none of the highly toxic species is indigenous to the United States. However, because of their size, scorpions can travel easily anywhere in the world as stowaways in cargo. Scorpions are more active at night.

The stings of most scorpions are harmless to humans and require no specific care, except when young children are stung. In the United States, the venom of the scorpion species *Centruroides* (which includes the bark scorpion) is potent enough to cause systemic toxicity in humans. It is found on or near trees in California, Arizona, Texas, and Mexico.

Signs and Symptoms

Scorpion stings are painful, with an immediate tingling in the affected area and local erythema that usually resolves in a few hours. There may be heightened sensitivity to touch in the area of the sting. Severe envenomation may exhibit complicated neuromuscular and autonomic symptoms.

Therapeutic Interventions

In addition to basic wound care:
- Administer mild analgesia to relieve pain. Narcotics and barbiturates may increase the toxic effects of the venom.
- Benzodiazepines may be used for myoclonus and muscle spasms.
- Scorpion antivenin is available on an extremely limited basis (and is not approved by the U.S. Food and Drug Administration). Its use is associated with major allergic complications and efficacy has not been established.[12]

BEE, WASP, HORNET, AND FIRE ANT STINGS[13]

Bees, wasps, hornets, yellow jackets, and fire ants fall into the order of insects known as *Hymenoptera*. Reactions can include local irritation at the sting site, anaphylactic reactions, and a delayed reaction as a serum sickness–like syndrome 10 to 14 days later. Toxic reactions, which involve multiple stings by highly potent insects, are unusual in the United States. Most severe *Hymenoptera*-related illnesses result from allergic reactions.

Signs and Symptoms

Fire ants have a painful sting that forms a wheal, which eventually expands into a large vesicle. The area reddens and a pustule forms. Pustule reabsorption is followed by crusting and scar formation.

Therapeutic Interventions

Therapeutic interventions for *Hymenoptera* stings for mild reactions include wound care already discussed. These additional interventions are also indicated:
- If a bee stinger is still present in the wound, use a dull object (such as a credit card or dull knife) to scrape the stinger in the direction opposite the angle of penetration. Do not grasp or pull stingers from the skin; this can squeeze the attached sac and inject more venom.
- Administer oral antihistamines and nonsteroidal anti-inflammatory analgesics.

Removal Rules of Thumb
- Ticks: tweezers to grasp
- Bee stinger: dull object to scrape

Prevention

The effect of stings is cumulative and once exposed patients have greater potential for a future reaction. To prevent future stings and serious reactions, advise patients to do the following:
- Avoid wearing bright colors or perfumes while outdoors.
- Wear shoes when walking outside.
- Carry a self-injection of epinephrine (EpiPen) if allergic to bee stings.
- Wear a MedicAlert bracelet or some other type of allergy notification.
- Consider desensitization therapy (allergy shots) if allergy exists. This is an option for certain patients, and the efficacy rate has been reported to be as high as 95%.

MARINE BITES AND ENVENOMATIONS

There are a variety of aquatic creatures that can cause injury. These types of injuries may be seen in any emergency department, as some exotic animals may be kept in private collections.[9] Marine animals, such as seals, sea lions, and sharks, inflict bites and puncture wounds. These can be managed with basic wound care techniques depending on the nature of the wound. There are other sea creatures that sting, including jellyfish and corals. Others have spines that contain venom, such as stingrays, sea urchins, and scorpion fish.[11] With any envenomation, anaphylaxis is a possibility. See Chapter 20, Shock, for management of anaphylactic shock.

Stingrays

Stingrays are flat fish with tails that contain a venom-coated barb. The injury inflicted by stingrays is quite painful and is most commonly seen on the feet and lower extremities, although other areas of the body may be affected. Typical symptoms include the following[14]:
- Severe pain
- Swelling and bleeding at the site
- Possible systemic effects, including nausea, vomiting, muscle cramping, and limb paralysis, depending on the species
- Some species of stingray may cause hypotension, bradycardia, seizures, and death
- Direct injury to vital organs may be immediately fatal[9]

Therapeutic Interventions

- Airway, breathing, and circulation stabilization as indicated
- Hot water immersion, sometimes up to 2 hours
  - Take care to prevent scald injury
  - Provides analgesia and may deactivate the venom
- Pain management
- Tetanus prophylaxis
- Wound care, including barb removal if necessary
  - Decontamination by irrigation is recommended[14]
- Consider wound culture and prophylactic antibiotics for more serious wounds or in immunocompromised patients
  - Pathogens found in seawater may include *Streptococcus* species, *Escherichia coli*, and *Vibrio* species.[15]

Jellyfish

Jellyfish are coelenterates that have stinging capsules, called nematocysts, on their tentacles. These inflict venom with effects that vary by species. Typically, the type of envenomation is local and causes moderate to severe pain and reddened welts where the tentacles contacted the skin. Occasionally, patients may experience headache, vomiting, or abdominal pain. For common jellyfish stings, death is rare.[9] One species of jellyfish found in Hawaii, the box jellyfish, is particularly dangerous and an antivenin has been developed.[15]

Therapeutic Interventions

For most jellyfish encounters, therapeutic interventions are as follows:
- Immediately rinse the area with salt water or normal saline.
  - Do not rub or use freshwater, as this may stimulate more nematocysts to inject venom.[11,15]
- If tentacles are still present, remove carefully using a gloved hand or forceps.
- Pain management
  - Some sources recommend local application of a paste of meat tenderizer to relieve pain.[11]

Seabather's Eruption[15]

This condition occurs because of exposure to larvae of certain jellyfish or coelenterates. It is a pruritic maculopapular rash that appears to be a hypersensitivity reaction. The rash may present in the areas of the body covered by a wetsuit or swimsuit, because the larvae become trapped between the suit and the skin. This rash may appear up to 1 to 2 days after exposure and may last for up to 2 weeks.

Therapeutic Interventions

Treatment is based on symptoms and may include irrigation with hot water or vinegar, application of topical steroids, and oral antihistamines. It is recommended that the swimsuit or wetsuit be thoroughly washed to prevent reexposure.

REFERENCES

1. Langley, R. L. (2008). Animal bites and stings reported by United States poison control centers, 2001–2005. *Wilderness and Environmental Medicine, 19*(1), 7–14.
2. Otten, E. J. (2010). Venomous animal injuries. In J. A. Marx, R., Hockberger, & R., Walls, *Rosen's emergency medicine* (7 ed., pp. 743–757). St. Louis, MO: Mosby.
3. World Health Organization. (2010, September). *Rabies.* Retrieved from http://www.who.int/mediacentre/factsheets/fs099/en/
4. Manning, S. E., Rupprecht, C. E., Fishbein, D., Hanlon, C. A., Lumlertdacha, B., Guerra, M., … Hull, H. F. (2008). Human rabies prevention—United States, 2008: Recommendations of the Advisory Committee on Immunization Practices. *MMWR Recommendations and Reports, 57*(RR-3), 1–28.
5. Driver, C. (2010). Tick-borne diseases. *Practice Nurse, 39*(3), 24–27.
6. Centers for Disease Control and Prevention. (2011, January 18). *Stop ticks.* Retrieved from http://www.cdc.gov/features/stopticks
7. Shockley, L. W. (2006). Bites and stings. In V. J. Markovchick & P. T. Pons (Eds.), *Emergency medicine secrets* (4th ed., pp. 512–514). St. Louis, MO: Mosby.
8. Reuter-Rice, K. (2008). Bites that bleed: Crotalid envenomation. *Journal of Pediatric Health Care, 22*, 258–261.
9. Weinstein, S., Dart, R., Staples, A., & White, J. (2009). Envenomations: An overview of clinical toxinology for the primary care physician. *American Family Physician, 80*(8), 793–802.
10. Herr, R. D. (2006). Bites and stings. In P. G. Zimmermann & R. D. Herr (Eds.), *Triage nursing secrets* (p. 421). St. Louis, MO: Mosby.
11. Flarity, K. (2007). Environmental emergencies. In Emergency Nurses Association, *Emergency Nursing Core Curriculum* (6th ed., pp. 339–342). St. Louis, MO: Saunders.
12. Foex, B., & Wallis, L. (2005). Best evidence topic report. Scorpion envenomation: Does antivenom reduce serum venom concentrations? *Emergency Medicine Journal, 22*, 195–197.
13. Flarity, K. (2010). Environmental emergencies. In P. K. Howard & R. A. Steinmann (Eds.), *Sheehy's emergency nursing: Principles and practice* (6th ed., pp. 535–553). St. Louis, MO: Mosby.
14. Forrester, M. B. (2005). Pattern of stingray injuries reported to Texas poison centers from 1998 to 2004. *Human and Experimental Toxicology, 24*(12), 639–642.
15. Zoltan, T. B., Taylor, K. S., & Achar, S. A. (2005). Health issues for surfers. *American Family Physician, 71*(12), 2313–2317.

Genitourinary Emergencies

Susanne Quallich

This chapter discusses common genitourinary emergencies seen the emergency department. Problems of the urinary tract are covered, as well as problems unique to males and dialysis patients. See Chapter 47, Gynecologic Emergencies, for more information related to specific female genitourinary emergencies.

PROBLEMS OF THE URINARY TRACT

Acute Uncomplicated Pyelonephritis

Pyelonephritis is an inflammation of the kidneys that involves the tubules, glomeruli, and renal pelvis. It is more commonly seen in women. The usual cause is a bacterial infection with gram-negative bacilli such as *Escherichia coli*. Risk factors for the development of pyelonephritis include anatomical or functional genitourinary abnormalities and a new sexual partner in women.

Signs and Symptoms

- Severe flank or back pain at the costovertebral angle
- Tenderness over the affected flank
- Fever, chills, and headache that can progress to rigors
- Nausea, vomiting, and diarrhea
- Lower urinary tract symptoms: frequency and urgency, dysuria, and nocturia
- Pyuria, hematuria, and bacteriuria

Diagnostic Procedures

- Urinalysis
- Blood urea nitrogen (BUN) and creatinine with history suggestive of decreased function
- Urine cultures and gram stain
- Blood cultures do not contribute to diagnosis or management
- A complete blood count will show leukocytosis but is otherwise noncontributory
- Renal ultrasound

- Computed tomography (CT) without contrast to rule out presence of renal calculi as a cause of symptoms

Therapeutic Interventions

- Encourage fluid intake to maintain brisk diuresis.
- Encourage bed rest as needed.
- Drainage via nephrostomy tube (if indicated).
- Administer broad-spectrum antibiotics.
  - Patients with severe disease, immunosuppression, pregnancy, abscesses, gram-negative septicemia, age extremes, or significant comorbidities require hospital admission and parenterally administered antibiotics.
  - Most other patients can take antibiotics orally on an outpatient basis.

Gross Hematuria

Hematuria is a symptom of nephrological and urological diseases; gross hematuria is enough blood present in the urine to cause a noticeable color change. Blood may appear in the urine as a result of the following:
- Trauma
- Renal calculi
- Excessive exercise
- Blood dyscrasias
- Urinary tract infections
- Renal, ureteral, or bladder tumors
- Recent urological manipulation

Bleeding at the start of urination suggests a problem in the region of the anterior urethra. If blood is visualized at the end of the urinary stream, suspect bleeding from the posterior urethra or prostate. If bleeding is noted throughout urination, the most likely cause is a bladder or upper urinary tract source.

Important considerations for the patient with gross hematuria include the following:

- Do not assume that all red-colored urine indicates hematuria. Urine may be tinted as a result of the ingestion of food colorings, certain medications, or beets.
- In females, determine whether the bleeding is actually vaginal or menstrual.
- Anticoagulation within the therapeutic range does *not* result in hematuria.
- It is very rare to lose enough blood via the genitourinary tract to alter hemoglobin and hematocrit (except in the case of trauma).
- Patient may have a history of radiation treatment to pelvic and rectal area, resulting in radiation cystitis that can be a cause of gross hematuria.

Signs and Symptoms

- Gross or microscopic blood in the urine
- May or may not have urinary symptoms

Diagnostic Procedures

- Carefully obtain a patient history.
- Collect a urine specimen for dipstick testing and urinalysis. In menstruating females it may be necessary to obtain the sample via a catheter.
- If signs of infection are present, check a complete blood count.

Therapeutic Interventions

- Maintain adequate hydration by encouraging oral intake or by intravenous fluid administration.
- Specific therapeutic interventions will depend on the cause. See "Renal Calculi" and "Acute Cystitis."

Renal Calculi

The pain of renal colic typically radiates from the flank to the ipsilateral lower quadrant, the groin, and (occasionally) the leg. Men may also describe pain that radiates to the testicle on the affected side, while women may report pain in the labia on the affected side. This pain results from ureteral distension caused by the passage of renal calculi. The size of the stone or clot does not necessarily relate to pain severity. Important patient historical information includes the following:

- Previous stones
- Presence of an ileal conduit or hypercalcemia
- Recent travel that may have contributed to dehydration or poor fluid intake

Calcium stones account for 80% of all renal calculi.[8]

Signs and Symptoms

- Sudden onset of severe, colicky, radiating flank pain on affected side
- Restlessness; the patient is unable to find a position of comfort and often cannot remain on the stretcher
- Tenderness to the costovertebral angle on affected side
- Urinary urgency, frequency, and dysuria
- Nausea, vomiting, diaphoresis, and low-grade fever

Aortic and iliac aneurysms can mimic renal colic. Assess for abdominal bruits and pulsatile masses.

Diagnostic Procedures

- Gross or microscopic hematuria, with patient noting small clots in urine and possible stones.
- BUN and creatinine levels if compromise to kidney function is suspected.
- Abdominal radiographs and ultrasound may reveal calculi but are not sensitive.
- Helical CT has replaced intravenous pyelogram as the diagnostic procedure of choice.

Therapeutic Interventions

- Strain the urine for calculi.
- Initiate an isotonic, intravenous crystalloid infusion.
- Provide analgesics; narcotic analgesics are commonly prescribed.
- Administer an antiemetic such as ondansetron (Zofran) or promethazine (Phenergan) if the patient is nauseated or vomiting.
- If kidney function is determined to be adequate, consider administering non-steroidal anti-inflammatory drugs (NSAIDs) such as ketalorac (Toradol).
- For ongoing care, including pain management, patients may require hospital admission, pharmacological stone dissolution, extracorporeal shock wave lithotripsy, laser lithotripsy, or surgical intervention.[1]

Urinary Retention

Urinary retention is the inability to completely empty the bladder of urine; the problem may be acute or chronic. Urinary retention may be caused by a variety of conditions, including the following:

- Urethral strictures
- An enlarged prostate or acute prostatis
- Blood clots
- Renal calculi
- Neurogenic bladder
- Pelvic organ prolapse
- Multiple sclerosis or other neurologic compromise
- Bladder calculi

Urinary retention is also a side effect of parasympatholytic agents and certain other drugs such as over-the-counter cold medicines, especially in men. Risk factors include recent genitourinary instrumentation and back injury that may have compromised the lumbosacral spine.

Signs and Symptoms

- Lower abdominal discomfort
- Bladder distension (a mass may be palpable just above symphysis pubis)

Diagnostic Procedures

- An ultrasonic bladder scan can quickly confirm urine retention.

Therapeutic Interventions

- Insert an indwelling urinary catheter for immediate relief.
- In men with urinary retention secondary to benign prostatic hypertrophy, the insertion of a curved-tipped Coude catheter may be easier and cause less patient discomfort.
- In rare instances, a suprapubic catheter may be necessary.
- Determine the cause and treat as indicated.
- Consider urological consultation to investigate functional status of the bladder.

Urinary Tract Infection (Acute Cystitis)[1,2]

Acute cystitis is an infection of the lower urinary tract, primarily the bladder, that results from bacterial migration from the urethra. The most common organism is *E. coli*. Females are more likely to have this condition because of their shorter urethras. Acute cystitis may also be precipitated by women having a new sexual partner. Males may contract acute cystitis as a result of the incomplete bladder emptying secondary to an enlarged prostate or following acute prostatitis.

Signs and Symptoms

- Patient reports difficulty starting urinary stream, accompanied by pain and burning
- Other irritative voiding symptoms such as dysuria, urgency, frequency, and nocturia may be present
- The patient may void only small amounts of cloudy urine at a time
- Patients often report foul-smelling urine
- Normal temperature or low-grade fever
- Suprapubic pressure or pain or low back pain
- Prostate tenderness possible
- Urinary retention in males

- A change in mental status may be the only indication of urinary tract infection in the elderly

Diagnostic Procedures

- Urinalysis will confirm the clinical diagnosis and may reveal the following:
  - Microscopic or gross hematuria
  - Many white blood cells (WBCs)
  - Positive leukocyte esterase and nitrite
- CBC with differential to detect possible leukocytosis

Therapeutic Interventions

- Stable, uncomplicated patients can be seen in the emergency department and discharged with a short course of oral antibiotics, usually 3 to 5 days.
- Begin antibiotic therapy. Trimethoprim and sulfamethoxazole (Septra, Bactrim) and nitrofurantoin are the first-line drugs of choice for uncomplicated urinary tract infection.
- NSAIDs can also be recommended for symptom management.
- Phenazopyridine (Pyridium) is a urinary analgesic that reduces dysuria pain and bladder spasms. This drug can be prescribed or purchased over the counter. Warn patients that phenazopyridine will turn their urine bright orange.
- Encourage patients to increase fluid intake to promote bacterial excretion.
- Individuals, particularly the elderly, may develop sepsis. A high index of suspicion is necessary because the elderly and diabetic and immunosuppressed patients often present with atypical symptoms and their clinical course can deteriorate rapidly. Refer to Chapter 21, Sepsis, for more information.

GENITOURINARY PROBLEMS UNIQUE TO MALES

Testicular Torsion

Testicular torsion is one of the few true urological emergencies. It is the twisting of a testicle or the spermatic cord within the tunica vaginalis, causing strangulation of the blood supply to the testis. This condition is seen most commonly in adolescents. The great majority of cases of testicular torsion occur in boys between the ages of 12 and 18 years; it is suspected to result from this period of rapid growth. Infants are also susceptible, but in infants it is congenital. Torsion is rare after the age of 30 years. Failure to correct torsion of the testicle results in ischemia and necrosis.[3]

Signs and Symptoms

- Sudden onset of severe, unilateral scrotal pain and tenderness followed by scrotal swelling and edema
- Pain can begin during physical activity but also can occur spontaneously
- History of previous similar episodes that resolved spontaneously
- Absence of urinary symptoms
- Nausea and vomiting
- Tense scrotal mass (the epididymis cannot be palpated)
- A high-riding or horizontal testicle may be noted; absence of cremaster reflex
- Intense pain or minimal pain relief when the testicle is elevated

> The affected testis is usually firm, tender, and aligned in a horizontal rather than a vertical axis in testicular torsion. The presence of cremasteric reflex is helpful to rule out testicular torsion. (Elicit it by gently stroking the inner aspect of the involved thigh and observing more than 0.5 cm of elevation in the affected testis.)[8]

Diagnostic Procedures

- Doppler ultrasonography, which will demonstrate a lack of flow to the affected testes
- Radionuclide scan

Therapeutic Interventions

- Obtain urgent urological consultation.
- Bedside detorsion may be attempted. Most testes twist medially. To correct torsion, manually rotate the affected testis laterally. Relief of pain indicates successful detorsion.
- Immediate surgical exploration (within 4 to 6 hours of onset) with subsequent orchidopexy is routinely the treatment of choice. After 24 hours untreated, the testicle has sustained necrosis.

Testicular Tumor

Testicular tumors are most common in males 20 to 40 years of age. These patients come to the emergency department complaining of a scrotal mass with or without pain. This continues to be one of the most successfully curable types of malignancy, even if a patient's initial presentation is late stage with metastases. Unfortunately, it is common for men to delay seeking evaluation for 3 to 6 months.[4]

Signs and Symptoms

- Patient may have noted abnormality during self-examination or while showering. These abnormalities may include a change in testicle size, increasing asymmetry of the testes, and pain in or heaviness of the involved side.
- Men with a history of undescended testes at birth, even if surgically corrected, have an increased risk for testicular cancer (7% to 10%).[5]
- Most men are asymptomatic, but may have complaints of testicular ache.
- Scrotal swelling with a testicular mass that is firm and nontender.
- Decreased lung sounds, wheezing, and shortness of breath with exertion, back pain, lower extremity swelling, and palpable supraclavicular nodes are all possible if metastasis present.

Diagnostic Procedures

- Scrotal ultrasound
- Transillumination: mass will not transilluminate
- Tumor markers: lactate dehydrogenase, alpha-fetoprotein, beta-human chorionic gonadotropin
- If metastasis is suspected, a chest radiograph and CT scan of the abdomen and pelvis will be ordered

Therapeutic Interventions

- Obtain urological consultation for surgical evaluation and likely orchiectomy for tumor pathology.

Priapism[3]

Priapism is considered a urological emergency. It is a prolonged, painful erection that persists for hours and usually is unrelated to sexual stimulation.[5] Physiologic causes include spinal cord injury, tumors, sickle cell disease, or other hematologic disorders. Pharmacological agents injected into the corpus cavernosum for the treatment of erectile dysfunction can result in priapism; oral phosphodiesterase type 5 inhibitor medications have been implicated as well. While this condition can occur at any age, it is more common between the ages of 5 and 10 years (and is usually associated with sickle cell disease) and again during the 20- to 50-year-old age range.

Signs and Symptoms

- Persistent and painful erection (low-flow or veno-occlusive priapism) lasting more than 4 hours
- Erect but nontender penis (high-flow or nonischemic priapism)

Diagnostic Procedures

- Penile Doppler
- Arteriography
- Complete blood count if malignancy suspected

Therapeutic Interventions

- Provide analgesia and sedation as needed.
- Manage any underlying conditions.
- Epinephrine, phenylephrine, pseudoephedrine, or terbutaline can be injected into the penis to help reverse engorgement.[5] The corpora may also be irrigated with normal saline.
- Obtain urgent urological consultation.

Fournier's Gangrene[6]

Fournier's gangrene is a rapidly progressing necrotizing fasciitis of the male perineum and genitalia, caused by both anaerobic and aerobic species of bacteria simultaneously. It can be preceded by an infection of the rectum, lower urinary tract, or perineum or direct trauma to the genital area. Although generally seen in males, it has been described in females as well. Risk factors include diabetes mellitus, alcoholism, malnutrition, and immunocompromise. There may be a history of recent poor serum glucose control in the diabetic patient. Mortality rates can be up to 50% and are dependent on the depth of the infection.

> The diagnosis and treatment of Fournier's gangrene are similar to those of necrotizing fasciitis.

Signs and Symptoms

- Painful swelling, erythema, and induration of the genitalia
- Cellulitis, odor, and tissue necrosis
- Fever, chills, and other systemic complaints
- Pain that seems in excess of the visible skin changes.
- Patient may report a break in skin integrity within the past 48 hours.

Diagnostic Procedures

- Plain films or CT may demonstrate gas in the subcutaneous tissue
- CBC to evaluate for elevated white blood cell count

Therapeutic Interventions

- Administer broad-spectrum IV antibiotics.
- Provide analgesia and sedation as needed.
- This is a surgical emergency. Surgical consultation may involve general surgery, urology, and plastic surgery for extensive surgical debridement.

Paraphimosis

Phimosis refers to the inability to fully retract the foreskin of an uncircumcised male over the glans penis.

Paraphimosis occurs when the retracted foreskin becomes entrapped behind the coronal sulcus and blood flow to the glans is occluded. This results in edema and pain and eventual necrosis if not treated promptly. Men with a history of chronic inflammation of the foreskin and phimosis are at highest risk for paraphimosis.

Signs and Symptoms

- Swollen, painful edematous glans
- Tight ring of skin apparent behind glans on examination
- Discolored, necrotic areas may be noted to the glans
- History of increasing difficulty advancing the foreskin (phimosis)

Therapeutic Interventions

- Provide NSAIDs for pain management.
- Initiate antibiotic therapy as indicated.
- Manual reduction can be attempted by applying pressure with the thumbs to reduce the edema and advance the foreskin. If this is unsuccessful, a local anesthetic may be given so that a small incision can be made to correct the restriction.
- Patients should be strongly advised to consider a circumcision or dorsal slit to prevent further episodes.

Acute Prostatitis

Acute prostatitis is an inflammation of the prostate gland, most commonly the result of a bacterial infection that has ascended via the urethra or refluxed into the prostate from the bladder. Prostatitis usually is accompanied by acute cystitis. Causative agents are usually enterococci or gram-negative bacteria.

Signs and Symptoms

- Sudden onset of dysuria and general malaise.
- Complaints of perineal pain, which may worsen with ejaculation or bowel movements
- Vague lower abdominal, penile, or suprapubic discomfort
- Prostate tenderness
- Fever and chills
- Possible urinary retention and irritative bladder symptoms
- Hematospermia

> Acute bacterial prostatitis presentation can be dramatic and usually includes frequency, urgency, dysuria, and some obstructive voiding symptoms.

Diagnostic Procedures

- Obtain urine for urinalysis and cultures; gross hematuria may be present
- Prostate-specific antigen may be elevated
- Prostate examination may reveal a boggy prostate that is exquisitely tender

Therapeutic Interventions

- Provide analgesia as indicated.
- Patient may require a catheter to drain bladder; may require short-term indwelling catheter to maintain drainage.
- Initiate antibiotic therapy; fluoroquinolones are the first choice. Administer acyclovir for herpes proctitis. Most patients are treated on an outpatient basis.
- Encourage patients to increase their fluid intake to aid bacterial elimination and antibiotic excretion.

Acute Epididymitis

Acute epididymitis is an infection of the epididymis resulting from organisms that ascend from the lower urinary tract and is the most common cause of intrascrotal inflammation. It may follow cystoscopic examination, prostate surgery, or bladder catheterization. However, acute epididymitis most commonly is contracted by sexual contact. *Chlamydia trachomatis* and *Neisseria gonorrhoeae* are the two organisms responsible for the majority of epididymitis cases. Exposure may predate manifestations of symptoms by as much as 2 weeks. This disorder is rare in prepubertal boys. Epididymitis in elderly men often follows urological manipulation or catheter placement or is a result of prostatic obstruction.

Signs and Symptoms

- Gradual onset of mild to moderate testicular or scrotal pain that is usually unilateral and radiates up spermatic cord to inguinal region or flank
- Progressive scrotal warmth, swelling, tenderness, erythema, and edema
- History may include a new sexual partner
- History of a recent episode of prolonged sitting (e.g., long airline flight, extensive cycling)
- Dysuria
- Ureteral discharge
- Elevated temperature, sepsis (in severe cases)

Diagnostic Procedures

- Scrotal ultrasound to differentiate epididymitis from testicular torsion (Table 33-1)
- Urethral smear for Gram stain and culture
- Urinalysis may show white blood cells, bacteria
- Urine culture

Therapeutic Interventions

- Scrotal elevation may decrease pain.
- Initiate antibiotic therapy based on the suspected organisms, per current Centers for Disease Control and Prevention guidelines or clinical suspicions. Encourage notification of partner for treatment.
- NSAIDs can also be recommended for symptom management. Occasionally a short course of oral narcotics may be prescribed.
- Encourage patients to increase oral fluid intake and limit activity. Pain usually resolves in 1 to 3 days, while epididymal induration can take 2 to 4 weeks to resolve.

TABLE 33-1   EPIDIDYMITIS VERSUS TESTICULAR TORSION

	ACUTE EPIDIDYMITIS	TESTICULAR TORSION
Onset	Gradual; can escalate quickly	Sudden Pain often begins during physical activity but can occur during sleep as well
Pain character	Mild to severe testicular or scrotal pain that is usually unilateral	Severe, unilateral scrotal pain and tenderness followed by scrotal swelling and erythema
Cause	Infectious (usually *Chlamydia trachomatis* and *Neisseria gonorrhoeae*)	Congenital abnormality (bell clapper deformity) Undescended testicle Cold weather Sexual activity
Common age group	Postpubertal (sexually active) males	Boys between the ages of 12 and 18 years (but can occur at any age)
Ureteral discharge	Yes	No
Scrotal elevation	May decrease pain	Often causes intense pain
Treatment	Antibiotics, supportive symptomatic management	Manual detorsion Surgery

Penile Fracture

This is a condition in which the tunica albuginea or the corpus cavernosa of the penile shaft, or both, rupture as a result of unusual torque. Penile fracture occurs most commonly during sexual activity and can range from mild in nature to quite severe, resulting in pain and eventual erectile difficulties if untreated. It can also result after direct trauma or falls or during masturbation.

Signs and Symptoms

- Male patient (and partner) may report hearing a "pop" during sexual activity, followed by pain to the penile shaft and immediate loss of erection
- Bright red blood from urethra
- Ecchymosis to site of injury, which may extend to much of penile shaft, may result in deviation of the shaft
- Edema and pain in penis
- Urinary function typically unaffected

Diagnostic Procedures

- Penile Doppler

Therapeutic Interventions

- Immediate surgical repair of the tunica albuginea defect is necessary—ideally within 24 to 36 hours after injury.
- Many men do not present within this time frame, however, because of embarrassment or a belief that the injury is less severe.
- If the injury is minor (no loss of erection) and the hematoma is confined to the penile skin, supportive measures such as ice and NSAIDs are recommended, with reassurance that the condition will improve with time.

EMERGENCIES IN DIALYSIS PATIENTS

Because of the chronic and serious nature of their condition, dialysis patients make frequent emergency department visits with a variety of complaints ranging from loss of access to lethal hyperkalemia and fluid overload. These patients are less able to handle fluid and solute loads, with the result that routine over-the-counter medications can contribute to metabolism and excretion issues. Some of the problems unique to this population are addressed briefly in this section.

Clotted Vascular Access

Hemodialysis patients have one of two basic types of vascular access systems. An arteriovenous fistula is a surgically created connection between an artery and a vein and can be constructed from the patient's own vessels or from synthetic graft materials. Fistulas are contained completely under the skin, with the most common site being the forearm for ease of access. A patent fistula will have a strong, palpable thrill. The second type of access consists of a subclavian or femoral catheter, the distal end of which is external to the patient. Catheters can be inserted for short-term use, or a tunneled catheter may be placed surgically for long-term access.

Regardless of the type, all vascular access devices are subject to clotting. Most dialysis center personnel do *not* want emergency department providers accessing or manipulating these devices. Declotting is rarely an emergency procedure, unless there is loss of the fistula's thrill. Catheters and fistulas can be declotted with a fibrinolytic agent (alteplase, recombinant tissue plasminogen activator) or reopened by angioplasty or angiographic clot removal. Consultation with the patient's nephrologist is mandatory.[7]

Clots in the hemodialysis patient's access device can detach and embolize to the lungs. Consider the possibility of pulmonary embolism in any hemodialysis patient who has a complaint of acute-onset shortness of breath.

Infection

Infection should always be part of the differential diagnosis, even in the absence of "classic" indicators of infection. Dialysis patients may not manifest typical signs and symptoms of infection beyond a slight elevation in temperature, similar to the presentation that can be seen with patients that are immunocompromised. Atypical sites for the infection should be investigated, such as infected diabetic extremity ulcers, dental abscesses, and perirectal abscesses.

Bleeding

Patients can present with bleeding from their fistula within several hours after dialysis, but a number of conditions predispose hemodialysis patients to bleeding disorders. Uremia suppresses platelet function, dialysis causes hemolysis, renal failure limits erythropoietin production, and patients are heparinized during dialysis. Catheters and fistulas provide opportunities for significant hemorrhage. Moderate pressure is usually sufficient to stop the bleeding without causing damage to the fistula.

Fistula Infection

Bacteremia resulting from fistula infections in hemodialysis patients can be accompanied by signs of systemic infection, but fever may be the sole indication. The fistula can become contaminated at the time of access, and the organism is usually *Staphylococcus* species. Draw blood cultures and administer antibiotics in a timely manner. Synthetic grafts are more vulnerable to infection than are fistulas made from native vessels. Failure to control infection aggressively can lead to loss of the fistula.

REFERENCES

1. Neal, D. E. (2008). Complicated urinary tract infections. *Urologic Clinics of North America, 35*(1), 13–22.

2. Nicolle, L. E. (2008). Uncomplicated urinary tract infection in adults including uncomplicated pyelonephritis. *Urologic Clinics of North America, 35*(1), 1–12.

3. Tanagho, E., & McAninch, J. (Eds.). (2007). *Smith's general urology* (17th ed.). New York, NY: McGraw-Hill.

4. Mostafa, G., Cathey, L., & Greene, F. (2006). Urologic malignancy. In *Review of surgery: Basic science and clinical topics for ABSITE* (pp. 375–380). New York, NY: Springer Science+Business Media.

5. American Urological Association. (2003). *Management of priapism*. Retrieved from http://www.auanet.org/content/guidelines-and-quality-care/clinical-guidelines.cfm?sub=priapism

6. Sarani, B., Strong, M., Pascual, J., & Schwab, C. W. (2009). Necrotizing fasciitis: Current concepts and review of the literature. *Journal of the American College of Surgeons, 208*(2), 279–288.

7. Wolfson, A. B. (2009). Renal failure. In J. Marx, R. Hockberger, & R. Walls (Eds.), *Rosen's emergency medicine* (7th ed.). New York, NY: Mosby.

8. Fernandes, C. M. B. (2011). Renal colic and scrotal pain. In V. J. Markovchick & P. T. Pons, *Emergency medicine secrets* (5th ed.). St. Louis, MO: Mosby.

Sexually Transmitted Infections

Darcy Egging

Sexually transmitted infections (STIs) are a major public health care concern. Women as well as infants are at a great risk of bearing the long-term consequences of STIs. The effective assessment and management of these diseases are key in the emergency department (ED). The emergency nurse must be able to assess and provide care for this population as they present to the ED.[1-3] This chapter places a primary focus on female patients who present to the ED seeking treatment for gynecological problems.

The adolescent population has the highest reported incidence of STIs.[3] Adolescence is a time of sexual exploration through experimentation. Therefore the emergency nurse must learn to establish a trusting relationship rapidly to garner information pertinent to the care of adolescents. This is accomplished by being nonjudgmental and allowing for confidentiality as well as respect.[1,3]

PATIENT HISTORY AND ASSESSMENT

An accurate history is essential when dealing with the potential diagnosis of an STI. Key issues to ask about are:
- Sexual orientation
- Sexual activity
- The potential of sexual abuse or assault
- Number of partners
- Previous STIs
- Possibility of pregnancy
- Type of contraceptive practices being used
- Use of condoms[3]
  Additional information to obtain:
- Menstrual history
- Medication use
- Pain: time of onset, quality, what makes it better or worse, treatment prior to arrival
- Vaginal discharge
- Obstetrical history
- Last Papanicolaou (Pap) test[4]

If the patient presents with a gynecological complaint, the emergency nurse should:
- Perform a general assessment as well as a focused assessment of the abdomen and genital area
- Prepare for a pelvic exam
- If STI is suspected, prepare for specimen collection

All female patients of childbearing age should have at least a urine pregnancy test performed.

SELECTED EMERGENCIES

Human Papillomavirus

Human papillomavirus (HPV) is the most prevalent STI in both adolescents and adult women. HPV is usually asymptomatic but can cause benign warts or certain types of cancer.[5,6] There are more than 40 types of HPV that can infect both men and women.

Signs and Symptoms
- Often asymptomatic
- Genital warts (*Condylomata acuminata*): can occur on the vulva, perianal area, vaginal walls, and cervix (Fig. 34-1); can also occur in male patients

Therapeutic Interventions
- In the absence of genital warts no treatment is recommended.
- Topical medication (Podofilox 0.5% gel or Imiquimod 5% cream) as ordered if external warts are identified.
- Educate patient on treatment and prevention related to spreading the virus.
- HPV vaccine starting at age 11 or 12 years.
  - Series of three injections; the second and third injections are given 2 and 6 months after the first injection.

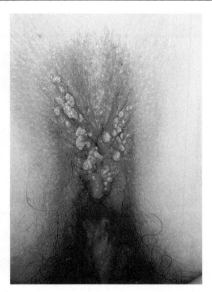

Fig. 34-1 Genital warts. (Reproduced with permission from Emergency Nurses Association. [2009]. *Sheehy's emergency nursing: Principles and practice* [6th ed.]. St. Louis, MO: Mosby.)

- The vaccine can be given to females 13 to 26 years of age who have not previously been immunized.
- Research is ongoing to determine the effectiveness of the vaccine in boys and young men.[7]
- Research is ongoing to determine the effectiveness of the vaccine in females older than 26 years.[8]
- Consistent use of condoms.
- Instruct patient to notify her obstetrician of HPV if pregnant, as HPV can worsen during pregnancy.
- Encourage routine Pap testing; HPV is associated with cervical dysplasia.

Herpes Simplex Virus

Herpes simplex virus (HSV) is a viral illness that is transmitted through oral, vaginal, and rectal intercourse. HSV is a chronic infection with remissions and exacerbations. It has been estimated that up to 70% of people with HSV are asymptomatic.[2,6]

Signs and Symptoms

- Multiple painful vesicles or ulcerations on the genital area
- Fever
- Malaise
- Myalgias
- Regional lymphadenopathy
- Dysuria

Diagnostic Procedures

- Obtain viral cultures and test for other STIs.

Therapeutic Interventions

- Antiviral therapy.
- Educate patient related to this chronic condition.
  - Viral shedding can occur even when asymptomatic.
  - Consistent use of condoms.
  - Take medications as directed.
  - Inform current and future sexual partners.
  - When lesions are present, abstain from sexual activities.
  - There is an increased risk of viral transmission to the fetus with vaginal delivery if lesions are present. Cesarean section is recommended.[9]

Gonorrhea

Gonorrhea, the second most common STI in the United States, is caused by *Neisseria gonorrhoeae*, a gram-negative diplococcus. Women under the age of 25 years are at greatest risk.[6] Gonorrhea is the leading cause of cervicitis and pelvic inflammatory disease (PID) in female patients and of urethritis in male patients.[6] Men will present symptomatically whereas women can remain asymptomatic. Untreated gonorrhea can lead to infertility, ectopic pregnancy, and chronic pelvic pain.[6,10]

Signs and Symptoms

- Urinary tract infection symptoms: frequency, urgency, and burning with urination
- Women will complain of mucoid discharge from cervix
- Men will complain of penile discharge

Diagnostic Procedures

- Cervical or penile cultures: gonorrhea and chlamydia deoxyribonucleic acid (DNA) probe
- Pelvic or penile examination
- Consider testing patient for syphilis and other STIs

Therapeutic Interventions

- Antibiotic therapy[9]:
  - Ceftriaxone (Rocephin) 250 mg in a single intramuscular (IM) dose *or if not an option*
  - Cefixime (Suprax) 400 mg in a single dose *or*
  - Single-dose injectible cephalosporin in regimens *plus* azithromycin 1 g orally in a single dose *or* doxycycline 100 mg orally twice daily for 7 days
- Patient education emphasizing the following:
  - All (recent and current) sexual partners need to be treated

- Follow up with primary care physician to ensure that treatment has been successful
- Consistent use of condoms

Chlamydia

Chlamydia is caused by *Chlamydia trachomatis* and is usually associated with gonorrhea and is the most frequently reported bacterial STI in the United States.[9] It is believed that 75% of all chlamydial infections are asymptomatic.[11]

Signs and Symptoms

- May be asymptomatic
- Later cases may present with:
  - Cervicitis
  - Endometriosis
  - Salpingitis
  - PID

Diagnostic Procedures

- Cervical or urine cultures
- Consider testing for other STIs

Therapeutic Interventions

- Antibiotic therapy[9]
  - Azithromycin (Zithromax) 1 g orally once *or*
  - Doxycycline 100 mg twice a day for 7 days
- Access the Centers for Disease Control and Prevention (CDC) for alternative treatments[10]
- Educate patient related to the following:
  - All sexual partners need to be treated
  - Take medication as directed
  - Follow up with primary care physician to ensure that treatment has been successful
  - Consistent use of condoms
  - No sexual intercourse for at least 7 days after Zithromax

Syphilis

Syphilis is a systemic STI caused by the spirochete *Treponema pallidum*. Syphilis is seen more commonly in the female population and in those who abuse drugs.[2]

Signs and Symptoms

- Three phases:
  - Primary: usually presents with a painless ulcer or chancre on the mouth or anogenital area[12]
  - Secondary:
    - Develops 4 to 10 weeks after primary infection
    - Myalgias
    - Lymphadenopathy
    - Flulike symptoms

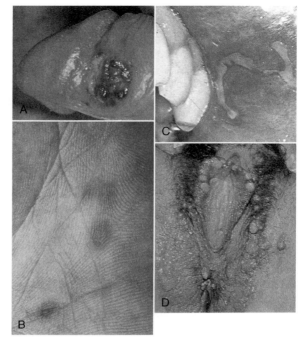

Fig. 34-2 Syphilis lesions. (Reproduced with permission from Goldman, L. [2007]. *Cecil medicine* [23rd ed.]. St. Louis, MO: Saunders.)

- May have skin rash on palms of hands and soles of feet (Fig. 34-2)
- Tertiary
  - Occurs 2 to 19 years after initial symptoms (such as, psychosis, delirium, and dementia) in an untreated patient
  - Rarely seen in the ED because of preventative programs and antibiotics[2,6]

Diagnostic Procedures

- Serology testing
  - Venereal Disease Research Laboratory (VDRL)
  - Rapid Plasma Reagin (RPR)[2,6]
- Syphilis should be considered in any sexually active patient with a genital ulcer or generalized rash
- Consider testing for other STIs

Therapeutic Interventions

- For all stages of syphilis: benzathine penicillin 2.4 million units IM once[9]
- If patient has penicillin allergy, alternative therapies include the following:

TABLE 34-1	**COMPARISON OF TYPES OF VAGINITIS**			
	SIGNS AND SYMPTOMS	**DIAGNOSTIC STUDIES**	**THERAPEUTIC INTERVENTIONS**	**PATIENT EDUCATION**
Vulvovaginal candidiasis	Vaginal irritation Vaginal itching Cottage cheese–like discharge Vulvar or vaginal inflammation	Wet prep looking for hyphae, pseudohyphae, or budding yeast[a,b]	Over-the-counter vaginal creams and vaginal suppositories Oral fluconazole (Diflucan) 150 mg orally once[c]	Fluconazole (Diflucan) is contraindicated in pregnancy Follow up with primary care physician
Trichomonas vaginalis	Vulvar irritation Dyspareunia: pain during sexual intercourse Urinary tract infection symptoms: frequency, pain on urination Vaginal odor some describe as "fishy" Vaginal discharge frequently yellow or green in color	Wet prep looking for motile trichomonads[d]	Metronidazole (Flagyl) 2 g orally in a single dose *or* Tinidazole 2 g orally in a single dose[c]	Take medication as directed Do not drink alcoholic beverages while taking metronidazole (Flagyl) Sexual partners need to be treated Follow up with primary care physician
Bacterial vaginosis (BV)	Vulvar irritation Vaginal odor with fishy characteristic Grayish vaginal discharge	Diagnosis requires 3 of the following 4 criteria: Homogenous, thin, white or gray discharge that smoothly coats the vaginal walls Presence of clue cells on microscopic examination pH of vaginal fluid >4.5 Positive amine test or "whiff test": fishy odor when potassium hydroxide is applied to vaginal discharge[a,b,d]	Metronidazole (Flagyl) 500 mg *bid* for 7 days *or* Metronidazole (Flagyl) gel, 0.75%, one applicator intravaginally once per day for 5 days *or* Clindamycin cream, 2%, one applicator intravaginally each night for 7 days	Sexual partners do not need to be treated Take medication as prescribed Follow up with primary care physician Avoid douching and bubble baths

[a]Jordan, K. S. (2008). Gynecologic emergencies. In P. K. Howard & R. A. Steinmann (Eds.), *Sheehy's emergency nursing: Principles and practice* (6th ed., pp. 578–589). St. Louis, MO: Mosby.
[b]Mollen, C. J. (2009). Sexually transmitted infections. In J. M. Baren, S. G. Rothrock, J. A. Brennan, & L. Brown (Eds.), *Pediatric emergency medicine* (pp. 543–559). Philadelphia, PA: Saunders Elsevier.
[c]Centers for Disease Control and Prevention (2010). Sexually transmitted diseases treatment guidelines, 2010. *Morbidity and Mortality Weekly Report, 59*(RR-12), 1–100.
[d]Biggs, W. S., & Williams, R. M. (2009). Common gynecologic infections. *Primary Care, 36*(1), 33–51.
bid, Twice a day.

- • Doxycycline 100 mg twice a day for 14 days *or*
- • Tetracycline 500 mg four times a day for 14 days[10]
- • Educate patient related to the following:
  - • All sexual partners need to be treated
  - • Follow up with primary care physician to ensure that treatment has been successful
  - • Consistent use of condoms

Vaginitis

Vaginitis is commonly caused by *Candida albicans*, *Trichomonas vaginalis*, or bacterial vaginosis (BV). People who are taking antibiotics or corticosteroids or who have a history of diabetes or pregnancy are more susceptible to vaginitis.[2] Three types of vaginitis are summarized in Table 34-1.

Pelvic Inflammatory Disease

Pelvic inflammatory disease is a polymicrobial infection of the upper female genital tract, including any of the following in combination: endometriosis, salpingitis, tubo-ovarian abscess, and pelvic peritonitis. The most common organisms that can cause PID are *N. gonorrhoeae* and *C. trachomatis,* but PID can be caused by a variety of bacterial sources.

Risk Factors for PID

- Use of intrauterine device (IUD)
- Previous STIs
- Multiple sexual partners
- Substance abuse
- Frequent vaginal douching

Signs and Symptoms

- Abdominal pain
- Dyspareunia
- Abnormal vaginal discharge
- Fever
- Positive cervical motion tenderness on vaginal examination

Diagnostic Procedures

- Abnormal white cells on saline smear of vaginal or cervical discharge
- Elevated erythrocyte sedimentation rate (ESR)
- Elevated C-reactive protein
- Positive cervical infection with *N. gonorrhoeae* or *C. trachomatis*
- Other diagnostics (not necessarily performed in the ED) that definitively identify PID:
  - Endometrial biopsy
  - Transvaginal sonography or magnetic resonance imaging (MRI) of pelvis shows thickened, fluid-filled fallopian tubes with or without free pelvic fluid or tubo-ovarian abscess
  - Laparoscopy[4]

Therapeutic Interventions

- Criteria for hospitalization
  - A surgical cause cannot be ruled out
  - Pregnancy
  - Patient not responding to antibiotic therapy
  - Severe illness: fever, vomiting
  - Tubo-ovarian abscess
- Parenteral and oral therapy
  - Parenteral treatment[9]
    - Regimen A: Cefotetan 2 g intravenously every 12 hours *or* Cefoxitin 2 g intravenously every 6 hours *plus* doxycycline 100 mg orally or intravenously every 12 hours
    - Regimen B: Clindamycin 900 mg intravenously every 8 hours *plus* Gentamycin loading dose intravenously or IM (2 mg/kg) followed by maintenance dose (1.5 mg/kg) every 8 hours
    - Alternative regimen: Ampicillin and sulbactam 3 g intravenously every 6 hours *plus* doxycycline 100 mg orally or intravenously every 12 hours
- Oral treatment[9]
  - Ceftriaxone (Rocephin) 250 IM in a single dose *plus* doxycycline 100 mg orally twice a day for 14 days. May add metronidazole (Flagyl) 500 mg twice a day for 14 days *or*
  - Cefoxitin (Mefoxin) 2 g IM single dose and probenecid 1 g orally *plus* doxycycline 100 mg twice a day for 14 days. May add metronidazole (Flagyl) 500 mg twice a day for 14 days.[4,9]
  - Other parenteral third-generation cephalosporin *plus* doxycycline 100 mg orally twice a day for 14 days. May add metronidazole 500 mg orally twice a day for 14 days.
- Patient education and discharge instructions related to the following:
  - Taking medication as directed.
  - Infertility may be a concern in the future.
  - Increased risk of ectopic pregnancy.
  - Follow up in 72 hours for reevaluation. If patient does not respond within 72 hours, she should be evaluated for possible hospital admission.

Tubo-Ovarian Abscess

Up to 30% of women with PID will develop the complication of tubo-ovarian abscess. The ovary becomes infected with purulent material from the fallopian tube.[13,14] If the abscess ruptures, this is considered a surgical emergency.

Signs and Symptoms

- Ill-appearing female
- Severe abdominal pain
- Peritoneal signs upon palpation
- Fever

Diagnostic Procedures

- Complete blood count
- Urinalysis
- C-reactive protein
- Cervical cultures and DNA probe
- Radiographic studies
  - Ultrasound
  - Computed tomography scan of abdomen and pelvis
- MRI[13,14]

Therapeutic Interventions

- Hospitalization.
- Parenteral therapy is the same as for PID.
- Possible surgical excision.
- Hysterectomy and bilateral salpingo-oophorectomy may be necessary in cases of overwhelming infection.

REFERENCES

1. Jordan, K. S. (2008). Gynecologic emergencies. In P. K. Howard & R. A. Steinmann (Eds.), *Sheehy's emergency nursing: Principles and practice* (6th ed., pp. 578–589). St. Louis, MO: Mosby.
2. Mollen, C. J. (2009). Sexually transmitted infections. In J. M. Baren, S. G. Rothrock, J. A. Brennan, & L. Brown (Eds.), *Pediatric emergency medicine* (pp. 543–559). Philadelphia, PA: Saunders.
3. Shafii, T., & Burstein, G. R. (2009). The adolescent sexual health visit. *Obstetrics and Gynecology Clinics of North America, 36*(1), 99–117.
4. Bayram, J., & Malik, M. (2008). Gynecologic infections. In J. G. Adams (Ed.), *Emergency medicine* (pp. 1371–1388). Philadelphia, PA: Saunders.
5. Hollier, L. M., & Workowski, K. (2008). Treatment of sexually transmitted infections in women. *Infectious Disease Clinics of North America, 22*(4), 665–691.
6. Frenkl, T. L., & Potts, J. (2008). Sexually transmitted infections. *Urologic Clinics of North America, 35*(1), 33–46.
7. Food and Drug Administration. (2009, October 16). *FDA approves new indication for Gardasil to prevent genital warts in men and boys* [press release]. Retrieved from http://www.fda.gov/NewsEvents/Newsroom/PressAnnouncements/ucm187003.htm
8. Markowitz, L. E., Dunne, E. F., Saraiya, M., Lawson, H. W., Chesson, H., & Unger, E. R.; Centers for Disease Control and Prevention; Advisory Committee on Immunization Practices. (2007). Quadrivalent human papillomavirus vaccine: Recommendations of the Advisory Committee on Immunization Practices (ACIP). *MMRW Recommendations and Reports, 56*(RR-2), 1–24.
9. Centers for Disease Control and Prevention. (2010). Sexually transmitted diseases treatment guidelines, 2020. *MMWR Recommendations and Reports, 59*(RR-12), 1–110.
10. Centers for Disease Control and Prevention. (2007). Update to CDC's sexually transmitted diseases treatment guidelines, 2006: Fluoroquinolones no longer recommended for treatment of gonococcal infections. *MMWR Morbidity and Mortality Weekly Report, 56*(14), 332–336.
11. Chiaradonna, C. (2007). The Chlamydia cascade: Enhanced STD prevention strategies for adolescents. *Journal of Pediatric and Adolescent Gynecology, 21*(5), 233–241.
12. Trigg, B. G., Kerndt, P. R., & Aynalem, G. (2008). Sexually transmitted infections and pelvic inflammatory disease in women. *The Medical Clinical of North America, 92*(5), 1083–1113.
13. Biggs, W. S., & Williams, R. M. (2009). Common gynecologic infections. *Primary Care, 36*(1), 33–51.
14. Lareau, S. M., & Beigi, R. H. (2008). Pelvic inflammatory disease and tubo-ovarian abscess. *Infectious Disease Clinics of North America, 22*(4), 693–708.

Trauma

Assessment and Stabilization of the Trauma Patient

Jeff Solheim

Trauma has far-reaching effects on society. Unintentional injury ranks as the fifth leading cause of death in the United States, claiming 41 of every 100,000 people.[1] When intentional injuries such as assaults and suicide attempts are added, the rate increases to 60.5 deaths per 100,000 people.[2] Yet death rates account for only a small portion of the effects of trauma. In 2004, 1.9 million hospitalizations were trauma related and trauma accounted for 6% of all hospital discharges.[3] Trauma also directly affects the health care system. For example, 42.2 million people visit emergency departments every year for treatment of unintentional injuries.[2] Annually, $33.7 billion is spent on inpatient trauma care, $31.8 billion dollars is spent on emergency department costs, and another $13.6 billion is spent on outpatient visits.[3]

Stabilization of the trauma patient is best implemented with a standardized approach that ideally involves a team of uniquely trained individuals. Emergency department staff need to be prepared to care for patients who are traumatically injured.

THE TRAUMA SYSTEM

Death from trauma has a trimodal pattern of distribution.
- The first morbidity peak occurs within seconds or minutes of injury. These deaths result from lacerations of the heart, large vessels, brain, or spinal cord. Because of the severity of such injuries, few patients are salvageable.
- The second morbidity peak takes place minutes or hours after the traumatic event. Deaths in this period generally result from intracranial hematomas or uncontrolled hemorrhage from pelvic fractures, solid organ lacerations, or multiple wounds. Care received during the first

hour after injury (the so-called "golden hour") is crucial to trauma patient survival.
- The third morbidity peak occurs days to weeks following trauma. Death during this period results from sepsis, multiorgan failure, or respiratory or other complications.

To maximize patient care, trauma systems have been developed to minimize the impact that this trimodal distribution of death has on traumatically injured patients. A trauma system is "an organized, coordinated effort in a defined geographic area that delivers the full range of care to all injured patients and is integrated with the local public health system."[4] Trauma systems begin with inclusive 9-1-1 emergency systems that activate trained prehospital providers. If patients are to survive the first morbidity peak, help must arrive in a timely fashion.

Minimizing death in the second trimodal peak requires a responsive prehospital system that can transport patients rapidly, providing stabilizing care in transit and delivering patients to the most appropriate facility that is capable of providing the needed care, preferably within that "golden hour." The American College of Surgeons as well as many state trauma systems have developed a trauma designation classification that assists prehospital personnel in determining which facility would be most prepared to receive a traumatically injured patient. Table 35-1 gives an overview of what resources exist at a facility based on the trauma designation it is given.

Regardless of the type of emergency department to which a trauma patient is taken, initial assessment and care of the trauma patient should be delivered in a standardized fashion by a coordinated team of health care providers trained in the delivery of trauma care. The team leader (or captain) oversees the course of patient resuscitation. Team

TABLE 35-1	TRAUMA VERIFICATION LEVELS
LEVEL	**CRITERIA**
Level I trauma center	• Highest level of care available in the trauma system • Has a full range of specialists and equipment available 24 hours per day • Admits at least 1200 trauma patients yearly with 240 of those admissions having an injury severity score exceeding 15 • Maintains an education, prevention, and outreach program • Is actively involved in trauma research • Acts as a referral source for communities in nearby regions[a]
Level II trauma center	• Works in collaboration with Level I trauma centers • Provides comprehensive trauma care supplementing the clinical expertise of the Level I institutions • 24-hour availability of all essential specialties, personnel, and equipment[b]
Level III trauma center	• Lacks 24-hour availability of specialists but maintains resources for emergency resuscitation, surgery, and intensive care of most trauma patients • Maintains transfer agreements with Level I or II trauma centers to transfer patients that exceed its capabilities[c]
Level IV trauma center	• This level is recognized by some states but is not verified by the American College of Surgeons • Provides initial evaluation, stabilization, and diagnostic capabilities until transfer to a higher level of care can be facilitated • Surgery and critical services may be used, but most patients are transferred to a facility with a higher trauma designation
Pediatric trauma center	The American College of Surgeons designates pediatric facilities as Level I and Level II pediatric trauma centers using similar criteria with an emphasis on being able to provide trauma care to pediatric patients[d,e]

[a]American College of Surgeons. (2010, April 22). *Level I requirements by chapter.* Retrieved from http://www.facs.org/trauma/vrc1.pdf
[b]American College of Surgeons. (2010, April 22). *Level II requirements by chapter.* Retrieved from http://www.facs.org/trauma/vrc2.pdf
[c]American College of Surgeons. (2010, April 22). *Level III requirements by chapter.* Retrieved from http://www.facs.org/trauma/vrc3.pdf
[d]American College of Surgeons. (2010, April 22). *Level I pediatric requirements by chapter.* Retrieved from http://www.facs.org/trauma/vrcped1.pdf
[e]American College of Surgeons. (2010, April 22). *Level II pediatric requirements by chapter.* Retrieved from http://www.facs.org/trauma/vrcped2.pdf

composition varies from facility to facility but usually consists of at least one physician, one nurse, and ancillary care personnel.

APPROACH TO CARE OF THE TRAUMA PATIENT

An easy way to remember the steps in assessing and caring for a trauma patient is to recall the first nine letters of the alphabet: A-B-C-D-E-F-G-H-I. These letters can serve as a reminder of the steps in early resuscitation of the traumatically injured patient.

• A—Airway (with consideration given to cervical spine injuries)
• B—Breathing
• C—Circulation
• D—Disability
• E—Exposure of the patient and environmental control
• F—Full set of vital signs, focused adjuncts, and family presence
• G—Give comfort measures
• H—History and head-to-toe assessment
• I—Inspect the posterior surface

THE PRIMARY ASSESSMENT

The first five letters in the mnemonic (A-B-C-D-E) represent the first part of trauma resuscitation: airway, breathing, circulation, disability, and exposure and environmental control. These first five steps include assessment of potentially life-threatening injuries and appropriate interventions. Potentially lethal conditions such as pneumothorax, hemothorax, pericardial tamponade, flail chest, and hemorrhage can be detected during the primary assessment. As each major problem is identified, appropriate interventions are initiated.

Airway

An adequate airway is required for breathing and circulation; therefore assessment and protection of the airway is always paramount in care of the trauma patient. Patients at particular risk of a compromised airway are those with

TABLE 35-2	**AIRWAY AND CERVICAL SPINE ASSESSMENT AND INTERVENTIONS**	
COMPONENT OF ASSESSMENT	**FINDINGS OF CONCERN**	**POTENTIAL INTERVENTIONS**
Airway	• Absence of breathing • Trauma to the face, mouth, pharynx, neck, or chest • Inability to speak (age appropriate) • Substernal or intercostal retractions • Depressed level of consciousness • Inspiratory or expiratory stridor • Pale, cyanotic, or dusky-gray skin color or ruddy or bright purple coloring	• Allow position that maximizes airway • Perform jaw thrust or chin lift • Remove or suction out loose objects • Insert a nasopharyngeal or oropharyngeal airway (Never insert a nasopharyngeal airway into patients with facial trauma. Consider the nasopharyngeal airway for conscious patients who require assistance to maintain their airway.) • Anticipate intubation or advanced airway techniques
Cervical spine	• Mechanism of injury consistent with possible cervical spinal injury • Inability to move or feel extremities • Pain on movement or palpation of the neck • Abdominal breathing (possible paralysis of the breathing muscles) • Bowel or bladder incontinence or retention • Signs of neurogenic shock • Priapism	• Initiate cervical spinal immobilization

altered levels of consciousness (Glasgow Coma Scale score of 8 or less) and those with maxillofacial and neck injuries. See Chapter 8, Airway Management, for further discussion of airway management techniques.

Most traumatic incidents place a patient at risk for spinal cord injury. In fact, it is estimated that there are 12,000 new cases of spinal cord injury every year associated with trauma.[5] It is also estimated that as many as 25% of spinal cord injuries occur after the initial insult as part of patient transport and initial management.[6] Therefore assessment and protection of the spinal cord should begin with the initial stages of trauma assessment and care, that is, with airway management. See Chapter 37, Spinal Cord and Neck Trauma, for further discussion of spinal cord injuries.

Table 35-2 summarizes assessment findings of concern and potential interventions associated with the airway and cervical spine.

Breathing

Even with an open airway, a patient must be able to exchange gases through the airway for effective breathing. Therefore assessment and interventions for breathing should always follow those for the airway. See Chapter 18, Respiratory Emergencies, for further discussion of respiratory assessments. Table 35-3 summarizes assessment findings of concern and potential interventions associated with breathing.

Circulation

The exchange of gases associated with breathing is useful only if the circulatory system can circulate those gases. Circulatory deficits in trauma are frequently related to the presence of shock, especially hypovolemic or obstructive shock. Chapter 20, Shock, reviews the assessment and treatment of shock. Table 35-4 summarizes assessment findings of concern and potential interventions associated with circulation.

Disability

The "D" in primary assessment is meant to remind caregivers to assess neurologic status. Profound alterations in neurologic function may indicate significant neurologic trauma. The negative long-term effects of neurologic trauma can sometimes be minimized with prompt interventions; therefore assess neurologic status early so that appropriate interventions can be initiated promptly. See Chapter 36, Head Trauma, for further information regarding head trauma and neurologic assessments. Table 35-5 summarizes assessment findings of concern and potential interventions associated with disability.

Exposure and Environmental Control

Clothing can obscure obvious injuries; therefore remove all clothing from the patient as part of the primary assessment. As part of this process, the trauma team should carefully

TABLE 35-3 BREATHING ASSESSMENT AND INTERVENTIONS

FINDINGS OF CONCERN	POTENTIAL INTERVENTIONS
• Blunt or penetrating trauma to the neck, chest, back, or abdomen • History of breathing diseases such as asthma or emphysema • Dyspnea, tachypnea, or apnea • Agonal breathing • Shallow respirations • Weak or gasping respirations • Cyanosis, diaphoresis • Respiratory distress • Decreased or absent breath sounds • Severe retractions • Open or sucking chest wounds • Paradoxical chest wall movement • Inability to converse in phrases or complete sentences • Pulse oximetry readings less than 95% (or below patient's baseline) • Abnormal arterial blood gas results	• Administer supplemental oxygen • Assist with ventilations using bag-mask device • Perform needle decompression or chest tube insertion as indicated • Cover any open chest wounds with a nonocclusive dressing

TABLE 35-4 CIRCULATORY ASSESSMENT AND INTERVENTIONS

FINDINGS OF CONCERN	POTENTIAL INTERVENTIONS
• Heart rate <60 beats per minute or >100 beats per minute in adults accompanied by indications of circulatory compromise • Heart rate >100 beats per minute or <80 beats per minute in small children accompanied by indications of circulatory compromise • Pulse with abnormal strength or quality (weak and thready, full and bounding) • Uncontrolled external bleeding • Pallor or cool, diaphoretic skin • Systolic blood pressure below normal for age (<90 mm Hg in adults) • Verbalization of sense of impending doom • Restlessness or anxiety • Capillary refill >2 seconds	• Begin chest compressions for absence of pulse (or inadequate perfusion in pediatric patients who may still have a pulse) • Control external bleeding through direct pressure, pressure dressings, and application of a tourniquet higher than systolic blood pressure if other measures fail • Begin fluid resuscitation

TABLE 35-5 NEUROLOGIC ASSESSMENT AND INTERVENTIONS

FINDINGS OF CONCERN	POTENTIAL INTERVENTIONS
• Unequal pupils or pupils that are sluggish to react or fail to react • Decreased Glasgow Coma Scale scores, altered level of consciousness • Weakness on one side or in one extremity or loss of function of one side or one extremity • Abnormal posturing	• Maintain head midline with the head or the bed flat or elevated 30 to 45 degrees • Consider mannitol (Osmitrol) for changes in level of consciousness associated with increased intracranial pressure • Decrease external stimuli

assess the exposed body for abnormalities that may require immediate intervention, such as open wounds or fractures, uncontrolled bleeding, or eviscerations.

Environmental control is meant to remind the trauma team of the importance of keeping a patient warm. Numerous factors increase the risk of a patient becoming hypothermic during trauma resuscitation, including:

- Ambient temperature of the resuscitation room (which is lower than body temperature)
- Infusion of large amounts of fluids or blood products that are below body temperature
- Elevated blood alcohol levels (resulting in vasodilation)
- Impaired thermogenesis secondary to shock and brain injuries

- Age (pediatric and older patients have decreased abilities to regulate body temperature)
- Moisture on the body from environmental conditions and bleeding
- Use of anesthetics and paralytics for intubation (which decreases internal heat production)
- Injuries to the pelvis, extremities, abdomen, and large blood vessels (which carry a greater risk of heat loss)[7]

If the core body temperature of a trauma patient drops below 95°F (35°C) during resuscitation, the patient has an increased risk of the following:

- Developing acidosis
- Tissue and cerebral hypoxia
- Increased diuresis with exacerbation of hypovolemia
- Infection due to suppression of the immune system
- Coagulopathies, including disseminated intravascular coagulation[8]

THE SECONDARY ASSESSMENT

Once the primary assessment is complete and issues involving the patient's airway, breathing, circulation, disability status, and exposure and environmental control have been addressed, proceed to the secondary assessment. This is not a final examination; it is a rapid, thorough inspection of the patient's entire body from head to toe. Unlike the primary assessment, issues noted on secondary assessment are not treated immediately. They are noted and then prioritized for later intervention. If the patient develops an airway, breathing, or circulatory problem at any time, return at once to the primary assessment and intervene as indicated. The last four letters of the mnemonic (F-G-H-I) make up the secondary assessment.

Full Set of Vital Signs

If a complete set of vital signs has not yet been obtained, it is appropriate to do so at this point. These vital signs will serve as a baseline for continued reassessment. Patients with suspected chest trauma should have apical and radial pulse rates documented and blood pressure assessed in both arms.

> Patients with chest trauma who are at risk for aortic trauma should have blood pressure and pulse measured in both arms and one leg. A difference of 10 mm Hg or more in blood pressure or a difference in pulse quality between sites should raise the index of suspicion for aortic trauma.

Focused Adjuncts

Interventions that should be considered at this point depend on the findings of the primary and secondary assessments and may include the following:

- Continuous cardiac and oxygen saturation monitoring
- Placement of a gastric tube
- Insertion of an indwelling urinary catheter (unless there is evidence of lower genitourinary trauma)
- Collection of appropriate laboratory studies
- Focused assessment with sonography for trauma (FAST)

> **Common Laboratory Tests Used During Assessment**
> - Type and crossmatch or type and screen
> - Complete blood count
> - Basic chemistry panel (electrolytes, glucose, and renal function tests)
> - Urinalysis
> - Pregnancy test
> - Ethanol level
> - Toxicology screen
> - Clotting studies
> - Serum lactate and base deficit

Family Presence

The presence of the family during the resuscitation of trauma patients has been shown to improve family members' ability to cope with the situation. There is strong evidence that it may also assist the patient who is aware of their presence during this stressful time. Based on this evidence, the Emergency Nurses Association has adopted a formal position statement encouraging family presence at the bedside of critically ill or injured patients.[9]

Give Comfort Measures

The trauma victim is often in physical and psychological distress. Pharmacologic and nonpharmacologic methods of reducing pain and anxiety are available for this population. The trauma team is obliged to recognize pain and intervene as necessary. See Chapter 11, Care of the Patient with Pain, for further information on pain management.

History

If the patient is awake, alert, and cooperative, try to elicit pertinent medication, allergy, and medical history information. Family members are also a resource for these data. If a patient is transported via prehospital personnel, they will also serve as an excellent resource, providing information regarding the mechanism of injury, injuries suspected, and treatment prior to arrival, including vital signs in the field.

Although each traumatic situation is unique, the trauma team may anticipate many injuries based on the mechanism of injury that is described by the patient, bystanders, or prehospital personnel. Injuries can be blunt, where the injuring force does not penetrate the skin, or penetrating, where an object penetrates the skin. Table 35-6 summarizes some injuries that can be anticipated based on common mechanisms of blunt trauma.

Obtaining any available details regarding the mechanism of a penetrating injury can be helpful in determining the extent of traumatic injury. Numerous considerations should also be taken into account when caring for patients with penetrating trauma:

- Penetrating trauma may appear less serious than it is, with minimal surface trauma but significant underlying trauma. A knife, for example, may create a very small wound on the skin surface, but if the assailant moved the knife up and down while it was in the body or if the victim moved while the knife was in the body, the underlying damage may be much greater than the surface trauma.
- When dealing with injuries as a result of firearms, consider the following facts:
  - Hollow point projectiles cause more extensive damage than solid projectiles.

TABLE 35-6 ANTICIPATED INJURIES ASSOCIATED WITH BLUNT TRAUMA

MECHANISM OF TRAUMA	ASSOCIATED INJURIES
Front impact motor vehicle crash	• The body tends to be thrown forward in the car, causing it to strike surfaces in front of it and leading to traumatic brain injury, facial trauma, spinal trauma, sternal injuries, pulmonary and cardiac injuries, hip and femur fractures, and ankle fractures.[a]
Side impact motor vehicle crash	• The frame of the car collapses in on the side of the patient and the patient is thrown toward the impact, resulting in rotational cervical spinal injuries, flail chest segments, pulmonary injuries, abdominal injuries (the spleen is affected more often in the driver and the liver is affected in the passenger secondary to the position of these organs against side of impact), and pelvic injuries.[a]
Rear-end impact motor vehicle crash	• The patient is often forced toward the top of the car and the seat reclines slightly and then springs forward, thrusting the patient to the front of the vehicle. This can cause intracranial injury (from the head being driven into the ceiling on initial impact) and flexion-extension injuries of the cervical spine. • Other patterns of injury are similar to those with front impact crash because the patient is thrown to the front of the vehicle.[a]
Rollover motor vehicle crash	• Axial loading with burst fractures of the spine or Jefferson fractures, and extremity trauma as extremities protrude out of broken windows. Nearly any injury is possible with this type of crash because of the multiple and varied points of impact.[a]
Motorbike crash	• Head injuries, especially when the rider is not wearing a helmet or the helmet is damaged. • Separation of the rider from the bike increases the risk of injury. • Riders who are crushed between their bike and another vehicle or other object can have significant trauma to the extremities. • Riders who are dragged or slide across surfaces sustain severe integumentary trauma.
Bicycle (nonmotorized) crash	• Injury considerations for bicycles are similar to those for motorbikes. • Heavier road bikes tend to propel the patient into the handlebars, increasing the risk of pancreatic, liver, splenic, and diaphragmatic injury. • Patients are more likely to be propelled over the handlebars with lighter speed bikes, sustaining head, face, shoulder, and upper arm trauma.
Fall	• A fall from three times a victim's height or greater should raise the concern for significant injury. • Patients who land on their feet tend to get calcaneus, lumbar spine, and wrist trauma as energy goes from the feet up the back and they fall forward on outstretched hands. • Patients who land on their sides usually put their hands out to protect themselves, resulting in arm trauma. As the arm buckles into the body, rib fractures, pulmonary trauma, and spleen or liver trauma can result. • The energy from landing on the buttocks results in energy being transmitted to the pelvis, abdominal organs, and chest organs with severe life-threatening injuries.

[a]Hazarika, S., Willcox, N., & Porter, K. (2007). Patterns of injury sustained by car occupants with relation to the direction of impact with motor vehicle trauma—evidence based review. *Trauma, 9*(3), 145–150.

- Firearms with longer barrels fire projectiles at greater speeds than firearms with shorter barrels and tend to produce more tissue damage.
- The closer the trauma patient was to the firearm, the more significant the trauma tends to be.

Patients involved in explosions can have a variety of different injuries:

- Primary injuries: When a solid or liquid changes to a gas, as happens in an explosion, it expands. The expansion causes a displacement of air that travels away from the blast site. When the blast of air strikes the body it can compress gas-filled organs, leading to injuries such as ruptured tympanic membranes, pneumothoraces, air emboli, and gastric or intestinal ruptures.
- Secondary injuries: As displaced air travels from the blast site, it carries small pieces of debris for long distances that can strike and imbed in bodies that may be a significant distance from the blast site. The resulting lacerations and impaled objects are referred to as secondary injuries.
- Tertiary injuries: Displaced air can hurl bodies away from the blast site and throw them into other objects, resulting in a variety of blunt traumatic injuries.

Head-to-Toe Examination

Items to be considered during a head-to-toe examination are addressed only briefly in this section. Refer to Chapters 36 through 41 for specific trauma information.

Head

- The head is inspected systematically and assessed for any obvious wounds, deformities, or asymmetry.
- Palpate the skull for depressed bony fragments, hematomas, lacerations, or tenderness.
- Note any areas of ecchymosis or discoloration. Ecchymosis behind the ears, over the mastoid process (Battle sign), or in the periorbital region (raccoon eyes) increases the suspicion for a basilar skull fracture.

Therapeutic Interventions

- Do not allow the patient to become hypotensive or hypoxic.
- Mannitol may be administered intravenously to decrease intracranial pressure.
- Facilitate surgical intervention or intracranial pressure monitoring.

Face

- Inspect the face for wounds and asymmetry.
- Note any drainage from the ears, nose, eyes, or mouth. Clear drainage from the nose or ears is assumed to be cerebrospinal fluid until proven otherwise.

- Reassess the pupils for symmetry, light response, and accommodation.
- Check gross visual acuity.
- Ask the patient to open and close the mouth to check for malocclusion, lacerations, loose or missing teeth, and foreign bodies.

Diagnostic Procedures

- Noncontrast computed tomography (CT) scans
- Panoramic radiographic views of the jaw

Neck

- While another team member provides cervical spine immobilization, partially remove the rigid cervical collar to assess the patient's neck.
- Palpate and inspect for obvious wounds, ecchymosis, neck vein distention, subcutaneous air, or endotracheal deviation.
- Auscultate the carotid arteries for bruits.
- Palpate for deformities, defects, or cervical vertebral tenderness before reapplying the collar.

The cervical spine cannot be cleared adequately in the presence of alcohol or drug intoxication or major distracting injuries. Conversely, the cervical spine of a low-risk, alert, oriented, nonintoxicated patient can be cleared based on clinical examination alone in the absence of pain, tenderness, or neurologic findings.[10]

Diagnostic Procedures. Four radiographic views are needed to visualize the cervical spine fully:

- Cross-table lateral (must visualize C1 to T1)
- Anterior-posterior
- Lateral
- Open-mouth odontoid

Obtain CT studies if plain radiographs are inconclusive. Flexion-extension views are used to check for soft tissue damage and are performed much less frequently.

Chest

- Visually inspect the chest for asymmetry, deformity, penetrating trauma, and other wounds.
- Auscultate the heart and lungs.
- Palpate the chest wall for deformities, subcutaneous air, and areas of tenderness.

Diagnostic Procedures

- Obtain a portable chest radiograph if the patient cannot sit upright for anterior-posterior and lateral views.
- Obtain a 12-lead electrocardiogram in patients with suspected or actual blunt chest trauma.
- Consider drawing arterial blood gases if the patient has any symptoms of airway obstruction or respiratory distress or has been placed on a mechanical ventilator.

Abdomen

- Inspect the abdomen for bruising, masses, pulsations, and penetrating objects.
- Observe for distension or evisceration of bowel contents.
- Auscultate for bowel sounds in all four quadrants.
- Gently palpate the abdomen checking for rigidity and areas of tenderness, rebound pain, or guarding.

Diagnostic Procedures

- FAST
- Diagnostic peritoneal lavage (used infrequently)
- CT scan of the abdomen (usually performed with a contrast medium)
- Abdominal or kidneys-ureter-bladder (KUB) radiographic series

Pelvis

- Visually inspect the pelvis for bleeding, bruising, deformity, and penetrating trauma.
- Inspect the perineum for blood, feces, and any obvious injury.
- A rectal examination is performed to assess sphincter tone, identify blood, and check the position of the prostate. A high-riding prostate, blood at the urinary meatus, or the presence of a scrotal hematoma are contraindications to bladder catheterization until a retrograde urethrogram can be performed.
- Gently press inward (toward the midline) on the iliac crests to assess pelvic stability. Also palpate over the symphysis pubis. *Stop* if pain or motion are elicited and obtain radiographic studies.

Extremities

- Inspect all four limbs for deformity, dislocation, ecchymosis, swelling, and other wounds.
- Check the sensory, motor, and neurovascular status of each extremity.
- Palpate for areas of tenderness, crepitus, and temperature abnormalities.
- If injuries are present, reassess distal neurovascular status regularly.

Diagnostic Procedures

- Radiographs of the affected extremities

Therapeutic Interventions

- Splinting
- Wound care

Inspect the Posterior Surface

It is essential to remember that 50% of the body's surface lies against the stretcher. Failing to roll the patient and inspect the back can result in numerous injuries being missed. Cervical spinal alignment must be maintained by using approved logrolling techniques.

- With the back exposed, look for bruising, discoloration, and any open wounds.
- Palpate the vertebral bony prominences for deformity, movement, and pain.
- Remove any clothing or wet items left under the patient.
- If the spine is cleared or the patient can lie still, remove the backboard (according to institutional protocol).

Therapeutic Interventions

- Consider padding or removing the backboard.
- Assess for signs of skin breakdown.

REEVALUATION AND ASSESSMENT

As long as the trauma patient is in the emergency department, assessment is never complete. Re-evaluate patients regularly to identify deterioration and injuries that were overlooked. Additionally, trauma patients may have underlying medical conditions that were not addressed during the initial resuscitation. Consider the following:

- Reassess pain and provide additional pain medication (as indicated) but watch for respiratory depression. Narcotic analgesics also may mask subtle signs of neurologic deterioration.
- Monitor urinary output and intervene as necessary.
- As in all aspects of health care, thorough documentation is essential. Because of the multiple assessments, interventions, and reassessments, recording trauma patient care in a timely fashion is crucial.
- The patient who has sustained a trauma requires consistent and uniform care from all members of the team. If life-threatening injuries are found, the team needs to intervene and correct them. Care of the trauma patient is enhanced by the use of a team approach and a consistent assessment technique such as the A-I mnemonic.

REFERENCES

1. Centers for Disease Control and Prevention. (2010, October 5). *Accidents or unintentional injuries.* Retrieved from http://www.cdc.gov/nchs/fastats/acc-inj.htm
2. Centers for Disease Control and Prevention. (2010, October 27). *All injuries.* Retrieved from http://www.cdc.gov/nchs/fastats/injury.htm
3. Bergen, G., Chen, L. H., & Fingerhut, L. A. (2008). *Injury in the United States: 2007 chartbook.* Hyattsville, MD: National Center for Health Statistics.
4. National Highway Transportation Safety Administration. (n.d.). *Trauma system: Agenda for the future.* Retrieved from

http://www.nhtsa.gov/People/injury/ems/emstraumasystem03/index.htm

5. The National Spinal Cord Injury Statistical Center. (2009, June). *Spinal cord injury statistics*. Retrieved from http://www.fscip.org/facts.htm

6. Consortium for Spinal Cord Medicine. (2008). Early acute management in adults with spinal cord injury: A clinical practice guideline for health-care professionals. *Journal of Spinal Cord Medicine, 31*(4), 403–479.

7. Hildebrand, F., Giannoudis, P. V., van Griensven, M., Chawda, M., & Pape, H. C. (2004). Pathophysiologic changes and effects of hypothermia on outcome in elective surgery and trauma patients. *American Journal of Surgery, 187*(3), 363–371.

8. Solheim, J. (n.d.). *Cold comfort: Treating hypothermia in the trauma patient*. Retrieved from http://ce.nurse.com/RetailCourseView.aspx?CourseNum=ce433&page=1&IsA=1

9. Emergency Nurses Association. (2010, September). *Family presence during invasive procedures and cardiopulmonary resuscitation* (position statement). Retrieved from http://www.ena.org/SiteCollectionDocuments/Position%20Statements/FamilyPresence.pdf

10. Stanford University School of Medicine. (n.d.). *C-Spine clearance algorithm*. Retrieved from http://scalpel.stanford.edu/2007-2008/c-%20Spine%20Protocol%20-%20McCall%20v2.pdf

Head Trauma

Jill C. McLaughlin

Head trauma and brain injury are not always synonymous. Differentiating between the two is important when considering assessment and care of patients with traumatic injuries. Head injuries usually present with more visible symptoms such as lacerations or deformities, while traumatic brain injuries (TBIs) may be present in a patient who appears neurologically intact. TBIs can range from mild to severe. Early diagnosis and intervention are paramount in minimizing adverse outcomes.[1]

Brain injury is a contributing factor in one third of all injury deaths. The Centers for Disease Control and Prevention (CDC) estimates that 1.7 million people sustain a TBI annually.[2] Of these, 52,000 die, 275,000 are hospitalized, and 1.365 million (nearly 80%) are seen in emergency departments.[2] TBI is most common in three age groups—birth to 4 years, 15 to 19 years, and over 65 years—with falls being the leading cause.[2] Motor vehicle crashes are the second leading cause but are responsible for the most deaths.[2]

Eighty percent of TBIs are classified as mild, but the effects can be long lasting and life changing. It has been estimated that 20% of military personnel involved in combat during the wars in Afghanistan and Iraq have sustained a TBI.[1] Depression, post-traumatic stress disorder, chronic traumatic encephalopathy, and personality changes have been linked to mild TBI.[3–5]

Common Causes of Traumatic Brain Injury[2]
- Falls (32.5%)
- Motor vehicle crashes (17.3%)
- Struck by or against events (16.5%)
- Assaults and interpersonal violence (10%)

PHYSICAL ASSESSMENT OF THE HEAD-INJURED PATIENT

Obtain an initial neurologic evaluation as soon as possible following head injury. Reevaluation should be performed frequently. Serial exams allow for the rapid detection of patient deterioration necessitating surgical intervention. The neurologic evaluation consists of the Glasgow Coma Scale (GCS) and assessment of cranial nerves, pupillary responses, and reflexes.

Glasgow Coma Scale

The GCS allows health care providers to perform a brief examination of level of consciousness in a precise, consistent manner. The GCS quantifies the eye opening, verbal responses, and motor responses of a patient with TBI to a set of standardized stimuli. Scoring is based on the patient's best response to stimuli. If necessary, noxious stimuli are used to elicit a response. For more information on using the GCS, refer to Chapter 25, Neurologic Emergencies.

Cranial Nerve Assessment

There are 12 cranial nerves. Table 36-1 summarizes the functions and assessment of the cranial nerves.

Pupillary Assessment

In addition to assigning a GCS score and assessing the patient's cranial nerves, the nurse should also assess the pupillary response using a bright, focused light. Tips for pupillary assessment include the following:
- Pupils normally constrict when exposed directly to light.
- Light shined into one pupil causes the other pupil to constrict as well (consensual response).

TABLE 36-1 FUNCTION AND ASSESSMENT OF CRANIAL NERVES

NUMBER	NAME	FUNCTION	PHYSICAL EXAMINATION	COMMENTS
I	Olfactory	Smell	With the patient's eyes closed, bring chewing gum to the patient's nose and ask him or her to identify the smell of the gum	Damage to the olfactory nerve (common in head injury) results in loss of sense of smell (anosmia) and an ability to discern only sweet and bitter tastes
II	Optic	Vision	Ask the patient to read the small print on the chewing gum wrapper	If the optic nerve is intact, the patient will be able to count fingers, perceive light, or blink when the eyes are threatened; the patient will also be able to read print
III	Oculomotor	Regulates pupil size and accommodation Extraocular eye movement	Assess direct and consensual papillary response to light Have patient follow movement of gum wrapper through the six positions of gaze without turning his or her head	The third cranial nerve passes through the tentorium; herniation through the tentorium puts pressure on this nerve, causing the pupil to dilate and become fixed on the side ipsilateral to the herniation. Even a 1 mm difference in pupil size may indicate significant pressure.
IV	Trochlear	Extraocular eye movement	Check the patient's pupil size, shape, reactivity, and extraocular movements	Cranial nerves III, IV, and VI are assessed together
V	Trigeminal	Swallowing	Have patient simulate chewing gum; check for strength of mastication muscles, jaw mobility, and facial sensation	Trigeminal nerve controls facial sensation and mandible movement
VI	Abducens	Extraocular eye movement	See cranial nerves III and IV	See cranial nerves III and IV
VII	Facial	Facial motor and taste	Have patient raise eyebrows, close eyelids tightly to resistance, show teeth, smile, frown, and puff out cheeks Place chewing gum on both sides of tongue to assess taste	The facial nerve controls facial expression as well as taste on the anterior two thirds of the tongue
VIII	Acoustic	Hearing and balance	With patient's eyes closed, open the package of chewing gum beside each ear to assess hearing Assess patient's response to voice or a loud clap	The eighth cranial nerve has two branches: the vestibular branch controls balance and the auditory branch is responsible for hearing. In the unconscious patient, this nerve can be assessed using the cold caloric (ice water) test
IX	Glossopharyngeal	Gag and swallowing	Assess swallowing of saliva and gag reflex Assess ability to discriminate between salty and sweet tastes	Cranial nerves IX and X are evaluated together because they are closely related anatomically and functionally Glossopharyngeal nerve controls taste on the posterior two thirds of the tongue and sensation in the pharynx and nostrils
X	Vagus	Gag and swallowing	Assess with cranial nerve IX	The vagus nerve controls the soft palate, pharynx, larynx, heart, lungs, and stomach
XI	Spinal accessory	Shoulder shrug	Have the patient turn head against resistance or shrug the shoulders	Do not assess this cranial nerve until cervical spine injury has been ruled out
XII	Hypoglossal	Tongue movement	Have patient stick out tongue to assess for deviation	If the tongue is midline, the nerve is considered intact

From Strickler, J., & Bonifacio, A. (2010). Assessing cranial nerves with a stick of gum. *Journal of Emergency Nursing*, *36*(5), 470–471.

- Allow at least 10 seconds between assessment of each eye for consensual response to diminish.

> Up to 20% of the population normally has slightly unequal pupils (anisocoria), highlighting the need for careful and ongoing assessment of pupillary response.[6]

- Fixed, pinpoint pupils indicate pons involvement or the use of opiates.
- A dilated, fixed pupil (unilateral) indicates (early) third cranial nerve involvement and possible transtentorial herniation.
- Bilateral, fixed pupils indicate severe brainstem injury and possible brain death. (Pupils also may be fixed and dilated in certain reversible conditions and toxic exposures.)
- Ptosis (a drooping eyelid) indicates third cranial nerve impairment.

Reflex Assessment

Assessment of the various reflexes is summarized in Table 36-2.

If present, abnormal posturing can be elicited using verbal, tactile, or noxious stimulation.
- Abnormal flexion (Fig. 36-1): Arms flex, wrists flex, and legs and feet extend. Abnormal flexion indicates a lesion above the midbrain.

- Abnormal extension (Fig. 36-2): Arms extend, wrists flex, and legs and feet extend. Abnormal extension indicates brainstem herniation.

DIAGNOSTIC PROCEDURES

Radiography

Plain radiographs of a patient's cervical spine including a cross-table lateral view can be obtained easily and rapidly but lack the diagnostic accuracy of computed radiographic studies. Skull radiographs can be useful for assessing penetrating head trauma (stab or gunshot wounds) but are rarely used in most situations as they do not offer significant useful information in terms of treatment interventions. Patients with significant head trauma may also have a concurrent spinal cord injury.

Health care providers must ensure that the cervical spine is immobilized and protected until radiographic studies or computed tomography (CT) scans and clinical examination have ruled out injury.

Computed Axial Tomography

Noncontrast CT scans are the standard diagnostic tool in the evaluation of TBI. CT allows for the visualization of injury to bone and tissue and intracranial hemorrhage.

TABLE 36-2 REFLEX ASSESSMENT

REFLEX	ASSESSMENT	NORMAL REACTION	ABNORMAL REACTION
Corneal (cranial nerves V and VII)	Touch cornea with wisp of cotton or a drop of normal saline solution	Eye blink	No response
Gag (cranial nerves IX and X)	Stimulate the back of throat with a swab, tongue depressor, or suction catheter	Intact gag	Loss of gag reflex
Deep tendon	Test deep tendon reflexes with a rubber reflex hammer Response is scored from 0 to 4: 0–absent 1–decreased 2–normal 3–increased 4–hyperactive	Score of 2	Hypoactivity or absence of reaction indicates cerebellar lesions, peripheral nerve or anterior horn disease Hyperactivity indicates pyramidal tract lesions or psychogenic disorders
Babinski	Apply brisk cutaneous stimulation to plantar surface of the foot	Negative reaction—great toe and other toes flex, curl downward	Positive reaction—great toe extends upward and other toes fan out toward the head This reaction is normal in children under 2 years of age No response at all is considered abnormal

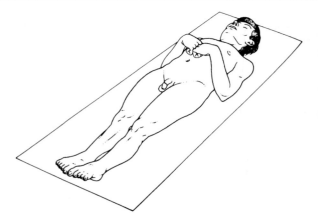

Fig. 36-1 Abnormal flexion.

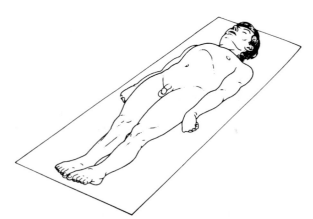

Fig. 36-2 Abnormal extension.

Magnetic Resonance Imaging

Magnetic resonance imaging (MRI) is a noninvasive method of obtaining excellent visual images of soft tissue. MRI may be used in the diagnosis of brain injury not clearly seen on CT. However, this method may not be feasible in the acute care setting for patients who are unstable, uncooperative, or otherwise unable to remain still. Any equipment (external or implanted) that contains ferrous material—such as pacemakers, ventilators, brain aneurysm clips, and retained bullet fragments—prohibits the use of MRI.

Angiography

Cerebral angiographic studies are the gold standard for diagnosing cerebrovascular abnormalities, but their use is limited in the acute care setting. However, if a patient presents with neurologic symptoms and a negative CT or

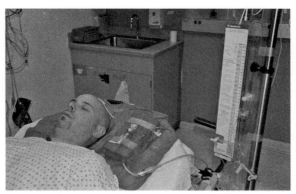

Fig. 36-3 A patient undergoing ICP monitoring in the emergency department. (From Fryman, L., Murray L. [2007]. Managing acute head trauma in a crowded emergency department. *Journal of Emergency Nursing.* 33(3), 208–213).

MRI, angiography should be considered for definitive diagnosis.[7]

Intracranial Pressure Monitoring

Intracranial pressure (ICP) monitoring is indicated for comatose patients with severe head injury (GCS score <8) postresuscitation and for those with abnormal CT scan findings or with a normal CT but two or more of the following:[8]

- Systolic blood pressure less than 90 mm Hg
- Age greater than 40 years
- Unilateral or bilateral posturing

ICP monitoring is useful as a guide to osmotic diuretic administration, patient positioning, sedation, analgesia, cerebrospinal fluid (CSF) drainage, and surgical intervention. In addition, ICP monitoring improves prognostic accuracy and may improve patient outcome. Normal ICP is 0 to 20 mm Hg.

Intracranial Pressure Monitoring Systems

- Intraventricular—catheter is placed in the ventricle, allows for CSF drainage, and is the reference standard for ICP monitoring[9]
- Intraparenchymal—fiber optic or electronic transducer inserted into the parenchyma
- Subarachnoid bolt—placed in the subarachnoid and uses a fiber optic transducer
- Epidural—uses an optical transducer that rests against the dura

Newer ICP monitoring probes measure cerebral tissue oxygen tension and temperature to better identify and prevent cerebral hypoxia. Figure 36-3 shows ICP monitoring in the emergency department.[10]

Cerebral Perfusion Pressure

Although ICP monitoring is important in patients with head trauma, an even more crucial number to track is cerebral perfusion pressure (CPP). CPP is defined as the mean arterial pressure (MAP) minus ICP. This number indicates the actual pressure of blood perfusing the brain. In head-injured adults, CPP should be maintained at greater than 60 mm Hg at all times.[8]

MANAGEMENT OF PATIENTS WITH SEVERE TRAUMATIC BRAIN INJURIES

Severe head injury is defined as a GCS score of 8 or less after resuscitation. In 2007 the Brain Trauma Foundation, the Joint Section on Neurotrauma and Critical Care of the American Association of Neurological Surgeons, and the Congress of Neurological Surgeons updated standardized, evidence-based practice guidelines that are applicable to the management of all patients with severe TBI. In 2003 pediatric guidelines were released. These interventions have been shown to minimize the extent and impact of secondary brain injury.[11]

Airway

- Orally intubate patients with a GCS score of 8 or less.
- Insert an oral gastric tube to decompress the stomach. Avoid nasogastric tubes.

Breathing

- Maintain PaO_2 greater than 100 mm Hg and oxygen saturation greater than 95%.
- Maintain eucapnia ($PaCO_2$ of 35 to 38 mm Hg), as carbon dioxide is a potent vasodilator and will lower CPP.
- Avoid hyperventilation unless signs of herniation are present.
- Initiate exhaled carbon dioxide monitoring.
- Consider neuromuscular blockade for patients who are difficult to ventilate.

Circulation

- Establish normovolemia. Keep MAP at 70 to 90 mm Hg. Hypotension must be avoided, as it is associated with increased mortality in patients with severe brain injury.[12]
- Maintain CPP greater than 70 mm Hg (an ICP catheter is required to monitor CPP).
- Restore volume as needed with isotonic fluids and blood products.
- Insert an indwelling urinary catheter. Maintain an hourly urine output of 0.5 to 1 mL/kg.
- Keep serum osmolality less than 320 mOsm.

Disability

- Perform and document serial neurologic examinations. The process of secondary injury can develop over a period of hours. Through serial exams, subtle changes in mental status can be observed. Interventions can be instituted to prevent further deterioration.
- Unilateral dilation of pupil is one of the first signs of impending herniation.

Facilitate Diagnosis and Neurosurgical Consultation

- Rapidly obtain a CT scan.
- Monitor ICP in all patients with a GCS score of 8 or lower and an abnormal CT scan. Abnormal CT scan refers to the presence of hematomas, contusions, swelling, herniation, or compressed basal cisterns.[8]
- Facilitate surgical intervention.
- Admit patient to a neurologic critical care unit or transfer to an appropriate facility.

Reduce Intracranial Pressure

- Provide sedation and analgesia.
- Infuse mannitol (an osmotic diuretic), 0.25 to 1 g/kg, in intermittent boluses to patients with signs of impending herniation or decreasing GCS scores not associated with extracranial causes.[8]
- Maintain the head in a neutral, midline (chin and umbilicus aligned) position.
- Keep the patient's head elevated 30 degrees, unless contraindicated by a spinal injury. (Most patients will benefit from this position, but some do better when the head rests flat.)
- Remove the cervical collar immediately after the patient has been cleared by a physician. Rigid collars have been shown to increase ICP.[13,14]
- Minimize external stimulation by keeping lights and noise to a minimum and limiting visitors.[9]
- Consider administration of pain medication and sedation before suctioning.
- Consider neuromuscular blockade for increased ICP unresponsive to treatment. Patients need particularly close monitoring once this therapy has been initiated

Other interventions that may be performed include the following:

- Hyperventilation as a temporary measure to quickly reduce ICP. Prolonged hyperventilation has been associated with less optimal outcomes.[14,15]
- Consider ventriculostomy placement for CSF drainage.
- Consider surgical decompression (i.e., hematoma evacuation, lobectomy, craniectomy) for increased ICP unresponsive to medical management.

- Hypertonic saline may be used in the treatment of increased ICP.[5]

General Care

- Assess for and manage other injuries.
- Perform toxicologic or alcohol screening as indicated. Do not assume that neurologic deficits are alcohol or drug related.[15]
- Regulate temperature to maintain normothermia. Cooling blankets are necessary, as antipyretics are ineffective because of damage to the neurologic regulation system.[9]
- Treat seizures. Consider seizure prophylaxis for the first week after injury.
- Do *not* use intravenous dextrose infusions.
- Do *not* give dextrose 50%, except in the presence of documented hypoglycemia.
- Do *not* give steroids.
- Consider organ donation in patients with a GCS score of 4 or less who remain unresponsive to treatment.

SPECIFIC HEAD INJURIES

Scalp Wounds

Scalp wounds, caused by blunt or penetrating trauma, are the most frequently seen head injuries. Because of its generous vascular supply, the scalp will bleed profusely when skin integrity is breached.

Signs and Symptoms

- Direct observation of the wound
- Bleeding (may be profuse)

Therapeutic Interventions

- Apply direct or peripheral pressure to stop bleeding. Clips or clamps may be used to control major blood loss.
- Palpate the underlying skull for fractures. Do not apply direct pressure over a depressed fracture.
- Immobilize and evaluate the cervical spine.
- Manage hypovolemia. Small children, in particular, are prone to significant volume loss from large scalp wounds.
- Cleanse the wound and debride devitalized tissue.
- Sutures, staples, hair ties, or wound glue may be used to close the scalp.
- Keep wound margins moist with an antibiotic ointment to promote healing.
- Apply a sterile dressing or leave the wound open to air.
- Systemic antibiotics are indicated for contaminated wounds such as bites.
- Ensure appropriate tetanus prophylaxis.
- Provide aftercare instructions for wound management and head trauma.

Skull Fractures

Examine the patient's head for bumps, depressions, bruises, lacerations, and other defects. The presence of a skull fracture does not necessarily indicate that intracranial injury has occurred.

Skull fractures commonly are classified by type (simple or linear and depressed) and location (cranial vault or basilar).

Simple (Linear, Nondisplaced) Skull Fractures

A simple skull fracture is a linear crack in the surface of the skull; the bone is not displaced and the fracture itself does not require any special care. Therapeutic intervention involves observation of the patient for potential intracranial injuries. If there are no other obvious findings and if a good support system (family or friends) is available, the patient may be discharged to his or her home with careful head trauma aftercare instructions.

Depressed Skull Fractures

A depressed skull fracture involves depression of a segment of the cranium. If the fragment is depressed below the table of the adjacent bone by more than 5 mm, surgical elevation must be performed to identify underlying brain contusions and reduce the incidence of intracranial infection. If the depression overlies one of the sinuses (sagittal or lateral), there may be profuse bleeding. Because of their softer skulls, young children are more prone to depressed skull fractures than are adults.

Signs and Symptoms

- Observation and palpation of the deformity
- Bleeding (either external blood loss or hematoma formation)
- Altered level of consciousness

Diagnostic Procedures

- Observation and palpation of the deformity
- CT scan

Therapeutic Interventions

- Provide airway management with cervical spine protection as needed.
- Control external bleeding.
- Place sterile dressings over open wounds.
- Repair lacerations.
- Consider administration of systemic antibiotics.
- Ensure tetanus prophylaxis if an open wound is present.
- Facilitate surgical intervention to do the following:
  - Elevate the depressed segment
  - Remove embedded fragments
  - Debride necrotic brain tissue
  - Evacuate hematomas

Basilar Skull Fractures

Basilar skull fracture describes a fracture location, not a type of fracture. Most basilar skull fractures are linear. Fractures may occur in any of the three fossae of the skull base: anterior, middle, or posterior.

Signs and Symptoms

- General
  - Headache
  - Nausea and vomiting
  - Altered level of consciousness
- Anterior fossa fracture
  - Periorbital ecchymosis or "raccoon eyes" (Fig. 36-4): Bilateral periorbital ecchymosis occurs as a result of blood seeping through the fracture and pooling in the soft tissues around the eyes. This finding may appear several hours after injury.
  - Rhinorrhea: Leaking of CSF into the nasal passages.
- Middle fossa fracture
  - Battle's sign: Ecchymosis formation behind the ear in the mastoid region; usually becomes obvious 12 to 24 hours after injury (Fig. 36-5).
  - Hemotympanum: Blood behind the eardrum caused by a fracture near the tympanic membrane.
  - Otorrhea: CSF leakage from the ear canal caused by a crack in the petrous portion of the temporal bone, with an associated meningeal tear. If the tympanic membrane is intact, CSF will exit via the eustachian tube (instead of through the ear canal), and the patient may complain of a salty taste in the mouth.
- Posterior fossa fracture
  - The posterior fossa is formed of thick, smooth bone that rarely is fractured. However, because of the proximity to the brainstem, even a small amount of bleeding into this fossa can put fatal pressure on the brainstem.
  - MRI may provide better visualization of the posterior fossa than CT scan.

> To check for the presence of CSF in blood draining from the nose or ear, perform the halo test:
> - Place a drop of the bloody fluid on a paper towel. If the substance contains CSF and blood, two distinct rings will form. Blood will pool in the center with a halo of CSF around it. If only blood is present, no such halo will form. This is also known as the "target" or "ring" sign.

Therapeutic Interventions

- Immobilize and evaluate the cervical spine.
- Do not attempt to plug CSF leaks; allow them to drain freely.

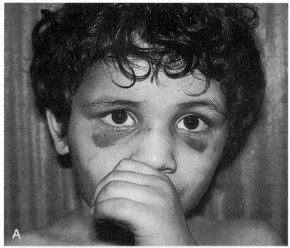
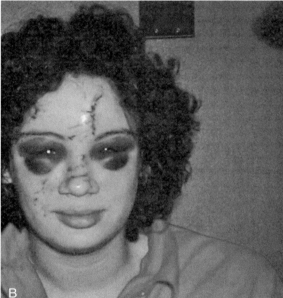

Fig. 36-4 Raccoon eyes. (Reproduced with permission from Roberts, J. R., & Hedges, J. R. [2009]. *Clinical procedures in emergency medicine* [5th ed.]. St. Louis, MO: Mosby.)

- Do not put gastric or endotracheal tubes through the nose; use the oral route.
- Perform baseline and serial neurologic examinations.
- Quickly obtain a CT scan of the head to identify intracranial injury.
- Provide tetanus prophylaxis.
- Admit the patient for observation.

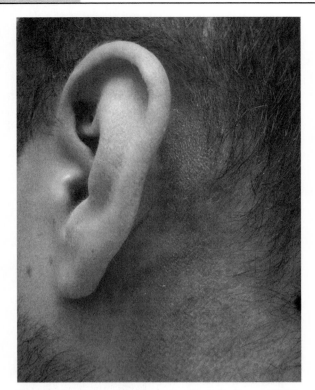

Fig. 36-5 Battle sign. (From Parrillo & Dellinger [2007]. *Critical Care Medicine* [3ʳᵈ ed.]. St. Louis, Mosby.)

Diffuse Brain Injuries

Concussion

Concussion results from acceleration, deceleration, or blast injuries that cause brain movement within the bony skull. A brief interruption of the reticular activating system occurs, causing a short period of diminished consciousness. There may or may not be a loss of consciousness. A concussion is a transient, limited process that usually requires no therapeutic intervention, although patients occasionally require months to recover fully. Concussion often accompanies other, more significant brain injuries. The CDC estimates that contact sports and recreational activities account for an estimated 3.8 million mild TBIs annually.[16] Children and adolescents are at particular risk because of their physiologic response and need for longer recovery after sustaining an impact to the head.[17]

Signs and Symptoms
- Loss or dimming of consciousness
- Flaccid paralysis (while unconscious)
- Delayed verbal response
- Confusion

- Slurred speech
- Fatigue
- Tinnitus[18]
- Dizziness, vertigo
- Headache
- Retrograde (post-traumatic) amnesia or anterograde amnesia
- Nausea, vomiting
- Visual disturbances
- Symptoms may not be immediately apparent

Other possible symptoms include:
- Behavior disorders
- Hypertension or hypotension
- Apnea
- Seizures

Diagnostic Procedures
- History of a recent head injury.
- Serial neurologic examinations.
- CT scan will be normal if concussion is the only injury.
- MRI may show subtle changes, but is rarely clinically indicated.

Therapeutic Interventions
- Immobilize and evaluate the cervical spine.
- Perform serial observations of level of consciousness.
- Administer nonnarcotic analgesics for headache.
- Admit the patient to the hospital for observation if the following are present:
  - Level of consciousness does not quickly return to normal
  - Severe vomiting
  - Skull fracture
- Discharge the patient home if a family member or friend can reliably follow careful verbal and written aftercare instructions.
- It is important to make the patient aware of the possibility of postconcussive symptoms so they can seek follow-up and treatment.[18]
- Children and adolescents should not return to sports until cleared by a physician.[19]

Postconcussive Syndrome

Late sequelae of concussion may include the following:
- Headache—up to 44% of patients report headache 6 months following mild TBI[18]
- Syncopal episodes
- Nausea
- Loss of coordination
- Memory loss
- Numbness
- Decreased concentration—children and adolescents may experience difficulty in school[18]

- Tinnitus
- Decreased organizational skills
- Diplopia (double vision)
- Difficulty handling multiple tasks
- Sleep disturbance
- Personality changes

Diffuse Axonal Injury

A diffuse axonal injury (DAI) is the most severe form of diffuse brain injury and differs from concussion in degree rather than in type of brain injury. Tension, shearing, and compression strains—created by rotational acceleration forces—cause widespread, microscopic axonal disruption throughout the brain. Severity and outcome depend on the extent and degree of structural damage. This injury is almost always associated with high-speed motor vehicle crashes.

Signs and Symptoms
- Immediate and prolonged coma lasting longer than 6 hours
- Abnormal posturing
- Confusion, amnesia, and behavioral problems following coma emergence
- Possible persistent vegetative state

Diagnostic Procedures
- History of sudden loss of consciousness following recent head injury.
- Serial neurologic examinations.
- Initial CT scan: Small hemorrhagic lesions may be visible, or the CT scan may be negative if DAI is the only injury. Subsequent CT scans (days to weeks following injury) will show diffuse cerebral edema, neuronal loss, and brain shrinkage.
- MRI will show lesions more effectively than CT, particularly in the early acute phase, but this study rarely is indicated emergently.

Therapeutic Interventions
- See "Management of Patients with Severe Traumatic Brain Injuries."

Focal Brain Injuries

Contusion

A contusion is a bruising of the surface of the brain. Findings and prognosis vary extensively based on contusion size, number, and location.

Signs and Symptoms
- Altered level of consciousness for more than 6 hours
- Nausea, vomiting
- Visual disturbances
- Neurologic dysfunction
- Weakness
- Ataxia

- Hemiparesis
- Confusion
- Speech problems
- Post-traumatic seizures

Diagnostic Procedures
- Clinical signs and symptoms
- CT scan
- MRI

Therapeutic Interventions
- Immobilize and evaluate the cervical spine.
- Admit to the hospital for observation.
- Administer antiemetics as needed.
- See "Management of Patients with Severe Traumatic Brain Injuries."
- Surgical intervention may be performed as indicated.

Intracranial Bleeding

The three meningeal layers of the brain (from outer to proximal) are the dura mater, the arachnoid mater, and the pia mater. Bleeding sites in the head are named according to their location with respect to these meningeal layers (Fig. 36-6). Bleeding (intracerebral hemorrhage) can occur directly into the brain tissue as well.

Epidural (Extradural) Hematomas. An epidural hematoma is a collection of blood between the skull and the dura mater (Fig. 36-7). Epidural hematomas occur in only 0.5% to 1% of all traumatic brain injuries.[19] This bleeding is usually arterial, caused by a rupture or tear of the middle meningeal artery that runs directly beneath the fractured temporal bone. Venous bleeding is rare and may be managed medically. Deterioration is generally rapid because accumulating arterial blood causes increasing pressure on the brain tissue, resulting in uncal herniation.

Signs and Symptoms
- Agitation and complaint of severe headache *or*
- Sudden loss of consciousness *or*
- Progressive loss of consciousness *or*
- Short period of unconsciousness (concussion) followed by a lucid interval (as the concussion resolves) and then a subsequent deterioration of consciousness caused by accumulating pressure from the bleed
- Contralateral (opposite side) weakness or hemiparesis
- Ipsilateral (same side) dilated pupil
- Bradycardia
- Increased blood pressure
- Abnormal respiratory patterns

Therapeutic Interventions
- See "Management of Patients with Severe Traumatic Brain Injuries."
- Emergent surgical evacuation may be required.

Subdural Hematoma. A subdural hematoma results from hemorrhage between the dura and the arachnoid

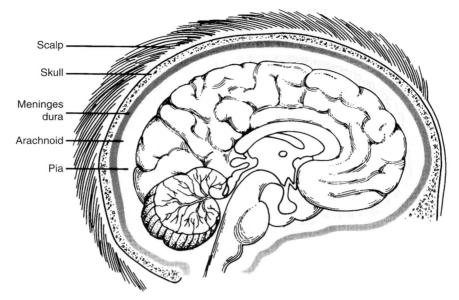

Fig. 36-6 Cross-section of the head.

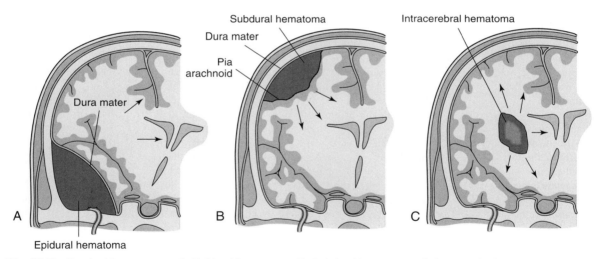

Fig. 36-7 Cerebral hematomas. **A,** Epidural hematoma. **B,** Subdural hematoma. **C,** Intracerebral hematoma. Arrows indicate the direction of pressure generated by the hematoma. (From Phipps, W., Monahan, F., Sands, J., Marek, J., & Neighbors, M. [2003]. *Medical-surgical nursing: Health and illness perspectives* [7th ed.]. St. Louis, MO: Mosby.)

mater in the subdural space (Fig. 36-8). The cause of acute bleeding is generally severe blunt trauma, such as an acceleration-deceleration incident, in which cortical tissue is lacerated, bridging veins between the cortex and venous sinuses are torn, or a dural tear into a venous sinus occurs. Subdural hematomas are much more common than epidural hematomas. They are reported to occur in 12% to 29% of severe TBIs and have the highest mortality rate (40% to 60%).[19] Subdural hematomas may develop rapidly (acute) or over a period of days or weeks (subacute or chronic). In alcoholics and the elderly, chronic subdural bleeds may develop atraumatically or following minor

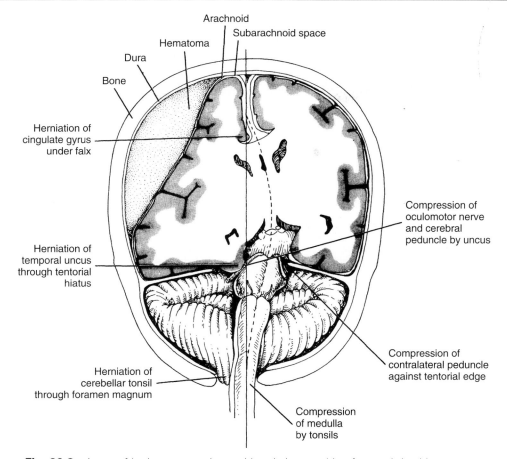

Fig. 36-8 Areas of brain compression and herniation resulting from subdural hematoma.

injury because of cerebral atrophy. Anticoagulant use increases the risk of developing a subdural hematoma following head trauma. The most common cause of subdural hematoma in persons less than 1 year of age is child maltreatment (shaken baby syndrome). If bleeding is not surgically controlled in a timely manner, pressure from an acute expanding subdural hematoma can cause transtentorial herniation and death.

Signs and Symptoms
- Acute subdural hematoma
  - Headache
  - Sudden or progressive loss of consciousness
  - Positive Babinski reflex
  - Fixed and dilated pupils (first ipsilateral and then bilateral)
  - Contralateral hemiparesis
  - Progression from hyperreflexia to abnormal flexion to abnormal extension to flaccidity

- Abnormal respiratory patterns (type depends on the level of involvement)
  - Elevated temperature
  - Increased ICP
  - Nausea and vomiting
- Subacute (24 hours to 2 weeks after injury) and chronic (2 weeks to months after injury) subdural hematoma
  - Headache
  - Ataxia
  - Incontinence
  - Increasing confusion or dementia
  - Decreasing level of consciousness
  - Worsening nausea and vomiting

Diagnostic Procedures
- Clinical findings
- Emergent CT scan—the old (isodense) blood of chronic subdural hematomas may be difficult to visualize on CT (Fig. 36-9)

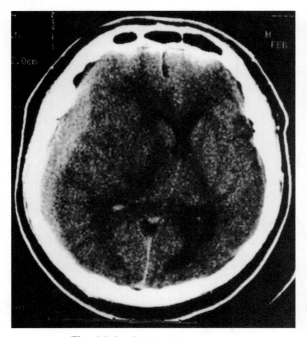

Fig. 36-9 Subdural hematoma.

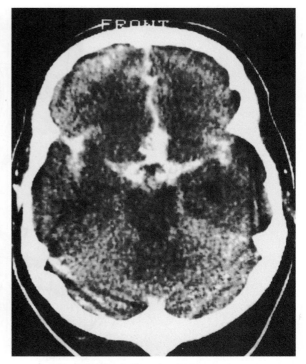

Fig. 36-10 Subarachnoid hemorrhage.

Therapeutic Interventions
- See "Management of Patients with Severe Traumatic Brain Injuries."
- Surgical evacuation of the clot or burr holes with gradual drainage of the hematoma to prevent recurrence.

Traumatic Subarachnoid Hemorrhage. A subarachnoid hemorrhage occurs between the arachnoid membrane and the pia mater. This can result from head injury, severe hypertension, or aneurysm or arteriovenous malformation (AVM) rupture. The most common cause is trauma,[20] but the most devastating bleeds are generally aneurysmal. In the trauma population, subarachnoid hemorrhage is usually an incidental finding associated with other, more serious brain injuries.

Signs and Symptoms
- Signs of meningeal irritation:
  - Headache
  - Vomiting
  - Photophobia
  - Nuchal rigidity

Diagnostic Procedures
- Clinical signs and symptoms
- CT scan (Fig. 36-10)
- Blood in the CSF

Therapeutic Interventions
- Because traumatic subarachnoid hemorrhage is rarely the primary brain injury, treatment focuses on associated conditions.
- Bloody CSF, which can lead to the development of obstructive hydrocephalus, may be drained through a ventriculostomy or shunt.

Intracerebral (Brain) Hemorrhage. Traumatic intracerebral hemorrhage (Fig. 36-11) involves bleeding into brain tissue or the ventricles. Bleeding may result from penetrating wounds, diffuse brain injury, or laceration of brain tissue, particularly in the basilar area of the skull where the bony prominences of the skull tend to tear delicate brain tissue during acceleration-deceleration events. In addition to the area of hemorrhage, an even larger surrounding zone of edema and tissue ischemia forms. Overall prognosis is poor.

Signs and Symptoms
- Presenting signs and symptoms vary dramatically based on the size, location, and number of hemorrhagic sites and on the presence of concomitant injuries.
- Loss of consciousness

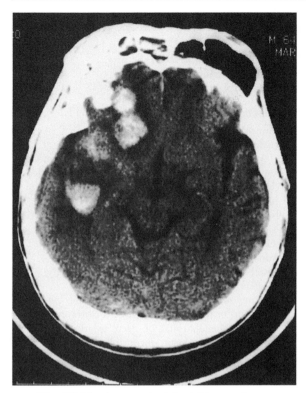

Fig. 36-11 Intracerebral (brain) hemorrhage.

- Abnormal size of pupils
- Abnormal respiratory patterns
- Abnormal motor function

Therapeutic Interventions
- See "Management of Patients with Severe Traumatic Brain Injuries."

Penetrating Injuries

Penetrating trauma to the head includes gunshot wounds, stab wounds, missile wounds, and impalement injuries. Because of their high velocity, bullets have a devastating effect on extensive areas of fragile brain tissue. Objects impaled in the cranial vault commonly travel at much lower velocities. Consequently, they may or may not produce severe injury. The extent of trauma depends on the location of the wound and on the size (caliber) and velocity of the penetrating object.

Diagnostic Procedures

- Direct observation
- Skull radiography
- CT scan

Therapeutic Interventions

- See "Management of Patients with Severe Traumatic Brain Injuries."
- Impaled objects:
  - Do not attempt to remove impaled objects.
  - Stabilize impaled objects to prevent movement or dislodgment.
  - Control associated bleeding.
  - Apply a sterile dressing around the impaled object.
- Ensure tetanus prophylaxis.

SPECIAL CONSIDERATIONS

Increased Intracranial Pressure

The brain, along with its CSF and blood, are contained within a rigid skull that allows little space for expansion. When one of these components increases, the others attempt to compensate by reducing their volume, thereby maintaining a constant ICP. Such compensation is effective only for slight or gradual increases in volume. If volume increase is extensive or rapid, ICP will rise. When ICP exceeds MAP, all blood flow to the brain ceases. Therefore management of brain-injured patients focuses heavily on avoiding or moderating increases in ICP and subsequent secondary brain trauma as a result of hypoxia, hypotension, hypercapnia, and hypocapnia.[11,19] Hypotension has been shown to nearly double the mortality rate in patients with TBIs.[19]

Herniation

Herniation occurs whenever portions of the brain extend beyond their normal location and impinge on other areas of brain tissue. Herniation can result from an expanding hematoma, cerebral edema, or a mass (e.g., tumor or impaled object) that propels brain tissue toward the path of least resistance.

Uncal (or Lateral, Transtentorial) Herniation

Uncal transtentorial herniation occurs when a lesion in the temporal lobe region causes the uncus (inner portion of the temporal lobe) to be pushed toward the midline and then over the edge of the tentorium.[15] Pressure builds at the tentorial notch, forcing brain tissue to the contralateral side and through the foramen magnum. This entraps the third (oculomotor) cranial nerve and the posterior cerebral artery between the herniated uncus and the edge of the tentorial notch, producing severe neurologic deficits.

Early Signs of Transtentorial Herniation
- Decreasing level of consciousness
- Ipsilateral pupil dilation
- Cheyne-Stokes respirations

- Contralateral hemiparesis
- Positive Babinski reflex
- Elevated ICP

Late Signs of Transtentorial Herniation
- Unconsciousness
- Bilateral fixed and dilated pupils
- Central neurogenic breathing or other abnormal respiratory patterns
- Flexion or extension posturing
- Elevated ICP unresponsive to therapy
- Bradycardia

Central Herniation

When ICP increases and is fairly uniformly distributed throughout the supratentorial region of the brain (e.g., cerebral edema), brain tissue begins to shift. This compresses the ventricles and forces both hemispheres of the cerebrum downward through the tentorial notch.[15]

Early Signs of Central Herniation
- Restlessness progressing to lethargy
- Pupils: constricted but equal and reactive
- Cheyne-Stokes respirations with yawns and sighs
- Elevated ICP

Late Signs of Central Herniation
- Loss of consciousness (coma) from reticular activating system impairment
- Pupils: midpoint or dilated, and fixed
- Decreased or abnormal motor response: posturing or flaccidity
- Cheyne-Stokes, central neurogenic, or ataxic respirations
- Elevated ICP unresponsive to therapy
- Bradycardia

Diagnostic Procedures

- Clinical observation
- CT scan
- Insertion of an ICP monitor

Therapeutic Interventions

See "Management of Patients with Severe Traumatic Brain Injuries."

Seizures After Head Trauma

Patients often develop seizures following a head trauma incident. These seizures can manifest within minutes, hours, days, or months of the incident. Early post-traumatic seizures result from direct injury to the brain or increased ICP. Late post-traumatic seizures occur with areas of tissue damage.[14] Seizure activity greatly increases metabolic demands. This can significantly aggravate preexisting cerebral hypoxia and edema in patients who are still in the acute phase of injury.[12]

Signs and Symptoms

- Loss of consciousness
- Generalized or focal seizure activity
- Autonomic findings
- Bowel or bladder incontinence

Diagnostic Procedures

- Clinical observation.
- History of TBI.
- Electroencephalography (intermittent or continuous) is required to diagnose seizures in the heavily sedated or chemically paralyzed patient.

Therapeutic Interventions

- Airway management with spinal immobilization (if there is a history of falling).
- Administer supplemental oxygen.
- Give benzodiazepines to control seizure activity; titrate to effect.
- For ongoing seizure control, administer phenytoin (Dilantin) or fosphenytoin (Cerebyx) intravenously.
- Consider phenobarbital or deep sedation (e.g., propofol) if seizures remain uncontrolled.

REFERENCES

1. Jagoda, A. S., Bazarian, J. J., Bruns, J. J., Jr., Cantrill, S. V., Gean, A. D., Howard, P. K., ... Whitson, R. R.; American College of Emergency Physicians; Centers for Disease Control and Prevention. (2008). Clinical policy: Neuroimaging and decisionmaking in adult mild traumatic brain injury in the acute setting. *Annals of Emergency Medicine, 52*(6), 714–748.
2. Faul, M., Xu, L., Wald, M. M., & Coronado, V. G. (2010). *Traumatic brain injury in the United States: Emergency department visits, hospitalizations and deaths 2002–2006.* Atlanta, GA: Centers for Disease Control and Prevention, National Center for Injury Prevention and Control.
3. Nicholl, J., & LaFrance, W. C., Jr. (2009). Neuropsychiatric sequelae of traumatic brain injury. *Seminars in Neurology, 29*(3), 247–255.
4. Lafferty, B. (2010). Traumatic brain injury: A factor in the causal pathway to homelessness? *Journal for Nurse Practitioners, 6*(5), 358–362.
5. Watanabe, T., Elovic, E., & Zafonte, R. (2010). Chronic traumatic encephalopathy. *PM&R, 2*(7), 671–675.
6. Eggenberger, E. R. (2010, November 18). *Anisocoria.* Retrieved from http://emedicine.medscape.com/article/1158571-overview
7. McInnis, L. A., Parsons, L., & Krau, S. D. (2010). Angiography: From a patient's perspective. *Critical Care Nursing Clinics of North America, 22*(1), 51–60.
8. Bullock, M. R., Chesnut, R., Ghajar, J., Gordon, D., Hartl, R., Newell, D., ... Wilberger, J. E. (2006). Guidelines for the

management of severe traumatic brain injury. *Neurosurgery*, *58*(Suppl 3), S2-S1–S2-62.

9. Inoue, K. (2010). Caring for the perioperative patient with increased intracranial pressure. *AORN Journal*, *91*(4), 511–515.

10. Fryman, L., & Murray, L. (2007). Managing acute head trauma in a crowded emergency department. *Journal of Emergency Nursing*, *33*(3), 208–213.

11. Stiver, S. I., & Manley, G. T. (2008). Prehospital management of traumatic brain injury. *Neurosurgical Focus*, *25*(4), E5.

12. Noble, K. A. (2010). Traumatic brain injury and increased intracranial pressure. *Journal of Perianesthesia Nursing*, *25*(4), 242–248.

13. Abram, S., & Bulstrode, C. (2010). Routine spinal immobilization in trauma patients: What are the advantages and disadvantages? *The Surgeon*, *8*(4), 218–222.

14. Mcilvoy, L., & Meyer K. (2008). *Nursing management of adults with severe traumatic brain injury*. Glenview, IL: American Association of Neuroscience Nurses.

15. Chestnut, R. M. (2007). Care of central nervous system injuries. *Surgical Clinics of North America*, *87*(1), 119–156.

16. Centers for Disease Control and Prevention. (2007). Nonfatal traumatic brain injuries from sports and recreation activities—United States, 2001–2005. *MMWR Weekly*, *56*(29), 733–737. Retrieved from http://www.cdc.gov/mmwr/preview/mmwrhtml/mm5629a2.htm

17. McCory, P., Meeuwisse, W., Johnston, K., Dvorak, J., Aubry, M., Molloy, M., & Cantu, R. (2009). Consensus statement on concussion in sport—The 3rd International Conference on Concussion in Sport held in Zurich, November 2008. *Journal of Science and Medicine in Sport*, *12*(3), 340–351.

18. Bergman, K., & Bay, E. (2010). Mild traumatic brain injury/concussion: A review for ED nurses. *Journal of Emergency Nursing*, *36*(3), 221–230.

19. Heegard, W., & Biros, M. (2007). Traumatic brain injury. *Emergency Medicine Clinics of North America*, *25*(3), 655–678.

20. Edlow, J. A., Malek, A. M., & Ogilvy, C. S. (2008). Aneurysmal subarachnoid hemorrhage: Update for emergency physicians. *Journal of Emergency Medicine*, *34*(3), 237–251.

Spinal Cord and Neck Trauma

Faye P. Everson

SPINAL CORD INJURIES

Every year in the United States, 11,000 to 15,000 new spinal cord injuries (SCIs) occur.[1] Motor vehicle crashes account for 41.3% in those patients younger than 44 years.[2] Falls, by patients over 45 years of age, are responsible for 27% of SCIs in this population.[2] Other causes of SCI include violence (15%) and sports (8%) along with vascular disorders, tumors, infections, spondylosis, and developmental disorders.[2] Extreme sports, which often epitomize the ultimate in risk-taking behavior, increase the incidence of SCI in males between the ages of 15 and 30 years.[2]

Mechanisms of Injury

Trauma may cause injury to the vertebral column, spinal nerves, or spinal cord. Blood supply may be impaired, causing damage to many other structures. Cord trauma may be caused through fracture or dislocation of the vertebrae. Transection or disruption of the cord or other extradural processes can also cause injury.

- Rapid acceleration-deceleration forces cause the vertebral column to be moved beyond its usual range of motion. Injuries can be the result of hyperextension, hyperflexion, rotation, and axial loading (Table 37-1).[3]
- Most SCIs result from blunt trauma; penetrating injuries from bullets affect the cord and column. Less frequently, stab wounds lacerate the cord or nerve roots.
- Concurrent injuries may include injuries to the head, chest, abdomen, and long bones.
  - Rib fractures and other chest injuries often occur with thoracic vertebral trauma.
  - Lumbar and pelvic fractures may occur simultaneously.
  - Axial loading, resulting from a blow to the head or from jumping or falling from a height, results in a specific pattern of injury with compression along the lumbar spine and fractures to the calcaneus.

- SCI should always be suspected in trauma patients who are intoxicated, demonstrate altered level of consciousness, or have distracting injuries such as open fractures.
- SCI is frequently associated with near drowning or diving incidents. In these situations, consider alcohol or drug use, seizure disorder, and unknown depth of water.

> Because of the flexibility of their spines, pediatric patients under 8 years of age may experience a phenomenon called SCIWORA (spinal cord injury without radiographic abnormality). However, this term is becoming outdated since magnetic resonance imaging on children with SCIWORA has demonstrated various spinal cord injuries, including ligament damage, spinal cord hemorrhage, and complete cord transection.

Consequences of Spinal Cord Injury

Spinal cord injuries may be primary or secondary. Primary cord injury occurs at the time of injury as a result of an initial mechanism (Table 37-1). Secondary injury is a progressive, pathologic response that may be caused by hypoperfusion and hypoxia of the spinal cord from:
- Respiratory depression or failure
- Systemic hypotension and shock
  - Hemorrhagic shock from multiple injuries
  - Neurogenic shock
- Cord injury or ischemia leading to neurologic deficits

Respiratory Depression or Failure

Spinal cord injuries, particularly injury to the upper cervical region, can result in alterations in respiratory function. The degree of respiratory impairment results in part from the level of injury, as noted in Table 37-2. Additional considerations related to respiratory function include the following:

TABLE 37-1   MECHANISMS OF INJURY TO THE VERTEBRAL COLUMN

MECHANISM OF INJURY	ETIOLOGY OF INJURY (CAUSE)	RESULT OF INJURY (EFFECT)	EXAMPLE	LOCATION OF INJURY[a,b]
Hyperextension	Backward thrust of the head beyond the anatomical capacity of the cervical vertebral column	Damage to anterior ligaments ranging from stretching to ligament tears and bony dislocations	Rear-end MVC resulting in "whiplash"	Cervical spine
Hyperflexion	Forceful forward flexion of the cervical spine with the head striking an immovable object	Wedge fractures; facet dislocations; subluxation (due to ligament rupture); teardrop, odontoid or transverse process fractures	Head-on MVC with head striking windshield creating a "star burst" effect	Cervical spine
Rotational	A combination of forceful forward flexion with lateral displacement of the cervical spine[c]	Rupture of the posterior ligament and/or anterior fracture or dislocation of the vertebral body	MVC to front or rear lateral area of vehicle resulting in conversion of forward motion to a spinning-type motion[c]	Cervical spine
Axial loading	Direct force transmitted along the length of the vertebral column	Deformity of the vertebral column; secondary edema of the spinal cord, resulting in neurologic deficits	Diver striking head on bottom of pool	T12 to L2

Reprinted with permission from Emergency Nurses Association. (2007). *Trauma nursing core course provider manual* (6th ed.). Des Plaines, IL: Author.
[a]Boss, B. J. (2002). Concepts of neurologic dysfunction. In K. L. McCance & S. E. Huether (Eds.), *Pathophysiology: The biologic basis for disease in adults and children* (4th ed., pp. 438–486). St. Louis, MO: Mosby.
[b]Boss, B. J. (2002). Alterations of neurologic function. In K. L. McCance & S. E. Huether (Eds.), *Pathophysiology: The biologic basis for disease in adults and children* (4th ed., pp. 487–549). St. Louis, MO: Mosby.
[c]Jackson, A. B., Dijker, S. M., Deviv, O. M., & Poczatek, R. B. (2004). A demographic profile of new traumatic spinal cord injuries: Change and stability over 30 years. *Archives of Physical Medicine and Rehabilitation, 85*, 1740–1748.
MVC, Motor vehicle crash.

TABLE 37-2   CERVICAL SPINE INJURIES AND RESPIRATORY IMPAIRMENT

LEVEL OF INJURY	VITAL CAPACITY	COUGH REFLEX	MUSCULAR INVOLVEMENT
Above C3	<5%–10% of normal	Absent	Paralysis of diaphragm, intercostals, and abdominal muscles Respiratory arrest and death unless interventions are immediate
C3–C5	20% of normal	Weak and ineffective	Weakness of diaphragm Intercostal and abdominal muscles paralyzed
C6–T1	30%–50% of normal	Weak	Intercostal and abdominal muscles paralyzed

- Concurrent lung injury (pneumothorax, pulmonary contusion)
- Medical history of respiratory dysfunction (chronic obstructive pulmonary disease)
- Associated head injury
- Presence of intoxication

Shock

Shock in the patient with SCI may be hemorrhagic (lose of intravascular volume), neurogenic (loss of sympathetic outflow), or spinal (loss of reflexes).

- *Hemorrhagic shock*—as in any trauma patient, hemorrhagic hypovolemic shock can lead to inadequate perfusion of vital organs. Hypoperfusion of the spinal cord is a common cause of secondary injury in the patient with SCI.

> In acute SCI, shock may be neurogenic, hemorrhagic, or both. Bleeding must be ruled out as a cause of hypotension before a diagnosis of neurogenic shock is made.

- *Neurogenic shock* can occur with an injury at the level of T6 or higher. Descending sympathetic paths are affected, resulting in loss of vasomotor tone and sympathetic stimulation.
  - Peripheral vasodilation results in maldistribution of blood volume; blood volume is maintained but the vascular bed is enlarged.
  - Classic signs of neurogenic shock are:
    - Hypotension
    - Bradycardia
    - Peripheral vasodilation
  - Additional signs may include hypothermia and loss of sweating below the level of injury.
  - This loss of sympathetic outflow prevents reflex tachycardia and vasoconstriction; expected signs of hypovolemic (hemorrhagic) shock may be absent, making its diagnosis difficult.
- *Spinal shock* is the temporary loss of motor, sensory, and reflex function below the level of damage.
  - Onset is usually immediate but may occur up to several days after the injury and last for days to weeks.
  - The level of the damage will determine the intensity and duration of the spinal shock.
  - Clinical presentation includes flaccid paralysis, areflexia, and loss of bowel and bladder function.

Neurologic Deficits

Neurologic deficits can be the result of both primary and secondary injury; they may be permanent or transient. Familiarity with the anatomic landmarks for the body's dermatomes (Fig. 37-1 and Table 37-3) will help the emergency nurse identify the level of SCI and anticipate complications related to the level of injury.

Helmet Removal

There are many different styles of helmets that offer varying degrees of protection to the head while participating in a wide variety of sports. When the helmet is in place, airway management is limited at best and it is difficult to maintain spinal immobilization. Removal of a helmet requires two or three trained staff members working as a team. See Figure 37-2 for the steps in removing a helmet.

Spinal Immobilization

Spinal immobilization is not a benign procedure. In addition to the pain of immobilization, there are concerns related to skin breakdown resulting from pressure and the potential for aspiration if the patient vomits. Therefore the first decision to be made, both in the field and in the emergency department, is whether the patient actually requires spinal immobilization. Various protocols exist to guide this decision; Table 37-4 is an example of one acronym that can be used.

General Assessment

- Ensure that spinal immobilization is maintained throughout the assessment process to minimize the potential for further injury. Table 37-5 lists considerations while applying spinal immobilization.
- Assessment and treatment of airway, breathing, and circulation problems take precedence over other assessments.
- Airway management is often complex and difficult because the spine must be maintained in neutral alignment at all times.
- Evaluate breathing by assessing respiratory rate, rhythm, and depth.
  - Determine if the patient can take a deep breath and cough.
  - Increased work of breathing or use of abdominal muscles may indicate deterioration of the patient's condition.
  - Patients with SCI may appear to breathe well initially but tend to decompensate over time. Continued reassessment is necessary.
- Circulatory assessment includes measurement of blood pressure and heart rate. Hypotension may be neurogenic or hemorrhagic in origin.
  - Search for occult signs of hemorrhage in the chest, abdomen, or retroperitoneal areas.
  - Pelvic or long bone fractures may be a source of blood loss.
  - Check skin signs, such as color, temperature, and moisture, as an indication of perfusion.
- Assess level of consciousness; concurrent head injury is common.
- Perform secondary assessment as for any trauma patient (see Chapter 35, Assessment and Stabilization of the Trauma Patient).
- Logroll patient, maintaining spinal alignment, to examine the patient's back.
  - Check for point tenderness, ecchymosis, and open wounds.

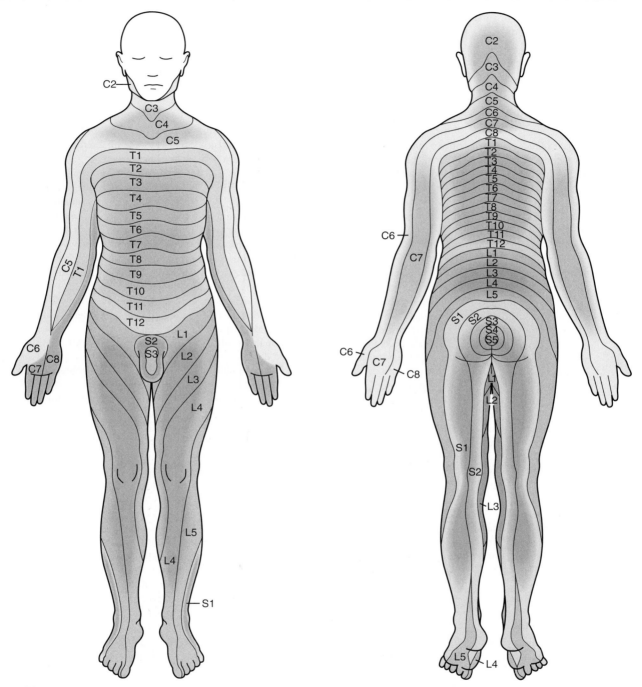

Fig. 37-1 Sensory dermatomes. (From Marx, J. A. [2010]. *Rosen's emergency medicine: Concept and clinical practice* [7th ed.]. Philadelphia, PA: Mosby Elsevier.)

TABLE 37-3 ANATOMIC LANDMARKS AND DERMATOME LEVELS

ANATOMIC LANDMARK	DERMATOME LEVEL	MOTOR FUNCTION PRESENT
Top of shoulder	C5	Flexion and extension of arms
Nipple line	T4	Respiratory muscles function
Umbilicus	T10	None
Great toe	L4	Flexion of foot, extension of toes
	S4	Positive sphincter tone

Data from Emergency Nurses Association. (2007). *Trauma nursing core course provider manual* (6th ed.). Des Plaines, IL: Author.

- Assess sphincter tone and the presence of "anal wink" (contraction of the sphincter in response to proximal pinprick).
- Determine patient's body temperature; with SCI, the patient's body temperature may be that of the ambient environment (poikilothermy).
- Observe for priapism in males (indicates vasodilation of blood vessels and strongly indicative of neurogenic shock).

Neurologic Assessment

Assessment of Motor Function

- Rate motor function using the six-point American Spinal Injury Association scale.[4]
  - 0—No contraction or movement
  - 1—Minimal movement
  - 2—Active movement, but not against gravity
  - 3—Active movement against gravity
  - 4—Active movement against resistance
  - 5—Active movement against full resistance

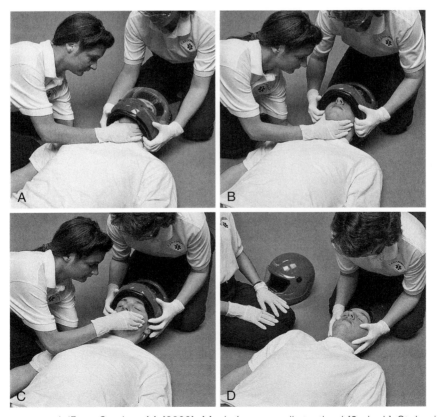

Fig. 37-2   Helmet removal. (From Sanders, M. [2000]. *Mosby's paramedic textbook* [2nd ed.]. St. Louis, MO: Mosby.)

TABLE 37-4	NSAIDs ACRONYM TO DETERMINE NEED FOR SPINAL IMMOBILIZATION*

N—Neurological examination: Any focal deficits such as tingling, numbness, or decreased strength in an extremity?

S—Significant traumatic mechanism of injury?

A—Alertness: Any alteration in the patient's level of consciousness? Is patient oriented to person, place, time, and situation?

I—Intoxication: Presence indicates impaired decision-making ability.

D—Distracting injury: Is there any injury that may distract the patient from the pain of cervical spine or back injury?

S—Spinal examination: Any point tenderness over spine or pain on movement of neck (if patient has no midline tenderness)?

Data from North Carolina College of Emergency Physicians & North Carolina Office of Emergency Medical Services. (2009). *Protocol 12, Spinal immobilization clearance.* Retrieved from http://www.ncems.org/pdf/Pro12-SpinalImmobilizationClearance.pdf

*If any of these findings is positive, the patient requires initial spinal immobilization.

- Compare right and left and upper and lower extremities.
- Assess rectal tone.
- Repeat assessment at frequent intervals to detect possible progression of deficit because of secondary injury.

Assessment of Sensory Function

- Determine lowest level of sensation to light touch (wisp of cotton) and gentle pinprick (pin or tip of broken cotton swab).
- Have the patient close his or her eyes during this assessment.[5]
- Assess proprioception (awareness of the body in space) by moving the big toe up or down and asking the patient to identify its position.
- Document any complaints by the patient of "electric shock" along the spine.

Assessment of Deep Tendon and Pathologic Reflexes

- Deep tendon reflexes are generally absent initially in the patient with SCI so examination of these is generally not useful in the emergency department.[6]
- Note the presence of pathologic reflexes.

TABLE 37-5	CONSIDERATIONS WHILE APPLYING SPINAL IMMOBILIZATION

- Spinal immobilization requires a team approach. A leader who will direct the process must be identified beforehand.
- Assess the patient's motor and sensory status prior to immobilization.
- The leader maintains in-line stabilization (not traction) with both hands on either side of the patient's head, stabilizing the head and neck in a neutral, vertical position. The patient's nose should be in line with his or her umbilicus.
- Remove earrings, necklaces, other sharp objects, and bulky clothing that could cause soft tissue pressure injury.
- Following the manufacturer's recommendations for sizing, apply the collar to fit between the point of the chin and the suprasternal notch, resting on the clavicles and supporting the lower jaw.
- Check motor and sensory status after application of the collar.
- At the leader's direction, gently logroll the patient onto a long board while the team leader maintains head and neck stabilization.
- Secure the patient to the long board using straps at the chest, hips, and knees. Straps should be snug but not restrict chest wall or abdominal movement.
- The patient's head is then secured using head blocks (not sandbags) and tape. Manual stabilization may then be released.
- Recheck motor and sensory status.
- Follow the institution's policy for removal of spinal immobilization, especially in the elderly patient, as soon as feasible.

- Hoffman sign—Positive if tapping or flicking the nail of the middle finger results in contraction (flexion) of the index finger and thumb.[7]
- Babinski reflex—Big toe flexes upward and other toes fan out in response to stroking the bottom of the foot.

Diagnostic Procedures

- Cervical spine radiograph
  - Three standard radiographic views are recommended: cross-table lateral, anterior-posterior, and odontoid.
  - All seven cervical vertebrae and the C7-T1 junction must be clearly visualized.
  - To help visualize C7 and T1, pull the arms downward while shooting the film, as this forces the shoulders to drop downward, especially in muscular patients.

TABLE 37-6	**NATIONAL EMERGENCY X-RADIOGRAPHY UTILIZATION STUDY'S (NEXUS) LOW-RISK CRITERIA**

If a patient meets all five of the following criteria, the probability of cervical spine injury is low and cervical radiography is probably unnecessary.
- No midline cervical tenderness
- No focal neurologic deficit
- Normal alertness and level of consciousness
- Absence of intoxication
- No painful, distracting injury

Data from Greenbaum, J., Walters, N., & Levy, P. D. (2009). An evidence-based approach to radiographic assessment of cervical spine injuries in the emergency department. *Journal of Emergency Medicine*, *36*(1), 64–71.

- Cervical spine radiographs may not be indicated in a subset of patients. See Table 37-6 for the National Emergency X-Radiography Utilization Study's (NEXUS) low-risk criteria.[8]
- Radiographs of the thoracic and lumbar spines should be obtained as indicated.
- Computed tomography (CT) scanning, if available, should be used if all cervical vertebrae and T1 are not visualized on standard radiograph, and to delineate bony abnormalities or fractures.
- Magnetic resonance imaging (MRI) is useful to evaluate ligament or cord damage and edema, compression injuries, and extradural spinal hematomas.

Contraindications to MRI include the presence of pacemakers or internal cardioverter defibrillators, metallic foreign bodies, MRI-incompatible monitoring systems, and cervical traction.

- Lactate level to monitor perfusion status in shock.
- Arterial blood gases (ABGs) to detect hypoxia or hypercapnia, especially in patients with suspected cervical injury.
- Urinalysis to assess for associated genitourinary injuries.

Therapeutic Interventions

- Prevent further injury to the spine by preserving spinal alignment in supine position.
- Anticipate airway difficulties, especially with injuries above the level of C5.
- Associated face, neck, and head injuries may contribute to airway problems.
- Anticipate vomiting. Have suction equipment available and be prepared to quickly turn patient to his or her side while maintaining spinal immobilization.
- A modified jaw thrust and insertion of an oral pharyngeal airway may be necessary if patient cannot protect his or her own airway; endotracheal intubation may be necessary.
- Prepare for rapid sequence intubation (RSI) if difficulty maintaining a patent airway and adequate ventilation is likely. Maintain spinal immobilization (not traction) during intubation.
- Do not delay intubation because of concerns about the stability of the spine.
- Frequently reassess the adequacy of ventilator effort.
  - Continuously monitor pulse oximetry.
  - Obtain ABGs as indicated.
- Obtain intravenous access with two large-bore catheters.
  - Initiate fluid resuscitation with crystalloids.
  - Hypotension resulting from neurogenic shock may require vasopressors to maintain an adequate mean arterial pressure.
  - Insert an indwelling urinary catheter to monitor hourly output.
- Insert a gastric tube to prevent distension resulting from ileus and decreased peristalsis.
- Maintain patient's body temperature with warm blankets and warming devices and by increasing the room temperature.
- Provide emotional support for both patient and family; offer realistic hope.
- Initiate skin assessment and care early. Pad pressure points and remove patients from backboard as soon as feasible.
- Assist with application of halo ring, skeletal tongs, and cervical traction.
  - Ensure that traction weights are hanging freely at all times.
  - If halo has been applied, tape the wrench used to remove the chest piece to the vest.
- Combative or uncooperative patients may require sedation or restraints to prevent further injury to themselves.
- Administer tetanus prophylaxis, analgesics, and antibiotics as indicated.
- Use of high-dose steroids (methylprednisolone) remains highly controversinal.[9]
- Anticipate possible transfer to tertiary care facility.

SPECIFIC VERTEBRAL AND SPINAL CORD INJURIES

Cervical Spine Dislocations and Fractures

A cervical spine dislocation occurs when one vertebra is displaced, overriding another vertebra.[5] This is an unstable injury and may occur in conjunction with cervical fracture.[10] The trauma that causes a cervical dislocation or fracture may also damage the spinal cord, resulting in devastating irreversible neurologic deficits.

Signs and Symptoms

- Vary with degree of SCI
- Cervical tenderness and muscle spasm
- Ecchymosis and swelling of neck
- Weakness and numbness of extremities
- Diminished (or absent) sensation in extremities

Diagnostic Procedures

- See "Diagnostic Procedures" above.

Therapeutic Interventions

- Manage patient as if injury to the spinal cord is present.
- Prepare for and assist with application of skeletal traction or halo vest or with internal fixation.

Incomplete Spinal Cord Lesions

The patient with incomplete spinal cord lesions maintains some degree of motor or sensory function below the level of the injury. However, SCI is a dynamic process; the full extent of the injury may not be apparent in the initial hours following the traumatic event.[4] For this reason, frequent repeated neurologic examinations should be performed to detect progression of deficits.

Signs and Symptoms

- Table 37-7 lists common syndromes and associated signs and symptoms that can result from incomplete spinal lesions. Figure 37-3 further illustrates these common syndromes.

Diagnostic Procedures

- Diagnosis is based mainly on clinical presentation and neurologic examination.
- Spinal radiographs should be obtained to determine fracture or damage to the vertebrae.
- Normal plain radiographs and CT scans do not rule out spinal cord damage.
- CT or MRI may be necessary to further delineate bony or cord damage.

Therapeutic Interventions

- Early treatment goals are related to preventing secondary injury and the progression of an incomplete lesion to a complete lesion.
- Airway maintenance and adequate tissue perfusion are the highest priorities.
- In the presence of hypotension, first consider occult hemorrhage as the cause.
- Prevent hypothermia.

Complete Spinal Cord Lesions

A complete spinal cord lesion may occur at any level. The patient loses all motor and sensory function below the level of the injury; there is no chance of recovering function if it has not returned within 24 hours after injury.

Signs and Symptoms

- Loss of motor function below the level of the injury with flaccid paralysis of all voluntary muscles
- Loss of sensory function below the level of the injury, including loss of pain, touch, temperature, pressure, vibration, and proprioception
- Loss of reflexes below lesion
- Possible neurogenic shock
- Loss of bowel and bladder function
- Paralytic ileus with abdominal distension
- Priapism

Diagnostic Procedures

- Diagnosis is based mainly on clinical presentation and neurologic exam.
- Spinal radiographs should be obtained to determine fracture or damage to the vertebrae.
- Normal plain radiographs and CT scans do not rule out spinal cord damage.
- CT to visualize bony anatomy, including fracture.
- MRI may show compression of the spinal cord.

Therapeutic Interventions

- Assess for and treat neurogenic shock.
- Provide emotional support as patient responds to loss of function.
- Initiate skin care, respiratory hygiene, venous thromboembolism prophylaxis, and other measures to prevent complications of immobility.

Autonomic Dysreflexia

Also known as hyperreflexia, autonomic dysreflexia is a potentially life-threatening condition that can occur in patients with a spinal cord injury at or above the level of T6. A strong sensory input, often pain or discomfort below

TABLE 37-7   INCOMPLETE SPINAL CORD SYNDROMES

SYNDROME	CAUSE	CLINICAL PRESENTATION
Central cord syndrome	Hyperextension Bleeding into center of cord	Loss of motor and sensory function below level of injury Greater loss in arms than legs Varied degrees of bladder dysfunction Dysesthesia (sensation of burning) in arms and hands is common
Anterior cord syndrome	Acute hyperflexion Compression of anterior spinal artery	Loss of motor function, pain, and temperature below injury Crude touch, deep pressure, proprioception, and vibration are intact Worst prognosis of all cord syndromes
Brown-Séquard syndrome	Transverse hemisection of cord Usually resulting from penetrating trauma Uncommon injury	Ipsilateral (same side) loss of motor function, proprioception, and vibration below level of injury Contralateral (opposite side) loss of pain and temperature Ipsilateral paralysis or paresis below injury
Cauda equina syndrome	Injury at lumbosacral nerve roots	Varying degrees of motor and sensory function loss in lower extremities Bowel and bladder dysfunction such as urinary hesitancy or retention, urinary or bowel incontinence, constipation

Data from Emergency Nurses Association. (2007). *Trauma nursing core course (TNCC) provider manual* (6th ed.). Des Plaines, IL: Author; and Schreiber, D. (2009, April 8). *Spinal cord injuries.* Retrieved from http://emedicine.medscape.com/article/793582-overview

the level of the injury, leads to massive reflex sympathetic response. This uncontrolled sympathetic outflow results in vasoconstriction and dangerously elevated blood pressure.

Common causes of autonomic dysreflexia in the emergency patient include:

- Pain
- Bladder distension
  - Urinary retention
  - Blocked urinary catheter
- Invasive diagnostic procedures
- Contact with hard or sharp objects[11]
- Fractures or other trauma
- Constipation, bowel distension or irritation
- Less common causes:
  - Decubitus ulcers
  - Tight or restrictive clothing or dressings
  - Ingrown toenails
  - Menstrual cramps
  - Labor and delivery

Signs and Symptoms

- Sudden increase in blood pressure, possibly as high as 200/100 mm Hg
- Pounding headache caused by vasodilation of intracranial vessels
- Piloerection ("goose bumps")
- Sweating and flushing above level of injury
- Cool, clammy skin below level of injury
- Bradycardia (reflexive attempt to lower blood pressure)
- Nasal congestion
- Sense of anxiety
- Blurred vision or spots in visual field

Diagnostic Procedures

- Diagnosis based on clinical presentation

Therapeutic Interventions

- Treatment must be initiated quickly to prevent complications.
- Place patient in upright position.
- Identify offending stimulation and stop or remove it as quickly as possible.
  - If a urinary catheter is in place, check for kinked tubing, blocked drainage, or location of drainage bag above the level of the bladder.
  - If the tubing is not kinked or a urinary catheter is not in place, insert or change the catheter.
  - If a procedure is being performed, terminate the procedure until the symptoms subside.
- Medications are indicated if the offending trigger or stimulus cannot be identified or removed, or if the episode persists after removal of the stimulus.[12]
  - Nifedipine (Procardia) 10 mg orally or sublingually
  - Nitroglycerine 0.4 mg sublingually or 0.5 inch topically
  - Clonidine 0.1 to 0.2 mg orally

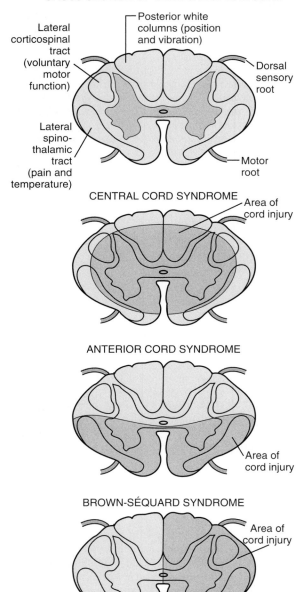

CROSS SECTION OF CERVICAL SPINAL CORD

Lateral corticospinal tract (voluntary motor function)

Posterior white columns (position and vibration)

Dorsal sensory root

Lateral spinothalamic tract (pain and temperature)

Motor root

CENTRAL CORD SYNDROME

Area of cord injury

ANTERIOR CORD SYNDROME

Area of cord injury

BROWN-SÉQUARD SYNDROME

Area of cord injury

Fig. 37-3 Incomplete spinal cord lesions: central cord syndrome, anterior cord syndrome, and Brown-Séquard syndrome. (From Marx, J. A. [2010]. *Rosen's emergency medicine: Concept and clinical practice* [7th ed.]. Philadelphia, PA: Mosby Elsevier.)

- Hydralazine 10 to 20 mg intramuscularly or intravenously
- Monitor blood pressure and heart rate as frequently as every 5 minutes.
- Additional medications may be required to prevent recurrent episodes.

TRAUMA TO THE NECK

The neck is protected from injury to some degree by the spine posteriorly, the head superiorly, and the chest inferiorly. This leaves the anterior and lateral aspects most susceptible to both blunt and penetrating trauma.[13]

Neck trauma accounts for 5% to 10% of all serious trauma, and 3500 people die each year from neck trauma.[13] Mortality rate is 2% to 6% and is most common in males, adolescents, and young adults.[13] The etiology of neck trauma is varied and includes the following:
- Motor vehicle crashes
- Sports-related injuries such as from a clothesline tackle
- Blows from feet or hands
- Strangulation from hanging or manual choking
- Penetrating trauma

The neck contains a large concentration of important structures relative to its small size. Because airway compromise is always a concern with trauma to the neck, these injuries are considered to be potentially life-threatening. The neck can be divided into three anatomic zones that can be used to anticipate which structures are likely to be injured (Table 37-8).

Penetrating Neck Wounds

Penetrating injuries are generally the result of gunshot wounds, stabbings, punctures, or impalements. The depth of the injury, the amount of force used, the type of penetrating instrument, and the location and angle of penetration will determine the extent of injury. Penetrating neck injuries occur in 5% to 10% of trauma cases and as many as 30% of these patients have concurrent injuries outside the neck zones.[14]

Signs and Symptoms

- Specific signs and symptoms will depend on which structures have been injured
- Dysphagia and hoarseness (suspect endotracheal or esophageal injury)
- Oronasopharyngeal bleeding
- Neurologic deficits if vascular or spinal cord injuries are present
- Respiratory distress
- Subcutaneous emphysema
- Expanding hematoma in the neck

TABLE 37-8 ZONES OF THE NECK

	ANATOMIC BOUNDARIES	STRUCTURES WITHIN ZONE
Zone I	Extends from the sternal notch and clavicle to the cricothyroid cartilage	Great vessels (subclavian and jugular veins, carotid arteries, aortic arch)
	Injuries to Zone I have the highest mortality and morbidity	Trachea and esophagus
		Upper lung tissue
		Cervical spine, cord, and nerve roots
Zone II	From the cricoid cartilage to the angle of the mandible	Carotid and vertebral arteries, jugular veins
		Pharynx and larynx
		Esophagus
		Cervical spine and cord
Zone III	The angle of the mandible to the base of the skull	Salivary and parotid glands
		Carotid arteries and jugular veins
		Trachea and esophagus
		Cervical spine
		Cranial nerves IX to XII

Diagnostic Procedures

- Anterior-posterior and lateral neck radiographs to identify bony injuries and presence of foreign bodies
- CT or helical CT of neck to define anatomy of injury
- Esophagography if injury to esophagus is suspected
- Laryngoscopy for direct visualization of injury
- Cerebral angiography to identify vascular damage
- Baseline hematocrit, type, and crossmatch in addition to routine trauma laboratory studies

Therapeutic Interventions

- Obtaining and maintaining a patent airway is especially important in the patient with neck injuries. The fascial compartments of the neck limit the amount of external bleeding but an expanding hematoma can obstruct the compressible trachea.
- Concurrent cervical spine injury is relatively uncommon with penetrating neck injuries.[14] If a cervical collar is deemed necessary, assess beneath the collar for hidden potentially life-threatening injuries.
- Fluid resuscitation and management of hypotension follow the general guidelines for care of a trauma patient. See Chapter 35, Assessment and Stabilization of the Trauma Patient.
- Frequently assess neurologic status to detect deficits because of vascular injury.

- Prepare the patient for possible surgical exploration of the penetrating wound.
- Provide tetanus immunization based on patient's immunization status.

Fractured Larynx

The most common cause of a fractured larynx is blunt trauma, often occurring when the larynx strikes the steering wheel in a motor vehicle crash. Other causes include a direct blow to the neck during sports or an altercation, manual strangulation, hanging, or a clothesline injury. Fractured larynx is a rare injury, occurring in less than 1% of all blunt trauma.[15] Its incidence continues to decrease because of the use of seat belts and restraint systems.

Signs and Symptoms

- Alteration in quality of voice
  - Hoarseness
  - Dysphonia or aphonia
- Pain or tenderness in anterior neck
- Ecchymosis of anterior neck
- Hemoptysis
- Dysphagia
- Stridor
- Drooling
- Subcutaneous emphysema or crepitus
- Dyspnea

Diagnostic Procedures

- History and clinical presentation are important in making a diagnosis
- Chest and cervical spine radiographs to rule out other significant injuries
- CT scan
- Endoscopy or esophagoscopy
- Direct laryngoscopy

Therapeutic Interventions

- Obtaining and maintaining a patent airway is the highest priority.
- Anticipate early tracheostomy or possible cricothyrotomy.
- Administer humidified air; supplemental oxygen may be administered if the patient is hypoxic.[15]
- Elevate the head of the bed to 30 to 45 degrees.
- Restrict the patient to nothing by mouth.
- Instruct the patient to "voice rest."
- Use of systemic corticosteroids (to decrease inflammation) is controversial.
- Administer antireflux medications (H_2 receptor antagonists and proton pump inhibitors).
- Surgical intervention may be necessary.

REFERENCES

1. *Spinal cord injury facts and statistics.* (2010, November 8). Retrieved from http://www.sci-info-pages.com/facts.html

2. National Spinal Cord Injury Statistical Center. (2010, February). *Spinal cord injury facts and figures at a glance.* Retrieved from https://www.nscisc.uab.edu/public_content/pdf/Facts%20and%20Figures%20at%20a%20Glance%202010.pdf

3. Emergency Nurses Association. (2007). *Trauma nursing core course provider manual* (6th ed.). Des Plaines, IL: Author.

4. Schreiber, D. (2009, April 8). *Spinal cord injuries.* Retrieved from http://emedicine.medscape.com/article/793582-overview

5. Nayduch, D. A. (2010). Acute spinal cord injury. *Nursing 2010, 40*(9), 25–34.

6. Hockberger, R. S., Kaji, A. H., & Newton, E. (2010). Spinal injuries. In J. A. Marx (Ed.), *Rosen's emergency medicine: Concepts and clinical practice* (7th ed.). Philadelphia, PA: Mosby.

7. Goodrich, J. A., & Riddle, T. (2010, May 14). *Lower cervical spine fractures and dislocations.* Retrieved from http://emedicine.medscape.com/article/1264065-overview

8. Greenbaum, J., Walters, N., & Levy, P. D. (2009). An evidence-based approach to radiographic assessment of cervical spine injuries in the emergency department. *Journal of Emergency Medicine, 36*(1), 64–71.

9. American College of Surgeons Committee. (2008) *Advanced trauma life support for doctors* (8th ed.). Chicago, IL: Author.

10. University of Southern California Center for Spinal Surgery. (n.d.). *Cervical spine fractures and dislocations.* Retrieved from http://www.uscspine.com/conditions/neck-fractures.cfm

11. Campagnolo, D. I. (2009, July 2). *Autonomic dysreflexia in spinal cord injury.* Retrieved from http://emedicine.medscape.com/article/322809-overview

12. Spinal Injury Network. (n.d.). *Autonomic dysreflexia.* Retrieved from http://www.spinal-injury.net/autonomic-dysreflexia.htm

13. Levy, D. B., & Gruber, B. S. (2010, December 7). *Neck trauma.* Retrieved from http://emedicine.medscape.com/article/827223-overview

14. Alterman, D. M., & Daley, B. J. (2009, November 19). *Penetrating neck trauma.* Retrieved from http://emedicine.medscape.com/article/433306-overview

15. Pancholi, S. S., Robbins, W. K., Desai, A., & Desai, T. (2010, January 9). *Laryngeal fractures.* Retrieved from http://emedicine.medscape.com/article/865277-overview

Chest Trauma

Faye P. Everson

Chest trauma, whether blunt or penetrating in nature, is a significant source of morbidity and mortality in the United States. Because the chest contains major organs responsible for ventilation, oxygenation, and circulation, traumatic injuries to the chest may disrupt the body's most vital functions. Chest injuries can affect any one or all components of the chest wall and thoracic cavity. Direct injury to bony structures alters the mechanics of ventilation, and damage to the lung parenchyma interferes with gas exchange or oxygenation. Cardiac output is adversely affected because of primary cardiac damage or dysfunction, changes in intrathoracic pressure and diminished venous return, or disruption of major vessels and massive blood loss.

The most common cause of chest trauma is motor vehicle crashes (MVCs). Acts of violence, falls, blast injuries, and pedestrian versus automobile collisions are other etiologies of chest injuries. Chest or thoracic injuries can be categorized as immediately life-threatening, potentially life-threatening, or non–life-threatening (Table 38-1).

In any trauma patient, rapid initial assessment and identification and treatment of life-threatening conditions are immediate priorities; many life-threatening conditions are a result of chest trauma. Table 38-2 lists some abnormal findings on initial assessment and the life-threatening conditions to be considered and ruled out. See Chapter 35, Assessment and Stabilization of the Trauma Patient, for a detailed discussion of the approach used with any trauma victim.

IMMEDIATELY LIFE-THREATENING CHEST INJURIES

Tension Pneumothorax

Tension pneumothorax occurs when air enters the pleural space during inspiration and is unable to escape during exhalation. Air accumulates in the thoracic cavity causing life-threatening hemodynamic compromise. The increasing intrathoracic pressure initially causes collapse of the lung on the injured side. As pressure from the accumulating air continues to rise, the opposite lung collapses and the mediastinum shifts, compressing the heart and great vessels. Venous return, and thus cardiac output, is markedly decreased. Immediate intervention is needed.

Tension pneumothorax is caused by blunt or penetrating trauma or is a complication of mechanical ventilation. A patient with a small pneumothorax may develop a tension pneumothorax shortly after positive pressure ventilation, with either bag-mask or mechanical ventilator, has been initiated.

Signs and Symptoms

- Severe respiratory distress: dyspnea, restlessness, and tachypnea
- Signs of decreasing cardiac output: tachycardia, hypotension, poor peripheral perfusion, cyanosis, and restlessness
- Jugular vein distension because of mediastinal shift and "kinking" of the great vessels
- Deviated trachea, away from the affected side (points to the "good" lung) and possible mediastinal deviation
- Hyperresonance with percussion of chest wall on affected side
- Distant heart sounds
- Symptoms such as jugular vein distension, tracheal shift and cyanosis will become increasingly worse as the condition worsens, and the patient may show signs of continued hypoxic deterioration such as decreasing levels of consciousness.

Diagnostic Procedures

- Clinical findings may indicate need for needle decompression (see "Therapeutic Interventions" below) of the affected lung before performing specific diagnostic procedures, such as a chest radiograph

TABLE 38-1	CLASSIFICATION OF CHEST TRAUMA	
IMMEDIATELY LIFE-THREATENING CHEST INJURIES	**POTENTIALLY LIFE-THREATENING CHEST INJURIES**	**NON–LIFE-THREATENING CHEST INJURIES**
Tension pneumothorax	Aortic disruption	Simple pneumothorax
Cardiac tamponade	Blunt cardiac trauma (cardiac contusion)	Rib fracture
Open pneumothorax	Pulmonary contusion	Sternal fracture
Massive hemothorax	Tracheobronchial disruption	Clavicular fracture
Flail chest	Diaphragmatic tear	Scapular fracture
	Esophageal disruption	

TABLE 38-2	ABNORMAL ASSESSMENT FINDINGS RELATED TO LIFE-THREATENING CHEST INJURIES
ASSESSMENT FINDING	**POSSIBLE INJURY OR CAUSE**
Breathing	
Unequal breath sounds, unequal chest expansion	Pneumothorax
	Hemothorax
	Foreign body obstruction
	Misplacement of endotracheal tube
	Tension pneumothorax
Paradoxical chest movement	Flail chest
Chest wall wound	Open ("sucking") chest wound
Subcutaneous air	Tracheobronchial disruption
Bowel sounds auscultated in chest	Ruptured diaphragm
Circulation	
Signs of shock	Massive hemothorax
• Poor skin perfusion	Tension pneumothorax
• Altered level of consciousness	Aortic disruption
	Cardiac tamponade
• Tachycardia	
• Hypotension	
Muffled heart sounds	Cardiac tamponade
Jugular venous distension, elevated central venous pressure	Cardiac tamponade
	Tension pneumothorax
Difference in blood pressure in arms	Incomplete aortic transection

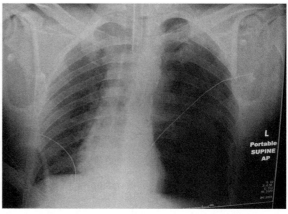

Fig. 38-1 Tension pneumothorax seen in intubated patient. (From Marx, J., Hockberger, R., & Walls, R. [Eds.]. [2009]. *Rosen's emergency medicine* [7th ed.]. St. Louis, MO: Mosby.)

- Chest radiograph: tracheal deviation and mediastinal shift may be evident (Fig. 38-1)

> Do *not* delay needle decompression of a clinically evident tension pneumothorax to obtain a confirming chest radiograph.

Therapeutic Interventions

- Support the patient's airway, breathing, and circulation; administer supplemental oxygen.
- Perform immediate needle decompression if severe hemodynamic compromise is present.
  - Use 14- or 16-gauge over-the-needle catheter, 3 to 6 cm in length (18- or 20-gauge for pediatric patient).
  - Insert needle just above the third rib into the second intercostal space (ICS), midclavicular line, on the affected side.
  - Air under pressure will be released. Remove needle stylet, leaving the catheter in place until chest tube

can be inserted. Connect to Heimlich flutter valve if unable to insert chest tube immediately.
- Prepare for immediate chest tube insertion.
- Provide pain control.

Cardiac Tamponade

Cardiac tamponade is the collection of blood or blood clots in the pericardial sac; the accumulating blood exerts pressure on the heart, limiting ventricular filling and decreasing cardiac output. The decrease in cardiac function is directly related to both rate and amount of fluid accumulation. If accumulation is rapid, as little as 100 to 150 mL of blood in the pericardial sac can adversely affect cardiac output. The leading cause of cardiac tamponade is penetrating chest injuries (80% to 90%) such as stab wounds.[1]

Signs and Symptoms

- Chest pain
- Tachycardia, tachypnea, and dyspnea
- Beck's triad (present in only about one third of patients with tamponade)[2]
  - Hypotension
  - Distended neck veins (may be absent with severe hypovolemia)
  - Muffled or distant heart sounds
- Altered mental status
- Pulsus paradoxus—a decrease in systolic blood pressure greater than 10 mm Hg during inspiration, caused by a decrease in venous return

Diagnostic Procedures

- Electrocardiogram (ECG) may show:
  - Low-voltage QRS complexes
  - Pulseless electrical activity
  - Electrical alternans—alternating amplitude of QRS complexes
- Chest radiograph may be normal initially; possibly widened mediastinum or enlarged heart shadow
- Focused Assessment with Sonography for Trauma (FAST) during the primary and secondary assessments has a significant false negative rate
- Bedside echocardiography
- Chest computed tomography (CT) scan if patient is hemodynamically stable

Therapeutic Interventions

- Support airway, breathing, and circulation; administer supplemental oxygen.
- Rapid infusion of intravenous fluids to increase cardiac filling pressures.
- In the hemodynamically unstable patient, needle pericardiocentesis may be needed to temporarily

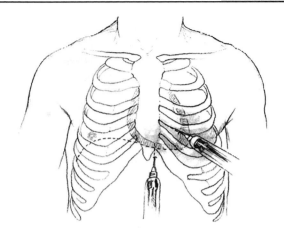

Fig. 38-2 Pericardiocentesis for acute cardiac tamponade. (From Davis, J. H., Foster, R. S., & Gamelli, R. L. [1991]. *Essentials of clinical surgery.* St. Louis, MO: Mosby.)

decompress the heart, "buying time" for transfer to the operating room or tertiary center (Fig. 38-2).
- Surgical intervention is generally needed.

Open Pneumothorax

If a penetrating chest wound communicates with the plural space, room air enters the thorax and normal negative intrathoracic pressure is lost. As with a closed pneumothorax, the lung on the affected side collapses. Air continues to enter and exit the chest cavity through the wound as the patient breathes, producing a "sucking" sound. If the chest wound is approximately two thirds the diameter of the trachea, air may preferentially enter the plural space with inspiration rather than via the patient's upper airways. This situation results in severe hypoxia and hypercapnea.[3]

Signs and Symptoms

- History of penetrating chest trauma; visible chest wound (may be as small as an ice pick hole)
- Signs of respiratory distress: dyspnea, tachypnea, restlessness, and cyanosis
- "Sucking" sound heard with respiration
- Asymmetric chest expansion (Fig. 38-3)
- Bubbling of blood around a chest wound with exhalation. Subcutaneous emphysema may also develop

Diagnostic Procedures

- Clinical assessment findings
- Chest radiograph will show evidence of a pneumothorax

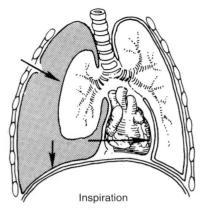
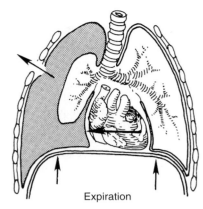

Inspiration   Expiration

Fig. 38-3 Open pneumothorax. (From Marx, J. A., Hockberger, R. S., & Walls, R. M. [Eds]. [2006]. *Rosen's emergency medicine: Concepts and clinical practice* [6th ed.]. St. Louis, MO: Mosby.)

Therapeutic Interventions

- Support airway, breathing, and circulation; administer supplemental oxygen.
- Immediately cover the wound with an occlusive dressing taped on three sides.

> Taping the occlusive dressing on three sides creates a flutter valve effect with an open pneumothorax. As the patient breathes in, the dressing prevents air from entering the pleural space; on exhalation, air is allowed to escape through the open end of the dressing thus preventing the development of a tension pneumothorax.[3]

- Observe patient closely for development of tension pneumothorax (increasing respiratory distress, jugular venous distension, hypotension). If tension pneumothorax occurs, remove dressing immediately to relieve tension.
- Prepare for immediate chest tube insertion.

Hemothorax

Hemothorax is the accumulation of blood in the pleural space and may result from either blunt or penetrating trauma (Fig. 38-4). Often accompanied by a pneumothorax, bleeding is the result of laceration of the intercostal vessels or internal mammary arteries, or from direct lung parenchymal damage. Massive hemothorax results from the rapid accumulation of more than 1500 mL of blood in the chest cavity and leads to respiratory and circulatory failure.

Signs and Symptoms

- Signs of respiratory distress: dyspnea and tachypnea
- Pain on inspiration
- Asymmetric chest wall movement

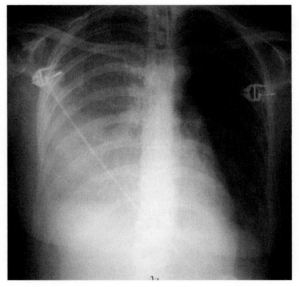

Fig. 38-4 Hemothorax. (From Adam, A., & Dixon, A. K. [Eds.]. [2008]. *Grainger & Allison's diagnostic radiology* [5th ed.]. Philadelphia, PA: Churchill Livingstone.)

- Clinical signs of hypovolemic shock: tachypnea, tachycardia, hypotension, cool clammy skin, decreased capillary refill, restlessness, and confusion
- Decreased breath sounds on the affected side
- Dullness to percussion on the affected side

Diagnostic Procedures

- Draw serial complete blood counts: may show a decreasing hemoglobin and hematocrit

TABLE 38-3	ADVANTAGES AND DISADVANTAGES OF AUTOTRANSFUSION	
ADVANTAGES	**DISADVANTAGES**
Immediately available	Limited to noncontaminated wounds
No incompatibility concerns	Requires special equipment and some operator training
Elimination of complications related to storage of blood (hyperkalemia, hypocalcemia, metabolic acidosis)	Cannot be used with wounds >4 to 6 hours old
Blood is at body temperature, minimizing secondary hypothermia	
May be acceptable to patients with religious objections to blood transfusion	

- Obtain a chest radiograph: may show blunting of the costophrenic angle in the upright position

Therapeutic Interventions

- Support airway and breathing; administer supplemental oxygen.
- Restore circulating blood volume with intravenous crystalloids and blood products.
- Assist with chest tube placement.
  - Large-size (36 to 38 French) tube should be inserted just anterior to midaxillary line, at the fourth or fifth ICS.
  - Attach chest tube to suction.
  - Keep the drainage unit below the level of the chest to facilitate flow of drainage.
  - Keep the unit upright to prevent loss of the water seal.
  - Assess and document **f**luctuation of drainage in the tubing, amount of **o**utput, **c**olor of drainage, and presence or absence of **a**ir leak, also referred to as FOCA assessment.
- Consider autotransfusion (Table 38-3).
- Prepare for emergent surgery if initial drainage is more than 1500 mL or initial drainage of 1000 mL is followed by 200 mL per hour for 2 to 4 hours.

Flail Chest

Flail chest occurs when two or more adjacent ribs are fractured in two or more places or when the sternum is detached. The flail segment loses continuity with the rest of the chest

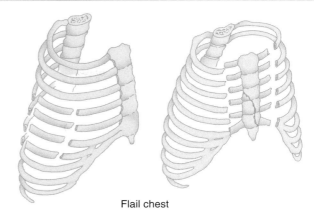

Flail chest

Fig. 38-5 Flail chest. (From Marx, J., Hockberger, R., & Walls, R. [Eds.]. [2009]. *Rosen's emergency medicine* [7th ed.]. St. Louis, MO: Mosby.)

wall and responds to changes in intrathoracic pressure in a paradoxical manner (Fig. 38-5). Paradoxical motion refers to movement of the flail segment in the direction opposite that of the intact chest wall. Instead of moving outward on inspiration, the flail segment is drawn inward; on exhalation, the flail segment is pushed outward. Often the flail segment is not observed initially, only becoming evident as the patient tires from the increased work of breathing. Pulmonary mechanics are disrupted by flail chest but the underlying pulmonary injury is of greater significance.

Signs and Symptoms

- Chest pain and bony crepitus
- Respiratory distress: dyspnea, tachypnea, and eventual respiratory failure
- Hemothorax and pneumothorax
- Asymmetric or paradoxical movement of chest wall
- Possible subcutaneous emphysema

Diagnostic Procedures

- Chest radiograph and CT scan show rib or sternal fractures
- Arterial blood gases (ABGs) to determine ventilation status

Therapeutic Interventions

- Pain management with systemic narcotics, intercostal nerve block, or epidural block.
- Administer supplemental oxygen to maintain pO_2 of 80 to 100 mm Hg; continuous pulse oximetry monitoring.
- Possible endotracheal intubation with mechanical ventilation and positive end expiratory pressure (PEEP).

- Insert chest tube if pneumothorax or hemothorax is present.
- Correct hypovolemia; judiciously administer further intravenous crystalloid fluids because of the probable underlying pulmonary contusion.
- Consider arterial catheter placement for frequent ABG determination.
- Prepare for admission or transfer to a tertiary facility.
- Anticipate possible surgery for internal fixation of the flail segment.
- Do not attempt to stabilize the flail segment by applying sandbags; splinting the flail segment with rolled towels may be beneficial if it increases the patient's tidal volume.[1]

> *Commotio cordis* refers to sudden cardiac death resulting from ventricular fibrillation following a seemingly insignificant blow to the chest. It occurs most often in young, healthy athletes during a sporting event. If defibrillation is performed immediately, survival is possible. Preventive measures include wearing chest protection during sports and making automatic external defibrillators available in schools and at sporting events.

Myocardial Rupture

Traumatic myocardial rupture may involve perforation of the ventricles (most commonly) or atria or laceration or rupture of the ventricular septum or valvular apparatus (leaflets, chordae tendineae, papillary muscle). Not surprisingly, the most common cause of myocardial rupture is a high-speed MVC. It is almost always immediately fatal with death resulting from exsanguination or cardiac tamponade. If the pericardium remains intact, bleeding may be temporarily contained, allowing the patient to survive immediate transport to the emergency department.

Signs and Symptoms

- Signs and symptoms consistent with exsanguination or cardiac tamponade
  - Severe hypotension unresponsive to fluid resuscitation
  - Distended neck veins; may be absent with hypovolemia
  - Distant heart sounds
- Loud, harsh murmur
- Cyanosis of upper torso, arms, and head
- May be little evidence of thoracic trauma or massive chest injuries

Diagnostic Procedures

- Chest radiograph to detect other chest injuries such as hemopneumothorax
- FAST examination, transthoracic echocardiogram (TTE), and transesophageal echocardiogram (TEE)

Therapeutic Interventions

- Minimize prehospital on-scene time ("load and go"), particularly in urban settings.
- Immediate surgical intervention is the treatment of choice.
- Pericardiocentesis may be performed as a temporary measure until surgery can be performed.
- If patient arrives at the emergency department with vital signs and then experiences cardiopulmonary arrest, open thoracotomy (resuscitative thoracotomy) should be considered.

POTENTIALLY LIFE-THREATENING CHEST TRAUMA

Injuries to the Aorta

Injuries to the aorta can range from a small intimal tear (partial transection) to complete aortic rupture that results in rapid exsanguination and an early mortality rate of 60% to 90%.[4] If the transection is partial, the patient may survive transfer to the hospital, but nearly all of these patients have associated serious injuries.[4] The most common sites of aortic injury are distal to the left subclavian artery (aortic isthmus) and the aortic root.

Signs and Symptoms

- History of sudden deceleration injury (MVC without seat belt, ejection from vehicle, fall from great height)
- Signs of significant chest wall trauma (scapula fracture, first or second rib fracture, sternal fracture, steering wheel imprint)
- Chest pain
- Back pain
- Signs of respiratory distress: dyspnea and tachypnea
- Signs of circulatory compromise: tachycardia, hypotension, altered level of consciousness, and poor peripheral perfusion
- Loud murmur in left parascapular region
- Unequal blood pressure in upper extremities
- Paraplegia resulting from ischemia distal to the aortic injury

Diagnostic Procedures

- Chest radiograph
  - Widened mediastinum
  - Blurring or obliteration of aortic knob
  - Hemothorax
  - Elevation of right main stem bronchus
- Chest CT if the patient is hemodynamically stable
- FAST examination of the chest, TEE, or TTE

- Aortography is the gold standard for detecting aortic injuries, allowing visualization of the aorta and any tears or occlusions[1]

Therapeutic Interventions

- Support airway and breathing; administer supplemental oxygen.
- Control hemorrhage regardless of source (hemopneumothorax, unstable pelvis or long bone fractures, intracranial bleeding).[4]
- Volume resuscitation with crystalloids and blood products.
- If transection is partial, administer short-acting beta-blockers (labetalol, esmolol) to decrease heart rate and decrease mean arterial pressure to approximately 60 mm Hg. This therapy may allow for transfer to a tertiary care facility.
- Endovascular stent placement at site of partial transection is often possible.[5]
- Open surgery with cardiopulmonary bypass may be necessary.

Blunt Cardiac Injury

Blunt cardiac injury (BCI) occurs more often than is diagnosed; it may be overlooked because of the presence of other more obvious injuries. BCI should be considered when the mechanism of injury is an MVC with acceleration-deceleration injuries (particularly when the chest strikes the steering wheel), a crush injury, or a fall from heights. BCI may also be caused by chest compressions during cardiopulmonary resuscitation (CPR).

The myocardial changes associated with BCI can range from scattered areas of petechiae and microscopic contusion to lacerations and full thickness wall damage. These injuries result in some degree of myocardial dysfunction.[2]

Signs and Symptoms

- Chest pain may be mild to severe, generally does not radiate to the arm or jaw, and is unrelieved by nitroglycerin[6]
- Chest wall contusions and abrasions
- Tachycardia and hypotension
- Dyspnea
- Possibly signs of cardiac tamponade

Diagnostic Procedures

- High index of suspicion based on mechanism of injury
- Continuous cardiac monitoring may reveal sinus tachycardia, premature ventricular or atrial contractions, atrial fibrillation

- 12-lead ECG may show elevated ST segments in V1, V2, and V3 and right bundle branch block pattern
- Transesophageal or transthoracic echocardiogram to identify abnormal left ventricular wall motion
- Creatine kinase MB and troponin may be elevated but this finding is not an accurate predictor of BCI[7]

Therapeutic Interventions

- Management is similar to that for patients experiencing acute myocardial infarction, with the exception of fibrinolytic therapy.
- Administer supplemental oxygen.
- Place patient in the semi-Fowler's position and allow bed rest.
- Administer analgesia for chest pain.
- Transfer patient to intensive care unit admission for hemodynamic and cardiac monitoring.
- If there are signs of cardiac failure, use vasopressors to maintain systolic blood pressure of 90 mm Hg and inotropes to improve contractility.

Pulmonary Contusion

Pulmonary contusion is the most common potentially life-threatening chest injury[7] and can occur with any severe blunt chest trauma (MVC, fall from heights), high-velocity missile wounds, or significant barotrauma from an explosion. Bruising of the lung parenchyma results in damage to the alveolar-capillary membrane and alveolar edema and hemorrhage. The resulting respiratory failure may develop over several hours and thus becomes apparent once the patient is in the intensive care unit rather than in the emergency department. Therefore a high index of suspicion should guide the assessment and management of these patients.

Signs and Symptoms

- Signs of respiratory distress: dyspnea, tachypnea, restlessness, and agitation
- Chest pain and chest wall bruising
- Ineffective cough or hemoptysis
- Decreased breath sounds, crackles, and wheezes
- Presence of other severe chest injuries

Diagnostic Procedures

- Chest radiograph may reveal infiltrates but these may not be present until 12 hours or more after injury
- ABGs to monitor for progressive hypoxemia
- Continuous SpO_2 monitoring

Therapeutic Interventions

- Administer high-flow supplemental oxygen; advanced airway management may become necessary if hypoxemia is significant or progressive.

- Be cautious with fluid resuscitation to minimize development of interstitial pulmonary edema.
- Consider arterial line placement for frequent ABG determinations.
- Consider noninvasive ventilatory support to avoid endotracheal intubation and mechanical ventilation, which are associated with increased morbidity (ventilator-associated pneumonia, sepsis) and length of stay in hospital.[8]
- Provide for adequate pain control.

Tracheobronchial Disruption

Traumatic disruption of the tracheobronchial tree is a rare injury resulting from blunt or, more likely, penetrating chest trauma. Disruption occurs most commonly within 2 cm of the carina.[1] Consider tracheobronchial injury in the presence of a karate-type kick or clothesline injury, or when the mechanism of injury includes hitting the neck on the steering wheel in a MVC. If the patient has sustained a direct blow or penetrating injury to the neck, assess for concomitant cervical or thoracic injuries.

Signs and Symptoms

- Signs of airway obstruction: may be immediate or progressive
- Signs of respiratory distress: dyspnea and tachypnea
- Hoarseness
- Hemoptysis
- Subcutaneous emphysema in neck, face, or suprasternal area
- Hamman's sign (crunching or bubbling sound, synchronous with the heartbeat, auscultated over the precordium) indicating mediastinal air
- Decreased or absent breath sounds
- Possible tension pneumothorax
- Persistent air leak in chest drainage system

Diagnostic Procedures

- Chest radiograph to look for mediastinal air, pneumothorax, concurrent rib fractures
- Bronchoscopy to detect the disruption

Therapeutic Interventions

- Maintaining a patent airway may necessitate endotracheal intubation or tracheostomy.
- Administer high-flow supplemental oxygen.
- Anticipate chest tube and mediastinal tube placement.
- If no contraindication from associated injuries, place patient in semi-Fowler's position.
- Anticipate possible surgical repair.

Diaphragm Rupture

Diaphragmatic rupture can result from penetrating trauma, such as gunshot or stab wounds, or blunt trauma caused by high-speed MVCs. Most ruptures occur in the left hemidiaphragm because the right diaphragm is structurally stronger and is partially protected by the liver.[9] A rupture or tear in the diaphragm allows abdominal contents to herniate into the chest cavity. This causes interference with adequate respiration and ventilation. Injuries to the lower thoracic or upper abdomen should raise the index of suspicion for this injury. Rupture of the diaphragm is not often diagnosed in the initial resuscitation period; mortality rate is increased by delayed identification.

Signs and Symptoms

- Dyspnea and orthopnea
- Dysphagia (difficulty swallowing)
- Bowel sounds in thoracic cavity
- Abdominal pain, may radiate to left shoulder (Kehr's sign)
- Decreased breath sounds on affected side
- Undigested food or fecal matter in chest tube drainage

Diagnostic Procedures

- Chest radiograph (Fig. 38-6) initially may be normal but assess for:
  - Elevated left diaphragm
  - Herniation of bowel into the chest

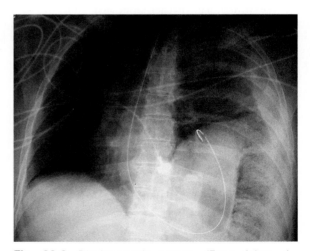

Fig. 38-6 Diaphragmatic rupture. (From Adam, A., & Dixon, A. K. [Eds.]. [2008]. *Graigner & Allison's diagnostic radiology* [5th ed.]. Philadelphia, PA: Churchill Livingstone.)

- Orogastric or nasogastric tube coiled in chest cavity
- Absence of costophrenic angle on the side opposite the injury
- CT of chest and abdomen
- FAST examination may indicate elevation of the diaphragm

Therapeutic Interventions

- Maintenance of airway, breathing, and circulation
- Orogastric or nasogastric tube to decompress the stomach
- Emergent surgical intervention or prompt transfer to tertiary facility for repair

Esophageal Disruption

The esophagus is well protected by its location in the posterior mediastinum and traumatic esophageal disruption is rare. It is usually not an isolated injury and may be the result of blunt or penetrating trauma.[10] Esophageal rupture should always be considered with first and second rib fractures, cervical spine fracture, and laryngotracheal tears.

Signs and Symptoms

- Sudden onset of severe chest or neck pain following injury
- Tachypnea, dyspnea, stridor, and airway compromise
- Pain on swallowing and dysphagia
- Subcutaneous emphysema
- Hamman's sign: crunching sound heard with each heartbeat caused by accumulation of air in the mediastinum
- Pneumothorax and hemothorax
- Gastric contents or bile in chest tube drainage
- Intra-abdominal free air
- High mortality due to sepsis if diagnosis is delayed more than 24 hours[11]

Diagnostic Procedures

- Chest radiograph may show:
  - Elevation of the hemidiaphragm
  - Possible bowel pattern in the chest
  - Nasogastric tube passing into the abdomen and curling up into the chest
- If patient is stable, upper gastrointestinal series, esophagoscopy, or gastroscopy may be performed
- Bedside endoscopy

Therapeutic Interventions

- Support airway, breathing, and circulation; endotracheal intubation may be necessary.
- Obtain intravenous access and begin fluid administration.

- Anticipate emergent surgery or transfer to a tertiary facility for repair.

NON–LIFE-THREATENING CHEST TRAUMA

Simple Pneumothorax

A simple, or closed, pneumothorax occurs when a leak in the lungs, bronchi, or lower trachea allows air to accumulate in the pleural space. This causes a loss of negative pressure within the thorax and partial or total collapse of the lung. A closed pneumothorax is often caused by puncture of the lung by a rib or compression of the chest against a closed glottis (similar to blowing up and popping a paper bag); iatrogenic causes include attempts at subclavian or internal jugular venous cannulation. Occasionally pneumothorax results from barotrauma following a high-energy shock wave or explosion. Atraumatic spontaneous pneumothorax can occur as the result of a ruptured bleb or cyst.

Signs and Symptoms

- History of blunt chest trauma or blast injury
- Sudden onset of sharp, pleuritic chest pain
- Signs of respiratory distress: dyspnea and tachypnea
- Diminished breath sounds on the affected side
- Asymmetric chest wall movement

Diagnostic Procedures

- Evidence of pneumothorax on chest radiograph

Therapeutic Interventions

- Administer supplemental oxygen; continuous SpO_2 monitoring.
- If no contraindications, place patient in semi-Fowler's position to promote chest expansion.
- Prepare for chest tube insertion as indicated.

Rib Fractures

Rib fractures are the most commonly seen thoracic injury. Fractures often result from a direct blow to the chest but also can be caused by penetrating objects such as a fence post or a bullet. Iatrogenic rib fractures occur as a consequence of chest compressions or abdominal thrusts.

Ribs generally fracture at the angle junctures, their weakest point. The most frequently fractured are ribs 4 through 9. Fractures of the sternum or first or second rib indicate that significant force has impacted the body; consider concomitant cardiac or vascular injuries. On the other hand, lower rib fractures may result in diaphragmatic tears or liver and spleen injuries and subsequent bleeding.

Always consider the possibility of serious injury to underlying structures if a first rib fracture, multiple rib fractures, or a flail chest is present. Fractures of the first, second, and third ribs are associated with higher mortality given their proximity to the subclavian vessels, aorta, and tracheobronchial tree.

Signs and Symptoms

- Pain that increases with motion and inspiration
- Point tenderness (the patient can point to the exact location of the pain)
- Splinting of chest muscles to decrease chest wall motion with inspiration
- Abrasions, redness, or ecchymosis at site of injury and pain
- Palpable deformity (step-off defect) if the fracture is displaced
- Bony crepitus at fracture site
- Subcutaneous emphysema possible if associated lung or tracheobronchial injury

Diagnostic Procedures

- Chest radiograph to identify fractures and to rule out additional thoracic injuries
- Chest CT to evaluate soft tissue injuries
- Arteriography if vascular injuries are suspected

Therapeutic Interventions

- Provide pain management with oral analgesics, intercostal nerve block, or epidural anesthesia to promote adequate chest expansion and ventilation.[3]
- Restrict activity.
- Administer cold therapy for the first 2 hours, then heat therapy.
- Elderly patients and those with comorbidities have decreased pulmonary reserves and may require hospitalization.
- Monitor respiratory status closely to detect early deterioration.
- Instruct patient in the proper use of incentive spirometer.
- The ribs of small children are cartilaginous and generally bend rather than break; consider maltreatment in any child with unexplained rib fractures.
- Rib belts or binders may restrict chest movement, promoting atelectasis, and are contraindicated.

Sternal Fractures

A tremendous amount of force is needed to fracture the sternum; it is rarely an isolated injury. The most common site of fracture is the junction of the manubrium and the body of the sternum (angle of Louis) at the second ICS. A totally detached sternum is considered a flail segment requiring treatment as described earlier in this chapter (see "Flail Chest").

Sternal fractures are generally the result of a direct blow, often from high-speed impact against the steering wheel in a MVC. Particularly in elderly patients, sternal fracture may be a complication of CPR.

Signs and Symptoms

- Chest pain, especially with inspiration
- Ecchymosis of the sternal area and soft tissue swelling
- Palpation of the fracture
- ECG changes and arrhythmias: premature ventricular contractions, atrial fibrillation, right bundle branch block, and ST segment changes

Diagnostic Procedures

- Chest radiograph and chest CT to view fracture (Fig. 38-7)
- 12-lead ECG and continuous cardiac monitoring to detect dysrhythmias and conduction disturbances
- Cardiac biomarkers to rule out concomitant blunt cardiac trauma

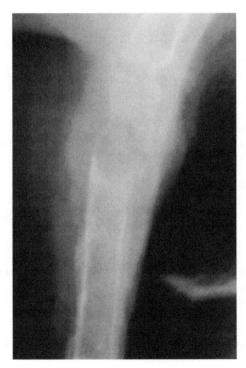

Fig. 38-7 Fracture of the sternum. (From Resnick, D. & Kransdorf, M. [2005]. *Bone and joint imaging* [3rd ed.]. Philadelphia, PA: Saunders.)

Therapeutic Interventions

- Frequent reassessment to detect possible pulmonary contusion or blunt cardiac trauma
- Pain control to facilitate adequate ventilation
- Possible surgery for sternal fixation

Clavicular Fractures

The clavicles are frequently and easily fractured. Clavicular fractures can result from almost any blunt force and are typically seen in athletic injuries from a lateral blow or a fall on an outstretched hand. These fractures are the most common among all pediatric fractures and generally not considered serious.[12] Clavicular fractures are usually closed injuries and are categorized based on the location of the break: distal (15%), middle (80%), and medial (5%).[12] Medial fractures (near the sternum) can be associated with other injuries, such as first rib fracture, sternal fracture, and great vessel injuries.

Signs and Symptoms

- Pain, swelling, and bruising over fracture site
- Palpable step-off defect
- Inferior and anterior displacement of shoulder secondary to loss of support
- Decreased pulses, sensation, and motor weakness

Diagnostic Procedures

- Chest radiograph to visualize fracture and rule out pneumothorax
- Consider arteriogram to rule out vascular injury

Therapeutic Interventions

- Ice packs to the affected area.
- Nonsteroidal anti-inflammatory drugs or narcotics for pain management.
- Immobilization with a simple sling or sling and swath.
- Carefully assess pulses in arm on side of injury to identify possible subclavian or other vessel injuries.
- Check neurologic status in arm on side of injury to detect possible damage to brachial plexus.
- Anticipate closed reduction of displaced fractures or surgery for open reduction of open fractures.

Scapular Fractures

A great deal of force and energy are required to fracture the scapula. A rare injury, it is usually the result of a high-speed MVC or a fall from height and is generally associated with other significant chest and lung injuries.

Signs and Symptoms

- Significant pain with movement
- If conscious, the patient may hold arm close to body
- Tenderness, crepitus, swelling, and hematoma over fracture site

Diagnostic Procedures

- Chest or shoulder radiograph; fractured scapula initially may be overlooked because of associated life-threatening injuries

Therapeutic Interventions

- Treatment of possible concomitant life-threatening injuries
- Pain management
- Immobilization with sling
- Surgery for open reduction of severely displaced fractures

REFERENCES

1. Yamamoto, L., Schroeder, C., Morley, D., & Beliveau, C. (2005). Thoracic trauma: The deadly dozen. *Critical Care Nursing Quarterly*, 28(1), 22–40.
2. Jones, L. B., & Lome, B. (2006). Delayed cardiac tamponade following blunt chest trauma. *Advanced Emergency Nursing Journal*, 28(4), 275–283.
3. American College of Surgeons. (2008). *Advanced trauma life support for doctors* (8th ed.). Chicago, IL: Author.
4. Cook, J., Salerno, C., Krishnadasan, B., Nicholls, S., Meissner, M., & Karmy-Jones R. (2006). The effect of changing presentation and management on the outcome of blunt rupture of the thoracic aorta. *Journal of Thoracic and Cardiovascular Surgery*, 131, 594–600.
5. Tehrani, H. Y., Peterson, B. G., Katariya, K., Morasch, M. D., Stevens, R., DiLuozzo, G., ... Eskandari, M. K. (2006). Endovascular repair of thoracic aortic tears. *Annals of Thoracic Surgery*, 82, 873–878.
6. Rauen, C. A., & Wolfe, A. C. (2009). Cardiac contusion and the 12-lead ECG. *AACN Advanced Critical Care*, 20(3), 301–304.
7. Velmahos, G. C., & Butt, M. U. (2008). Cardiac and pulmonary injury. *European Journal of Trauma and Emergency Surgery*, 34, 327–337.
8. Hernandez, G., Fernandez, R., Lopez-Reina, P., Cuena, R., Pedrosa, A., Ortiz, R., & Hiradier, P. (2010). Noninvasive ventilation reduces intubation in chest trauma-related hypoxemia: A randomized clinical trial. *Chest*, 137(1), 74–80.
9. Mihos, P., Potaris, K., Gakidis, J., Paraskevopoulos, J., Varvatsoulis, P., Gougoutas, B., ... Lapidakis, E. (2003). Traumatic rupture of the diaphragm: Experience with 65 patients. *Injury*, 34, 169–172.
10. Eckstein, M., & Henderson, S. O. (2010). Thoracic trauma. In J. A. Marx (Ed.), *Rosen's emergency medicine: Concepts and clinical practice* (7th ed.). Philadelphia, PA: Mosby.
11. Brinster, C. J., Singhal, S., Lee, L., Marshall, M. B., Kaiser, L. R., & Kucharczuk, J. C. (2004). Evolving options in the management of esophageal perforation. *Annals of Thoracic Surgery*, 77, 1475–1483.
12. Estephan, A., & Gore, R. J. (2010, September 28). Clavicle fracture in emergency medicine. Retrieved from http://emedicine.medscape.com/article/824564-overview

Abdominal Trauma

Catherine Harris

Abdominal injuries account for 13% to 15% of traumatic deaths, making this the third leading cause of trauma mortality.[1] Knowing the mechanism of injury, conducting a diligent physical examination, maintaining a high degree of suspicion, and performing serial evaluations are essential for reducing the morbidity and mortality related to abdominal trauma. The two mechanisms of injury most commonly associated with abdominal trauma are blunt and penetrating; each of these forces produces distinctive patterns of organ damage.

> Many blunt abdominal injuries are not evident on initial physical examination. Frequent reassessment is needed to detect injuries that manifest over time.

BLUNT TRAUMA

Blunt abdominal trauma (BAT) results when force is applied to the abdominal wall without creating an open wound.

- In the United States, motor vehicle crashes are the leading cause of BAT, responsible for 50% or more of significant injuries.[2]
- Other mechanisms of BAT are contact sports, falls, and physical abuse.[3]
- The abdominal viscera and other structures are injured by direct blows, compression, or deceleration.
  - Compression injuries occur from direct blows against a fixed object (lap belt, steering wheel, or the spine).
  - Deceleration forces between relatively fixed and free objects cause a shearing or tearing type of injury; part of the tissue continues to move forward while another part remains stationary.[4]
- The solid organs—most frequently the spleen, liver, and kidneys—are likely to rupture in response to blunt force.
- Although seat belts save lives, they are nonetheless associated with their own constellation of injuries, including visceral rupture, organ compression, orthopedic fractures, and abdominal vessel tears.
- The placement of the seat belt above the bony pelvic area can cause momentary trapping of the underlying tissue against the spine and lead to shearing and compression injuries.
- A red mark or bruise with the imprint of a seat belt may indicate underlying damage and requires frequent monitoring.
- Symptoms of seat belt injury may develop slowly.

PENETRATING TRAUMA

Penetrating trauma results when an object—such as a bullet, a knife blade, or projectile fragments—pierces the abdominal wall, entering the abdominal cavity.

- In the United States, the leading cause of penetrating abdominal trauma is interpersonal violence, particularly in urban settings.[1]
- Stab wounds most commonly produce intestinal injury, but many do not penetrate the peritoneal cavity. Thus they are associated with a lower mortality rate and may not require surgery.
- On the other hand, 96% to 98% of abdominal gunshot wounds involve significant damage to intra-abdominal organs and vessels, necessitating emergent operative intervention.[3]

PHYSICAL ASSESSMENT OF THE ABDOMEN

While penetrating injuries may be restricted to the abdomen, BAT is rarely an isolated event. Head and chest trauma, and other life-threatening injuries, routinely complicate assessment and care.

Perform a thorough physical examination with diagnostic procedures when assessing patients, particularly

TABLE 39-1	CLINICAL SIGNS ASSOCIATED WITH ABDOMINAL TRAUMA	
SIGN	**DESCRIPTION**	**INDICATION**
Ballance sign[a]	Fixed dullness to percussion in left flank and dullness in right flank that disappears with change of position	Presence of fluid blood on right side but coagulation on left side
Cullen sign	Bluish purple bruise or ecchymosis around the umbilicus	Retroperitoneal bleeding
Grey-Turner sign	Bluish purple bruise or ecchymosis over flank or back area	Retroperitoneal bleeding
Kehr's sign	Pain that radiates to the left shoulder	Intra-abdominal blood, fluid, or air irritating the phrenic nerve at the diaphragm
Rebound tenderness	Pain on release of deep palpation	Peritoneal irritation

[a]Seidel, H. M., Ball, J. W., Dains, J. E., Flynn, D. A., Soloman, B. S., & Stewart, R. W. (2010). *Mosby's physical examination handbook* (7th ed.) St. Louis, MO: Mosby.

individuals who are unconscious, are intoxicated, have altered level of consciousness at baseline, or have experienced a head injury. A person with concomitant spinal cord injuries will have altered sensations that will affect the abdominal examination. The absence of clinical findings does not rule out the presence of abdominal injury, especially in patients who are pregnant or have concurrent neurologic deficits.

Inspect the abdomen for the following:
- Obvious penetrating wounds
- Ecchymosis and abrasions
- Flank bruising
- Distension
- Rectal bleeding
- Testicular swelling
- Ballance, Cullen, or Grey-Turner signs (Table 39-1) Auscultate for bowel sounds in all four quadrants.
- Check for presence of a bruit, which may indicate traumatic arteriovenous fistula.[5]
- Auscultation should be done prior to percussion and palpation.

> Abdominal findings, particularly bowel sounds, are most useful when they are normal initially and change over time.

Percuss over the abdomen and costovertebral area for:
- Tympany indicating air in the abdomen as a result of bowel perforation
- Dullness related to blood, fluid, or a solid mass in the abdomen
Palpate the most painful area last to minimize distracting pain in other areas of the abdomen. Palpate for the following:
- Tenderness
- Rigidity
- Rebound tenderness

- Involuntary guarding is a reliable sign of peritoneal irritation[5]
- Pelvic instability

DIAGNOSTIC PROCEDURES

Laboratory Tests

- Complete blood count and complete metabolic and chemistry panels
- Serial hematocrit and hemoglobin levels
- Type and crossmatch
- Serum lactate and base deficit levels
- Coagulation studies and bleeding times
- Liver function tests, amylase, and lipase
- Urinalysis
- Pregnancy test in all females of childbearing age
- Possibly alcohol levels and toxicology screen
- Gastric contents and stool for occult blood determination

Focused Assessment with Sonography for Trauma

A focused assessment with sonography for trauma (FAST) examination is a rapid, bedside ultrasound of four to six specific abdominal areas (pericardial, perihepatic, perisplenic, and pelvic) (Fig. 39-1). This examination is used to identify free intraperitoneal or pericardial fluid in trauma. The FAST examination is extremely sensitive and can detect fluid volumes of 100 to 200 mL. Additionally, it is noninvasive, can be done concurrently with resuscitation, and takes less than 5 minutes. Unfortunately, the FAST examination cannot adequately assess the retroperitoneum or colorectal areas, nor is it very sensitive for evaluating solid organ and visceral damage. Indications for FAST examination include the following:
- Evidence of blunt or penetrating abdominal trauma
- Any patient with a mechanism highly suspicious for blunt injury

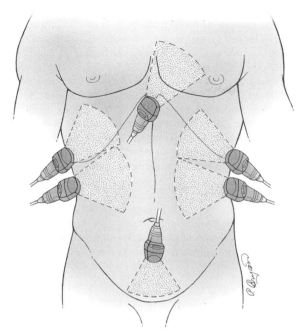

Fig. 39-1 FAST ultrasound examination. (From Rothrock, J. C. [2007]. *Alexander's care of the patient in surgery* [13th ed.]. St. Louis, MO: Mosby.)

Additional diagnostic studies should be performed if the FAST examination is negative.

Abdominal Computed Tomography

Abdominal computed tomography (CT) is a fast and accurate way to evaluate a large number of intra-abdominal injuries with high sensitivity for detecting solid organ lesions, vascular injuries, and intraperitoneal hemorrhage. Additionally, with the current trend toward nonoperative management of abdominal trauma, serial CT scans offer an excellent way to perform ongoing evaluation of intra-abdominal structures.[6]

Indications for abdominal CT include the following:

- Persons with obvious abdominal injuries or suggestive physical findings
- Hemodynamically stable patients whose FAST examination revealed intraperitoneal fluid
- Patients with a mechanism of injury highly suspicious for intra-abdominal trauma

Abdominal CT has limited use in the hemodynamically unstable patient because it is time-consuming, may involve the use of contrast media, and requires transport of the patient to the scanner.[5]

Diagnostic Peritoneal Lavage

Once common practice, diagnostic peritoneal lavage (DPL) has been largely replaced by CT scans for assessing abdominal injuries. It retains a place in the assessment of patients with blunt abdominal trauma who are hemodynamically unstable and when traveling to the CT scanner places a patient at risk for complications. As with the FAST examination, DPL does not access the retroperitoneum. DPL is not indicated in penetrating injury; these wounds require surgical exploration.

Indications for DPL include the following:

- Rapid assessment of the multitrauma patient who requires immediate surgery for severe head or chest injuries in whom abdominal trauma has not yet been ruled out. DPL can be quickly performed in the emergency department or operating room while other interventions are in progress.
- Evidence of blunt trauma to the abdomen in hemodynamically unstable patients with an equivocal FAST exam.[7]
- Hemodynamically stable patients in whom it is impossible to elicit reliable signs of BAT and for whom no CT scan available. This would include patients who are unconscious or intoxicated or who have sustained a spinal cord injury.

THERAPEUTIC INTERVENTIONS

A basic knowledge of injury mechanism can guide initial care of the abdominal trauma patient. It is not essential to determine immediately which specific abdominal structures have been injured.[2] The primary focus of care is on airway, breathing, and circulation assessment and basic stabilization, frequent assessment and reassessment, and diagnostic procedures. Signs of abdominal injuries can be subtle; ongoing assessment of the abdomen is needed to identify changes.

- Consider the possibility of concurrent thoracic injury (see Chapter 38, Chest Trauma) or spinal trauma (see Chapter 37, Spinal Cord and Neck Trauma) based on an abnormal breathing pattern. For example, abdominal breathing may be associated with spinal cord injury.[2]
- Administer supplemental oxygen.
- Assist ventilation as needed with a bag-mask or mechanical ventilation.
- Frequently assess circulatory status (heart rate, skin color and temperature, pulses, capillary refill, blood pressure), as patients with abdominal injuries can lose a large volume of blood.
- Insert two large-bore (14- to 16-gauge) intravenous (IV) catheters. Placement of a central line (by jugular,

subclavian, or femoral approach) may be necessary to infuse large volumes of fluid and to monitor central venous pressure.

- Infuse isotonic crystalloid solutions (lactated Ringer solution, normal saline). Warm all IV fluids to prevent hypothermia and acidosis.
- Because of the potential for fluid boluses to displace newly formed clots, the role of fluid resuscitation in the abdominal trauma patient is controversial. A judicious approach to volume replacement is recommended. Titrate IV fluids to a systolic blood pressure of 90 mm Hg to maintain vital organ perfusion.[2]

TABLE 39-2 INDICATIONS FOR EXPLORATORY LAPAROTOMY

Evidence of shock without obvious external blood loss	Free air in the abdomen
Evidence of peritonitis, particularly in the elderly and patients with severe head injury	Positive DPL results—aspiration of >10 mL frank blood or red cell count of peritoneal aspirate >100,000/mm³
Altered level of consciousness no matter the cause	Continuing decrease in hematocrit or hemoglobin

DPL, Diagnostic peritoneal lavage.
Data from Salomone, J. A., & Salomone, J. P. (2011, March 16). *Blunt abdominal trauma*. Retrieved from http://emedicine.medscape.com/article/821995-overview; Yanar, H., Ertekin, C., Taviloglu, K., Kabay, B., Bakkaloglu, H., & Guloglu, R. (2008). Non-operative treatment of multiple intra-abdominal solid organ injury after blunt penetrating abdominal trauma. *Journal of Trauma, 64*(4), 943–948.

- Transfuse packed red blood cells, fresh frozen plasma, and platelets as needed. Monitor serum calcium levels and replace as needed since transfusion of large amounts of banked blood can lead to hypocalcemia.
- Identify the mechanism of injury (e.g., crash speed, restraint use, fall height, type and size of weapon, time since the injury, estimated external blood loss, etc.) and prehospital treatment (oxygen, IV fluids, pain medication, vital signs). A history of prehospital hypotension is a predictor of significant intra-abdominal injury.[2]
- Maintain cervical spine control and logroll the patient to inspect the posterior abdomen for wounds and signs of injury.
- Consider placing an orogastric or nasogastric tube for stomach decompression and an indwelling urinary catheter to monitor output.
- Cover open abdominal wounds with sterile saline dressings. Do not allow exposed viscera to dry.
- Stabilize, but do not remove, objects impaled in the abdomen.
- The trend is toward nonoperative management of patients with solid organ injury. See Table 39-2 for indications for exploratory laparotomy.

SPECIFIC ORGAN INJURIES

Table 39-3 provides a comparison of specific abdominal organ injuries.

THE PREGNANT PATIENT WITH ABDOMINAL TRAUMA

Trauma in the pregnant patient is specifically addressed in Chapter 43, Obstetrical Trauma. Nonetheless, a few considerations related to abdominal injury warrant emphasis.

TABLE 39-3 COMPARISON OF SPECIFIC ABDOMINAL ORGAN INJURIES

ORGAN	INCIDENCE AND IMPLICATIONS OF INJURY	SIGNS AND SYMPTOMS OF INJURY	THERAPEUTIC INTERVENTIONS
Spleen	Commonly injured following BAT
Dense, encapsulated organ that stores approximately 200 mL blood
Splenic rupture causes acute hemorrhage	History of blunt trauma to LUQ
LUQ tenderness
Kehr's sign
Signs of peritoneal irritation (rebound tenderness and guarding)
Hypotension	Hemodynamically stable patients may be managed nonsurgically
Close observation and frequent reassessment of abdomen
Serial hematocrits and repeat CT scans

TABLE 39-3   **COMPARISON OF SPECIFIC ABDOMINAL ORGAN INJURIES—cont'd**

ORGAN	INCIDENCE AND IMPLICATIONS OF INJURY	SIGNS AND SYMPTOMS OF INJURY	THERAPEUTIC INTERVENTIONS
Liver	Along with the spleen, the liver is the most frequently injured abdominal organ[a] Largest internal solid organ in body Commonly injured because of: • Anterior location • Large size • Denseness • Relatively unprotected status Contains several major blood vessels and stores up to 500 mL blood, making it a major source of potential blood loss	History of blunt trauma to right lower chest ribs 8–12 or upper central abdomen RUQ pain Involuntary guarding and rebound tenderness Abdominal wall muscle spasm and rigidity Hypoactive or absent bowel sounds Signs of hypovolemic shock	50% to 60% of liver injuries stop bleeding spontaneously[b] Large stellate (star-shaped) lacerations with hemodynamic instability require surgical intervention
Stomach	Hollow, fairly mobile organ Seldom injured in blunt trauma; often injured with penetrating abdominal trauma	Bloody drainage on nasogastric tube insertion Free air under diaphragm on abdominal radiograph	Nasogastric tube to decompress stomach and monitor bleeding Surgical intervention
Pancreas	Rarely injured following BAT (incidence 2% to 12%) because of its relatively protected retroperitoneal position[c]	Pancreatic damage may be undetected initially; often only apparent when complications arise or during treatment of other injuries[c] Negative peritoneal lavage Epigastric pain, abdominal distension	Obtain serial amylase levels
Kidneys	Injured in as many as 10% of patients who sustain abdominal trauma[d] Three types of renal injuries[d]: • Laceration • Contusion • Vascular injury	Diagnosis begins with high index of suspicion Hematuria (frank or microscopic) Ecchymosis over flank Flank or abdominal tenderness	Contusions may be treated with bed rest, observation, and increased fluid intake Surgical intervention for lacerations associated with hemorrhage and urine extravasation Nephrectomy possible if serious parenchymal or vascular injury
Bladder	Injury may consist of contusion or rupture Mechanisms of injury for bladder rupture: • Bladder may "pop" in response to a direct blow (similar to a water balloon) • Bony fragment from pelvic fracture may puncture the bladder Full bladder rises into abdominal cavity, making it more susceptible to injury	Lower pelvic pain Inability to void Abdominal distension Lack of urine from indwelling urinary catheter following adequate fluid resuscitation Cystogram nearly 100% sensitive for bladder rupture	Bladder contusions are usually self-limiting[e] Urethral or suprapubic catheter for 7–10 days post bladder rupture Broad spectrum antibiotics

Continued

TABLE 39-3   COMPARISON OF SPECIFIC ABDOMINAL ORGAN INJURIES—cont'd

ORGAN	INCIDENCE AND IMPLICATIONS OF INJURY	SIGNS AND SYMPTOMS OF INJURY	THERAPEUTIC INTERVENTIONS
Urethra	Because of its external location, male urethra more commonly injured than female urethra Trauma commonly because of straddle injury, impact with crossbar of motorcycle or bicycle, or pelvic fracture In females, injury involves shearing of the urethra away from the symphysis pubis and can be associated with significant vaginal and bladder trauma	Presence of blood at urinary meatus High-riding prostate on rectal exam Hematuria (frank or microscopic) Scrotal swelling Pelvic or suprapubic pain Abdominal wall rigidity, spasm, or guarding Rebound tenderness	Often seen in patients with multiple injuries; life-threatening injuries should be corrected first Placement of suprapubic catheter and delayed surgical repair
Intestines	Both small and large intestines susceptible to injury follow blunt and penetrating trauma because: • They fill most of the abdominal cavity • Anterior position • Points of fixation • Vascularity	High index of suspicion in the presence of lap belt marks on abdomen Hypoactive or absent bowel sounds Vague, generalized abdominal pain or epigastric burning Rebound tenderness Abdominal rigidity, spasm, or guarding Obvious evisceration Blood in rectum (positive occult blood) Positive peritoneal lavage	Anticipate surgical intervention
Pelvis	Unstable and open pelvic fractures carry a mortality rate as high as 30%; 10% to 12% of these deaths result from blood loss[f] Traumatically fractured pelvis is seldom an isolated injury Associated injuries may include trauma to the bladder, urethra, vagina, and prostate	Severe hypotension Pelvic pain Hematuria Inspection may reveal rotation of the iliac crests[f] Perineal ecchymosis or hematoma See above for signs and symptoms of associated injuries	The main goal of management is to stop the bleeding Fluid resuscitation may require large amounts of crystalloids and blood products Temporary stabilization of the pelvis can be accomplished by placing a bedsheet underneath the patient, crossing the sheet over the anterior pelvis, and securing the sheet snugly[f] Anticipate angiography with embolization, external fixation in the emergency department, or surgical intervention for internal fixation of the unstable pelvis

BAT, Blunt abdominal trauma; *CT*, computed tomography; *LUQ*, left upper quadrant; *RUQ*, right upper quadrant.

[a]Udeani, J., Salomone, J. A., Keim, S. M., Legome, E. L., & Salomone, J. P. (2011, September 20). *Blunt abdominal trauma*. Retrieved from http://emedicine.medscape.com/article/1980980-overview#aw2aab6b2b4

[b]Zargar, M., & Laal, M. (2010). Liver trauma: Operative and non-operative management. *International Journal of Collaborative Research on Internal Medicine and Public Health, 2*(4), 96–107.

[c]Wolf, A., Bernhardt, J., Patrzyk, M., & Heidecke, C. D. (2005). The value of endoscopic diagnosis and the treatment of pancreas injuries following blunt abdominal trauma. *Surgical Endoscopy, 19*(5), 665–669.

[d]Geehan, D. M., & Santucci, R. A. (2010, January 27). *Renal trauma*. Retrieved from http://emedicine.medscape.com/article/440811-overview

[e]Rackley, R., & Vasavada, S. P. (2009, August 17). *Bladder trauma*. Retrieved from http://emedicine.medscape.com/article/441124-overview

[f]Kobziff, L. (2006). Traumatic pelvic fractures. *Orthopaedic Nursing, 25*(4), 235–241.

- Trauma in pregnancy is relatively unusual. However, blunt abdominal injury can produce placental abruption and uterine rupture.
- Fetal survival is completely dependent on maternal survival. Therefore resuscitative efforts must always focus on the mother.
- After 20 weeks gestation, the combined weight of the fetus, placenta, and amniotic fluid is sufficient to compress the abdominal vena cava and produce obstructive hypovolemia when the patient is supine. Whenever possible, elevate the female patient's right hip, tilt the backboard to the left, or manually displace the uterus to promote venous return to the heart.
- Shield the uterus with a lead apron as much as possible during radiograph procedures. However, never defer necessary procedures for fear of fetal irradiation.

REFERENCES

1. Emergency Nurses Association. (2007). *Trauma nursing core course provider manual* (6th ed.). Des Plaines, IL: Author.

2. Udeani, J., Salomone, J. A., Keim, S. M., Legome, E. L., & Salomone, J. P. (2011, September 20). *Blunt abdominal trauma*. Retrieved from http://emedicine.medscape.com/article/1980980-overview#aw2aab6b2b4

3. Isenhour, J. L., & Marx, J. A. (2010). Abdominal trauma. In J. A. Marx (Ed.), *Rosen's emergency medicine: Concepts and clinical practice* (7th ed.). Philadelphia, PA: Mosby.

4. McQuillan, K., Makic, M., & Whalen, E. (2009). *Trauma nursing: From resuscitation through rehabilitation* (4th ed.). Philadelphia, PA: Saunders.

5. American College of Surgeons. (2008). *Advanced trauma life support for doctors* (8th ed.). Chicago, IL: Author.

6. Yanar, H., Ertekin, C., Taviloglu, K., Kabay, B., Bakkaloglu, H., & Guloglu, R. (2008). Non-operative treatment of multiple intra-abdominal solid organ injury after blunt penetrating abdominal trauma. *Journal of Trauma, 64*(4), 943–948.

7. Whitehouse, J. S., & Weigelt, J. A. (2009). Diagnostic peritoneal lavage: A review of indication, technique, and interpretation. *Scandinavian Journal of Trauma, Resuscitation, and Emergency Medicine, 17*, 13. Retrieved from www.sjtrem.com/content/17/1/13

Musculoskeletal Trauma

Judith S. Halpern

According to the Centers for Disease Control and Prevention, approximately 53% of all hospitalized injuries are because of fractures.[1] Trauma to the bony skeleton produces pain, affects a person's ability to do activities of daily living, and in some cases can be life threatening or limb threatening. The goals of caring for any trauma patient are to prioritize care to protect life, preserve function, and reduce long-term disability. All trauma patients should have a primary assessment to rule out problems with airway, breathing, circulation, and disability before attention is focused on injury-specific conditions. See Chapter 35, Assessment and Stabilization of the Trauma Patient, for a description of the primary assessment of the trauma patient. The purpose of this chapter is to provide an overview of initial and specific assessments and emergency care for musculoskeletal injuries.

INITIAL ASSESSMENT

Focused History

- The history helps the health care provider do a more thorough assessment by following a general rule as stated below. Always examine the joints above and below the obvious injury.
- Ask the patient to identify areas of pain, altered nerve function, and loss of extremity motor function.
- Mechanism of injury is used to direct primary and secondary assessments. It is important to distinguish low-energy forces (e.g., falls from level heights) from high-energy forces (e.g., motor vehicle crashes, falls from distance, high-velocity gunshots). In the latter, the force from the point of impact can be transmitted to distal structures and produce patterns of multiple injuries.

Inspection

Inspect the injured extremity for general appearance, deformity, and motion.

- Skin signs suggestive of a musculoskeletal injury include ecchymosis, pallor, dusky color, edema, and any open soft tissue wounds.
- Always examine the joints above and below the obvious injury.
- Note obvious deformities such as changes in size, shape, or alignment. It is helpful to compare an injured extremity with the uninjured one. Observe hand position in patients with hand injuries and decreased level of consciousness. Turn hand with palm up and note if all fingers are flexed in a gentle cascade. If any one finger remains extended, suspect tendon injury.[2]
- Loss of range of motion and subtle signs and symptoms suggestive of an extremity injury include the person favoring or hesitating to move the extremity (e.g., limping, holding the injured part).

The following guidelines can be used to guide the triage nurse in determining the necessity of ankle or knee radiographs.[3]

- Ottawa ankle rules
  - Tenderness on palpation at (posterior) tip of lateral malleolus
  - Tenderness on palpation at (posterior) tip of medial malleolus
  - Inability to bear weight (four steps) at the time of injury or the time of physical examination
- Pittsburgh knee rules
  - Blunt trauma or fall as mechanism of injury plus either of the following:
    - Age younger than 12 years or older than 50 years
    - Inability to walk four weight-bearing steps in the emergency department

---

Palpation

- Determine skin temperature, which is a rough estimate of arterial perfusion. Compare an injured extremity to the uninjured extremity.
- Put the extremity through active range of motion. Check motor strength distal to the injury, rating it on an objective scale and comparing it to the uninjured side. This allows for more consistent interrater assessments and identification of subtle changes.
- Palpate the limb or joint for tenderness and crepitus.
- Assess for limb or joint instability.

Assessing Neurovascular Status

Major peripheral blood vessels and nerves tend to lie in close proximity to bones and share joint space with other structures. Because extremity injuries may affect these structures, carefully evaluate the distal neurovascular status, not only to protect the patient but also to reduce liability. Documenting "neurovascular status intact" in the patient's chart is considered medical-legal proof that the patient's functions were assessed and intact on admission. Any deficits identified after that documentation can be presumed to have occurred while the patient was under the care of that staff.

- Assess function at the time of admission, after any manipulation, when the injured part is immobilized, and at intervals until after swelling has minimized.
- Check the patient's ability to feel light touch in the injured extremity. It may be necessary to check for two-point discrimination. Assess response to pain if the patient has decreased level of consciousness.
- Assessment includes inspecting and palpating the involved structures. Significant findings are known as the Six P's:
  - **Pain** can result from the initial injury or a complication that produces nerve or vascular compromise. Ask the patient to describe the pain (e.g., burning, throbbing, knifelike), if it is localized (i.e., "point tenderness") or more generalized, and to rate the severity on a scale such as 0 to 10 (10 being the worst). Serial assessments help identify potential causes, significant changes, and response to interventions. See Chapter 11, Care of the Patient with Pain, for further discussion of pain and pain management.
  - Absence of a **pulse** in the injured extremity or joint is a serious complication and must be identified immediately. The pulses distal to the injury should be palpated for strength and quality. If unable to palpate the pulse, an ultrasound device (e.g., Doppler) may be used to auscultate over the vessel.

Injuries that produce severe angulation or distal neurovascular compromise need to be reduced promptly to prevent ischemic complications.

- **Pallor** is reflected in a quick check of skin perfusion. Pale, cool skin can result from obstructed arterial flow or capillary vasoconstriction. It is helpful to do a blanch test to check perfusion status (press on the area distal to the injury and count until the skin color returns). Normal refill should occur in less than two seconds. The blanch test for capillary refill is a rough estimate since other factors, such as ambient temperature, use of vasoconstrictive medications, and ice packs, can also affect refill time.
- **Paresthesias** indicate abnormal sensory nerve responses, such as tingling, burning, or numbness. The major peripheral nerves supplying the extremities conduct both sensory and motor impulses. Damage can occur to the entire nerve or to partial fibers. Therefore it is important to evaluate both motor and sensory functions to identify or rule out nerve injury. Table 40-1 lists the functions of peripheral nerves, how to assess their function, and common mechanisms of injury.
- **Paralysis** refers to the loss of voluntary motor function and may result from nerve injury or the patient guarding a painful extremity. Any decrease in motor activity in an injured extremity needs to be carefully assessed for potential nerve injury.
- **Pressure** or a tense feeling of the extremity on palpation could be an indication of compartment syndrome or muscle spasms.

> Reevaluate neurovascular status after repositioning or immobilization of an injured extremity.

Age-Specific Considerations

Patients at extremes of age can present more challenges in diagnosing and treating musculoskeletal injuries.

- The bones of young children are more cartilaginous and tend to sustain fractures that do not extend through the bone cortex. The epiphyseal growth plates, located on the ends of long bones, remain open until after puberty and are areas of weakness. Fractures in these areas may arrest healing and subsequent bone growth.
- Geriatric patients are prone to injury because of osteoporosis, decreased muscle mass to protect them during a fall, and limited mobility because of joint disease. They tend to require increased healing time and have fewer physiologic reserves to protect against acute blood loss or prolonged immobilization.

TABLE 40-1   PERIPHERAL NERVE FUNCTIONS, HOW TO ASSESS FUNCTION, AND COMMON MECHANISMS OF INJURY

PERIPHERAL NERVE	ASSESSING MOTOR FUNCTION	SENSORY DISTRIBUTION: CHECK FOR SENSATION AT	COMMON MECHANISMS OF INJURY
Radial	Wrist and finger extensors; ask patient to extend thumb ("hitchhike")	Dorsum of hand from thumb to middle of ring finger	Fractures of humerus, elbow, distal radius
Median	Oppose thumb to other fingers	Palmar aspect of hand from midthumb to middle of ring finger, tips of index, long, and ring finger	Elbow dislocation, wrist or forearm injury
Ulnar	Innervates intrinsic muscles of hand; ask patient to abduct (fan out) fingers	Innervates dorsum of hand in the middle of ring finger and small finger	Fracture of medial humeral epicondyle
Peroneal (a division of the sciatic nerve)			Fibular fractures, direct trauma to the region near the head of the fibula
Deep	Foot and toe dorsiflexors; weakness or inability to flex foot upward	Web space between first and second toes	
Superficial	Foot everter; weakness or inability to abduct feet	Sensory of the lateral area of lower leg and dorsum of foot	
Tibial (a division of the sciatic nerve)	Weakness or inability to push the foot downward (plantar flexion)	Supplies the muscles and skin of the calf and sole of the foot, and the toes	Fractures or other injury to the back of the knee or the lower leg, direct trauma, prolonged pressure on the nerve, and compression of the nerve

EMERGENCY CARE OF AN INJURED EXTREMITY

Splinting

Once life-threatening and limb-threatening complications are ruled out, immobilize the injured extremity to reduce blood loss, pain, and potential for further injury. Principles of splinting include the following:

- Follow the rule "splint the injury as it is lies." It is not necessary to realign an extremity unless there is severe angulation that compromises circulation or makes it difficult to apply a splint.
- Ensure that joints above and below the injury are also immobilized.
- Splints should be well padded and secured to the extremity. Because injured extremities tend to continue to swell, check and document the distal circulation after a splint has been placed.

Edema

Edema is a physiologic response to injury and can be increased with blood loss into tissues. Efforts should be made to reduce the swelling and pain associated with injuries, including:

- Elevate the affected extremity.
- Apply ice packs. Do not apply them directly to the skin.
- Remove items that will become constrictive with swelling, such as tight clothing, rings, jewelry, boots or shoes, and athletic equipment.

Pain Management

- Medication is generally needed in addition to splinting and edema control to manage pain in the patient with a musculoskeletal injury. See Chapter 11, Care of the Patient with Pain, for more information.

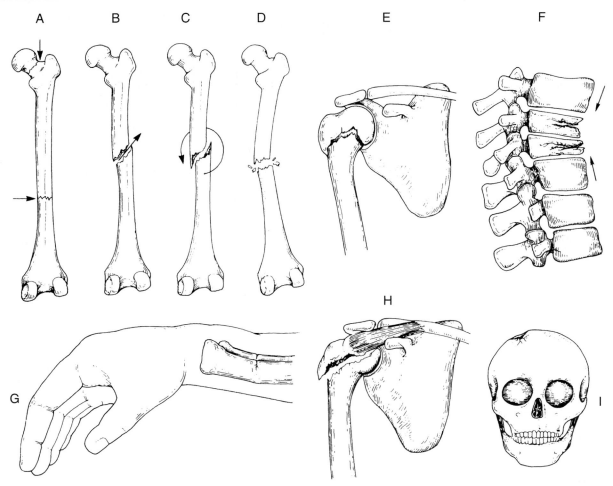

Fig. 40-1 Types of fracture: transverse through depressed. **A,** Transverse. **B,** Oblique. **C,** Spiral. **D,** Comminuted. **E,** Impacted. **F,** Compressed. **G,** Greenstick. **H,** Avulsion. **I,** Depressed. See Table 40-2 for descriptions.

• Procedural sedation may be necessary to reduce dislocation injuries. See Chapter 15, Procedural Sedation, for more information.

ACUTE MUSCULOSKELETAL INJURIES

The musculoskeletal system is composed of the bones, joints, muscles, ligaments, tendons, and cartilage. Any portion of the system can be injured alone or in combination with other structures. This section describes common types of injuries seen in the emergency department.

Fractures
Types of Fractures

Figure 40-1 and Table 40-2 illustrate various types of fractures. The type of break produced is a result of mechanism of injury and patient characteristics. Patient-specific factors that can affect bone structure and composition are as follows:
• Normal growth and development
• Nutritional intake
• Repetitive trauma
• Hormonal changes
• Disease processes

TABLE 40-2 TYPES OF FRACTURES

TYPE	ETIOLOGY
Transverse	Sharp, direct blow
Oblique	Twisting force
Spiral	A force directed along the axis of a limb or shaft; for example, the twisting force with a firmly planted foot
Comminuted	Severe direct trauma causes more than two bone fragments
Impacted	Severe trauma causing bone ends to jam together
Compressed	Severe force to the top of the head, sacrum, or os calcis (axial loading), forcing vertebrae together
Greenstick	Compression force; usually occurs in children under 10 years old
Avulsion	A muscle mass contracts forcefully, causing a bone fragment to tear off at the muscle insertion site; ligaments also can tear fragments from bone
Depressed	Blunt trauma to a flat bone; usually involves extensive soft tissue damage

See Figure 40-1 for illustrations.

By matching characteristics of the patient with the mechanism of injury, it is possible to anticipate patterns of fractures and help the health care provider focus assessment.

Open Versus Closed Fractures

Fractures are further classified according to the status of the soft tissue around the break.

- If the skin remains intact, the fracture is classified as closed or simple.
- If an open skin wound communicates with the fracture site, the break is distinguished as open or compound.
  - Compound fractures have an increased risk of neurovascular compromise, blood loss, and infection. Treatment consists of surgical debridement, irrigation, and soft tissue repair.
  - An injury will be classified as an open fracture if a penetrating foreign body enters the bone or creates an opening in the tissue over the bone. Do not remove penetrating objects until it is determined if the object affected the structures underneath.

Assess the patient's tetanus immunization status if open injury or penetrating or impaled objects are present.

Table 40-3 lists common fractures, their mechanism of injury, clinical findings, and treatment options.

Joint Injuries

The peripheral skeleton is constructed of joints that connect bones by fibrous connective tissue and cartilage. These structures work together to provide mobility, strength, and motion (e.g., flexion, extension, rotation, abduction, and adduction). Peripheral blood vessels and nerves share the joint space.

The soft tissues that surround the exterior of the joint provide stability and protection. These include tendons that attach muscles to bones and ligaments that attach bones to bones. When excessive force is applied to a joint, the joint structure can separate. There are two main classifications for joint injury:

- Dislocation—a complete disruption of the bony articulating surfaces in the joint
- Subluxation—a partial joint disruption that maintains some contact between the surfaces

Table 40-4 lists common types of joint injuries, their mechanism of injury, clinical findings, and treatment options.

Soft Tissue Injuries

When a joint is forced out of its normal position, the ligaments, tendons, and muscles can be injured. There are two main categories of injury: sprains and strains.

Sprains

A sprain is defined as an injury to the ligaments that have been stretched or torn by an excessive force. Sprains are graded according to the degree of damage and instability.

- Grade I injuries have microdamage but the joint is stable.
- Grade II sprains have partial tears and are still stable.
- Grade III sprains have significant tears and result in significant joint instability.

Strains

A strain refers to the stretching or tearing of a muscle or tendon as a result of excessive force. Strains tend to be seen in individuals with physically demanding occupations, those who engage in atypical activities (e.g., "weekend warrior" activities, shoveling heavy snow), and athletes who participate in contact sports or use extensive gripping actions. Strains are graded in a manner similar to that used for grading sprains.

- Grade 1 strains are a result of stretching a few muscle fibers.

Text continued on page 436.

TABLE 40-3 **COMMON FRACTURES**

BONE	USUAL MECHANISM OF INJURY	UNIQUE CLINICAL FINDINGS	TREATMENT
Clavicle	80% of fractures occur in middle third; usually because of direct force to shoulder (e.g., fall, sports, MVC); more common in younger patients. 15% involve distal or lateral third; usually because of force from top of shoulder; more common in the elderly. Less than 5% involve proximal or medial third; because of force to anterior chest, which can cause intrathoracic trauma.[a]	• Skin tenting over fracture • Inability to raise arm • Associated neurovascular injuries are rare except with proximal or medial fractures • First rib and cervical spine can be injured with same mechanism	Mid and proximal fractures treated with sling, rest. Athlete should avoid sports until preinjury strength and range of motion are regained.
Scapula	Fractures are rare and tend to be associated with significant, high-energy force.	• Serious associated injuries common and include fractured ribs, humerus, skull; soft tissue injuries of the lungs, spleen; central and peripheral nervous system[b] • Pulmonary, brachial plexus, and vascular injuries can be produced with same mechanism	Sling while symptomatic.
Humerus—head and neck	*Young:* Athletes involved in high-energy impact or involved in sports that use overhead throwing (i.e., affects the open epiphysis in proximal humerus) *Elderly:* Osteoporotic, falls on shoulder	• Unable to use shoulder[c] • Loss of motion can remain for over a year	Sling immobilization with nondisplaced fracture. Surgical repair may be option in approximately 20% of cases.[c]
Humerus—shaft	*Proximal:* Falls *Midshaft:* Falls, twisting force that produces spiral fractures *Distal:* Falls, more common in children	• Poor perfusion of forearm. Radial nerve lies close to midshaft and is easily injured • Patients often prefer to have arm hang at side	Allowing arm to hang at side acts to help reduce fracture. Sling, brace. Surgery, if vascular compromise, fracture extends into elbow.
Humerus—distal • Supracondylar	Fall on outstretched hand (most common elbow fracture in children)	• Unable to straighten, bend elbow • Pain around joint	Displaced fracture an emergency because of neurovascular compromise. May use splints with negative radiographs but positive clinical signs.
• Lateral condyle	Fall on arm or elbow, break through epiphyseal plate and joint.		

TABLE 40-3   COMMON FRACTURES—cont'd

BONE	USUAL MECHANISM OF INJURY	UNIQUE CLINICAL FINDINGS	TREATMENT
Radius—head and neck	Fall on outstretched hand, extended elbow	• Nondisplaced fracture hard to see on radiograph • Suspect if radial head tenderness, pain with rotation	Nondisplaced, minimally displaced fractures treated conservatively. Surgery for large, displaced, comminuted fractures. Early motion encouraged.
Monteggia's fracture or dislocation: • Radius—dislocation of radial head • Ulna—fracture of proximal third	Falls on an outstretched hand with forced pronation Direct blow ("nightstick fracture") to ulna	• Elbow pain • Shortening, angulation of elbow • Ulna fracture usually apparent; radial head dislocation can be overlooked • Always radiograph joints above and below injuries to find this injury	Immediate reduction of radial head ORIF for open ulna fracture Posterior arm splint with arm flexed 90 degrees for closed fracture
Ulna—Olecranon	Fall on tip of elbow Athletic stress fracture (e.g., baseball pitchers)	• Unable to straighten elbow	Posterior splint, sling ORIF for displaced fractures
Wrist • Colles fracture (distal radius fracture with ulna injury)	Fall on outstretched hand most common injury to wrist	• "Silverfork deformity" because of displaced radius	Closed reduction, cast
• Distal radius	Fall on outstretched hand, direct impact, MVC		May be treated closed or open, depending on pathology
• Scaphoid (carpal bone)	Fall on outstretched hand	• Tenderness in "anatomic snuff box" region of wrist	Thumb spica cast for 8 to 12 weeks if nondisplaced, ORIF if displaced
Hand • Metacarpals	"Boxer's fracture": neck of fifth finger injured while punching with fist	• Swelling over fracture, depression of affected knuckle • Angulation on lateral radiograph view • May require reduction	*Undisplaced:* Compression dressing for 1 week Ulnar splint for minimally displaced fracture ORIF for severe displacement
• Phalanges	*Young:* Sports related *Adult:* Falls, machinery, crush, axial blow	• Check digit for rotational deformity; ask patient to flex fingers and view the nails on end, compare with other hand • Malrotation often missed on radiograph	*Undisplaced transverse fracture:* Buddy tape to adjacent finger *Nondisplaced spiral or oblique fracture:* Splint *Unstable:* May need ORIF
Pelvis	*Stable fracture:* Ring broken at only one point; low-energy forces (e.g., fall from standing, especially in elderly) *Unstable fracture:* Ring broken in two or more places; high-energy forces (e.g., MVC)	• *Stable:* Pain with compression or movement of pelvic bones • *Unstable:* May be life threatening; can involve vascular, GU, and visceral injuries	*Stable:* Short-term rest *Unstable:* Life support, angiography and embolize bleeding vessels, external fixation

Continued

TABLE 40-3   COMMON FRACTURES—cont'd

BONE	USUAL MECHANISM OF INJURY	UNIQUE CLINICAL FINDINGS	TREATMENT
Femur • Head	Osteoporotic elderly, fall on hip	• Muscle spasms, shortening, external rotation of affected leg	ORIF
• Femur shaft	*Multisystem trauma:* High-energy forces (e.g., MVC, GSW, direct blow) *Isolated injuries:* Repetitive stress (e.g., running, baseball, basketball) Chronic diseases (e.g., metabolic bone disease, metastatic diseases)[d]	• May have significant blood loss, swollen thigh • *Isolated:* Swollen thigh, limited range of motion, pain radiates to groin	Traction splint to reduce pain, blood loss Protected crutch-assisted, touch-down weight bearing for 1 to 4 weeks, avoid running for 8 to 16 weeks[d]
Tibia and Fibula	*Low-energy injuries:* Ground-level falls *Athletic injuries* *High-energy injuries:* MVC, GSW, fall from height on bended knee or with foot fixed, rotational forces *Tibial plateau fractures:* Axial loading with valgus or varus forces (e.g., fall from a height or collision with bumper of a car) *Tibial shaft:* Major force *Stress fracture:* Athletics[e]	• Able to ambulate with isolated fibula fracture • Monitor for compartment syndrome	Treatment depends on type and location of injury, if open vs. closed, if neurovascular compromise present, mechanism of injury
Ankle • Talus, malleolus	Eversion, lateral rotation forces	• Sprained ankles more often associated with inversion forces	*Undisplaced:* Splint, cast *Displaced:* Immediate reduction, avoid weight bearing
Foot • Metatarsals	Compression forces		*Displaced:* Short leg walking cast, may need ORIF
• Phalanges	Direct trauma, kicking, stubbing toes, athletics, crush injuries		*Undisplaced:* Buddy tape to adjacent toes *Displaced:* Reduce in ED
Calcaneus	Fall from height	• Look for injuries to lumbar spine, leg, other foot; pain increases with hyperflexion	Compression dressing, crutches

ED, Emergency department; *GSW,* gunshot wound; *GU,* genitourinary; *MVC,* motor vehicle crash; *ORIF,* open reduction internal fixation.

[a]Estephan, A., & Gore, R. J. (2010, September 28). *Clavicle fracture in emergency medicine.* Retrieved from http://emedicine.medscape.com/article/824564-overview

[b]Goss, T. P., & Cantu, R. V. (2010, September 30). *Scapula fracture.* Retrieved from http://emedicine.medscape.com/article/1263076-overview

[c]McMahon, P. J., & Kaplan, L. D. (2006). Sports medicine. In H. B. Skinner (Ed.), *Current diagnosis & treatment in orthopedics* (4th ed., pp. 163–220). New York, NY: Lange Medical Books/McGraw Hill.

[d]Aukerman, D. F., Deitch, J. R., Ertl, J. P., & Ertl, W. (2008, October 30). *Femur injuries and fractures.* Retrieved from http://emedicine.medscape.com/article/90779-overview

[e]Norvell, J. G., Steele, M., & Cooper, T. M. (2009, October 1). *Tibia and fibula fracture.* Retrieved from http://emedicine.medscape.com/article/826304-overview

TABLE 40-4 COMMON JOINT INJURIES

JOINT	COMMON MECHANISM	CLINICAL FINDINGS	CLINICAL INTERVENTIONS
Shoulder			
AC separation	Direct blow to top of shoulder or fall on outstretched hand, causing ligaments to rupture	Tenderness, swelling over AC joint Inability to raise arm or adduct across chest Tenting of skin over fracture	Sling, if needed for pain, but active range of motion should be encouraged as tolerated Surgery rarely indicated
Glenohumeral dislocation	*Anterior:* Athletic injury, fall on extended arm	Visible deformity in joint with abduction and external rotation of the arm. The patient will be unable to bring the affected arm high enough to touch the ear on the opposite side of the dislocation.	Splint in position of comfort; reduction done in ED, may need sedation to overcome muscle spasms
	Posterior: Rare, arm forced while extended, may be seen after grand mal seizure	Arm held in adduction with internal rotation with visible deformity over the joint	
Elbow			
Dislocation	*Posterior:* Fall on outstretched hand with elbow extended	Need to rule out associated fracture Carefully assess neurovascular function in affected hand	Reduction done in ED, check elbow for stability, range of motion If stable postreduction, may rest in sling but increase range of motion as soon as possible Never force motion
Wrist			
Dislocation	Fall on outstretched hand, repeated stress on carpal ligaments, athletes involved in high-speed activities, falls from heights	Sensation of clicking, decreased grip strength, localized tenderness worse with dorsiflexion Positive ballottement test	Splint for initial evaluation, immobilize for 10 to 14 days
Sprain	Fall on outstretched hand		Radiograph to rule out fracture or subluxation
Hand and Fingers			
Thumb	Rare except in athletes	Thumb deformity at MP joint	Reduce, buddy tape for 2 to 3 weeks
Fingers	PIP joint posterior dislocations more common than volar DIP joint dislocations rare	Deformity of PIP joint	Dorsal PIP joint dislocations can be reduced with closed traction, often with digital block Volar PIP joint dislocations should be referred to hand surgeon
Hip			
Dislocation	*Posterior:* Requires significant force; knee struck while hip and knee are flexed, force along femur drives femoral head out of posterior joint ("dashboard knee syndrome") *Anterior:* Force on knee while thigh abducted	*Posterior:* Hip flexed, adducted, internally rotated *Anterior:* Hip flexed, abducted, externally rotated	Emergent reduction needed to prevent disrupted blood supply to femoral head for both types of dislocations

Continued

TABLE 40-4 COMMON JOINT INJURIES—cont'd

JOINT	COMMON MECHANISM	CLINICAL FINDINGS	CLINICAL INTERVENTIONS
Knee			
Patella dislocation	Direct blow to medial aspect or sudden valgus strain (distal part angulates away from midline)	Patella displaced laterally, knee held in flexion	Closed reduction in ED, crutches, knee immobilizer for 3 to 4 weeks
Knee dislocation	Major trauma, anterior dislocation most common	Joint may spontaneously reduce, decreasing signs of injury. Suspect if severe ligament injury present, neurovascular compromise especially loss of peroneal nerve or popliteal artery	Splint for comfort; emergency reduction needed to prevent neurovascular injury; angiography to determine vascular status; ligament injury repair considered
Ankle			
Dislocation	Large amount of force required, ankle plantar flexed and foot inverted or everted under stress; occurs more frequently with children and adolescents. Posterior dislocation most common but can also have anterior, lateral, or superior dislocations	Associated injuries common: ankle fracture, ligament injuries. Neurovascular compromise possible. Evaluate for other injuries to leg, hip, or spine if force applied from directly above or below foot	Prompt reduction of dislocation or fracture; splint in neutral position
Sprain	Most common ankle injury, a common sports-related injury	May report feeling a "pop," significant swelling, ecchymosis, inability to bear weight	Splint for comfort, depending on joint stability. Rest, ice, compression, elevation of extremity, use of crutches as needed. Refer to physical therapy for rehabilitation
Achilles tendon rupture	Sudden forced plantar flexion of foot, unexpected dorsiflexion of foot, and violent dorsiflexion of a plantar-flexed foot. Other mechanisms include direct trauma, jumping, pushing off. Also a high incidence with use of fluoroquinolone medications (e.g., Levaquin, Cipro, Avelox) and direct steroid injections into tendons	Patient feels sharp pain or "pop" in heel. Walks flat-footed, unable to stand on ball of foot, unable to plantar flex foot	Use evidence-based criteria such as Ottawa ankle rules to determine if radiographs are necessary[a]. Ice acute injuries, splint foot in plantar flexion. Patient should use crutches for ambulation. Surgical repair as soon as possible
Foot			
Toe dislocation	Hyperextension	Obvious deformity over joint	Closed reduction with digital block; buddy tape for 4 weeks

AC, Acromioclavicular; *DIP*, distal interphalangeal; *ED*, emergency department; *MP*, metacarpophalangeal; *PIP*, proximal interphalangeal.
[a]Steill, I. G., Greenberg, G. H., McKnight, R. D., Nair, R. C., McDowell, I., Reardon, M., ... Maloney, J. (1993). Decision rules for the use of radiography in acute ankle injuries, refinement and prospective validation. *The Journal of the American Medical Association, 269*(9), 1127–1132.

- Grade 2 strains cause a partial tearing of the ligament and are characterized by bruising, moderate pain, and swelling.
- Grade 3 strains involve complete rupture of the muscle and possibly the overlying fascia.

Compartment Syndrome

Compartment syndrome is a pathologic process in which excessive pressure develops within a closed body space. Musculoskeletal trauma tends to affect extremities where closed spaces contain bones, muscles, vessels, and nerves.

These closed spaces, or compartments, are surrounded by nonelastic fascia that does not tolerate changes in volume or pressure from bleeding, edema, or excessive external pressure. As the intracompartmental pressure increases, microcirculation is compromised, causing more edema. Eventually the pressure within the muscle compartment exceeds the intra-arterial hydrostatic pressure, causing collapse of the small vessels, which leads to ischemia and necrosis. This pathologic process can be triggered by a fracture, soft tissue injury (e.g., crush injuries, snake envenomation), vascular injury, edema resulting from burns, or external compression, such as when an intoxicated person falls asleep on an arm or leg or when a cast has been applied too tightly.

Assessment

Anticipate compartment syndrome in extremity trauma, especially closed injuries of the forearm and calf. Serial neurovascular assessments are essential to recognize subtle changes.

- The most reliable indicator is severe pain with passive motion. The pain tends to be out of proportion to the injury and is unrelieved by pain medications.
- Capillary refill may be delayed.
- Patient may experience decreased distal sensation, paresthesia, or "burning."
- Pulses are usually present; pulselessness is a late finding.

Therapeutic Interventions

- Remove restrictive items, such as circumferential tape or elastic wraps, and ice bags in patients who are at risk for compartment syndrome.
- Maintain the extremity in a neutral position. Elevation further inhibits arterial perfusion to the affected tissue.
- Measure intracompartmental pressure when indicated. Various devices can be used to measure intracompartmental pressure, including a simple manometer attached to a syringe via tubing and a stopcock, or commercial devices.
- Use intracompartmental pressure along with the clinical presentation to determine if a fasciotomy is indicated.

Traumatic Amputation

Traumatic amputation, the loss of part of or the entire extremity, is commonly the result of external guillotine (sharp) or blunt (crushing) force. The fingers, toes, arms, or legs are affected most often. Emergency care of an amputation is directed toward two goals:

- Protect the person's life and limb
- Preserve the amputated part for potential replantation

Factors that inhibit good outcomes in the event of traumatic amputation include:

- Crush wounds
- Long ischemia times (>6 hours)
- Proximal amputations
- Nerve injuries
- Systemic hypotension
- Severe contamination
- Concomitant injuries
- Concurrent medical conditions
- Patient age
- Poor nutritional status
- Injuries associated with psychological disorders

Assessment

- Assess the patient for signs of hypovolemic shock related to blood loss.
- Determine the amount of soft tissue injury and degree of wound contamination.
- Obtain a history of mechanism of injury and timeline of events since the injury.

> Obtain radiographs of both the injured extremity and the amputated part to assess the degree of bony injury.

Therapeutic Interventions

- Because traumatic amputation may be associated with other major trauma, airway, breathing, and circulation are of primary concern.
- Inspect the injured extremity for active bleeding, cover with sterile dressings, and immobilize.
- Preserve and protect the amputated part by placing it in a watertight container labeled with the patient's information; the container is then placed in an iced saline bath. Keep amputated tissue dry and never place it directly on ice. The amputated part should be transported with the patient to a facility capable of replantation.

REFERENCES

1. Buie, V. C., Owings, M. F., DeFrances, C. J., Golosinskiy, A. (2010). National Hospital Discharge Survey: 2006 summary. *Vital and Health Statistics, 13*(168), 1–70.
2. Harrahill, M. (2006). A brief motor evaluation of the injured hand. *Journal of Emergency Nursing, 32*(3), 283–285.
3. Ebell, M. H. (2005). A tool for evaluating patients with knee injury. *Family Practice Management, 12*(3), 67–68.

Facial, Ocular, ENT, and Dental Trauma

Jeff Solheim

Trauma to the maxillofacial region of the body affects as many as 80% of patients with multiple traumatic injuries.[1] Common sources of maxillofacial trauma include the following:

- Motor vehicle crashes
- Intimate partner violence (IPV)
- Sporting injuries
- Penetrating trauma
- Falls

Traditionally, the majority of facial trauma cases were related to motor vehicle crashes (MVCs), but with the introduction and enforcement of prevention strategies such as airbags and seat belts, the incidence of maxillofacial trauma secondary to MVCs has declined significantly. As a result, IPV has overtaken MVCs as the leading cause of trauma to the face.[2]

The face is a frequent target in IPV, also known as domestic abuse. Between 34% and 73% of woman who present with trauma to the face will have sustained the injury because of IPV, but many of these victims will attempt to mask the source of their injury by providing false stories such as "I walked into a door" or "I hit my head on the corner of a coffee table."[3] The emergency nurse should always evaluate the degree of injury with the history provided, looking for inconsistencies, and use these opportunities to open a dialogue with these patients about breaking the cycle of violence. Refer to Chapter 50, Intimate Partner Violence, for more information.

Trauma to the facial region has far-reaching effects on an individual.

- The face is the beginning of both the respiratory and the gastrointestinal tract, and facial trauma often affects both of these systems.

- The face sits directly in front of the cranial vault and is held up by the neck; brain injury and spinal cord trauma are commonly associated with facial injuries.
- The face houses three of the five senses (taste, smell, and sight) and is closely associated with hearing and touch; as well, it plays an integral role in speech. Therefore interaction with the world can be negatively affected by maxillofacial trauma.
- The face is an important part of a person's identity, leaving a patient with facial trauma to deal with significant psychological impacts long after the initial injury.

PRIMARY ASSESSMENT

Assessing the patient with maxillofacial and ocular trauma is no different than assessing a patient with trauma to other body systems. The ABCs (airway, breathing, and circulation) of trauma assessment are a priority. Table 41-1 describes the primary assessment of the patient with facial trauma.

SECONDARY ASSESSMENT

After completing the primary assessment to rule out life-threatening injuries, a secondary assessment of the face should be undertaken. Specific assessments included in the secondary assessment include the following:

- Inspecting the face for asymmetry, performing a side-to-side comparison of the eyebrows, infraorbital rims, zygomatic arches, anterior sinus walls, jaw angles, bridge of nose, and lower mandibular borders. At times, a "bird's-eye" view of the patient, performed by standing at the head of the patient and looking across the patient's

TABLE 41-1	**PRIMARY ASSESSMENT OF THE PATIENT WITH FACIAL TRAUMA**		
	CATEGORY	**CONSIDERATIONS**	**INTERVENTIONS**
A	Airway and protection of the cervical spine	Numerous factors may make it difficult or impossible for the patient to maintain his or her own airway: • Fractures of the mandible may cause loss of ability to properly use the tongue, leading to difficulty swallowing or even obstruction of the throat by the tongue. • Fractures of the maxilla may lead to an unstable palate, decreasing the ability of the patient to swallow. A severely displaced palate may obstruct the airway. • Avulsed tissue, blood, tooth fragments, edema, and foreign objects such as dentures or shrapnel may occlude the airway. Alterations in the ability to swallow or spit will exacerbate these problems. • Neurologic involvement may result in a depressed level of consciousness, further decreasing the ability of the patient to protect his or her own airway. Significant force is required to cause maxillofacial trauma. This same force can cause the neck to be violently snapped. As much as 19.3% of patients with maxillofacial trauma will sustain concomitant neck and spinal cord injuries.[a]	Interventions to protect the airway should include the following: • Oral, endotracheal, and nasal suctioning as required. • Allowing the patient to remain upright when possible increases patient comfort, facilitates the patient's ability to maintain his or her airway, and provides a superior position for airway structures to remain open. • Decrease edema formation through application of ice to the face and allow the patient to maintain the upright position. • Early intubation if a patient is unlikely to be able to protect his or her airway or if edema in the airway is likely to increase. • Insertion of blind airway devices such as Combitubes, King airways, or laryngeal mask airways protects an airway until a definitive management plan is available. These devices carry the advantage of temporarily tamponading bleeding in the posterior nasopharynx. • Cricothyrotomy or tracheostomy if the upper airway is damaged to the point that it is no longer a patent airway. Measures to protect the cervical spine should be instituted, including in-line immobilization with cervical collars and head blocks as appropriate. The conscious patient with maxillofacial trauma may be unable to breathe in the supine position. In this case, protect the cervical spine in the position in which the patient finds it easiest to breathe until an alternate airway is available.
B	Breathing	Maxillofacial trauma may affect a patient's ability to breathe in numerous ways: • Swallowing of blood increases gastric contents and may increase the risk of aspiration. • Loss of tissue integrity or bony integrity of the lower face can make bag-mask assistance difficult or impossible. • Neurologic damage associated with maxillofacial trauma may alter the rate and depth of respirations.	Interventions to promote breathing include the following: • Administer supplemental oxygen as appropriate to the injury. • Provide bag-mask ventilations when appropriate. • Assist with insertion of blind airway devices, endotracheal intubation, cricothyrotomy, or tracheostomy as required.

	CATEGORY	CONSIDERATIONS	INTERVENTIONS
TABLE 41-1	**PRIMARY ASSESSMENT OF THE PATIENT WITH FACIAL TRAUMA—cont'd**		
C	Circulation	Although the face is highly vascular and trauma to this area can lead to significant blood loss, there are few blood vessels in the facial region large enough to cause hypovolemia. Therefore, if a patient with maxillofacial trauma presents with signs of hypovolemic shock, the emergency nurse should search for other concomitant injuries that may be causing heavy blood losses.[a]	Interventions to stabilize circulation should include the following: <ul><li>Application of direct pressure to areas of bleeding.</li><li>Elevation of the head of the bed when appropriate.</li><li>Initiation of large-bore intravenous catheters.</li><li>Treatment of hypovolemic shock as outlined in Chapter 20, Shock.</li></ul>
D	Disability (neurologic assessment)	The face and the brain are in close proximity to one another, separated by the skull and sinuses. For this reason, facial trauma is often associated with intracranial trauma. In one study, 24.5% of maxillofacial trauma patients had a closed head injury and 9.7% experienced intracranial bleeds.[b] The delicate cranial nerves are also easily injured in facial trauma.	Interventions to assess for concomitant neurologic trauma should include the following: <ul><li>Initial and sequential neurologic assessments, including measurement of a Glasgow Coma Scale score and pupillary reactions.</li><li>Assessment of the various cranial nerves.</li><li>Assessment of vital signs for indications of increasing intracranial pressure (i.e., bradycardia, widening pulse pressure, and abnormal respiratory patterns).</li></ul>

[a]Lynham, A., Hirst, J., Cosson, J., Chapman, P., & McEniery, P. (2004). Emergency department management of maxillofacial trauma. *Emergency Medicine Australasia, 16*(1), 7–12.
[b]Hohlrieder, M., Hinterhoelzl, J., Ulmer, H., Lang, C., Hackl W., Kampfl, A., ... Gassner, R. (2003). Traumatic intracranial hemorrhages in facial fracture patients: Review of 2,195 patients. *Intensive Care Medicine, 29*(7), 1095–1100.

forehead to the face, will reveal deformities that are not evident when looking directly at a patient.
- Palpating the face, noting areas of palpable tenderness, crepitus, or bony deformities while simultaneously assessing for areas of numbness on the face.
- Assessing for mandibular injury by asking the patient to open and close the mouth. Patients with mandibular fractures or temporomandibular joint injuries may have difficulty doing so.
- Asking the patient to follow fingers as they move in various directions. The eyes should move simultaneously through all visual fields. Inability to move the eyes in all directions may indicate orbital wall fractures; injuries to cranial nerves III, IV, or VI; or ocular injuries.
- Assessing the cranial nerves associated with the face (Table 41-2).

> Use the mnemonic "Three, four, and six makes the eyes do tricks" to remember that cranial nerves III, IV, and VI are all involved in the movement of the eyes in various directions.

FACIAL SOFT TISSUE TRAUMA

Numerous considerations are unique when dealing with soft tissue trauma to the face.
- Because the face is highly vascular and tends to bleed longer, wound closure may be delayed as long as 20 hours from the time of injury (as opposed to 4 to 6 hours on other parts of the body).
- "Road rash" to the face may result in permanent epidermal staining (tattooing) from imbedded grease or asphalt. Gunpowder can also permanently stain the face. Application of topical anesthetic followed by scrubbing with a hard brush over areas of road rash will minimize these effects.
- Lacerations involving the eyelids and eyebrows should receive a high triage priority to facilitate rapid closure before edema makes wound edge approximation difficult. Eyebrows should never be shaved, as they may not grow back. They also serve as an anatomic guide for proper wound closure.
- Because of the long-term psychological consequences of scarring, plastic surgery consultation may be considered

TABLE 41-2 ASSESSMENT OF THE CRANIAL NERVES

CRANIAL NERVE	ASSESSMENT TECHNIQUE
I	Have the patient identify a smell.
II	Perform a visual acuity test.
III, IV, and VI	Have the patient move their eyes through the various visual fields and test for pupil reactivity.
V	Touch a wisp of cotton to various areas of the patient's face looking for areas of altered sensation.
VII	Check symmetry and mobility of the face by having the patient frown, close the eyes, lift the eyebrows, and puff the cheeks.
VIII	Test hearing acuity.
IX and X	Listen to the sound of the patient's voice; it should be smooth. Assess for the presence of both the gag and the swallowing reflex.
XI	Have the patient rotate the head and shrug the shoulders against resistance.
XII	Ask the patient to stick out his or her tongue or say the sounds of the letters L, T, and D.

for facial wounds. This is especially true of lacerations through the lip border to assure that the vermilion border is aligned.

- Wounds inside the mouth, including those on the tongue, carry a higher risk of infection. Carefully inspect these wounds for debris and tooth fragments. Antibiotics are frequently prescribed.
- Lacerations of the cheek may be associated with injuries to the parotid gland and parotid ducts. Clear drainage from the wound is one indication that these glands or ducts are injured.
- Because vasoconstriction on small body parts can lead to significant tissue ischemia, lacerations of the ear and nose are generally closed using anesthetic *without* epinephrine.

> The vermilion border is the edge of the lip. It is the point where the red or pink area that makes up the lip merges with the regularly colored skin surrounding it.

Therapeutic Interventions

- Apply direct pressure and ice to actively bleeding facial wounds.
- Anesthetic with epinephrine is often used on facial wounds to decrease bleeding. Anesthetic without epinephrine is more likely to be used on wounds of the nose or ears.
- Elevate the head of the bed if cervical spinal injuries are not suspected.
- Assist with wound cleansing. Scrub abrasions to remove imbedded material, irrigate other wounds with copious amounts of wound irrigant. Bite wounds tend to be significantly contaminated and will require scrupulous cleansing.
- Apply sterile dressings.
- Consider the need for tetanus prophylaxis.
- Consider the possibility of abuse or crime as the underlying cause and report as per hospital policy and local reporting requirements.

Patient and Family Teaching

- Because of the vascularity of the face and its thin skin, it heals faster. Therefore instruct the patient to return for suture removal within 3 to 5 days.[4] Sutures in the ear are usually left in for 10 to 14 days.[5]
- If wound glue is used for wound closure, instruct the patient to keep the area clean and dry and avoid application of petroleum-based products (such as antibiotic ointment) that can break down the adhesive. The glue will slough off in 5 to 10 days.
- Instruct the patient to apply sunblock with a sun protection factor (SPF) of at least 15 to the wound for at least 6 months to prevent discoloration of the wound.[4]
- Teach the patient to return if there are signs of infection, including redness, swelling, warmth, or discharge from the area.

AURICULAR TRAUMA

The auricle or pinna is the portion of the ear that is visible outside of the skull. Because the pinna projects from the side of the head, it is an easy target for trauma. Piercings and dangling earrings further exacerbate this risk. Contact sports such as football, wrestling, and boxing are common sources of auricular trauma, as are dog bites. Injuries can range from hematomas of the pinna, to lacerations, to complete amputations.

Therapeutic Interventions

- Cleanse the wound, removing any obvious dirt or debris.
- Grossly contaminated wounds may require systemic antibiotics.

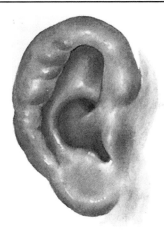

Fig. 41-1 Cauliflower ear. (From Gisness, C. M. [2010]. Maxillofacial trauma. In Emergency Nurses Association, *Sheehy's emergency nursing: Principles and practice* [6th ed., pp. 355–363]. St. Louis, MO: Mosby.)

- Lacerations are debrided prior to repair. A plastic surgeon may be asked to do the repair to ensure acceptable cosmetic results. The skin is carefully pulled over any exposed cartilage and care must be taken that sutures are not passed through cartilage because this can lead to further damage.
- Complete amputation of the ear will require surgical intervention for reattachment.
- Hematomas of the pinna are aspirated using a large-bore needle or a small stab incision. A drain may be placed to facilitate continued drainage of the area. After the area has been drained, a pressure dressing is applied to the area to prevent blood reaccumulation.
- Figure 41-1 shows "cauliflower ear," a deformity of the external ear that can result from auricular trauma.

> Failure to appropriately drain a hematoma on the pinna can result in a defect known as cauliflower ear.

RUPTURED TYMPANIC MEMBRANE

The tympanic membrane or eardrum is a delicate piece of tissue, not unlike the skin, that separates the middle ear from the outer ear. If the pressure between these two spaces is different, the thin membrane may rupture. Potential causes of pressure differences include infection in the inner ear (which causes a buildup of fluid on the internal surface of the membrane) and barotrauma from an explosion or during pressure changes associated with either diving or flying. Penetrating trauma from an object such as a cotton-tipped swab or even a slap over the ear are other potential causes of this trauma.

Signs and Symptoms

- Sudden sharp ear pain at the time of the rupture
- Blood or purulent drainage from the ear canal
- Hearing impairment (proportional to the size of the perforation)
- Possible tinnitus and vertigo

> Although patients may experience sharp pain at the time of an eardrum rupture, the pain is frequently less severe after the rupture because the pressure behind the eardrum has been relieved. This is especially true if the rupture is secondary to a middle ear infection.

Diagnostic Procedures

- Otoscopic examination

Therapeutic Interventions

- Provide analgesia.
- Do not irrigate the ear to prevent fluid from damaging the structures normally protected by the eardrum.
- Antibiotics are indicated if there is a history of ear contamination.
- Ninety percent of perforations will heal spontaneously but large perforations may require surgical repair.
- Instruct the patient and family:
  - Keep the affected ear dry. Avoid activities such as swimming and showering.
  - A cotton ball lightly coated with petroleum jelly will decrease the risk of moisture in the ear.
  - Wear ear protection as appropriate. Do not put instruments into the ear.

FACIAL FRACTURES

The amount of energy required to fracture many of the bones of the face is significant. When a patient presents with facial fractures, assess for other injuries, such as intracranial and spinal trauma.

Nasal Fractures

The most frequently fractured bones of the face are the nasal bones, accounting for 39% to 45% of all facial fractures.[6] While fractures of the nasal bones are typically less serious than other facial fractures, serious complications such as septal hematomas, epistaxis with excessive blood loss, and basilar skull fractures need to be ruled out.

Nasal septal hematomas need to be drained rapidly to prevent ischemia and destruction of the septum. These patients should receive a high triage priority.

Signs and Symptoms

- Nasal deformity, crepitus, ecchymosis, and edema
- Anterior or posterior epistaxis
- Periorbital ecchymosis
- Subconjunctival hemorrhage
- Visible swelling and purplish discoloration of the nasal septum if a hematoma is present
- Cerebrospinal fluid drainage if the fracture is associated with basilar skull fractures

Diagnostic Procedures

- Computed tomography (CT) scan
- Nasal bone radiographs (Waters' view)

Therapeutic Interventions

- Apply a cold pack.
- Control bleeding with direct pressure or pinching the nares. If this is unsuccessful, application of topical vasoconstrictors or packing may be considered.
- Splint the nose as indicated.
- Closed or open reduction may be necessary if fracture is displaced, but surgery is usually delayed until after the swelling has abated.

Zygomatic Fractures

The zygomatic bone sits under the eye and extends to the lateral aspect of the face. It is part of both the floor and the lateral aspect of the orbit and joins with the maxilla in the front of the face and the temporal bone at the side of the head. Externally, the most visible portion of the zygoma is the zygomatic arch, a rounded bony projection, which forms the cheekbone (also known as the malar eminence). Because of the prominent position of the zygoma on the face, it is the second most fractured facial bone, accounting for 13% of all craniofacial fractures.[7] Zygomatic fractures are frequently associated with both orbital wall fractures and trauma to the eye as illustrated in Figure 41-2.

Signs and Symptoms

- Trismus (if there is impingement on the coronoid process of the mandible)
- Infraorbital hypesthesia
- Diplopia with impaired upward gaze
- Epistaxis (on the same side as the fracture)
- Symmetrical abnormalities (cheekbone may appear flat on affected side)
- Periorbital and facial edema and ecchymosis

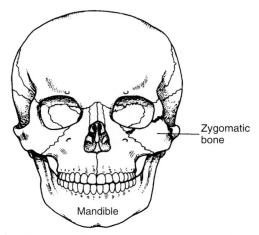

Fig. 41-2 Fracture of the zygomatic arch.

- Subconjunctival hemorrhage
- Palpable step defect and point tenderness
- Anesthesia of the cheek, upper lip, side of the nose, teeth, and gums (disruption of infraorbital nerve)
- Subcutaneous emphysema of the face (if the fracture involves the sinuses around the zygoma)

The first five symptoms of zygomatic fractures may be remembered using the mnemonic TIDES (trismus, infraorbital hypesthesia, diplopia, epistaxis, and symmetrical abnormality).

Diagnostic Procedures

- Radiographs (submental vertex, Waters', and Caldwell views)
- Facial CT scan

Therapeutic Interventions

- Apply a cold pack.
- Keep the head elevated to reduce edema.
- Instruct the patient not to sleep on the affected side and to avoid the Valsalva maneuver, straining, or blowing the nose, which can increase subcutaneous emphysema.
- Obtain ophthalmologic consultation as needed.
- Open reduction and internal fixation may be necessary if a cosmetic or functional deformity exists. Surgery is usually deferred until the edema subsides.

Orbital Rim Fractures

The frontal, zygoma, and maxillary bones form the orbit of the eye. The walls of the orbit are thin and can fracture when force is exerted on them. If the force is exerted externally, such as by a baseball hitting the side of the face, the

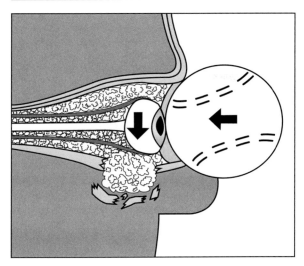

Fig. 41-3 Mechanism of a blow-out fracture caused by the impact of a baseball.

bones may fracture into the orbit toward the eye (blow-in fracture). If the force hits the front of the eyeball itself, such as by the baseball hitting directly into the globe (see Fig. 41-3), the eye may be pushed back so forcefully into the orbit that the orbital bones may fracture outward (blow-out fracture). Regardless of the mechanism of injury, orbital rim fractures can be associated with injuries to the brain, globe, optic nerve, and cranial nerves III, IV, and VI.

Signs and Symptoms

- Visible or palpable deformity around the orbit
- Ocular entrapment—the patient is able to move the uninjured eye but the injured eye remains fixed secondary to the ocular muscles being trapped in the fracture line
- Diplopia worse when looking up or laterally (associated with ocular entrapment)
- Enophthalmos (associated with blow-out fractures) or exophthalmos (associated with blow-in fractures)
- Infraorbital paresthesia
- Periorbital edema and ecchymosis
- Subconjunctival hemorrhage
- Subcutaneous emphysema if the fracture extends into neighboring sinuses

> *Enophthalmos* is a recession of the eyeball into the orbit.
> *Exophthalmos* is a bulging of the eyeball out of the orbit.

Diagnostic Procedures

- Radiographs (Waters' view)
- Facial CT scan

Therapeutic Interventions

- Apply a cold pack to the affected eye.
- Obtain an ophthalmologic consultation.
- Open reduction and internal fixation may be necessary if a cosmetic or functional deformity exists.
- Instruct the patient to avoid activities such as the Valsalva maneuver, straining, or blowing the nose, which can increase subcutaneous emphysema.

Maxillary (Midface) Fractures

In 1901 Dr. René Le Fort described various kinds of fractures to the maxilla, the bone that makes up the middle of the face, and his name is still used to describe these fractures. Maxillary fractures are numbered, and the higher the number, the more serious the fracture (Fig. 41-4). Although the Le Fort system is a convenient way to describe maxillary fractures, many midface fractures do not follow the exact pattern of the traditional Le Fort system. Table 41-3 describes the various Le Fort fractures and provides assessment findings for each.

A tremendous amount of force is required to fracture the maxilla, so careful assessment for concomitant intracranial and spinal cord trauma is essential. Airway compromise is another frequent complication of this fracture. The loss of bony stability can impede the upper airway and make swallowing difficult if not impossible. These factors, coupled with facial edema, blood, and other traumatic debris, will often require frequent oral suctioning and possibly intubation or a surgical airway.

Diagnostic Procedures

- Facial and head CT scans
- Facial radiographs with lateral Waters' and Caldwell views
- A chest radiograph to rule out tooth aspiration if any teeth are unaccounted for

Therapeutic Interventions

- Provide suction and assist with intubation or surgical airway as required.
- Elevate the head of the bed (if cervical spinal injuries have been ruled out) and apply ice to minimize edema.
- Administer antibiotics as prescribed by the health care provider.
- Obtain ophthalmologic and neurologic consultation for Le Fort II and III fractures.
- Surgery is required for reduction and internal fixation.

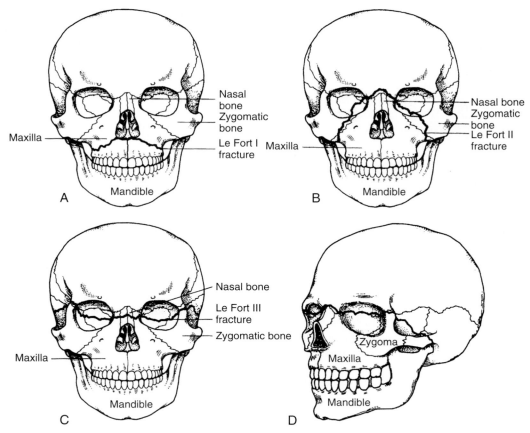

Fig. 41-4 **A,** Le Fort I fracture. **B,** Le Fort II fracture. **C,** Le Fort III fracture. **D,** Le Fort III fracture, lateral view.

TABLE 41-3	**TYPES OF LE FORT FRACTURES**	
FRACTURE	**DESCRIPTION**	**ASSESSMENT FINDINGS**
Le Fort I	A fracture above the front teeth but below the nose that separates the upper jaw from the face.	• If the upper teeth are manipulated, they will move but the nose will remain intact.
Le Fort II	A fracture that extends above the nose in a pyramidal fashion separating the nose and upper palate from the rest of the face.	• If the upper teeth are manipulated, both the nose and the upper palate will be mobile. • A basilar skull fracture with CSF leakage is commonly associated with this fracture.
Le Fort III	A complete craniofacial separation that extends through the orbits and may involve the maxilla, zygoma, mandible, nasal bones, ethmoids, and orbits.	• When the patient is upright, the face may appear elongated and deformed. When the patient is supine, the face will sink back into the skull, resulting in a spoonlike appearance. • A basilar skull fracture with CSF leakage is commonly associated with this fracture.

CSF, Cerebrospinal fluid.

Mandibular Fractures

It takes as much as 70 to 100 times the force of gravity to fracture the mandible.[8] Despite this fact, the prominent position of the mandible on the face, coupled with its U-shape, makes it a frequently fractured bone on the face. In the same way that maxillary fractures compromise the bony stability of the upper face, mandibular fractures can alter the bony stability of the lower face, decreasing the ability of the patient to maintain a patent airway.

Signs and Symptoms

- Malocclusion of the teeth
- Trismus
- Edema and ecchymosis of the lower face
- Lacerations, blood, and bony fragments in the mouth
- Sublingual hematomas
- Point tenderness
- Numbness in the lower lip (indicates involvement of the inferior alveolar nerve)

> One way to assess for malocclusion of the teeth is to ask the patient to bite down on a tongue blade placed between the front teeth. Patients with fractures will usually find this painful and may note that teeth on one side of the mouth come together while teeth on the other side of the mouth do not.

Diagnostic Procedures

- Facial CT scan
- Panoramic topography radiographs
- Plain radiographs: mandibular series with a reverse Towne's view

Therapeutic Intervention

- Suction as needed and be prepared to assist with intubation or a surgical airway as required.
- Elevate the head of the bed if cervical spine injuries are not suspected.
- Apply cold packs to the lower face.
- Administer analgesics and antibiotics (for open fractures) as prescribed by the health care provider.
- Surgery is frequently required for fractures with malocclusion.

Patient and Family Teaching

- Take antibiotics and analgesics as directed.
- "Jaw rest" (for fractures that are not surgically repaired) includes a soft diet and avoiding talking or other activities that require use of the jaw.
- If the patient's jaw is wired:
  - Leave intermaxillary fixation wires or rubber bands in place for 3 to 6 weeks.
    - During this time, maintain appropriate oral intake, consuming a high-calorie, high-protein liquid diet through a straw.
    - Brush the teeth and wires and rinse out the mouth several times per day.
    - Carry wire cutters at all times to open the jaws in case of an airway emergency.
- Avoid strenuous exertion because this makes it more difficult to breathe and places strains on the wires or bands.

DENTAL TRAUMA

Trauma to the teeth can range from a fractured tooth to an avulsed tooth. Patients with dental trauma require careful assessment to ensure that tooth fragments and other debris do not pose a threat to the airway. If tooth fragments or entire teeth are missing, a chest radiograph may be warranted to ensure that the missing pieces have not been aspirated. Careful assessment of any mouth wounds should be undertaken to rule out the possibility that missing tooth fragments are imbedded in these wounds, posing a threat for future infection. The anatomy of the tooth is illustrated in Figure 41-5.

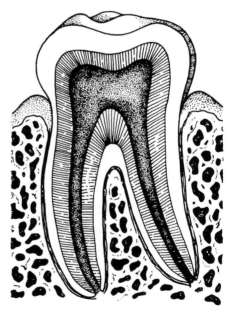

Fig. 41-5 Anatomy of the tooth. (From Gaudet Nolan, E. [2010]. Dental, ear, nose, throat, and facial emergencies. In Emergency Nurses Association, *Sheehy's emergency nursing: Principles and practice* [6th ed., pp. 590–601]. St. Louis, MO: Mosby.)

TABLE 41-4   CLASSIFICATION OF TOOTH FRACTURES

CLASSIFICATION	DESCRIPTION OF FRACTURE	SIGNS AND SYMPTOMS	TREATMENT
Ellis class I	Fracture affecting the outer enamel portion of the tooth	• The tooth takes on a chalky white appearance. It may also appear jagged. • Isolated Ellis I fractures are often painless.	Does not require emergent treatment. Jagged edges may be covered with dental wax to prevent irritation of the oral mucosa. The patient should be encouraged to see a dentist for cosmetic repair.
Ellis class II	Fracture through the enamel portion into the dentin	• The tooth may take on the yellowish appearance of dentin. • Nerve involvement with sensitivity to hot and cold is likely.	Application of calcium hydroxide gel to the fracture to reduce sensitivity and decrease the risk of infection. The patient should be instructed to see a dentist within 24 hours for repair of the tooth.
Ellis class III	A fracture through the enamel and dentin exposing the pulp and nerve of the tooth. The tooth may be broken off.	• The tooth may appear pink or blood-tinged. • Part of the tooth may be missing. • The exposed nerve causes this fracture to be very painful.	Cover the tooth with dental foil or gauze and facilitate an emergent dental referral.
Subluxed tooth	A loose tooth	• The affected tooth is mobile. Pulp may be exposed at the gum line of a severely subluxed tooth.	Minimally subluxed teeth (pulp is not visible, tooth has minimal mobility): The patient is discharged home on a soft diet. Severely subluxed tooth (significant mobility of the tooth in the socket or pulp exposed at the gum line): Facilitate dental referral and instruct the patient not to eat or drink until the dental visit.

The three main injuries affecting teeth are:

- Tooth fractures—Dr. Ellis first classified tooth fractures and his name continues to be used to describe these fractures. Fractures of the teeth are ranked from one to three; the higher the number, the more severe the fracture.
- Subluxed tooth—Trauma to a tooth can stretch the ligaments that hold the tooth in place, resulting in a "loose tooth," also known as a subluxed tooth.
- Avulsed tooth—A tooth that comes out of its socket is known as an avulsed tooth.

Table 41-4 describes various forms of dental trauma and appropriate treatment modalities for each.

OCULAR TRAUMA

There are an estimated 2.4 million eye injuries in the United States every year, 95% of them in males under the age of 30 years.[9] Fortunately, the majority of these injuries are not sight-threatening and do not require surgical intervention.[9]

Ocular injuries may be readily apparent, such as when a pencil or fish hook is impaled in the globe. Other injuries such as intraocular foreign bodies may be less evident and require careful assessment. Injuries that frequently involve the eye and should raise the index of suspicion for ocular trauma include zygomatic, orbital wall, maxillary, and nasal fractures as well as soft tissue injury to the eyelids or other surfaces around the globe.

General Principles

- Assess and provide interventions for the patient's airway, breathing, circulation, and disability status prior to assessment of ocular injuries.
- Check for and, if present, remove contact lenses in the unconscious patient to prevent corneal ulcerations. Figure 41-6 shows proper removal of hard and soft contact lenses.

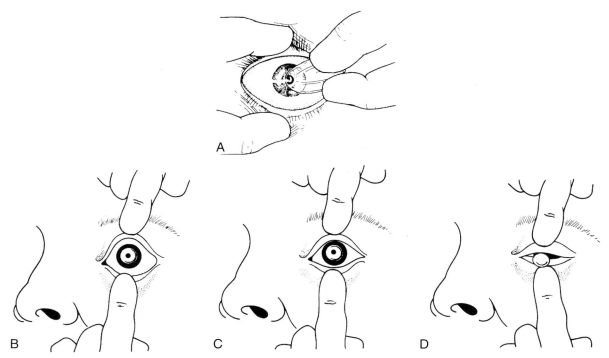

Fig. 41-6 A, Soft contact lens removal. Lift lens off cornea. **B-D,** Technique for removing hard contact lens from the eye. **B,** Spread eyelids apart. **C,** Push lids toward center of eye under contact lens. **D,** Remove lens. (From Egging, D. [2010]. Ocular emergencies. In Emergency Nurses Association, *Sheehy's emergency nursing: Principles and practice* [6th ed., pp. 602–618]. St. Louis, MO: Mosby.)

- Measure visual acuity on all conscious patients with ocular injuries.
- Assess pupillary size, response, and accommodation to light.
- Do not instill eye drops until evaluation of the ocular injury is complete.
- Based on the type of injury, consider bilateral patching to reduce further injury secondary to consensual movement.
- Consider the need for tetanus prophylaxis if the surface of the eye is injured or penetrated.

Subconjunctival Hemorrhage

A subconjunctival hemorrhage is a collection of blood under the conjunctiva that may involve only a portion of the sclera or the entire white of the eye. This finding is common after ocular trauma and, while an isolated subconjunctival hemorrhage is rarely serious, it may be an indication of more serious eye trauma; therefore careful ocular assessment should accompany this injury. Subconjunctival hemorrhages may also result from forceful coughing, sneezing, or straining; high blood pressure; bleeding disorders; and vomiting.

Signs and Symptoms

- Reddish discoloration to a portion of or the entire scleral layer

Patient and Family Teaching

- Avoid aspirin or nonsteroidal anti-inflammatory drugs unless approved by the health care provider.
- Follow up with the family care provider if the condition recurs or does not resolve in 2 weeks or if there are indications of a serious underlying disorder.

Eyelid Laceration

Common causes of eyelid lacerations include projectiles, automobile airbag deployment, falls, assaults, and gunshot injuries.[10] Because the eye is frequently injured with these lacerations, careful ocular assessment should be carried out.

Therapeutic Interventions

- Save any avulsed pieces.
- Reduce lid edema to increase the ability to approximate wound edges.
  - Apply cold pack to the lid.
  - Assign an appropriate triage categorization to facilitate movement to the treatment room before edema becomes problematic.
  - Assist with wound irrigation but remember that extensive irrigation can increase lid edema.
- Instruct the patient to keep the head elevated.

> If the lacrimal duct is involved, an ophthalmologic surgeon may need to be consulted. If an avulsion of the eyelid is present, a plastic surgeon may need to be consulted for reconstruction to protect the cornea.

Hyphema

Blunt or penetrating forces to the eye may cause blood to escape from the iris or ciliary body into the anterior chamber of the eye. A collection of blood in the anterior chamber is termed a hyphema. Frequently, as blood accumulates in the anterior chamber, the resulting increases in pressure will stem further bleeding. Activities such as coughing, sneezing, or leaning forward may cause the bleeding to resume. If the entire anterior chamber fills with blood, the outflow tracts that normally drain fluid from the eye may become obstructed with partially clotted blood, leading to secondary glaucoma and vision loss.[11]

> When the entire anterior chamber fills with blood that ultimately clots, the condition is termed an "eight-ball" hyphema.

Signs and Symptoms

- Visible blood in the anterior chamber
- Blurred vision or a reddish hue to vision
- Photophobia and ocular pain
- Possible elevation of intraocular pressure

Therapeutic Interventions

- If cervical spine injury is not suspected, elevate the head of the bed 30 to 45 degrees.
- Maintain bed rest.
- Administer analgesics as needed.
  - Aspirin and nonsteroidal anti-inflammatory drugs should be avoided to reduce the risk of further bleeding.

- Cycloplegics and topical steroids may be prescribed. If the intraocular pressure is elevated, topical beta-blockers may also be prescribed.
- Patch the affected eye with a rigid eye shield.
- Hospital admission is controversial but is frequently considered for patients with excessively high intraocular pressures or "eight-ball" hyphemas.

Patient and Family Teaching

- Restrict activity.
- Avoid activities that increase intraocular pressure (e.g., sneezing, coughing, bending forward, performing the Valsalva maneuver).
- Maintain eye shield over the affected eye.
- Seek medical care for any change in vision.
- Follow up with an ophthalmologist.

Foreign Bodies

Foreign bodies, such as eyelashes, dirt, sand, environmental debris, metal, glass, and wood, may be present on the surface of the eye, leading to irritation. This is referred to as an *extraocular foreign body*. If an object hits the eye at a high rate of speed, such as a piece of metal, it may penetrate the globe. A foreign body in the posterior chamber of the eye is referred to as an *intraocular foreign body*. Small pieces of debris that penetrate the eye may leave a very small entrance wound that is difficult or impossible to detect. Therefore a high degree of suspicion based on mechanism of injury, coupled with careful diagnostic testing, is required to locate foreign bodies and remove them to prevent potential vision loss. Vegetative matter on or in the eye carries a higher rate of infection than other objects.

> Metallic objects on the cornea can begin to rust within hours, leaving a permanent rust ring that can stain the cornea and result in future visual disturbances.

Signs and Symptoms

- Reddened conjunctiva
- Tearing
- Photophobia
- Pain, especially when opening or closing the eye
- Sensation of a foreign body in or on the eye

Diagnostic Procedures

- Visualize the eye for the presence of foreign bodies or rust rings
- Radiographs of the eye to visualize radiopaque objects
- Slit lamp examination
- B-scan ultrasound (ultrasound biomicroscopy)
- Computed tomography

Therapeutic Interventions

- Administer a topical anesthetic agent. If penetration of the globe is suspected, withhold topical anesthetics until approved by an ophthalmologist.
- Remove nonimbedded foreign bodies with eye irrigation using an isotonic solution such as normal saline or lactated Ringer solution.
- If objects cannot be easily removed with eye irrigation, a sterile foreign body removal device or needle may be used.
- Metal objects can be removed with a tuberculin needle or foreign-body spud and any rust staining can be extracted with an automated rust ring drill, brush, or burr.
- Intraocular foreign bodies usually require surgical removal.
- Topical or systemic antibiotics are often required.

Rupture of the Globe

The eyeball or globe can rupture secondary to numerous mechanisms of injury. Any sharp object, such as a fish hook, dart, pencil, or nail, can penetrate the outer surface of the eye, rupturing the globe (Fig. 41-7). Sudden traumatic increases in intraocular pressure, such as by a baseball directly hitting the eye, can also cause the globe to rupture. Always assess patients with orbital fractures for globe rupture. Regardless of the mechanism, rupture of the globe will always lead to some degree of visual disturbance or loss of vision. Without emergent treatment, permanent visual loss or even loss of the entire eye is likely.

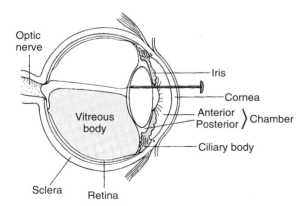

Fig. 41-7 Foreign bodies that penetrate the globe can cause a rupture of the globe. (From Cullen, M. M. [2007]. Facial and eye, ear, nose, and throat trauma. In D. M. Danis, J. S. Blansfield, & A. A. Gervasini [Eds.], *Handbook of clinical trauma care* [4th ed., p. 214]. St. Louis, MO: Mosby.)

Signs and Symptoms

- Unusually deep or shallow anterior chamber
- Obvious impalement (e.g., pencil imbedded in the eye)
- Diminished or absent vision
- Ocular pain
- Vitreous humor leakage from the eye
- Teardrop shape to the pupil

> When a pupil associated with a ruptured globe assumes a teardrop shape, the point of the tear points to the area of the rupture.

Diagnostic Procedures

- CT scan
- Radiographs including Waters' and Caldwell views to rule out associated orbital fractures
- Magnetic resonance imaging (unless metallic objects are suspected)

Therapeutic Interventions

- Provide analgesia, antiemetics, and sedation as appropriate.
- Do not instill topical medications into the eye.
- Secure impaled objects with gauze rolls or a paper cup over the object, being cautious not to put pressure on the object or manipulate it, both of which can lead to increased trauma.
- Do not apply external pressure to the eye.
- Elevate the head of the bed to decrease intraocular pressure.
- Administer systemic antibiotics.
- Obtain an emergent ophthalmologic consultation for surgical intervention.

> When securing a foreign object in an eye, always patch the unaffected side to prevent further damage due to consensual movement of the eyes.

Conjunctival and Corneal Lacerations and Abrasions

If a foreign object does not completely penetrate the globe but causes a disruption to the surface, it is referred to as a *laceration*, either of the conjunctiva or cornea. If the epithelium of the cornea is abraded or scraped, such as from a fingernail or contact lens, it is a *corneal abrasion*. All of these injuries carry a risk for infection. Conjunctival lacerations and corneal abrasions usually heal without intervention whereas corneal lacerations may require suturing or surgical repair.

Signs and Symptoms

- Photophobia
- Tearing
- Pain
- Impaired vision
- Reddened eye
- Corneal abrasions often have the same sensation as a foreign body in the eye

Diagnostic Procedures

- Slit lamp examination.
- Stain the eye with fluorescein dye and then evaluate the cornea with a cobalt light.
- Assess for foreign bodies in the wound.

Therapeutic Interventions

- A rigid shield may be placed over the eye for corneal lacerations. Eye patches are rarely used in conjunctival lacerations and corneal abrasions.
- Systemic or topical antibiotics.
- Systemic or topical anesthetics.
- Obtain ophthalmologic consultation as needed.

REFERENCES

1. Lynham, A., Hirst, J., Cosson, J., Chapman, P., & McEniery, P. (2004). Emergency department management of maxillofacial trauma. *Emergency Medicine Australasia, 16*(1), 7–12.

2. Zellweger, R. (2007). Maxillofacial fractures. *ANZ Journal of Surgery, 77*(8), 613.

3. Arosarena, O. A., Fritsch, T. A., Hsueh, Y., Aynehchi, B., & Haug, R. (2009). Maxillofacial injuries and violence against women. *Archives of Facial Plastic Surgery, 11*(1), 48–52.

4. Ramirez, E. G. (2007). Wounds and wound management. In K. S. Hoyt, & J. Selfridge-Thomas (Eds.), *Emergency nursing core curriculum* (6th ed., pp. 738–760). St. Louis, MO: Mosby.

5. Lee, S., & Bogdan, Y. (2009, December 29). *Facial soft tissue trauma.* Retrieved from http://emedicine.medscape.com/article/882081-overview

6. Smith, J. E., & Perez, C. L. (2009, November 23). *Nasal fracture imaging.* Retrieved from http://emedicine.medscape.com/article/391863-overview

7. Tadj, A., Kimble, F. (2003). Fractured zygomas. *ANZ Journal of Surgery, 73*(1–2), 49–54.

8. Widell, T. (2008, March 6). *Mandible fracture in emergency medicine.* Retrieved from http://emedicine.medscape.com/article/825663-overview

9. Kent, C. (2008). Managing serious cases of ocular trauma. *Review of Ophthalmology, 15*(11), 35–42.

10. *Eyelid laceration.* (2006, March 15). Retrieved from http://www.accessmylibrary.com/coms2/summary_0286-14880322_ITM

11. Kabat, A. G., & Sowka, J. (2007, October 27). *A bloody challenging situation.* Retrieved from http://www.revoptom.com/content/d/cornea/c/15321/

Burns

Kathleen A. Ribbens and Megan DeVries

Deaths from fires and burns are the fifth most common cause of unintentional injury deaths in the United States and the third leading cause of fatal home injury.[1,2] In 2008 someone in the United States died in a fire approximately every 158 minutes and was injured in a fire every 31 minutes.[3] Burn injuries account for an estimated 700,000 visits to the emergency department (ED) annually; of these, 45,000 require hospitalization in a burn center.[4] The high-risk, low-frequency exposure to burn-injured patients continues to be anxiety provoking to many emergency personnel. However, proper management in the ED is an essential first step in appropriately managing burn care and can have a significant impact on patient outcomes.

ETIOLOGY

Flame is the predominant cause of burns in patients admitted to burn centers, particularly in the adult age group.[5] Thirty percent of all burns requiring admission to the hospital are caused by scalding resulting from hot liquids.[5] Burn injury is caused by more than fire and scald, however. A burn can also occur from thermal exposure, chemicals, electric current, and radiation, as well as from inhalation of heat or smoke. Table 42-1 lists various types of burns and their possible etiologies.

PATHOPHYSIOLOGY

The body's response to burn injury varies with the degree of tissue damage, cellular impairment, and fluid shifts. Damage to burned tissue causes the release of mediators that initiate an inflammatory response. The release of these mediators is associated with vasodilation and increased capillary permeability, resulting in intravascular fluid loss and tissue edema.[6]

> Burn injury results in:
> - Vasodilation
> - Increased capillary permeability
> - Intravascular fluid loss
> - Tissue edema

Burn shock is the most significant component of burn pathophysiology. Direct thermal injury can result in dramatic changes in the microcirculation, particularly the increase in capillary permeability throughout the body. Burn shock is both hypovolemic shock and cellular shock.[5] Table 42-2 summarizes the pathophysiology of hypovolemic burn shock. Table 42-3 describes the extensive effects of burn injury on the body.

TRIAGE ASSESSMENT

Inadequate treatment and delays in treatment, particularly related to fluid resuscitation, lead to increased morbidity and mortality. Timely interventions and the application of principles of emergency resuscitation care are essential to minimize negative outcomes for the burn patient. Therefore the immediate assessment of the burn patient should focus on lifesaving measures of airway, breathing, and circulation management (ABCs). Mechanism of injury must always be considered, as concomitant traumatic injuries often accompany the burn injury.

In addition to addressing the ABCs, attention should be directed toward stopping the burning process if this has not been accomplished already by emergency medical services (EMS) personnel.

- Remove all clothing from any burned area, including shoes and jewelry that may retain heat.
- Flush all areas of the body that came in contact with chemicals with copious amounts of water.

TABLE 42-1 TYPES OF BURN INJURIES

TYPE OF BURN	EXAMPLES
Thermal	
Scald	Hot liquids (water, oil, beverages, bath water)
Flame	Flammable fabrics, campfire
Flash	Furnace blast, gasoline explosion
Contact	Hot burner, clothes iron
Tar	Work-related injuries
Steam	Radiator, steam pipes, hot water with cooking
Electrical	
Alternating current	Commercial appliances
Direct current	Car batteries, lightning
Chemical	
Alkaline	Cleaning supplies, household plumbing agents
Acid	Sulfuric acid, hydrofluoric acid
Radiation	Exposure to ultraviolet light (sun, tanning booths), radiation therapy, radioactive fallout, radiographs
Friction	
Tissue abrasion	"Road rash," as a result of motorcycle/bicycle crash

TABLE 42-2 PATHOPHYSIOLOGY OF BURNS

First 24 Hours Following Burn Injury
↓
Coagulation necrosis of soft tissue occurs
↓
Release of vasoactive substances
↓
Increased capillary permeability and vasodilation
↓
Formation of tissue edema
Increased fluid loss
↓
Hypovolemic shock, decreased cardiac output, cellular shock

The Next 18 to 24 Hours
↓
Capillary permeability returns to normal
↓
Third spacing resolves

• Tar that is part of burned, blistered tissue should be removed. Applying ointments, such as polymicrobial antibiotic ointment or petroleum jelly, or common household agents such as mayonnaise promotes tar removal.[4]

PRIMARY ASSESSMENT

Airway and Breathing

Airway, Airway, Airway!
• Assess it first, assess it often.
• When in doubt, intubate early.

All burn patients should receive supplemental oxygen by EMS personnel en route to the ED; its administration should be continued until deemed unnecessary. Intubation must be considered immediately in any patient with symptoms of a compromised airway.

Inhalation Injury

Assessment for inhalation injury should be completed on every burn patient on arrival at the ED. An inhalation injury cannot be ruled out until the components of the Inhalation Injury Triad have been considered (Fig. 42-1).

Mechanism of Injury
• Assess for burns that occurred in an enclosed space with heat or smoke exposure for an extended period of time. The likelihood of airway injury is greater in an enclosed space than it is outdoors.
• Consideration should be given to the toxins that can be produced when objects are burning in an enclosed space.
• Damaged cilia in the airway result in an inability to clear secretions and bacteria manifested by a tracheal bronchitis.[7]

Progressive airway edema should be expected in the first 24 hours in a patient with inhalation injury.

Assessment Data. Any of the following may be evident with an inhalation injury:
• Dyspnea
• Hoarse voice
• Cough
• Anxiety or agitation
• Stridor
• Wheezing
• Facial burns, singed nasal hairs[5,8]
• Presence of carbonaceous sputum

TABLE 42-3   IMPACT OF BURN INJURY ON BODY SYSTEMS

Cellular Response
- Direct thermal injury to endothelial cells with increased burn tissue osmolarity
- Decreased tissue oxygen tension
- Sodium and water shift into cell—intracellular swelling
- Possible cell death
- Shifting of potassium out of the cell resulting in increased serum potassium
- Decreased oxygen level
- Anaerobic metabolism begins
- Increased lactic acid levels
- Increased lactic acid levels lead to metabolic acidosis

Cardiovascular System—First 24 Hours
- Activation of the sympathetic nervous system and catecholamine release
  - Tachycardia
  - Vasoconstriction
- During early phase:
  - Classic signs and symptoms of compensated shock
  - Dramatic decrease in cardiac output
- Volume loss and decreased venous return
  - Decreased preload
  - Decreased cardiac filling pressure
  - Decreased central venous pressure and pulmonary artery occlusion pressure (PAOP)

Respiratory System
- Upper airway and parenchymal injury
  - Involves all airways to level of true vocal cords
  - Initially because of inflammation from heat of inspired smoke
  - Exacerbated by accumulation of excess interstitial fluid

Neurologic System
- Decreased cerebral perfusion
- Cerebral edema as a result of sodium shifts
- Carbon monoxide poisoning or associated head injury may cause neurologic changes

Gastrointestinal System
- Slowed peristalsis and possible ileus
- Increased hydrochloric acid production from stress response
- Narcotics for pain management further impair gastrointestinal function

Immune System
- Alters function of immune cells
  - Decreases "killing power" of neutrophils
  - Macrophages and lymphocytes ineffective

Hematologic System
- Destruction of red blood cells
- Hemoglobinuria
- Increased hemoglobin level and hemoconcentration
- Increased white blood cells
- Altered coagulation

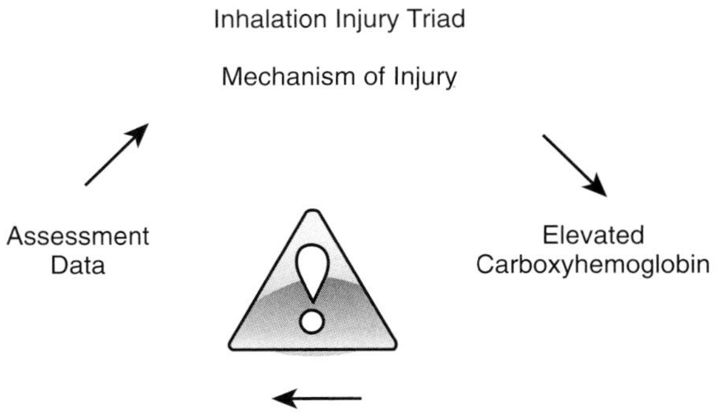

Inhalation Injury Triad

Mechanism of Injury

Assessment Data

Elevated Carboxyhemoglobin

Fig. 42-1   Inhalation Injury Triad.

Elevated Carboxyhemoglobin. Carboxyhemoglobin level may be as high as 50% to 70%. See Table 42-4 for signs and symptoms of elevated carboxyhemoglobin level.

Carbon Monoxide Poisoning

The majority of fatalities that occur at the scene of a fire are the result of asphyxiation or carbon monoxide poisoning. Carbon monoxide poisoning is also the most immediate threat to life in survivors of inhalation injury.

- Carbon monoxide binds to hemoglobin 200 times more effectively than oxygen does; tissue hypoxia occurs if sufficient hemoglobin is bound to carbon monoxide.[9]
- The skin of a patient with high carbon monoxide levels may appear cherry red in color, but this has been observed in only 50% of patients with severe carbon monoxide poisoning.

TABLE 42-4	SIGNS AND SYMPTOMS OF ELEVATED CARBOXYHEMOGLOBIN

Carboxyhemoglobin Saturation Percentage and Symptoms

5–10	Mild headache and confusion
11–20	Severe headache, flushing, dilation of skin vessels
21–30	Disorientation, nausea
31–40	Irritability, dizziness, vomiting, prostration
41–50	Tachypnea, tachycardia, prostration
51–69	Coma, seizures, convulsions, Cheyne-Stokes respiration. Death is possible
70–80	Slowing/stopping of breathing, death within hours
80–90	Death in less than 1 hour
90–100	Death within a few minutes

Data from Essig, M. G. (2008, March 18). *Carbon monoxide (CO)*. Retrieved from http://firstaid.webmd.com/carbon-monoxide-co

- Although the oxygen content of the blood is diminished, the amount of oxygen dissolved in the plasma (PaO_2) is unaffected by carbon monoxide poisoning; the arterial blood gas will appear normal.
- Pulse oximetry detects saturated hemoglobin and does not measure carbon monoxide, so the oxygen saturation usually appears normal.
- A serum carboxyhemoglobin level must be determined in any patient with potential exposure to carbon monoxide during a fire.

Management of Carbon Monoxide Poisoning or Inhalation Injury

- Immediately administer 100% oxygen if this has not been accomplished by EMS personnel prior to arrival at the ED.
- If the airway is compromised in any way, endotracheal intubation should be performed and difficult airway supplies should be available. See Table 42-5 for considerations for early intubation.
- Intubation can often be difficult in this patient population because of swelling of the face and hypopharynx.[9]

Circumferential Burns

- Assessment of chest expansion is essential in a full-thickness circumferential chest burn. Chest wall excursion may become compromised and ultimately will hinder the patient's ability to ventilate adequately. Full-thickness circumferential and near circumferential skin burns result in the formation of tough, inelastic burned tissue.

TABLE 42-5	CONSIDERATIONS FOR EARLY INTUBATION

- Agitation resulting from hypoxia, decreased level of consciousness
- Carbonaceous sputum
- Hoarseness, stridor
- Progressive edema
- Oral or nasal erythema
- Inability to handle secretions
- Crackles, rhonchi, diminished breath sounds
- Facial burns, singed nasal hairs

- Inelastic tissue (eschar) can result in a burn-induced compartment syndrome caused by the accumulation of extracellular and extravascular fluid within a confined anatomic space.
- Excessive fluid causes the intracompartmental pressures to increase, resulting in collapse of vascular and lymphatic structures and loss of tissue viability.
- A compartment pressure of 30 mm Hg is accepted as the level that requires intervention to prevent tissue death.[10]
- Escharotomy and fasciotomy are surgical procedures performed to restore circulation and avoid further complications of full-thickness circumferential burns and high-voltage electrical burns. Decisions to perform these procedures are often based on clinical examination of the burned area.[11]
  - Escharotomy is the surgical division of the nonviable eschar or burned tissue. When performed to relieve the pressure within the chest compartment it allows more effective chest expansion. Figure 42-2 demonstrates some common locations of escharotomy incisions.
  - Bleeding from escharotomy incisions should be controlled by use of the electrocautery.
  - The resulting wounds are a potential source of infection and should be treated, as is the burn wound, with application of a topical antimicrobial and dressings.[10]
  - Extravascular fluid accumulation generally occurs slowly over time, so it is rare that escharotomy will need to be performed in the first 4 to 6 hours after burn injury.
  - Fasciotomy is a surgical procedure in which the fascia is cut to relieve tension or pressure that limits circulation to an area of tissue or muscle.
  - A fasciotomy is a limb-saving procedure used to treat acute compartment syndrome, a potential

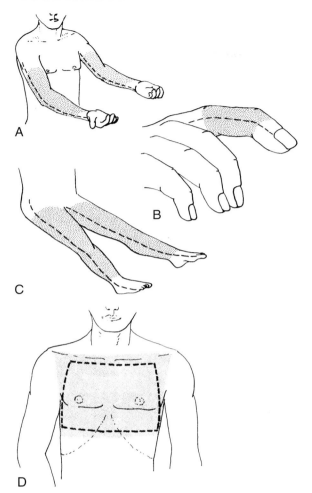

Fig. 42-2 Indications for emergency escharotomy include the presence of circumferential eschar with impending or established vascular compromise of the extremities **(A, C)** or digits **(B)** or impending or established respiratory compromise because of circumferential torso burns **(D)**.

complication of high-voltage injury with entrance or exit wounds in one or more extremities.[12]
- Although fasciotomy is seldom required, it may be necessary to restore circulation in burns involving tissue beneath the investing fascia.[9]

Circulation

Assessing and maintaining adequate circulation is an essential component of burn injury management. Failure to do so can contribute directly to the development of

burn shock. The following actions help ensure adequate circulation:
- Establish intravenous (IV) access.
  - Insert two large-bore peripheral IV catheters for fluid resuscitation and pain management, preferably through nonburned tissue. IV access through burned tissue is acceptable when no other option is available.
  - If unable to establish a peripheral IV catheter, intraosseous or central line catheters may be used.
- Fluid of choice for the adult is lactated Ringer solution. See "Fluid Resuscitation" below.
  - Because children have decreased glucose stores, lactated Ringer solution should be transitioned to dextrose 5% Ringer lactate to prevent life-threatening hypoglycemia. For this reason, bedside glucose testing should be assessed every 4 to 6 hours during the hypermetabolic state.[13]
- *Avoid* normal saline for IV fluid resuscitation.
  - Normal saline crosses the blood-brain barrier.
  - Its use can cause a shift in electrolytes that contributes to significant edema.
  - Its use can result in increased intracranial pressure and the development of abdominal compartment syndrome and can lead to significant morbidity and mortality.
- Monitor adequacy of fluid resuscitation by measuring urine output. Urine output target is adult = 0.5 to 1 mL/kg per hour; child = 1 to 1.5 mL/kg per hour.[13]
- Assess for effects of inadequate fluid resuscitation.
  - Decreased circulating volume because of increase in capillary permeability
  - Shock and organ failure, most commonly acute renal failure
  - Greatest risk in the immediate post-burn period and over the next 24 hours
- Assess for effects of excessive fluid resuscitation.
  - Compromised local blood supply to the tissues and burned area
  - Exaggerated edema formation
  - Compromised delivery of nutrients
- Monitor hemodynamic stability. A decrease in cardiac output and a subsequent drop in blood pressure after a burn injury is not uncommon. This is a result of decreased preload to the heart through volume loss into burned and nonburned tissues.
  - Blood pressure readings via cuff and arterial line may be unreliable in major burns secondary to peripheral vasoconstriction. If unrecognized, misinterpretation of blood pressure can lead to massive fluid overload from excessive fluid resuscitation.[9]

- The administration of vasopressors is controversial because of the vasoconstrictive properties of these medications, which can cause impairment of blood flow to burned tissue. Vasopressors are not recommended in the acute resuscitative phase of burn care. The end result of the redistribution in blood flow can cause conversion of partial-thickness skin injuries to full-thickness burns.[5]
- Elevate burn-injured areas above the level of the heart to help reduce edema formation.
- Assess for cardiac and circulatory problems in patients who have experienced lightning injuries.
  - Lightning injuries are not usually associated with deep burns but most often with superficial injury to the skin and underlying soft tissue. However, significant cardiac and neurologic damage may result.
  - The lightning flashes cause an immediate depolarization of the entire myocardium and leads to asystole.[9]

Disability

Unlike patients with other traumatic injuries, the burn patient is generally awake and alert despite the extent of severe burn injury. If loss of consciousness or impaired neurologic status is present, consider causes such as associated head injury, substance abuse, carbon monoxide poisoning, hypoxia, or preexisting medical conditions.[9] Conduct a more thorough neurologic assessment in the secondary assessment as indicated.

Exposure

- Remove all clothing and jewelry upon arrival at the ED.
- Cover the patient with a clean, dry sheet to maintain body temperature. Loss of skin integrity and increased capillary permeability will lead to hypothermia.
- Covering the burn with a clean, dry sheet will also decrease pain by reducing air currents over burned tissue.
- Do not place ice or iced saline on burn wounds.

SECONDARY ASSESSMENT

History and Physical

- Repeat head-to-toe assessment, including complete assessment of the back.
- Identify any missed injuries or burned areas.

- Obtain a more in-depth history using a mnemonic such as:
  - A—Allergies
  - M—Medications currently used, substances ingested
  - P—Past illness, Pregnancy
  - L—Last meal eaten
  - E—Events and Environment related to injury
- Obtain essential information from EMS personnel related to events surrounding the burn injury.
  - Location where patient was found
  - Duration of exposure to smoke and flame
  - Circumstances surrounding the burn injury
  - Concomitant injuries
  - Actual time of burn injury (not arrival at ED)
- Be alert to any discrepancies between history and extent and presentation of physical injury. Always consider the possibility of maltreatment, suicide, or homicide.

Diagnostic Procedures

The following diagnostic studies may be performed, as indicated by history:

- Arterial blood gases
- Carboxyhemoglobin level
- Hemoglobin and hematocrit
- Complete blood count
- Basic metabolic panel
- 12-lead electrocardiogram
- Chest radiograph
- Computed tomography of any obvious bony deformity

Determine Need for Transfer to Burn Center

Table 42-6 lists criteria indicating that the patient requires transfer to a burn center.

Determine Depth of Burns

A typical burn injury does not consist of only one depth. There will be areas that have a combination of all three depths of burn.[6] Burns that appear as superficial partial-thickness burns in the ED may evolve into deep partial-thickness burns, or even full-thickness burns, over the next 72 hours. Refer to Table 42-7 for a description of superficial and deep partial-thickness burns and full-thickness burns.

Determine Extent of Burns

There are two main methods of determining the extent of a burn. Most burn centers use the Lund and Browder formula to calculate the extent of burns.[5] It is also seen as

TABLE 42-6	**AMERICAN BURN ASSOCIATION TRANSFER CRITERIA**

- Partial thickness burns >10% total body surface area
- Burns that involve the face, hands, feet, genitalia, perineum, or major joints
- Full-thickness (third-degree) burns in any age group
- Electrical burns, including lightning injury
- Chemical burns
- Inhalation injury
- Burn injury in patients with preexisting medical disorders that could complicate management, prolong recovery, or affect mortality
- Any patient with burns and concomitant trauma (such as fractures) in which the burn injury poses the greatest risk of morbidity or mortality. In such cases, if the trauma poses the greater immediate risk, the patient may be initially stabilized in a trauma center before being transferred to a burn facility. Physician judgment will be necessary in such situations and should be in concert with the regional medical control plan and triage protocols.
- Burned children at hospitals without qualified personnel or equipment for the care of children.
- Burn injury in patients who require special social, emotional, or long-term rehabilitative intervention.
- Questions about specific patients can be resolved by consultation with the burn center.

Data from American Burn Association. (2005). *Advanced burn life support.* Chicago, IL: Author.

TABLE 42-7 **THE DEPTH OF BURNS**

Superficial Partial-Thickness (First-Degree) Burns
- Only the epidermis is involved
- Local redness and pain occur, similar to that of a sunburn
- Minimal or no edema and no blistering occur
- Skin blanches with pressure and refills when pressure is removed
- Wound heals within 7 days

Deep Partial-Thickness (Second-Degree) Burns
- The epidermis and some portion of the dermis are involved
- Sweat glands, hair follicles, capillaries, and nerves remain
- Burn appears mottled with pink, red, white, and tan areas
- The wound is moist and may form large, wet blisters
- Pain is intense
- Skin blanches with pressure and refills when pressure is removed
- Healing time is 5 to 35 days but may require excision and grafting
- Wound can convert to a full-thickness injury if undertreated or infected

Full-Thickness (Third-Degree) Burns
- Burn involves the epidermis, the dermis, and the subcutaneous tissues
- Burn can extend to muscles, tendons, ligaments, cartilage, vessels, nerves, and bone
- Charred vessels may be visible under the eschar
- Burn appearance depends on the cause; it can be white, brown, charred, or leathery
- Wound is dry; no blister formation occurs
- No blanching occurs with pressure
- Full-thickness burns may be insensate but usually are surrounded by painful partial-thickness burns
- Wound requires excision and grafting

the most accurate method to determine the extent of burns in children, as it compensates for variations in body shape.

The Rule of Nines is the most commonly used method outside of burn centers to determine the extent of burns and is illustrated in Figure 42-3.

- Important note: Children's body surface area distribution differs from that of the adult (see Fig. 42-3).
- Superficial partial-thickness (first-degree) burns are not to be included in estimating the extent or percentage of the burn injury.
- Another guideline to help estimate the extent of burns with irregular outlines or distribution is to use the palmar surface (including the fingers) of the patient's hand, which represents approximately 1% of the patient's body surface area.[14]

FLUID RESUSCITATION

The goal of fluid resuscitation is to maintain tissue perfusion and organ function. Over-resuscitation may lead to excessive edema, compromising blood flow to burned tissue. Under-resuscitation could result in shock and organ damage. The Parkland Formula is one method used to guide fluid resuscitation.

> Inadequate fluid resuscitation in the first 24 hours increases morbidity and mortality from hypovolemic shock.

> Urine output is the best indicator for adequacy of fluid resuscitation.

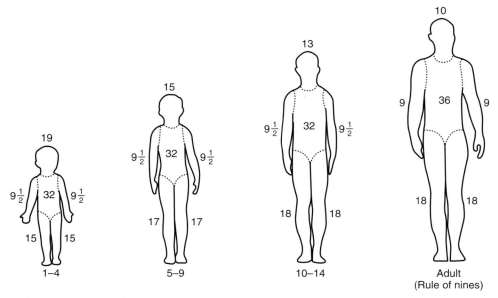

Fig. 42-3 Rule of Nines calculations from infancy through adulthood. (Reprinted with permission from Bryant, R., & Nix, D. [2007]. *Acute and chronic wounds: Current management and concepts* [3rd ed.]. St. Louis, MO: Mosby.)

Parkland Formula

- Used to calculate the amount of fluid to be given in the first 24 hours after burn injury.
  - Calculated from the time of actual injury, not arrival time at the ED.
  - One half of the calculated total volume for fluid resuscitation should be administered in the first 8 hours after burn injury.
  - The second half of the calculated total volume should be administered over the remaining 16 hours.
  - Recommended fluid of choice is lactated Ringer solution.
- Resuscitation volume is an estimate of the fluid that will be required; continuous evaluation of the patient's response to resuscitation efforts, including hourly urine output measurement, is essential in the evaluation of proper fluid resuscitation.
  - The single best monitor of fluid replacement is urine output.
  - Diuretics are generally not indicated during the initial resuscitation efforts.[5]
  - Placement of a urinary catheter is recommended with burns greater than 20% of total body surface area. Place the catheter with an hourly monitoring device and a temperature probe if possible.
- Parkland Formula Fluid Calculations[9]:

- Adults: 2 to 4 mL × kg body weight × total body surface area burned; urine output target: 0.5 to 1 mL/kg per hour
- Children: 3 to 4 mL × kg body weight x total body surface area burned; urine output target: 1 to 1.5 mL/kg per hour
- The decreased glycogen stores in infants and young children can easily lead to hypoglycemia. Pediatric patients weighing less than 30 kg should receive fluid with 5% dextrose at a maintenance rate in addition to the resuscitation fluid calculated above.[14]

Formula to determine volume requirements for fluid resuscitation during the first 24 hours after burn injury:

	Amount of Lactated Ringer Solution	**Urine Output Target**
Adults	2 to 4 mL × weight (kg) × %TBSA	0.5 to 1 mL/kg per hour
Children	3 to 4 mL × weight (kg) × %TBSA	1 to 1.5 mL/kg per hour

TBSA, Total body surface area.

- Infuse half of the calculated volume in first 8 hours.
- Infuse remaining half of calculated volume in next 16 hours.
- The first 24 hours begin with time of burn injury occurrence, not arrival at emergency department.

PAIN MANAGEMENT

Burns are one of the most intensely painful injuries. Pain in the burn patient is caused by direct tissue destruction. However, pain is also induced by stimulation of both inflammation and hyperalgesia (extreme sensitivity to painful stimuli). The inflammatory reaction of burns includes the secretion of histamine, bradykinin, and prostaglandin, irritating substances that stimulate the exposed peripheral nerve endings and produce additional pain.[15]

- Every burn patient will experience pain regardless of the size, depth, or mechanism of injury.
- Providing effective analgesia in the ED should be considered a priority once the primary and secondary assessments have been completed.
- Opioids provide rapid relief of pain and should be titrated to achieve the desired comfort level for each patient.
- IV administration of analgesics is the route of choice in the burn patient.
- Drugs of choice in the emergency setting include the following. Follow dosing guidelines as outlined by hospital formulary.
  - Morphine
  - Hydromorphone (Dilaudid)
  - Fentanyl (Sublimaze)
- Avoid intramuscular and oral pain medications in the acutely burned patient. Medication via these routes may not be metabolized adequately for pain control because of decreased perfusion in the burn-injured patient.
- Burn injuries may require high doses of analgesics. Vigilant monitoring for airway adequacy and respiratory depression is essential.
- Side effects from opioids can be reversed quickly if necessary. Reversal agents include the following. Follow dosing guidelines as outlined by hospital formulary.
  - Flumazenil (Romazicon)
  - Naloxone (Narcan)

WOUND CARE

If the burn-injured patient is to be transferred to a burn center:

- Wounds should be covered with a clean, dry sheet and blanket if needed to maintain temperature.
- Cold application should be avoided to prevent hypothermia and further damage to burned tissue.[9]

Do not delay transfer for debridement of the wound or application of antimicrobial agents. Burns that do not meet American Burn Association transfer criteria can be managed in the emergency setting if a burn specialist or burn clinic is not available.

- Clean the wound and apply silver sulfadiazine (Silvadene) as per institutional recommendations.
- Do not use Silvadene on facial burns; the use of bacitracin is preferred.
- Arrange for follow-up as appropriate.

ADDITIONAL INTERVENTIONS

- A patient undergoing resuscitation should have a urinary catheter placed.
- Nasogastric tubes should be considered in patients with burns greater than 20% of total body surface area, as they will experience gastroparesis and probable emesis.[16]
- Continuous cardiac monitoring may be necessary during the first 24 hours after an electric burn injury.[9]
- Update tetanus status as appropriate.
- Do not administer prophylactic antibiotics for burn injuries. Although prophylactic systemic antibiotics have no role in thermal injury, topical antimicrobial therapy is efficacious.[16]

ASSESSING FOR MALTREATMENT

Injured children and vulnerable adults need to be screened for indicators of abuse each time they encounter the health care system. Assessment for abuse and maltreatment should begin at the time of admission to the ED; see Chapter 49, Abuse and Neglect, for more information.

- When maltreatment is suspected, a report must be made to the proper governing protective agency for children and adults.
- Table 42-8 lists common indicators of abuse for both children and adults related to burn injuries.[5]

INTERACTION WITH PATIENTS AND FAMILIES

Shock and disbelief are early emotional responses to traumatic events. Anger can also be a component; some individuals move quickly to a stage of attrition, blame, or guilt. Nurses should provide general information to the family before their initial encounter with the burn patient. The nurse should answer the patient's questions honestly and provide emotional support, recognizing the psychological reactions to trauma.[9] Essential points during this interaction include the following:

TABLE 42-8	INDICATORS OF ABUSE IN THE BURN-INJURED PATIENT
PHYSICAL INDICATORS OF ABUSE	**PSYCHOSOCIAL INDICATORS OF ABUSE**
Scald burn with clear-cut immersion lines	History of burn injury inconsistent with injuries
Scald burn with no splash marks	History of burn injury inconsistent with developmental capacity of patient
Scald involving perineum, genitalia, buttocks	
Mirror-image burn injury of extremities	Historical account of injury differs with each interview
Other physical signs of abuse: bruises, welts, fractures	Unexplained delay in seeking medical treatment
	History of injuries to patient

- Introduction of personnel who will be caring for the patient.
- Reassurance that measures are being taken to provide for the patient's comfort.
- Identification of a family spokesperson.
- Explanations regarding smoke inhalation and compromise to the airway. Intubation and mechanical ventilation usually will cause a tremendous amount of anxiety in the patient and family members.
- Reinforce any information provided by the physician and instruct the patient to report any change in feelings of discomfort or difficulty breathing.
- Provide explanations for the appearance of the burn patient, especially if there are significant facial burns. The patient and his or her family should be prepared for facial edema and the subsequent swelling shut of the eyes. They should be informed that this is only temporary.
- Age-appropriate explanations of all procedures should be provided to the patient before performing them.

Caring for the burn-injured patient requires an ability to prioritize critical interventions immediately upon arrival at the ED. Careful attention to the patient's immediate needs and vigilant surveillance for complications of both the burns and the therapeutic interventions used to resuscitate the burn victim are necessary to improve patient outcomes.

REFERENCES

1. Centers for Disease Control and Prevention. (2010, October 1). *Fire deaths and injuries: Fact sheet.* Retrieved from http://www.cdc.gov/HomeandRecreationalSafety/Fire-Prevention/fires-factsheet.html
2. Runyan, C. W., & Casteel, C. (Eds.), (2004). *The state of home safety in America: Facts about unintentional injuries in the home* (2nd ed.). Washington, DC: Home Safety Council.
3. Karter, M. J. (2009). *Fire loss in the United States during 2008.* Quincy, MA: National Fire Protection Association. Retrieved from http://tkolb.net/FireReports/USFireLoss2008.pdf
4. Jenkins, J. A., & Schraga, E. D. (2011, September 26). *Emergent management of thermal burns.* Retrieved from http://emedicine.medscape.com/article/769193-overview
5. Herndon, D. (2007). *Total burn care* (3rd ed.). Philadelphia, PA: Saunders.
6. Howard, P. K., & Steinmann, R. A. (Eds.), (2010). *Sheehy's emergency nursing: Principles and practice* (6th ed.). St. Louis, MO: Mosby.
7. Demling, R. (2008). Smoke inhalation lung injury: An update. *Eplasty, 8,* e27. Retrieved from http://www.ncbi.nlm.nih.gov/pmc/articles/PMC2396464
8. Sheridan, R. L. (2000). Airway management and respiratory care of the burn patient. *International Anesthesiology Clinics, 38*(3), 129–145.
9. American Burn Association. (2005). *Advanced burn life support.* Chicago, IL: Author.
10. Pal, N. (2009, May 31). *Emergency escharotomy.* Retrieved from http://emedicine.medscape.com/article/80583-overview
11. Wong, L., & Spence, R. J. (2000). Escharotomy and fasciotomy of the burned upper extremity. *Hand Clinics, 16*(2), 165–174.
12. Demling, R. H., & DeSanti, L. (n.d.). *Initial management of the burn patient: Electrical burns.* Retrieved from http://www.burnsurgery.com/Modules/initial_mgmt/sec_7.htm
13. Oliver, R. I., (2009, June 19). *Resuscitation and early management burns.* Retrieved from http://emedicine.medscape.com/article/1277360-overview
14. American College of Surgeons. (2008). *Advanced Trauma Life Support for Doctors student manual* (8th ed.). Chicago, IL: Author.
15. Connor-Ballard, P. A. (2009). Understanding and managing burn pain: Part 1. *American Journal of Nursing, 109*(4), 48–56.
16. Latenser, B. (2009). Critical care of the burn patient: The first 48 hours. *Critical Care Medicine, 37*(10), 2819–2826.

43

Obstetric Trauma

Laura M. Criddle

EPIDEMIOLOGY AND PRIORITIES OF CARE

Five to ten percent of gravid women will sustain an injury for which they seek medical care.[1,2] Fortunately, most cases involve minor or moderate trauma, but life-threatening injuries complicate 3 in 1000 pregnancies.[3] As is true for nonpregnant women in their childbearing years, motor vehicle crashes are the primary mechanism of maternofetal trauma for pregnant women as well. Falls are the second most common cause of injury in pregnant patients.[1,2] Pregnancy is a time of increased interpersonal stress, which puts women at risk for abuse. The frequency of intimate partner violence during pregnancy is difficult to establish but has been estimated to be between 1.2% and 24%.[4] Following major trauma, the obstetric patient has about the same mortality rate as a nonpregnant woman with comparable wounds.[5] However, the vulnerable fetus is five to seven times more likely to die from an injury than is its mother.[1]

Care of the gravid trauma patient is complicated by the normal physiologic changes of pregnancy (Table 43-1) and by the presence of a second patient, the fetus. Pregnancy should never be permitted to divert attention from the rapid identification and appropriate management of maternal injuries.[6] Vigorous maternal resuscitation remains the initial care priority and provides the fetus with the best possible chance of survival. Virtually all diagnostic procedures and interventions routinely employed in the care of the trauma patient are equally appropriate for management of the pregnant patient, with the addition of a few diagnostic procedures, modifications, and simple safety measures.

ASSESSMENT OF THE OBSTETRIC TRAUMA PATIENT

Primary Assessment

The primary assessment of the pregnant trauma patient is conducted in the same manner and sequence as that of any other patient (see Chapter 35, Assessment and Stabilization of the Trauma Patient). Evaluation of airway, breathing, and circulation occurs simultaneously with interventions when a potentially life-threatening condition is identified. Importantly, the changes of pregnancy can mask normal physiologic responses to trauma, and these alterations must be considered carefully when managing the gravid patient. Table 43-2 summarizes the effects of these changes on the traumatized gravid patient.

Airway and Breathing

- Decreased functional residual capacity and increased oxygen demands leave the pregnant patient vulnerable to hypoxia, especially during endotracheal intubation.[6]
- Maternal oxygen supplementation is the only effective way to improve fetal oxygen levels.[5] The normal fetal PaO_2 is only 32 mm Hg, so any drop from this already marginal level is poorly tolerated by the fetus.
- Once the patient's spine has been cleared, raise the head of her bed to reduce diaphragm compression by the gravid uterus.

> **Chest Tube Placement in Pregnant Patients**
> The diaphragmatic elevation of late pregnancy necessitates chest tube placement and emergency thoracotomy be performed one to two intercostal spaces higher than in the nonpregnant patient.[6]

TABLE 43-1	MATERNAL CARDIOVASCULAR AND RESPIRATORY CHANGES DURING PREGNANCY		
CARDIOVASCULAR		**RESPIRATORY**	
Cardiac output	Increases 30%	Tidal volume	Increased 40%
Heart rate	Increases 15–20 beats/minute	Vital capacity	Decreased by 100–200 mL
Blood pressure	Decreases 15–20 mm Hg	Respiratory rate	Slightly increased
Venous pressure	Varies	$PaCO_2$	Decreased to 30 mm Hg
	Increased in lower extremities		
Hematocrit	Decreased to 31–34%	PaO_2	Increased to 101–104 mm Hg
White blood count	Increased to 15,000/mm^3	Arterial pH	Slightly increased
Electrocardiogram	Flattened or inverted T waves in leads III, aVF, aVL	Serum HCO_3	Increased
Fibrinogen, clotting factors VII, VIII, IX	Increased		

Data from Criddle, L. (2009). Trauma in pregnancy. *American Journal of Nursing, 109*(11), 41–47.
HCO_3, bicarbonate; $PaCO_2$, partial pressure of carbon dioxide; PaO_2, partial pressure of oxygen.

TABLE 43-2	THE IMPACT OF NORMAL PHYSIOLOGIC CHANGES OF PREGNANCY ON THE TRAUMA PATIENT
Airway	The risk of aspiration is increased because of cardiac sphincter laxity, stomach compression, and gastric hypomotility. Consider liberal gastric tube placement.
	Endotracheal intubation is complicated by increased upper airway vascularity. Epistaxis and oral bleeding are potential problems.
Breathing	Pregnancy causes the patient to exist in a state of compensated respiratory alkalosis. Therefore arterial blood gases suggestive of shock (lactic acidosis) will not be evident until shock is advanced.
	High metabolic demands and diaphragm elevation (which reduces functional residual capacity) predispose the patient to hypoxia.
Circulation	The pregnant patient's 40% increase in circulating volume can mask signs of shock until the patient has lost 1500 mL of blood.
	The pregnant patient (normally hot and flushed) may be slow to develop the cool, clammy skin characteristic of hemorrhagic shock.
	The physiologic anemia of pregnancy makes interpreting hemoglobin and hematocrit results difficult.
	The normal hypotension and tachycardia of pregnancy make interpreting vital signs difficult.
	After 20 weeks gestation, the combined weight of the fetus, uterus, placenta, and amniotic fluid will compress the vena cava, decreasing blood pressure and cardiac output when the patient is supine.
	In the presence of hypovolemia, the uterus (a nonvital organ) and the fetus inside it quickly become hypoperfused.
	Most clotting factor levels are elevated in pregnancy, making the pregnant patient prone to venous thromboembolic events and bleeding disorders.
	Because of a large circulating volume and hormonal changes, the pregnant patient does not concentrate urine efficiently and may produce normal amounts of urine output in the face of hypovolemia.
	Massively increased blood flow through the uterus predisposes the pregnant patient to major hemorrhage if the uterus or its vessels are damaged.

Data from Criddle, L. (2009). Trauma in pregnancy. *American Journal of Nursing, 109*(11), 41–47.
HCO_3, bicarbonate; $PaCO_2$, partial pressure of carbon dioxide; PaO_2, partial pressure of oxygen.

Circulation

- Mild hypotension (systolic blood pressure ≤100 mm Hg) and heart rate elevation (≥100 beats per minute) are expected findings during pregnancy.[2,6]
- Central venous pressure is unaffected by pregnancy (except during delivery) and therefore serves as an indicator of maternal volume status.[7]
- A dramatic increase in circulating volume (starting at the tenth week of pregnancy) provides a significant maternal buffer against shock but masks gradual blood losses of 30% to 35% (approximately 1500 mL) or the acute loss of 10% to 15%.[4]
- As a result of shunting blood from the fetus, placenta, and uterus, signs of hemorrhage in the pregnant patient are often absent until volume deficits are severe.[6,8]
  - The gravid patient needs early, vigorous fluid replacement to support herself and her fetus.
  - Establish vascular access with two or more large-bore (14 to 16 gauge) intravenous catheters and anticipate early and aggressive red blood cell transfusion—using O-negative or type-specific blood—until crossmatched units are available.[6]
- By 24 weeks gestation the combined weight of the uterus, fetus, placenta, and amniotic fluid will compress the inferior vena cava, obstructing venous return to the heart, when the mother is placed in a supine position.[7] This phenomenon is known as vena caval compression syndrome or supine hypotension of pregnancy.
  - The simple intervention for this problem is to tilt the mother to her left side, shifting uterine weight off of the vena cava.[1,6]
  - For the patient in spinal immobilization, manually displace the uterus or tilt the backboard 15 degrees to the left.[5]

Secondary Assessment

Secondary assessment of the pregnant trauma patient involves the usual head-to-toe examination along with a detailed evaluation of the abdomen and pelvis. Consult Chapter 35, Assessment and Stabilization of the Trauma Patient, and Chapter 46, Obstetric Emergencies, for more information. This section will address evaluation and intervention considerations specific to the pregnant trauma patient.

Obstetric Assessment

Many pregnancies are obvious, but one of the most important interventions when caring for the gravid trauma patient is simply identifying that a pregnancy exists.

- Query any injured woman of childbearing age regarding the date of her last menstrual period and ask if there is any possibility she may be pregnant.
- Perform a pregnancy test if gestational status is in question.[6]
- Obtain an obstetric history. Determine the patient's estimated date of delivery and her number of previous pregnancies and births.
- In the noncommunicative patient, gestational age can be estimated by assessing fundal height.
  - By 12 weeks gestation the top of the uterus is normally palpable just over the rim of the pelvis.
  - At 20 weeks the fundus approximates the level of the umbilicus.
  - After that, the uterus rises about 1 cm (or one finger's breadth) per week, reaching maximal fundal height at the level of the xiphoid at 36 to 38 weeks.[1,6,8]
- Inquire about complications related to the pregnancy such as contractions, bleeding, or backache. Each of these findings is potentially an indicator of impending delivery.
- Evaluate uterine activity by palpating the uterus, noting fundal height and resting tone as well as contraction frequency, intensity, and duration. Specific contraction patterns are associated with various conditions that can adversely affect fetal outcome and require emergent intervention.
- Inspect the perineum for blood, amniotic fluid, meconium, a prolapsed cord, crowning, or other presenting parts.

Fetal Assessment and Management

- Gestational age and most fetal injuries can be identified by ultrasound. Ultrasonographic evaluation can also be used to determine whether fetal cardiac activity is present or absent.
- For ongoing fetal assessment, use Doppler ultrasound to auscultate heart rate intermittently (<20 weeks gestation) or initiate continuous electronic fetal monitoring (>20 weeks gestation).
- Any patient with a viable pregnancy should be monitored for a minimum of 4 hours after injury. To detect late-onset complications, continue electronic fetal monitoring for up to 48 hours if the woman is symptomatic.[4]
  - Collaboration with obstetric nursing staff is imperative. Interpretation of electronic fetal monitor tracings requires extensive training and practice to identify fetal distress and provide appropriate interventions. Emergency nurses rarely have the requisite skill and should not routinely be delegated this task.

- For a discussion of delivery and newborn resuscitation see Chapter 46, Obstetric Emergencies.

Indicators of Fetal Stress and Distress
- Fetal heart rate greater than 160 or less than 110 beats per minute
- Absence of fetal heart rate accelerations
- Periodic fetal heart rate decelerations
- Lack of beat-to-beat variability
- Decreased fetal movement noted by the mother

Interventions for Fetal Distress
- Administer oxygen to the mother via a nonrebreather mask at 12 to 15 L/min.
- Position the mother on her side or displace the uterus to the side with a wedge under the left hip.
- Infuse a bolus of lactated Ringer solution or normal saline solution.
- Consider emergent cesarean delivery if the fetus is potentially viable.
- Consider maternal steroid injection (betamethasone, [Celestone]) to stimulate fetal surfactant production if delivery of a preterm infant appears inevitable.

Maternal Management

- The gravid patient needs to receive all indicated imaging studies (e.g., radiographs, computed tomography, ultrasonography, magnetic resonance imaging, angiography, intravenous pyelography), invasive procedures (e.g., emergent thoracotomy, needle decompression, surgery), and medications.
  - Shield the uterus during radiographic procedures except when abdominal or pelvic imaging is in progress.[1]
  - Bedside ultrasonographic examination of both the mother and the fetus is an excellent evaluation tool.[2,6]
- Medication administration is always a concern in the pregnant patient. Check with a pharmacist for contraindications prior to administering any pharmaceutical agents. Many drugs are teratogenic. Others—including tetanus toxoid, heparin, narcotic analgesics, acetaminophen, contrast dyes, and some antibiotics—can be safely administered during pregnancy.[6]

SPECIFIC OBSTETRIC EMERGENCIES

Placental Abruption

Placental abruption (also called *abruptio placentae*) is the most common cause of fetal demise following trauma.[3] Abruption involves shearing of the placenta from the uterine wall, typically caused by rapid deceleration or a blunt abdominal blow. The placenta becomes completely or partially detached from the uterus, disrupting maternal-fetal circulation. Fetal effects depend on the amount of functional placenta remaining. Early identification of this condition is important because placental bleeding also threatens maternal survival by precipitating disseminated intravascular coagulation (DIC).

Signs and Symptoms
- Abdominal pain and tenderness
- Uterine rigidity
- Depressed or absent fetal heart rate
- Maternal backache
- Vaginal bleeding (may be minimal or concealed)
- A clot noted behind the placenta on ultrasound
- Port wine–colored amniotic fluid
- Maternal shock

Therapeutic Interventions
- Administer oxygen via a tight-fitting face mask at 10 to 15 L/min.
- Infuse a bolus of lactated Ringer solution or normal saline solution.
- Obtain an obstetric consultation to evaluate the patient for emergent cesarean delivery or other interventions.
- Draw and send laboratory studies, including a complete blood count, Kleihauer-Betke test, type and crossmatch, and coagulation studies (i.e., prothrombin time and international normalized ratio, activated partial thromboplastin time, fibrinogen, and D-dimer).

Preterm Labor

Preterm labor (regular contractions occurring before 37 weeks gestation) puts the fetus at risk for preterm birth and is the most common obstetric complication following trauma.

Signs and Symptoms
- Uterine contractions that occur every 10 minutes or less
- Abdominal cramping
- Backache
- Pelvic pressure
- An increase or change in vaginal discharge or onset of vaginal bleeding

Therapeutic Interventions
- Assist with a pelvic examination (sterile speculum) to evaluate the cervix and assess for membrane rupture.
- Initiate tocolytic therapy (terbutaline [Brethine]) for patients with a potentially viable fetus between 20 and 35 weeks gestation.
- Admit the patient to an obstetric unit for continuous electronic fetal monitoring and ongoing assessment of uterine activity.

Uterine Rupture

Uterine rupture is a rare injury that occurs in less than 1% of pregnant patients with major trauma. The uterus is a strong, flexible muscle that requires a great deal of force to rupture. This condition is associated with sudden deceleration or severe abdominal compression (e.g., patient run over by a vehicle). Rupture is more likely in women with prior uterine scarring. The fetus is almost invariably dead.

Signs and Symptoms

- Sudden onset of severe abdominal pain related to major trauma
- Vaginal bleeding (may be minimal or concealed)
- Fetal parts that can be palpated outside of the uterus
- Fetal bradycardia or asystole
- Maternal hypovolemic shock

Therapeutic Interventions

- Initiate volume replacement with crystalloids and blood products.
- Prepare for emergent cesarean delivery; hysterectomy may be required.

Fetal Injuries

The fetus can sustain injuries to any body part but the probability of trauma is related to the relative size of the part.

- Because the fetal head is the largest body region, skull fractures and intracranial insults account for a significant percentage of the injuries seen.
- The large fetal liver is also at risk.[3]
- Other etiologies of fetal demise include the following:
  - Preterm labor
  - Premature rupture of the membranes

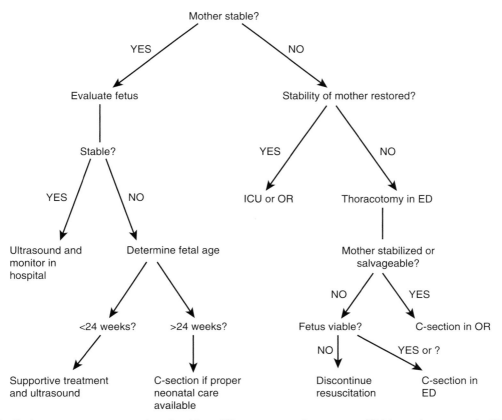

Fig. 43-1 Perimortem cesarean section algorithm. *ED*, emergency department; *ICU*, intensive care unit; *OR*, operating room.

- Placental lacerations
- Umbilical cord injuries
- Penetrating trauma
- Early evaluation by an obstetrician or perinatologist and continuous electronic fetal monitoring contribute to good fetal outcome.[5]
  - Because most fetal demise occurs within hours of injury, electronic monitoring is indicated for a minimum of 4 hours, even following minor trauma.[1,5,6]

Perimortem Cesarean Delivery

In the rare event of maternal cardiopulmonary arrest or imminent demise, perform all standard basic and advanced life support interventions, including defibrillation and medication administration, and consider emergent cesarean delivery. The fetus must be alive and of a viable gestational age (minimum age of 24 weeks).

- Cesarean section performed within 5 minutes of maternal death offers the greatest chance of delivering a neurologically intact infant.
- The only deviation from standard care involves manually displacing the gravid uterus off of the vena cava to facilitate perfusion.
- In rare instances, maternal resuscitation efforts are enhanced by fetal removal.[1,5,6]
  - Perimortem delivery can occur in the emergency department. However, a team capable of resuscitating and stabilizing the neonate must be present with the appropriate equipment and supplies.
- Continue maternal cardiopulmonary resuscitation until the fetus is delivered.
- See Figure 43-1 for a sample perimortem cesarean section algorithm.

REFERENCES

1. Mattox, K. L., & Goetzl, L. (2005). Trauma in pregnancy. *Critical Care Medicine, 33*(10), S385–S389.
2. Tsuei, B. J. (2006). Assessment of the pregnant trauma patient. *Injury, 37*(5), 367–373.
3. El Kady, D. (2007). Perinatal outcomes of traumatic injuries during pregnancy. *Clinical Obstetrics and Gynecology, 50*(3), 582–591.
4. Criddle, L. (2009). Trauma in pregnancy. *American Journal of Nursing, 109*(11), 41–47.
5. Sosa, M. E. (2008). The pregnant trauma patient in the intensive care unit: Collaborative care to ensure safety and prevent injury. *Journal of Perinatal and Neonatal Nursing, 22*(1), 33–38.
6. Tweddale, C. J. (2006). Trauma during pregnancy. *Critical Care Nursing Quarterly, 29*(1), 53–67.
7. Fujitani, S., & Baldisseri, M. R. (2005). Hemodynamic assessment in a pregnant and peripartum patient. *Critical Care Medicine, 33*(10 Suppl), S354–S361.
8. Kerr, M. (2005). Obstetrical trauma. In Emergency Nurses Association, *Sheehy's manual of emergency care* (6th ed., pp. 773–778). St. Louis, MO: Mosby.

Pediatric Trauma

Diana Ropele

Traumatic injuries continue to be the leading cause of death and disability in pediatric patients (ages 1 to 18 years).[1] Approximately one in every six pediatric patients in the United States is treated in emergency departments for injury each year, with an average of 12 pediatric patients under age 15 years injured every minute.[2,3] This represents nearly 10 million pediatric patients, of which 10,000 die annually because of an injury-related event. For every pediatric patient who dies, four survive but are permanently disabled.[2–4]

Children have a smaller body mass, so there is more force per unit area, creating a propensity toward multiple injuries. Morbidity and mortality from trauma surpasses all major diseases in children and young adults.[2]

The most common mechanism of death and injury in this population is motor vehicle crashes, whether associated as an occupant, pedestrian, or cyclist. Other mechanisms for death and injury include falls, drownings, recreational injury, homicides, suicide, and burns.[3–5] The vast majority of pediatric patients sustain blunt trauma (about 80%) as opposed to penetrating wounds (about 20%).[6] Factors that influence the mechanism of injury include age and stage of development, gender, behavior, and environment.

ASSESSMENT AND TREATMENT OF THE PEDIATRIC TRAUMA PATIENT

The principles of trauma assessment and management are the same for pediatric and adult patients (see Chapter 35, Assessment and Stabilization of the Trauma Patient, for more information). Some aspects unique to the pediatric population are discussed below.

Primary Assessment
Airway[7]

The pediatric patient's airway is smaller and more easily obstructed than an adult's. Remember that infants under 3 months may still be obligate nose breathers and may require more aggressive methods to ensure that the airway remains patent.

Therapeutic Interventions

- Use jaw thrust to open the airway; the tongue is large compared to the oral cavity and can easily obstruct the airway.
- Maintain full spinal immobilization for any known mechanism of injury, symptoms, or physical findings that suggest a spinal injury or any unknown mechanism of injury in the unconscious pediatric patient (e.g., abusive head trauma).
- If the pediatric patient is unable to maintain a patent airway, place a nasopharyngeal airway (in the conscious patient) or an oropharyngeal airway (in the unconscious patient and those who may have a possible basilar skull fractures).
  - Select the appropriate-sized oropharyngeal airway by measuring from the corner of the mouth to the angle of the jaw.[5]
  - Using a tongue blade to depress and displace the tongue forward, gently insert the oral airway from the side.
- As with adults, endotracheal intubation is recommended for any pediatric patient with respiratory distress, poor ventilation, or a Glasgow Coma Scale score less than or equal to 8. See also Chapter 8, Airway Management.

- Traditionally an uncuffed tube is used in pediatric patients less than 8 years old to avoid vocal cord trauma, subglottic edema, and pressure necrosis because the narrowest portion of a pediatric patient's airway is the cricoid cartilage. Use of a cuffed tube is becoming more common. Do not inflate the cuff unless an air leak is detected. A half-size smaller tube can be used if the tube is cuffed.[8]
- Perform ongoing assessment of tube placement. The trachea is shorter in children, and it is easy to unintentionally extubate. (It is also easier to place a tube in the main stem bronchus.)
- Choose an appropriate-sized tube using one of the following methods:
  - Use a length-based resuscitation tape and follow the suggestion for the correct size of endotracheal tube.
  - Calculate tube size using the following formula:
    - Tube size (mm) = (Age in years + 16)/4
    - Example: (4 years old + 16)/4 = 5. Therefore, a size 5 tube is recommended.

> Do not invert the oropharyngeal airway or rotate it 180 degrees as is commonly done in adults. This practice can traumatize the pediatric patient's oral soft tissues.

Breathing[7]
Assessment
- A pediatric patient's chest wall is smaller and thinner so breath sounds can be transmitted easily from one location to another. Auscultate breath sounds for equality and the presence of adventitious sounds in the midaxillary region.
- Observe for respiratory fatigue. The pediatric patient's intercostal muscles are more poorly developed.

Therapeutic Interventions
- Administer high-flow oxygen to all patients during the initial resuscitation phase.[3]
- Minimize metabolic stressors (e.g., pain, stimulation, hypothermia). An infant's metabolic rate is about two times that of an adult.
- Prepare to perform optimal bag-mask ventilation. The pediatric patient has a small functional residual capacity and can desaturate rapidly despite preoxygenation.
- Hypoxemia, airway stimulation, and medications (especially succinylcholine for rapid sequence intubation) may result in a vagal response, such as bradycardia; therefore have atropine readily available to treat this potential reaction.
- Avoid overly aggressive ventilation. Pediatric patients are more prone to barotraumas so use the lowest possible tidal volume to achieve a gentle chest rise.

> Use the "squeeze, release, release" method when bagging to allow exhalation time, avoid breath stacking, and prevent barotraumas.[8]

Circulation[7]
Assessment
- Check capillary refill time. Less than 2 seconds is considered normal; greater than 2 seconds is delayed.
- Palpate the quality and effectiveness of central and peripheral pulses. The pediatric patient's circulating blood volume is 80 mL/kg and is proportionally greater than that of an adult. Hypovolemia can occur more quickly than in an adult.
- Observe skin color and feel for temperature; mottling and cool extremities are abnormal.

> Elevated heart rate is an early indicator of circulatory failure; hypotension is a late sign (loss of at least 25% of blood volume) resulting from compensatory vasoconstriction.[7]

Therapeutic Interventions
- If the pediatric patient's heart rate is less than 60 beats per minute and perfusion is ineffective, initiate cardiopulmonary resuscitation following the American Heart Association's Pediatric Advanced Life Support (PALS) guidelines.[9]
- Administer crystalloid fluid resuscitation by the 3:1 rule (e.g., crystalloid resuscitation to blood loss). Therefore, for a 20 mL/kg blood loss, a replacement should be 60 mL/kg.[11]
- If a pulse is present but circulation is inadequate, obtain vascular access by inserting two large-bore intravenous catheters or intraosseous needles.
  - Administer a 20 mL/kg bolus of warmed lactated Ringer solution or 0.9% sodium chloride and repeat as needed.
  - After two boluses, consider switching to warmed type-specific or O negative packed red blood cells for female patients or type-specific as well as O positive or O negative packed red blood cells for male patients at 10 mL/kg for ongoing fluid resuscitation.[6,10]

Disability (Neurologic Evaluation)
Assessment
- Assess the fontanel. The anterior fontanel does not close until 12 to 18 months of age. A bulging fontanelle may indicate increased intracranial pressure; a depressed fontanel suggests volume insufficiency.[5,10]
- Assess pupillary size, shape, and response to light.

- Determine the patient's level of consciousness using the pediatric Glasgow Coma Scale or the AVPU scale:
  - *A:* alert
  - *V:* responds to verbal stimuli
  - *P:* responds to painful stimuli
  - *U:* unresponsive

Therapeutic Interventions

- Keep the head in neutral alignment (nose and navel in line).[5]
- Assist with endotracheal intubation of any patient with a Glasgow Coma Scale score of 8 or less.[10,12]

Secondary Assessment

After completing the primary assessment (with concomitant resuscitation), conduct a secondary examination to identify any other injuries. Reassess the pediatric patient's respiratory, circulatory, and neurologic status frequently.[5,10]

The secondary assessment includes the following:

- Completely undress and expose the patient.
- Maintain normothermia by warming with the use of blankets, increased room temperature, radiant heaters, convective air warmers (e.g., Bair Hugger), and warmed intravenous fluids. An immature thermoregulatory system and a high body surface area to fluid volume ratio makes pediatric patients more susceptible than adults to hypothermia.[13]
- Obtain a full set of vital signs, including blood pressure, oxygen saturation, and a core temperature (rectal temperature preferred over axillary). Facilitate family presence.
  - Ensure that weight in kilograms has been established.
  - Obtain initial blood pressure manually, as many electronic devices continuously cycle when sensing low blood pressure or pulse not detected.
- Obtain a history, including mechanism of injury, treatments before arrival, medical history, allergies, current medications, tetanus immunization status, and the time of last oral intake. It is important to determine specific information related to the mechanism of injury such as time, whether the event was witnessed, activity before and after, and environment.
- Perform a detailed head-to-toe assessment, inspecting and palpating the anterior and posterior body surfaces, making sure to logroll when inspecting the posterior.

Therapeutic Interventions

- Diagnostic procedures
- Wound care
- Fracture care
- Insert an indwelling urinary catheter and maintain output between 1 and 2 mL/kg per hour. Urine output

combined with specific gravity is an excellent method of determining the adequacy of volume resuscitation.[5,6]

- Urethral catheterization is contraindicated for patients with a suspected injury to the urethra, which may be indicated by[7]:
  - Blood at the urethral meatus
  - Blood in the scrotum
  - Suspicion of an anterior pelvic fracture
- Place a nasogastric or orogastric tube and attach it to intermittent suction to decompress the stomach. Pediatric patients are known abdominal breathers so gastric distension can impede adequate ventilation. (Air is swallowed when crying.)
- Provide analgesics and other comfort measures.

Diagnostic Procedures

Not all patients need all radiographic studies, but traditionally major trauma patients receive computed tomography (CT) evaluation of the head, neck, thorax, abdomen, and pelvis. Many studies now suggest that in an alert and cooperative pediatric patient, radiographs can be limited to those indicated by physical examination.[1]

- Always obtain an image of injured extremities.
- Pediatric patients are prone to spinal cord injuries without radiographic abnormalities (SCIWORA).[5,6] Plain spine radiographs are normal in two thirds of children with spinal cord injury. A CT, followed by magnetic resonance imaging, may be needed. Continued immobilization and appropriate consultation are warranted if there is suspicion of spinal cord injury, particularly if neurologic deficits are present.[11,14]
- Consider skeletal survey in any suspected intentional trauma.

> Maintain fluids at two thirds of the usual maintenance rate once the patient has been volume resuscitated and is hemodynamically stable.

SPECIFIC PEDIATRIC INJURIES

Head Trauma

Head injuries (and cervical spine injuries) are common in pediatric patients primarily because of their proportionally large head size, weak skull bones, and lax neck muscles.[6,12] Intracranial trauma is the leading cause of death and disability in pediatric patients. Head injuries are present in nearly 80% of all significant pediatric patient trauma cases, and most are blunt injuries.[5,6,10] Pediatric patient maltreatment in the form of abusive head trauma is the leading cause of head injury in infants and young pediatric patients[5,6,10] (see Chapter 49, Abuse and Neglect). Traumatic brain injury occurs in approximately 100 per 100,000 pediatric patients.[1]

Care Considerations

- The injured brain is profoundly sensitive to hypoxia and hypotension. Ensure that the pediatric patient is well oxygenated and volume resuscitated.[12]
- Significant blood can be lost via a scalp laceration. Control bleeding with direct pressure.
- Unlike the skulls of adults and older pediatric patients, the infant's skull can accommodate a blood volume sufficient to cause hypotension and shock. Observe the infant for bulging anterior fontanels (up to age 12 to 18 months).[10,12]
- Herniation is less common in the young pediatric patient than in the older pediatric patient because of the nonfused fontanels.
- Palpate the skull for depressed fractures and other injuries. A boggy, crepitant swelling (associated with subgaleal hematoma) often can be felt over linear skull fractures.
- Anticipate seizures following head injuries. Strong evidence for prophylactic anticonvulsant medications does not exist but can be considered for pediatric patients with significant intracranial bleeds or diffuse cerebral edema.[12] Administer benzodiazepines to control active seizures.
- Pediatric patients often sustain cerebral hyperemia following significant head injuries. The precise cause of this increased cerebral blood flow is unknown so measures to maintain cerebral perfusion pressure and oxygenation are critical.[12]
- Hyperventilation is no longer considered an appropriate, routine practice when caring for the brain-injured patient. Maintain exhaled carbon dioxide in the normal range (35 to 45 mm Hg).[12,15]
- CT scan is the most efficient assessment. Consider it for obvious signs of trauma, if loss of consciousness is longer than 1 minute, if the pediatric patient is less than 2 years of age, or if emesis begins 4 to 6 hours after injury.[1]

> Lack of rib fractures does not rule out underlying organ damage. Rib fractures strongly suggest intrathoracic or abdominal injury.[7]

Blunt Abdominal Trauma

A child has an immature cartilaginous rib cage and weak abdominal musculature and chest walls are thinner and compliant. Therefore a pediatric patient's intra-abdominal organs are less protected than those of an adult[5,6] (see Chapter 39, Abdominal Trauma). Abdominal contents can be as high as the nipple line because children have a large abdominal cavity and a proportionally small pelvis.

> Gross hematuria associated with abdominal symptoms is a reliable marker for intra-abdominal injury. In a child, the bladder is an intra-abdominal organ and is thus exposed to injury.[1]

Care Considerations

- Suspect abdominal injury in the presence of shoulder- or lap-belt abrasions or bruising.[6] The seat belt complex consists of ecchymosis of the abdominal wall, a flexion distraction injury of the lumbar spine, and intestinal or mesenteric injury.[11]
- Consider an injury (typically a duodenal hematoma or pancreatic injury) resulting from a bicycle handlebar mechanism. An elbow striking the right upper quadrant or epigastrium can cause a similar injury.[11]
- Inspect for visceral injuries. Pediatric patients are more prone to visceral injuries. The most commonly injured intra-abdominal organs are the liver, spleen, and intestines.
- In the absence of blood at the urinary meatus, insert an indwelling catheter to monitor hourly urine output.
- Growing evidence suggests that a focused assessment with sonography for trauma (FAST) in children can replace peritoneal lavage for the unexamined patient.[16,17]

> Six findings have a high association with intra-abdominal injuries[1]:
> - Low systolic blood pressure
> - Femur fracture
> - Aspartate aminotransferase (AST) more than 200 units/L or alanine aminotransferase (ALT) more than 125 units/L
> - Urinalysis with more than five red blood cells per high-power field
> - Initial hematocrit less than 30%

Extremity Trauma

Sprains, strains, and limb fractures are among the most frequent pediatric injuries. See Chapter 40, Musculoskeletal Trauma, for more information.

Care Considerations

- Compare the uninjured extremity when assessing extremities. When performing radiographic studies, views of the injured and uninjured sides can be helpful.
- Treat fractures occurring near the epiphyseal (growth) plates with specialized attention and interventions that provide optimal tissue perfusion such as early immobilization, elevation, and cold therapy.

- Because young pediatric patients are not able to pinpoint pain and to communicate well, ensure radiographs of the joint above and below a suspected fracture site to assess the extent of injury.
- Assess and document peripheral neurovascular assessment (five P's: pallor, pain, pulse, paresthesia, and paralysis) before and after any manipulation or splinting of an injured extremity.[5]

PREVENTION OF PEDIATRIC TRAUMA

Simple strategies, such as the use of protective equipment and supervision, can prevent up to 80% of pediatric injuries.[2–4] Health care providers have a responsibility to integrate injury prevention into practice. Recommendations on injury prevention include the following:

- Establish and support injury prevention laws such as child passenger safety, helmet use, and firearm safety.
- Promote safety education such as farm safety to families.
- Develop and provide community education in the use of safety equipment such as helmets and car seats.[3,5,6,18]

REFERENCES

1. Davis, M., Gruskin, K., Chiang, V. W., & Manzi, S. (Eds.). (2006). *Signs and symptoms in pediatric patients*. St. Louis, MO: Mosby.
2. National Safety Council. (2007). *Injury facts*. Itasca, IL: Author.
3. Safe Kids USA. (n.d.). *Safety fact sheets*. Retrieved from http://www.safekids.org
4. Centers for Disease Control and Prevention. (2008, November). *Unintentional injuries, violence, and the health of young people*. Retrieved from http://www.cdc.gov/HealthYouth/injury/pdf/facts.pdf
5. Emergency Nurses Association. (2004). *Emergency nursing pediatric course provider manual* (3rd ed.). Des Plaines, IL: Author.
6. American College of Surgeons. (2008). *Advanced trauma life support for doctors* (8th ed.). Chicago, IL: Author.
7. Emergency Nurses Association. (2007). *Trauma nurse core curriculum provider manual* (6th ed.). Des Plaines, IL: Author.
8. Braude, D. (2009). *Rapid sequence intubation and rapid sequence airway: An Airway 911 guide* (2nd ed.). Albuquerque, NM: Department of Emergency Medicine, University of New Mexico.
9. Ralston, M., & Hazinski, M. (Eds.), (2006). *Pediatric patient advanced life support provider manual*. Dallas, TX: American Heart Association.
10. Rupp, L., & Day, M. (2003). Pediatric patients are different: Differences and the impact on trauma. In P. Maloney-Harmon & S. Czerwinski (Eds.), *Nursing care of the pediatric trauma patient*. St. Louis, MO: Saunders.
11. Kim, D. S., & Biffl, W. L. (2006). Pediatric trauma. In V. J. Markovchick & P. T. Pons (Eds.), *Emergency medicine secrets* (4th ed.) St. Louis, MO: Mosby.
12. Carney, N., Chestnut, R., & Kochanek, P. (2003). Guidelines for the acute medical management of severe traumatic brain injury in infants, children, and adolescents. *Pediatric Critical Care Medicine, 4*(3), S1.
13. Moore, E., Mattox, K., & Feliciano, D. (Eds.), (2003). *Trauma manual* (4th ed.). New York, NY: McGraw-Hill.
14. Pang, D. (2004). Spinal cord injury without radiographic abnormality in children, 2 decades later. *Neurosurgery, 55*(6), 1325–1343.
15. American College of Emergency Physicians, American Academy of Pediatrics, & Emergency Nurses Association. (2009, September). *Guidelines for care of children in the emergency department*. Retrieved from http://aappolicy.aappublications.org/cgi/reprint/pediatrics;124/4/1233.pdf
16. Soudack, M., Epelman, M., Maor, R., Hayari, L., Shoshani, G., Heyman-Reiss, A., et al. (2004). Experience with focused abdominal sonography for trauma (FAST) in 313 pediatric patients. *Journal of Clinical Ultrasound, 32*, 53–61.
17. Suthers, S. E., Albrecht, R., Foley, D., Mantor, P. C., Puffinbarger, N. K., Jones, S. K., & Tuggle, D. W. (2004). Surgeon-directed ultrasound for trauma is a predictor of intra-abdominal injury in children. *American Surgeon, 70*, 164–167.
18. American College of Emergency Physicians. (2008, June). *Role of the emergency physician in injury prevention and control for adult and pediatric patients*. Retrieved from http://www.acep.org/content.aspx?id=29820

Geriatric Trauma

Laura M. Criddle

THE IMPACT OF TRAUMA

The number of Americans aged 65 years and over is expected to increase from the current level of 36.3 million to 86.7 million by 2050.[1] Trauma, once considered predominately a disease of the young, has long been the leading cause of death in the United States for individuals between the ages of 1 and 44 years.[2] Although the incidence of major traumatic injury remains lower in the geriatric population than in any other group, dramatic longevity gains and increasingly active lifestyles have contributed to rising injury rates among senior citizens.[3] In some areas of the United States, the number of elderly women hospitalized for injury now exceeds that of young men.[4] These trends are substantially altering long-standing patterns of injury demographics. More than 900,000 seniors require hospitalization for trauma each year, and half of these patients have one or more fractures.[5] As the population continues to age, trauma care providers need to be cognizant of these trends and shift care to match.

There are significant differences between older and younger patients related to both injury patterns and the frequency and type of complications experienced following trauma. Despite a typically less severe mechanism of injury, older adults experience a greater number of post-injury complications than do their younger counterparts.

In older adults, poor outcomes following traumatic injury are related to both the normal changes of aging and the prevalence of preexisting comorbid conditions. As a consequence of reduced physiologic reserves and chronic disease, injured geriatric patients are hospitalized for trauma at a rate twice that of the general population.[6] On average, trauma care expenditures for geriatric patients are two and a half times those for younger individuals.[6] These higher costs are attributed to greater frequency and duration of critical care admissions, an increased number of complications, and overall longer hospital stays.[7] It

is difficult to determine whether the incidence of trauma is a surrogate for preexisting fragility in the elderly or the actual cause of decline, but studies of isolated single-system trauma in older individuals have documented serious outcomes after injuries as minor as a closed radial fracture.[8]

The incidence of fatal injury increases markedly with aging. Trauma is the eighth leading cause of mortality in those over the age of 55 years and the ninth most common cause of death in persons 75 years and older.[9] Although seniors comprise only 12.5% of the population, almost one third of injury deaths occur in the 65-years-plus age group.[6] Following major trauma, geriatric patients experience in-hospital mortality rates two to six times greater than younger adults with equivalent injuries.[10] Even minor trauma may result in substantial mortality among older adults.

BARRIERS TO TRAUMA CARE IN THE OLDER ADULT

Researchers examining prehospital data have identified high rates of geriatric trauma center undertriage compared to younger adults. A statewide Pennsylvania study found that 47% of younger patients were correctly identified in the field and triaged to a designated trauma center but only 36% of those over age 65 years were triaged to the appropriate level of care.[11]

> In-hospital trauma team activation criteria (e.g., heart rate >100 beats per minute; systolic blood pressure <90 mm Hg) are not sensitive to the physiology of injured elders. Seniors often fail to exhibit the same vital signs, symptoms, and pain levels found in their younger counterparts.[6]

Trauma team activation criteria have been deliberately selected to overtriage patients in order to avoid missing those in need of special care. However, one study documented 16% mortality among geriatric trauma patients who failed to meet even a single activation criterion and an alarming 50% mortality in those who met only one.[12] Such findings have prompted some authors to argue that older individuals with apparently minor or moderate injuries should be initially triaged as trauma patients and given the benefits of full trauma team activation at a designated center.[12]

MECHANISMS OF INJURY

Falls

Falls, most of which occur at home, are the leading trauma mechanism among persons over age 65 years.[6,9] In this population even low-energy, same-level falls frequently produce significant fractures, craniocerebral trauma, and visceral injury. In the 75-years-plus age group, falls outnumber motor vehicle crashes as the primary cause of traumatic death.[2] Many factors associated with aging contribute to the high incidence of falling:

- Decreased visual acuity
- Obesity
- Neurologic and musculoskeletal impairments (dizziness, seizure disorders, arthritis)
- Cardiac dysrhythmias
- Gait and balance disturbances
- Age-associated fragility
- Medication use
- Dementia
- Urinary urgency
- Alcoholism
- Environmental factors—floor surfaces, footwear, furniture, stairways, poor lighting, and unfamiliar surroundings[6]

Motor Vehicle Crashes

Currently, motor vehicle crashes account for 21.5% of injuries in the geriatric population,[9] but this number is likely to climb. By 2020, the number of drivers in the United States over age 65 years will total 33 million.[10] Age-related declines in cognitive function, decreased auditory acuity, changes in direct and peripheral vision, impaired coordination, limited neck mobility, and increased reaction time all contribute to crashes involving elderly motorists.[7] Although the annual number of miles driven decreases after age 55 years, seniors have a total motor vehicle crash rate second only to that of 16- to 25-year-olds.[6] Unfortunately, the elderly (particularly those 75 years or older) sustain a post-crash fatality rate greater than any other age group.[13]

In contrast to younger motorists, seniors are more likely to crash during daylight hours, in good weather, and close to home. Older adults are also more prone to crashes involving another vehicle, intersections, left turns, traffic sign violations, and right-of-way decisions. Yet, compared to younger cohorts, the older driver is less likely to have ingested alcohol.[6]

Motor Vehicle versus Pedestrian Incidents

Motor vehicle versus pedestrian incidents are a major source of musculoskeletal and head injury in older patients and are the third most common cause of trauma-related mortality in those over age 65 years. In fact, seniors have the highest pedestrian fatality rate of any age group.[6] Factors that contribute to geriatric pedestrian injury include:

- Slowed ambulation
- Increased reaction time
- Vision and hearing losses
- Limited neck rotation
- Medication use
- Substance abuse
- Poor judgment
- Kyphosis, which is experienced by many elders and produces a stooped posture that makes it difficult to raise the head to see oncoming traffic[7]

Burns

Diminished sensation, psychomotor delays, and impaired vision and hearing can leave older adults unaware of (or unable to escape from) the hazards of heat and flames. Basic resuscitation and treatment goals remain the same for geriatric burn victims. (See Chapter 42, Burns, for more specific information.) Nonetheless, the older adult with a thermal injury deserves careful consideration because the physiologic changes of aging significantly compromise recovery time and substantially increase mortality. Burns in this population are commonly more severe than they initially appear because of thinning skin, diminished blood flow, and poor wound-healing capabilities.

Elder Abuse

In the injured geriatric patient the possibility of abuse, maltreatment, or neglect must always be considered. See Chapter 49, Abuse and Neglect, for a general discussion of abuse but suggestive findings in the trauma patient include the following:

- Unexplained fractures, bruises, burns, or internal injuries.
- A history of multiple emergency department visits or reports of being "accident prone."
- Unexplained delays in seeking treatment and differing explanations of the events surrounding injury.
- Unusual injury locations on the body.

- Distinct pattern injuries.
- Findings inconsistent with the history offered.

If abuse is suspected as the proximate cause of injury, follow standard hospital procedures as well as state and local laws for notification and referral.

APPROACH TO THE GERIATRIC TRAUMA PATIENT

Diagnosis and care of the geriatric trauma patient is complicated by normal age-associated changes, comorbidities, and polypharmacy. Assessment and intervention priorities remain essentially the same as for younger individuals, but the structural and functional changes associated with aging affect patient management strategies and nursing care. Trauma teams have long understood the benefit of including pediatric and obstetric specialists on an as-needed basis. Similarly, geriatricians are now being incorporated in trauma teams at several centers to lend their expertise to the care of this complex population.

> More diagnostic procedures are necessary with the geriatric trauma patient because of the increased likelihood of problems and the importance of accurate diagnosis.

Older adults exist in a tenuous state of homeostasis. Following injury, seniors are likely to exhibit findings that are subtle, delayed, atypical, or difficult to assess.

The physiologic changes of aging and concomitant medication use can limit the geriatric patient's ability to compensate, making it difficult to interpret vital signs. For example, a healthy young adult in hypovolemic shock exhibits tachycardia, vasoconstriction, and increased cardiac contractility. An elderly patient with compromised cardiac function and daily beta-blocker use may be unable to mount an adequate compensatory response. Likewise, blood pressure and body temperature norms in older adults are subject to considerable variation.

Despite fluid overload concerns, an aggressive approach to resuscitation is recommended because shock represents the primary cause of death in the injured geriatric patient.[8]

ASSESSMENT

For a detailed discussion of age-associated changes, comorbidities, and assessment of the older adult, see Chapter 53, Geriatric Considerations in Emergency Nursing. Refer to Chapter 35, Assessment and Stabilization of the Trauma Patient, for general information regarding care of the injured patient. This section focuses specifically on geriatric trauma concerns.

Primary Assessment

- Begin with a standard primary assessment and initial interventions. Assess the patient's airway, breathing, and circulatory status.
- Loose dentures require removal since they may compromise the airway. Kyphosis, chronic lung disease, musculoskeletal changes, pain, and supine positioning commonly limit breathing.
- Perform a brief neurologic examination.
- Impaired hearing and dementia may limit patient responsiveness. Evaluate pupil size, shape, and reaction to light, but cataracts, ophthalmologic surgery, other ocular conditions, and various medications may greatly affect pupillary findings in the elderly.

History

- Identify the mechanism of injury and estimate the amount of energy (high, low) involved. Bear in mind that even low-energy mechanisms (e.g., a same-level fall) can produce significant trauma.
- In older adults injury is frequently secondary to a medical condition. Analyze symptoms proximate to the event (such as light-headedness, confusion, palpitations, or chest pain) that suggest that a possible dysrhythmia, transient ischemic attack, seizure, or hypoglycemic episode may have precipitated the event.
- Ask about a history of previous injuries; recidivism is a common finding in geriatric trauma patients.

Secondary Assessment

Conduct a rapid but thorough secondary ("head-to-toe") examination to identify injuries. The following are special considerations for the geriatric trauma patient.

Head

- Inspect and palpate the scalp and face examining for pain, bleeding, hematomas, or bony deformities.
- The anticoagulated patient can lose significant amounts of blood from a scalp wound or from a large subgaleal hematoma. Anticoagulated individuals may also develop hyphema or experience epistaxis and oral bleeding.
- As a result of age-associated neuronal atrophy and increased space in the cranial vault, subdural hematomas are common in the older adult. These intracranial hemorrhages may be acute, subacute (symptoms appear 3 or more weeks after injury), or chronic.
- Prepare the head-injured patient for computed tomography, surgery, or transfer to an intensive care unit.

- Intracerebral hemorrhage in the warfarin-anticoagulated patient is a very serious problem. In-hospital mortality approaches 50%.[14] Emergent interventions include intravenous fresh frozen plasma and vitamin K (phytonadione). Prothrombin complex concentrate (Octaplex) and recombinant factor VIIa administration are additional potential interventions to limit hematoma expansion.

Spinal Cord and Spinal Column

- To minimize skin breakdown, remove backboards and cervical collars from older adults as soon as possible.
- Assess motor and sensory status by checking for movement, motor strength, paralysis, and paresthesias in the extremities. Compare findings side to side and document the level of injury.
- Palpate the entire spine for any deformities, defects, pain, or swelling.
- Seniors are prone to intravertebral disc and ligamentous injuries that are not readily apparent on routine radiographs. Emergent magnetic resonance imaging is indicated if deficits are present.
- Older adults have the highest incidence of central cord syndrome.[15] Because edema plays a large role in this condition, symptoms commonly progress, causing the level of deficit to rise over time.

Chest

- Assess respiratory rate, depth, and effort.
- Hypoventilation (carbon dioxide retention) may be the patient's norm.
- Inspect the thorax for symmetry, respiratory excursion, defects, and abnormalities differentiating acute from chronic disorders.
- Auscultate the chest for diminished, absent, or adventitious breath sounds. Assess heart tones; an S_3 sound suggests volume overload.
- Atrial fibrillation and occasional ventricular complexes are common.
- Determine if the patient has a pacemaker or an implanted defibrillator.
- Monitor oxygen saturation status; levels in the low 90s may be normal even for geriatric patients without underlying pulmonary disease. Therefore this population requires aggressive oxygen supplementation.
- Observe for accessory muscle use.
- Hypoventilation is very common in the geriatric patient with chest injury and in those who have received narcotic analgesics. Consider exhaled carbon dioxide monitoring for continuous assessment of ventilatory status.

- Evaluate the patient's ability to clear secretions effectively and check for the presence of adequate gag and cough reflexes prior to giving anything by mouth.
- Fracture of two or more ribs is an indication for hospitalization in elderly individuals. Surgical rib plating, thoracic epidural catheter placement, and local anesthetics delivered through a tunneled catheter (e.g., a "pain ball") can dramatically reduce the incidence of pulmonary complications in the geriatric patient with thoracic injury.[16]

Abdomen and Genitals

- Observe the abdomen for surgical scars, bruising, and distension. Abdominal pain in older adults is often vague but may signal serious pathology.
- Auscultate bowel sounds; slowed peristalsis is both a normal age-associated finding and an indicator of bowel hypoperfusion in the trauma patient.
- Prostate hypertrophy, noted on rectal exam, is common in elderly males.
- Test stool for occult blood.
- Anemia secondary to gastrointestinal (GI) losses may be the event that precipitated injury. Additionally, GI bleeding makes assessing acute traumatic blood losses more difficult.
- Intravenous contrast dye administration can have serious renal consequences in older adults.

Extremities

- Palpate distal pulses and evaluate capillary refill, skin temperature, and skin condition. However, it may be normal for the geriatric patient not to have a capillary refill response.
- Splint suspected fractures for comfort and hemorrhage reduction. Fracture-associated bleeding can quickly progress to hypovolemic shock in older adults.
- Assess limbs for pain, tenderness, and guarding. Range-of-motion limitations may be chronic. Compare joints side to side.
- Leg shortening and external rotation of the foot strongly suggest hip fracture.
- Consider the possibility of elder abuse in patients with fractures.

Skin

- Assess skin turgor, temperature, and color. Identify areas of skin tears, bruising (old and new), burns (old or recent), rashes, and breakdown.
- Pad bony areas to promote perfusion to the skin and deep tissues.

- Remove splints, backboards, and cervical collars as soon possible to reduce discomfort and skin breakdown.
- Use paper tape and nonadhesive dressings to minimize skin tears.
- If bruising and tears appear suspicious, consider the possibility of elder abuse.

DIAGNOSTIC PROCEDURES

Diagnostic procedures for evaluation of the elderly trauma patient consist of all standard laboratory tests (e.g., complete blood count, lactate, electrolytes, glucose, blood urea nitrogen, and creatinine) but are also likely to include magnesium and calcium levels, troponin I, and arterial blood gases.

- Consider coagulation studies, especially if the patient takes an anticoagulant medication such as aspirin or warfarin (Coumadin).
- Check serum levels of any medication that may be considered a contributing cause or precipitating factor (such as aspirin or digoxin toxicity). Perform drug and alcohol screens as indicated.
- Obtain echocardiograms, abdominal ultrasound studies, computed tomography scans, and other diagnostic studies as warranted.
- All geriatric trauma patients should have a 12-lead electrocardiogram.

THERAPEUTIC INTERVENTIONS

There are several general considerations regarding interventions in the geriatric trauma patient.

- Determine whether the patient has completed an advance directive.
- Administer intravenous fluids cautiously to prevent volume overload yet do not under-resuscitate patients.
- Monitor the patient's temperature; decreased amounts of body fat and muscle and lower metabolic rates make elderly individuals prone to hypothermia.
- Keep the patient warm; infuse warmed intravenous fluids and apply warming devices to the patient.
- Monitor vital signs, repeat the primary survey, reassess level of consciousness, and check urine output frequently.
- Evaluate glycemic status in the patient with altered level of consciousness or a history of diabetes.
- Administer analgesics as prescribed, preferably small intravenous doses; repeat as needed.
- Provide diphtheria and tetanus immunization, if indicated. Many older adults are not adequately vaccinated.
- Perform meticulous wound care.

INJURY PREVENTION

Although substantial gains have been made in reducing the incidence and severity of trauma among young adults, similar reductions in the incidence of geriatric trauma have not been noted.[4] Injury prevention education has long been a mandatory criterion for trauma center designation, yet prevention campaigns aimed at motorcycle helmet use, diving injuries, and drinking and driving have little impact on the older population. Information about preventing crosswalk injuries, falls, suicide, and motor vehicle crashes at intersections should be specifically tailored to older persons.

REFERENCES

1. Vincent, G. K., & Velkoff, V. (2010). *The next four decades: The older population in the United States: 2010 to 2050.* Washington, DC: US Census Bureau. Retrieved from http://www.census.gov/prod/2010pubs/p25-1138.pdf
2. Centers for Disease Control and Prevention. (2010, June 28). *Death and mortality.* Retrieved from http://www.cdc.gov/nchs/fastats/deaths.htm
3. Clark, D. E., & Chu, M. K. (2002). Increasing importance of the elderly in a trauma system. *American Journal of Emergency Medicine, 20*(2), 108–111.
4. Shinoda-Tagawa, T., & Clark, D. E. (2003). Trends in hospitalization after injury: Older women are displacing young men. *Injury Prevention, 9*(3), 214–219.
5. McGwin, G., Jr., May, A. K., Melton, S. M., Reiff, D. A., & Rue, L. W., III (2001). Recurrent trauma in elderly patients. *Archives of Surgery, 136*(2), 197–203.
6. Criddle, L. M. (2009). Caring for critically ill elderly patient. In K. Carlson (Ed.), *AACN Advanced Critical Care Nursing* (pp. 1372–1400). St. Louis, MO: Saunders.
7. Richmond, T. S., Thompson, H. J., Kauder, D., Robinson, K. M., & Strumpf, N. E. (2006). A feasibility study of methodological issues and short-term outcomes in seriously injured older adults. *American Journal of Critical Care, 15*(2), 158–165.
8. Kuhne, C. A., Ruchholtz, S., Kaiser, G. M., & Nast-Kolb, D. (2005). Mortality in severely injured elderly trauma patients—when does age become a risk factor? *World Journal of Surgery, 29*(11), 1476–1482.
9. Centers for Disease Control and Prevention. (2010, June 1). *WISQARS leading causes of death reports, 1999–2007.* Retrieved from http://webappa.cdc.gov/sasweb/ncipc/leadcaus10.html
10. Criddle, L. M. (2009). 5-year survival of geriatric patients following trauma center discharge. *Advanced Emergency Nursing Journal, 31*(4), 323–336.
11. Richmond, T. S., Kauder, D., Strumpf, N., & Meredith, T. (2002). Characteristics and outcomes of serious traumatic injury in older adults. *Journal of the American Geriatrics Society, 50*(2), 215–222.

12. Demetriades, D., Sava, J., Alo, K., Newton, E., Velmahos, G. C., Murray, J. A., … Berne, T. V. (2001). Old age as a criterion for trauma team activation. *Journal of Trauma, 51*(4), 754–757.

13. Carr, D. B. (2004). The older adult driver. In K. Moylan (Ed.), *The Washington Manual of Geriatrics* (pp. 59–65). Philadelphia, PA: Lippincott Williams & Wilkins.

14. Mayer, S. A., Brun, N. C., Begtrup, K., Broderick, J., Davis, S., Diringer, M. N., et al. (2008). Efficacy and safety of recombinant activated factor VII for acute intracerebral hemorrhage. *New England Journal of Medicine, 358*(20), 2127–2137.

15. Chaudhry, S., Sharan, A., Ratliff, J., & Harrop, J. S. (2007). Geriatric spinal injury. *Seminars in Spine Surgery 19*(4), 229–234.

16. Stawicki, S. P., Grossman, M. D., Hoey, B. A., Miller, D. L., & Reed, J. F., III. (2004). Rib fractures in the elderly: A marker of injury severity. *Journal of the American Geriatrics Society, 52*(5), 805–808.

Special Populations

Obstetric Emergencies

Judith H. Poole and Joanne E. Thompson

Patients with obstetric problems are frequently seen and receive treatment in emergency departments (EDs). These are anxiety-filled times for the mother, her significant other, and family members as the well-being of both the mother and her unborn child may be threatened. Emergency care providers must care for these women and their loved ones with compassion and competence.

Nurses and patients frequently are confused by some of the terminology used to describe obstetric and gynecologic conditions. Table 46-1 provides some definitions for obstetric and gynecologic conditions.

COMPLICATIONS OF PREGNANCY

Ectopic Pregnancy

Two percent of all pregnancies in the United States are ectopic. An ectopic pregnancy occurs when a fertilized egg implants outside the endometrial cavity, usually in a fallopian tube (95% of the time). Less common sites of implantation include the cervix (<1%), in a cesarean scar (<1%), within the peritoneal cavity (1%), or within the ovary (3%). If the fetus continues to grow, the fallopian tube inevitably will rupture.[1] Symptoms commonly present around the sixth week of gestation.

Signs and Symptoms

- Late or irregular period
- Abnormal vaginal bleeding
- Severe sudden onset of unilateral pelvic pain
- Abdominal tenderness and guarding
- Palpable pelvic mass
- Positive pregnancy test
- Sensation that a bowel movement would help relieve discomfort
- Nausea and vomiting

If a rupture has occurred, additional signs and symptoms are as follows:

- Shoulder pain (Kehr's sign)
- Tachycardia
- Cold, clammy skin
- Hypotension, delayed capillary refill, narrowed pulse pressure
- Decreasing level of consciousness

Diagnostic Procedures

- Human chorionic gonadotropin (hCG) level (pregnancy test) indicative of pregnancy
- Serum progesterone level (greater than 25 ng/mL)
- Complete blood count (CBC) and type and crossmatch with Rh
- Transabdominal or transvaginal sonography

Therapeutic Interventions

- Initiate intravenous (IV) therapy with lactated Ringer solution or normal saline.
- Give Rho(D) immune globulin (human RhoGAM) if the mother is Rh negative.
- Prepare the patient for surgery if rupture is suspected.
- Consider intramuscular injection of methotrexate for unruptured ectopic pregnancies.
  - Methotrexate is a cytotoxic, antimetabolite agent that interferes with DNA synthesis and disrupts cell multiplication.[2]
  - A candidate for methotrexate therapy must be hemodynamically stable with no signs of bleeding and must be reliable, compliant, and able to return for follow-up.[2]
  - Methotrexate can be administered as multiple doses or as a single injection.
  - Follow institutional policy and procedure for methotrexate administration; administration of this drug may be limited to specially trained nurses in some institutions.

TABLE 46-1	OBSTETRIC AND GYNECOLOGIC DEFINITIONS

Labor: The process by which the fetus, placenta, and membranes are expelled from the uterus. This usually occurs 40 weeks after conception.

Spontaneous abortion: The natural termination of pregnancy before viability (<20 weeks gestation).

Miscarriage: The term commonly preferred by laypersons, who use *abortion* to denote induced pregnancy loss.

Gravida: The total number of pregnancies, including a current pregnancy.

Para: The number of pregnancies that have progressed to at least 20 weeks gestation, regardless of whether the infant was dead or alive at birth. Multifetal gestations (i.e., twins, triplets) are counted as one para.

Primigravida: Pregnant for the first time.

Nullipara: A woman who has not carried a pregnancy to viability.

Primipara: A woman who has carried one pregnancy to viability.

Multipara: A woman who has carried more than one pregnancy to viability.

Examples

Gravida 3, Para 1: A woman who has been pregnant three times and delivered one viable child.

Gravida 4, Para 0: A woman who has been pregnant four times but has carried none of the pregnancies to viability.

Gravida 2, Para 2: A woman who has been pregnant twice and has delivered two viable children.

Gravida 1, Para 1: A woman who has been pregnant once but has delivered two viable children (twins).

- Pregnant nurses or those of childbearing age should not handle methotrexate.
- Refer the patient for follow-up care with a gynecologist.

Abortion

The term *abortion* is defined as the death or expulsion of the fetus (or products of conception) before the age of viability. About 15% to 20% of all known pregnancies end in spontaneous abortion.[3] The major complications are hemorrhage and infection. Pregnancy loss in the first trimester is largely the result of embryonic chromosomal defects. Loss after the first trimester more frequently is associated with infections, maternal endocrine disorders, or anatomic abnormalities of the mother's reproductive tract. Spontaneous abortions are classified as threatened, inevitable, incomplete, complete, missed, and septic. See Table 46-2 for a comparison of these types of abortion.

General Post-Abortion Care

- If procedural sedation was administered for uterine evacuation, ensure that the patient is fully recovered before discharge; follow institutional policy and procedures regarding discharge.
- Explain potential medication effects.
- Assess amount and characteristics of vaginal bleeding.
- Many women (and men) find the loss of their child devastating, even when it occurs early in pregnancy.
- Comfort the patient and significant others as appropriate. (See Chapter 17, End-of-Life Issues for Emergency Nurses, for more specific information.)
- Determine what information is needed regarding the cause of abortion. Refer the patient to experts (e.g., obstetrician, geneticist) for evaluation, as indicated.
- Provide the names of local support groups such as Compassionate Friends and Share. The hospital's obstetric unit may have a list of resources.
- Refer patients for psychological counseling as needed, especially if the patient has a history of depression or significant concurrent stressors.

Septic Abortion

Patients with septic abortion resulting from *Clostridium* infection are of particular concern. This anaerobic organism may produce gas gangrene, tissue necrosis, and uterine tissue sloughing. To avoid significant morbidity and mortality, treatment of septic abortion must be immediate and aggressive. If the patient does not improve after dilation and curettage, hysterectomy is indicated.

Discharge Instructions

- Vaginal bleeding may last 1 to 2 weeks. The bleeding should get progressively lighter until it subsides.
- Slight cramping for several days is normal.
- Avoid douching, tampons, or intercourse for at least 2 weeks (or until after a follow-up visit with a gynecologist).
- Bed rest is not necessary but exertion should be minimal for 2 to 3 days.
- Monitor body temperature in the morning and evening for 5 days.
- Seek medical care for the following:
  - Temperature above 37.7°C (100°F)
  - Chills
  - Severe nausea and vomiting
  - Severe cramps
  - Excessive bleeding, which can be defined for the patient as:
    - Consistently soaking a pad in less than 1 hour
    - Bleeding more than a normal heavy period
    - Clots larger than a quarter

TABLE 46-2   **TYPES OF ABORTION**

TYPE	DESCRIPTION	THERAPEUTIC INTERVENTIONS
Threatened abortion	Early symptoms of abortion include episodic, painless uterine bleeding and mild cramping The cervical os is closed and the uterus is enlarged and soft Quantitative beta hCG (serum) test provides better indicator of fetal development than qualitative beta hCG (urine) test	Bed rest Pelvic rest—no tampons, douches, or sexual intercourse Mild sedatives Ultrasound confirmation of pregnancy
Inevitable abortion	A threatened abortion may progress to inevitable abortion Signs and symptoms include increased pain, cramping, and bleeding The cervical os is dilated 3 cm or more	Bed rest Analgesics Uterine evacuation (dilation and curettage or dilation and evacuation) performed at discretion of provider and patient
Incomplete abortion	Bleeding is heavy, cramping is severe, and the cervical os is open Patient has a positive pregnancy test and an enlarged uterus Tissue has been passed but some products of conception are retained	Obtain intravenous access and infuse lactated Ringer solution Oxytocin (Pitocin, Syntocinon) in lactated Ringer solution to induce uterine contractions Facilitate surgery for uterine evacuation Administer Rho(D) immune globulin as needed
Complete abortion	A small amount of bleeding occurs, cramping is mild, all tissue has been passed (often in an intact amniotic sac), and the cervical os is closed	Observation Ultrasound may be indicated to determine if all products of conception have been passed If mother is Rh negative, administer RhoGAM according to institutional guidelines to prevent Rh incompatibility in future pregnancies
Missed abortion	A pregnancy loss in which the products of conception remain in the uterus for an extended period after fetal demise Characteristic symptoms of bleeding and cramping are absent	Uterine evacuation may be performed Patient may be sent home for expectant management or scheduled evacuation
Septic abortion	May occur in patients who have a complete abortion without surgical uterine evacuation More frequently the result of an elective abortion or delayed treatment for an incomplete abortion Common causative bacteria include: • Alpha- and beta-hemolytic streptococci • Gram-negative aerobes such as *Escherichia coli*, *Clostridium perfringens* Signs and symptoms include: • Foul vaginal discharge • Constant pelvic pain • Uterine tenderness • Fever, chills	Initiate an oxytocin infusion to expel uterine contents Administer appropriate antibiotics Prepare the patient for dilation and curettage Observe for signs of toxic shock: • Hypotension • Renal failure • Tachycardia

hCG, Human chorionic gonadotropin.

Gestational Hypertension

Gestational hypertension is the current global term for hypertension complicating pregnancy and has replaced the term *pregnancy-induced hypertension* (PIH).[4] Any patient presenting with signs and symptoms consistent with a hypertensive disorder of pregnancy should receive an obstetric consult as soon as possible. Both the woman and her fetus can change status quickly and need intensive obstetric management.

Classification of the Hypertensive Disorders of Pregnancy

Gestational Hypertension

- New onset of hypertension, generally after the twentieth week of gestation
- Hypertension is defined as a systolic blood pressure (SBP) 140 mm Hg or greater or a diastolic blood pressure (DBP) of 90 mm Hg or greater

Preeclampsia

- Gestational hypertension plus gestational proteinuria in a previously normotensive woman
- Gestational proteinuria is defined as greater than 300 mg proteinuria on a random specimen or 1+ or more on dipstick
- In the absence of proteinuria, suspect preeclampsia if any of the following are present:
  - Headache
  - Blurred vision
  - Abdominal pain
  - Abnormal laboratory values, especially thrombocytopenia, elevated liver enzymes, or early findings of disseminated intravascular coagulation (DIC)
- HELLP syndrome
  - Variant of severe preeclampsia
  - Diagnosis based on presence of **H**emolysis, **E**levated **L**iver enzymes, and **L**ow **P**latelets
    - Hemolysis diagnosed in the presence of an abnormal peripheral smear, lactate dehydrogenase (LDH) greater than 600 units/L, or a total bilirubin 1.2 mg/dL or greater
    - Elevated liver enzymes include aspartate aminotransferase (AST) and alanine transaminase (ALT)
    - Thrombocytopenia significant when platelet count is less than 100,000

Eclampsia

- Occurrence of seizure in patient with no other possible etiology for seizure
- At highest risk of morbidity and mortality, especially cerebral hemorrhage

Chronic Hypertension

- Hypertension that is present and observable before pregnancy or diagnosed prior to 20 weeks gestation
- Preeclampsia or eclampsia can be superimposed on chronic hypertension

Preeclampsia

Preeclampsia is the second leading cause of maternal mortality. This condition is far more than just chronic elevated blood pressure. Preeclampsia is a multisystem disorder associated with decreased oxygenation and perfusion deficits. At times, coagulopathies and liver function abnormalities are present as well. Preeclampsia can be mild or severe; preeclampsia and HELLP syndrome can also occur in the postpartum period.

Signs and Symptoms

- Elevated blood pressure
  - SBP greater than 140 mm Hg *or*
  - DBP greater than 90 mm Hg
- Proteinuria
- Oliguria
- Edema of the face, hands, and sacrum
- Weight gain of 2 pounds or more per week
- HELLP syndrome (defined above)
- Visual changes
- Headaches
- Nausea
- Epigastric or right upper quadrant pain
  Severe preeclampsia is present when at least one of the following is present:
- SBP 160 mm Hg or greater
- DBP 110 mm Hg or greater
- Proteinuria greater than 2 g per 24 hours
- Serum creatinine greater than 1.2 mg/dL
- Platelets less than 100,000
- Elevated LDH as evidence of hemolysis
- Elevated ALT or AST
- Persistent headache
- Persistent visual disturbances
- Persistent epigastric pain
  Additional criteria for the diagnosis of severe preeclampsia may include:
- Oliguria less than 500 mL per 24 hours
- Pulmonary edema
- Impaired liver function of unclear etiology
- Intrauterine growth restriction of fetus
- Oligohydramnios (deficiency of amniotic fluid)
- Eclampsia

Therapeutic Interventions

- Provide supportive care to maintain mother's hemodynamic stability.
- Obtain urgent obstetric consultation.

- Institute continuous electronic fetal monitoring.
- Minimize external stimulation by darkening room and limiting visitors.
- Give hydralazine (Apresoline) or labetalol (Normodyne, Trandate) intravenously for hypertension after consultation with obstetric specialist.
- Infuse magnesium sulfate intravenously to prevent seizures after consultation with obstetric care unit.
  - Generally a 4 g loading dose, followed by a continuous infusion of 2 g per hour as a secondary infusion
  - Monitor vital signs every 5 minutes during administration of loading dose
  - Assess hourly for neurologic changes (i.e., headache, blurred vision, spots before eyes)
  - Monitor hourly urine output since magnesium is excreted by the kidneys
  - Monitor for signs and symptoms of magnesium toxicity:
    - Check for loss of patellar reflexes every 2 to 4 hours
    - Shortness of breath
    - Oxygen saturation less than 95%
    - Nausea
  - Have calcium gluconate readily available to treat respiratory depression
- Arrange for admission to an obstetric care unit.

Eclampsia

In the continuum of hypertensive disorders of pregnancy, eclampsia represents preeclampsia that has progressed to the convulsive phase. Ultimately, delivery is the only cure for eclampsia. Nonetheless, patients are at risk for this disorder for up to 3 weeks postpartum; those with late presentation eclampsia often have atypical presentations.[5]

Signs and Symptoms
- Symptoms of preeclampsia
- Generalized seizures with an associated postictal period that may last as long as 15 to 20 minutes
- Significantly elevated blood pressure (SBP 140 to 200 mm Hg, DBP >90 mm Hg)
- Decreased fetal heart rate as noted on fetal monitor, particularly during seizures

Therapeutic Interventions
- Maintain a patent airway.
- Administer high-flow supplemental oxygen.
- Place the patient in a left lateral position.
- Initiate continuous electronic fetal monitoring.
- Administer a 4 to 6 g IV bolus of magnesium sulfate over 15 minutes, followed by a maintenance infusion of 2 g per hour.[5]
- Administer hydralazine (Apresoline) or labetalol (Normodyne, Trandate) intravenously for hypertension.[4]
- Monitor blood pressure, respiratory rate, and deep tendon reflexes every hour or as indicated.
- Arrange for admission to a high-risk obstetric care unit.

Bleeding in Pregnancy
Placenta Previa

Placenta previa is defined as implantation of the placenta in the lower uterine segment or over the internal os. The incidence of placenta previa varies in the literature. Placenta previa is categorized based on the extent of internal cervical os involvement. The cervical os can be totally covered by the placenta or only partially covered. A marginal placenta previa is one that is within 2 to 3 cm of the internal cervical os but does not cover it (Fig. 46-1). As the fetus grows and the uterus expands, implantation may be disturbed, causing the placenta to bleed through the cervical os. Placenta

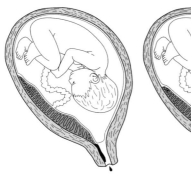 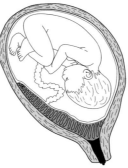 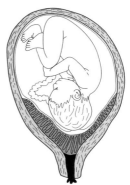

Marginal implantation   Partial implantation   Complete implantation

Fig. 46-1 Placenta previa.

previa is associated with potentially life-threatening hemorrhage and fetal loss.

Signs and Symptoms

- Sudden *painless* bleeding (usually after 7 months gestation)
- Bright red (versus dark) blood from the vagina
- Maternal hemorrhagic shock (hypotension, tachycardia, poor capillary refill)

Therapeutic Interventions

- Call obstetric team to co-manage the care of the patient with placenta previa. If emergent delivery is required, consult neonatal and nursery staff capable of emergency resuscitation of the neonate.
- Insert one or more large-bore IV catheters and administer a bolus of lactated Ringer solution or normal saline solution.
- Send blood for CBC and type and crossmatch with Rh.
- Keep the patient in a left lateral recumbent position to increase blood return to the heart.
- Defer a vaginal examination until an ultrasound has indicated the placental location. (Manual examination can disrupt the placenta further.)
- Anticipate cesarean section depending on the gestational age, extent of bleeding, and maternal condition.

Placental Abruption

Placental abruption (*abruptio placentae*) is a major cause of obstetric hemorrhage and hypovolemic shock. Placental abruption is the most common cause of fetal demise following maternal trauma. The rupture of small arterial vessels causes separation of the placenta from the uterine wall. This ultimately inhibits the supply of oxygen and nutrients to the fetus. The area of separation can be small or large. If separation occurs at the placental margin, vaginal bleeding will be present. However, areas of separation toward the placental center are concealed and do not cause obvious blood loss. Maternal and fetal death can occur as a result of this condition.

Signs and Symptoms

- Backache
- Painful uterine contractions
- Uterine rigidity or high-frequency, low-amplitude contractions
- Sudden, colicky abdominal pain
- Frank, dark red vaginal bleeding *or* bleeding concealed behind a partially separated placenta
- Maternal hemorrhagic shock (hypotension, tachycardia, poor capillary refill)
- Disseminated intravascular coagulopathy is a potential complication

- Bleeding from venipuncture sites
- Microemboli evidenced by tissue ischemia
- Elevated D-dimer and fibrin split products
- Decreased platelet count
- If a large portion of the placenta has separated, fetal heart tones can be abnormal or absent
- Patients with small, concealed bleeds may be asymptomatic

Therapeutic Interventions

- Call obstetric team to co-manage the care of the patient with placental abruption. If emergent delivery is required, consult neonatal and nursery staff capable of emergency resuscitation of the neonate.
- Consider transport to tertiary care facility if appropriate.
- Administer high-flow oxygen.
- Insert one or more large-bore IV catheters and give the patient a bolus of lactated Ringer solution or normal saline solution.
- Send blood for CBC and type and crossmatch with Rh.
- Consider transfusion with crossmatched or O negative packed red blood cells.
- Rapidly transport the patient to an operating room or obstetric unit (depending on fetal viability and the degree of maternal shock).
- Unless the patient is delivered emergently, continuous electronic fetal monitoring is required. This procedure must be performed by skilled obstetric nurses.

EMERGENT DELIVERY

Emergency department births are rare and considered to be high-risk deliveries. Patients should be transported to a facility that has obstetric and neonatal resources as appropriate. However, delivery during transport can be disastrous for both the mother and the neonate.[6] Careful assessment of the imminence of delivery (head is crowning, mother has urge to push) must be the basis for the transfer decision.

Although a natural process, childbirth is by definition an emergent condition. Add any complications and the process can jeopardize two (or more) lives. The following provides a concise, step-by-step approach to caring for the delivering mother and the neonate. Table 46-3 outlines the stages of labor; Table 46-4 lists information to elicit from the laboring mother or a family member.

If the signs and symptoms listed below are present, prepare for immediate delivery. Birth in a sterile environment is desirable. However, if delivery is imminent, do not risk endangering the mother and neonate while attempting to create a sterile situation.

TABLE 46-3 STAGES OF LABOR

STAGE	DESCRIPTION	AVERAGE DURATION	
		PRIMIPARA	MULTIPARA
Stage 1: Dilation	From the onset of regular uterine contractions to complete cervical dilation	12.5 hours	7 hours
Stage 2: Expulsion	From the time of complete cervical dilation until the baby is delivered	80 minutes	30 minutes
Stage 3: Placental	From the time immediately following delivery of the baby until expulsion of the placenta	5 to 30 minutes	5 to 30 minutes

TABLE 46-4 QUESTIONS TO ASK THE LABORING PATIENT

- How many weeks along are you? What is your due date?
- When did your labor (pain) start?
- How close together are your contractions?
- Has your water broken?
- Are you bleeding now?
- Have you had any complications with this pregnancy?
- How many babies have you delivered before?
- Is there more than one baby?
- Do you feel the need to push or move your bowels?
- Have you taken any medications?

Signs and Symptoms of Impending Delivery

The following are indications of impending delivery:
- Findings that can occur days or minutes before delivery:
  - Bloody show: A mucous discharge that is tinged with blood
  - Amniotic membranes rupture ("my water broke"): A trickle or gush of amniotic fluid
  - Frequent, painful contractions
- A desire by the mother to bear down
- The mother states that she is going to defecate or that "the baby is coming"
- Bulging membranes are visible at the vulva
- Crowning of the fetal head (Fig. 46-2)

Necessary Equipment for Emergent Delivery

Except for the Isolette, the following equipment can be stored together easily in an emergent delivery kit for ready access. Consider having a kit in the triage area and in several of the emergency department treatment rooms. The kit should contain:
- Basin or plastic bag
- Scissors or a scalpel (sterile)
- Two cord clamps or two Kelly clamps (sterile)
- One bulb syringe
- Fluid-absorbent pads (large)
- Sterile gloves
- Clean baby blankets
- Sanitary pad or towel
- One infant hat (stockinette material can be used to make a hat)
- Identification bands for the mother and infant
- Heated Isolette (if possible) or warm blankets
- Copy of the Apgar score

Procedure for Emergent Delivery

1. If there is time and qualified personnel are located within the facility, call for assistance with delivery and resuscitation of the neonate.
2. Place the mother in the low Fowler's position with a wedge on either side of the lower back or upper abdomen, with the knees bent up, or in a side-lying position (Fig. 46-3). Delivery of the anterior shoulder is often easier if the mother is side-lying. However, this position requires someone to support the mother's upper leg.
3. Check vital signs (including fetal heart tones) if time permits.
4. Offer ongoing verbal support and explanations.
5. Place a fluid-absorbent pad under the mother.
6. Don sterile gloves.
7. Have the mother pant or lightly push with each contraction.
8. When the head appears, place gentle pressure on the crown to prevent rapid fetal expulsion. Support the perineum to reduce tearing (Fig. 46-4).
9. Hold the neonate's head with both hands and allow it to rotate naturally (Fig. 46-5 and Fig. 46-6).
10. Feel for the umbilical cord around the neonate's neck. If the neonate is entangled, do the following:
    - Attempt to slip the cord over the neonate's head.
    - If the cord is wound too tightly, immediately clamp the cord in two places and cut between the clamps. Call personnel capable of neonatal resuscitation.

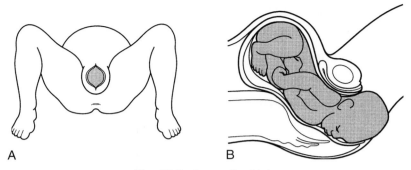

Fig. 46-2 Impending birth.

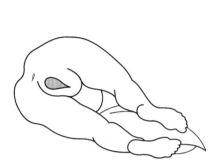

Fig. 46-3 Side-lying position.

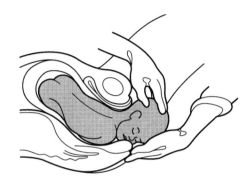

Fig. 46-4 Perineal support.

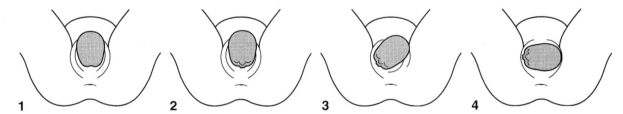

Fig. 46-5 Rotation of the head.

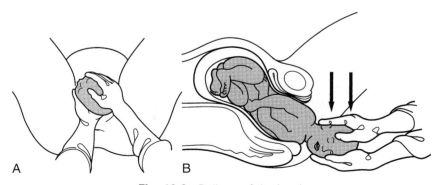

Fig. 46-6 Delivery of the head.

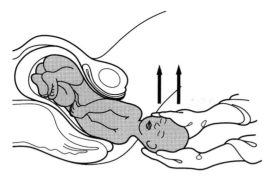

Fig. 46-7 Delivery of the rest of the body.

TABLE 46-5   APGAR SCORE CHART

	0	1	2
Appearance (color)	Blue, pale	Pink body, blue extremities	Pink
Pulse (heart rate)	Absent	<100 beats/min	>100 beats/min
Grimace (muscle tone)	Limp	Some flexion	Good flexion
Activity (reflex irritability)	Absent	Some motion	Good motion
Respiratory effort	Absent	Weak cry	Strong cry

From Mason, D. L. (2009). Obstetric emergencies. In P. K. Howard & R. A. Steinmann, *Sheehy's emergency nursing: Principles and practice* (6th ed., pp. 619–629). St. Louis, MO: Mosby Elsevier.

11. If the amniotic sac is still intact, make a quick snip at the newborn's nape and peel the membranes away from the face.

12. Suctioning at the perineum is no longer considered standard of care, and non-suctioning has been shown to be as safe as suctioning.[7]

13. Deliver the shoulders by guiding the head downward (to deliver the anterior shoulder) and then upward (to free the posterior shoulder).

14. Once the head and shoulders are free, the remaining parts will deliver quickly. Gentle traction may need to be applied (Fig. 46-7).

15. Note the time of birth.

16. After delivery, the newborn should be held at the level of the uterus and the oropharynx should be suctioned again to prevent aspiration.

17. Clamp the cord at two sites 4 to 5 cm from the baby. Be sure that the clamps are closed firmly. Using sterile scissors, cut between the clamps.

18. Dry the neonate immediately and thoroughly. While drying the neonate, assess for evidence of respiratory effort. Discard wet blankets or towels.

19. The newborn should make an effort to breathe by crying spontaneously. If spontaneous breathing does not occur following gentle stimulation (back rub, foot tapping), initiate neonatal resuscitation.

20. Determine Apgar score at 1 minute and again at 5 minutes (Table 46-5).[8]

21. Keep the newborn warm by placing the neonate in a heated Isolette. If a prewarmed Isolette is not readily available, the mother can hold the newborn on her chest or abdomen to provide skin-to-skin body heat. Wrap the mother and newborn well. If available, place a hat on the newborn.

22. Transport mother and newborn to the obstetric unit for further care and evaluation.

Delivery of the Placenta

Placental separation generally occurs within minutes of birth but can be delayed as long as 30 minutes. There is no reason to hurry this process. Allow the placenta to expel naturally. Never tug on an umbilical cord to speed expulsion because it may cause uterine inversion. Gentle fundal massage can aid placental separation from the uterine wall. Again, transport mother and neonate to the obstetric unit for further evaluation and care.

Signs and Symptoms of Impending Placental Delivery

- The umbilical cord advances 2 to 3 inches further out of the vagina
- The fundus rises upward in the abdomen
- The uterus becomes firm and globular
- A large gush of blood comes from the vagina (this bleeding is normal)

Procedure for Delivering the Placenta

1. Instruct the mother to bear down.

2. Do *not* exert traction on the umbilical cord. Allow the placenta to deliver spontaneously.

3. Massage the fundus immediately after placental delivery. The fundus should feel firm, similar to a grapefruit. Provide support for the lower uterine segment while performing fundal massage.

4. After the placenta is expelled, inspect it for missing sections.

5. Save the placenta in a basin or plastic bag and send it with the mother to the obstetric unit.

6. Closely observe the mother for signs of hemorrhage. Once the placenta has delivered, bleeding should slow significantly.

Care of the Mother

- If available in the facility, call obstetric team to assist with care and evaluation.
- To involute the uterus and expel clots, massage the fundus while applying moderate suprapubic pressure.
- Gently wipe the perineal area with a clean towel.
- Remove the soiled fluid-absorbent pad and any soiled linen from underneath the mother.
- Place a sanitary pad or towel over the perineum.
- Infuse IV fluids (usually lactated Ringer solution) at approximately 125 mL per hour (faster if bleeding is excessive).
- Administer oxytocic agents as indicated. Oxytocin (Pitocin) in lactated Ringer solution can reduce bleeding effectively.
- Keep the mother warm.
- Observe the mother closely; monitor vital signs frequently (every 15 minutes) until they are stable.
- Put an infant identification band on the mother's wrist.
- Transport mother to obstetric unit or women's hospital.

Care of the Newborn

- Initial care of the newborn is always per current neonatal resuscitation program guidelines.[9]
- Call neonatal and obstetric team to assist with care and evaluation of the neonate.
- Dry the newborn.
- Keep the newborn warm. If a preheated Isolette or warming lamps are not available, place the infant directly on the mother's skin. If this is impractical (e.g., resuscitation is in progress), a large chemical warming pad works well. However, *never* place a neonate directly on a warming pad. Always put several layers of blanket between the chemical pad and the neonate. Check the temperature of the pad frequently to avoid burns.
- Once the newborn is pink and breathing well, continuously monitor respirations.
- Observe the cord stump for bleeding. Ensure that the clamp is closed tightly.
- Put an identification band on the newborn's wrist or ankle (or both).
- Observe the neonate closely and monitor vital signs.
- Prepare to transfer the mother and neonate to an obstetric or neonatal unit.

Normal Newborn Vital Signs
Pulse: 100 to 160 beats per minute
Respirations: 40 to 60 breaths per minute
Temperature: >36.5°C (97.7°F)

COMPLICATIONS OF DELIVERY

Meconium-Stained Fluid

Care of the neonate with meconium-stained fluid should always be per current neonatal resuscitation guidelines. Unless delivery is imminent, transfer the mother to a tertiary facility or an obstetric unit or page obstetric staff members to the ED.

Signs and Symptoms

- Fluid will be green or dark yellow. It may be "pea soup" thick.
- Possible indeterminate or abnormal fetal heart rate. All fetal monitoring should be done only by the obstetric team experienced in interpretation of the fetal heart rate.

Therapeutic Interventions

- Administer oxygen to the mother.
- If possible, have a neonatal nurse, respiratory therapist, and physician present.
- Initiate neonatal resuscitation as needed. See Table 46-6 for initial steps in resuscitation of a newborn when meconium-stained fluid is present.

Breech Position of the Fetus

Three percent of all fetuses present in the breech position. This can be buttocks first (frank or full breech) or foot first (footling breech) (Fig. 46-8). These positions are dangerous for the fetus because of the increased likelihood of a difficult delivery and cord prolapse. Optimally, breech fetuses will be delivered by cesarean section. Nevertheless, a woman may have an obvious breech delivery in progress.

Therapeutic Interventions

- Notify obstetric and neonatal specialists immediately.
- Support the neonate's legs and buttocks. Do not allow them to hang freely.
- Do *not* pull on the neonate. This may cause the cervix to clamp tighter around the neonate's head. Work with the mother's contractions.
- When the mother has a contraction, place gentle traction on the fetus. Wrapping a towel around the neonate makes the newborn easier to grasp.
- Insert a gloved finger into the vagina to help deliver first one shoulder and then the other (Fig. 46-9).

TABLE 46-6	INITIAL STEPS IN NEONATAL RESUSCITATION

1. Place infant under radiant warmer to provide easy access to infant and to reduce heat loss.
2. Position baby in "sniffing" position (neck slightly extended, not hyperextended or flexed) to open airway.
3. If newborn has depressed respirations, poor muscle tone, and/or heart rate <100 beats/minute, directly suction mouth and trachea.
4. Endotracheal intubation may be required to assist in tracheal suctioning. Obtain 3.5–4 mm (or less if infant is preterm) and 8F–12F suction catheter.
5. Once airway has been cleared, stimulate breathing by thoroughly drying the baby (which also minimizes heat loss), repositioning the head, and gently slapping or flicking the soles of the newborn's feet or rubbing the back, trunk, or extremities.
6. Administer warmed and humidified supplemental oxygen by mask or "blow-by".
7. Positive pressure ventilation will be required if the baby remains apneic.
8. Continue to evaluate respirations (good chest movement), heart rate (>100 beats/minute), and color (pink lips and trunk).

Data from Kattwinkle, J. (2006). *Textbook of neonatal resuscitation* (5th ed.). Elk Grove Village, IL: American Academy of Pediatrics and American Heart Association.

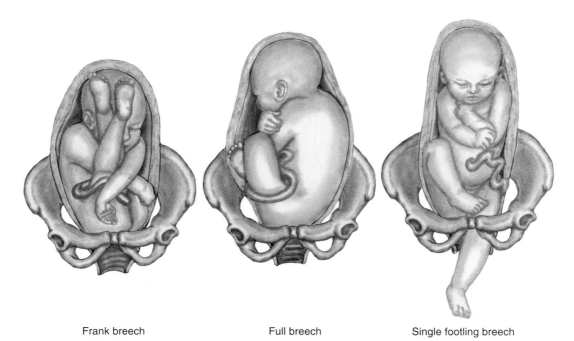

Frank breech   Full breech   Single footling breech

Fig. 46-8 Breech presentation. (Reprinted with permission from Gorrie, T. M., McKinney, E. S., & Murray, S. S. [1998]. *Foundations of maternal-newborn nursing*. Philadelphia, PA: W.B. Saunders.)

- To deliver the head, do the following:
  - Support the fetus's chest with your arm and hands.
  - Place a finger into the posterior vagina and find the newborn's mouth.
  - As the mother pushes with contractions, reach into the newborn's mouth, grasp the chin, and apply gentle upward pressure to the head and shoulders (Fig. 46-10).

- Have an assistant apply pressure to the suprapubic area to aid head expulsion.

Prolapsed Cord

A prolapsed cord is a state in which the umbilical cord precedes the neonate out of the vagina. This is an acute emergency because the cord will be compressed between the fetus's and the mother's bodies, reducing or eliminating blood flow (Fig. 46-11).

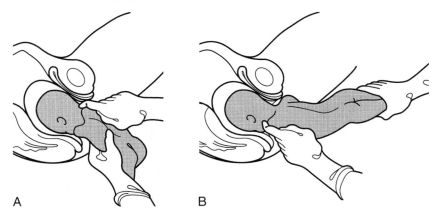

Fig. 46-9 Breech—shoulder delivery.

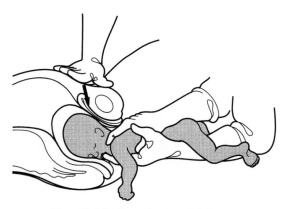

Fig. 46-10 Breech—head delivery.

Signs and Symptoms

- Visible cord protruding from the vagina
- Fetal heart rate frequently less than 100 beats per minute (palpate the cord to check for pulsations)

Therapeutic Interventions

- Notify obstetric and neonatal specialists immediately if available at the facility.
- Place the mother in a knee-chest position (face and knees on the stretcher, buttocks in the air).
- Administer high-flow oxygen.
- Keep the mother warm.
- Put a gloved hand into the vagina and elevate the fetus's head (or other body part) to relieve pressure on the cord; *once this has been accomplished, leave the hand in place.*
- Do not attempt to return the cord to the vagina.

- Feel for cord pulsations but handle the cord as little as possible to prevent spasm of the cord vessels.
- Transport the patient for immediate cesarean section. If transport time is prolonged, keep the cord moist.

Postpartum Hemorrhage

Postpartum hemorrhage is defined as excessive vaginal bleeding any time after delivery (or abortion) for up to 6 weeks. Hemorrhage that occurs within 24 hours is called primary postpartum hemorrhage. Blood loss with delivery is normal and the mother has an excess blood supply available. However, losses in excess of 500 mL are considered postpartum hemorrhage. The "four T's" should guide the consideration of possible causes of bleeding.[6]

- Tone—Uterine atony is the most common cause of serious immediate postpartum hemorrhage.
- Trauma—Common sites of tears resulting from maternal birth trauma are the vagina, perineum, and rectum.
- Tissue—Retained product of conception.
- Thrombin—Disseminated intravascular coagulopathy can occur as a consequence of placental abruption, eclampsia, or amniotic fluid embolism.

Signs and Symptoms

- Steady flow of bright red blood
- Nausea
- Pale, clammy skin
- Palpation of uterus reveals soft, boggy mass
- Signs of hypovolemia and hemorrhagic shock (see Chapter 20, Shock, for more information)

Therapeutic Interventions

- Call the obstetric team for evaluation and treatment.
- Massage the uterus while applying suprapubic pressure to promote involution and expulsion of clots. Fundus

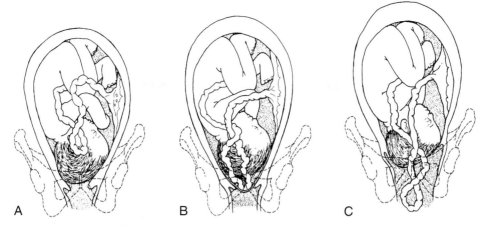

A   B   C

Fig. 46-11 Prolapse of the umbilical cord. (Modified from Lowdermilk, D. L., Perry, S. E., & Bobak, I. M. [2000]. *Maternity and women's health care* [7th ed.]. St. Louis, MO: Mosby).

should feel firm, similar to a grapefruit. It should also be centrally aligned at the umbilicus.

- Apply manual pressure to perineal tears, if present.
- Provide appropriate interventions for hemorrhagic shock.
- Administer high-flow oxygen.
- Insert two large-bore IV catheters and administer a bolus of lactated Ringer solution or normal saline.
- Draw blood for type and crossmatch. Transfuse blood products as indicated.
- Give oxytocic agents. Oxytocin (Pitocin, Syntocinon) 20 units per 1000 mL of lactated Ringer solution (250 to 500 mL per hour) can reduce bleeding effectively.

REFERENCES

1. Callen, P. W. (2008). *Ultrasonography in obstetrics and gynecology* (5th ed.). Philadelphia, PA: Saunders.
2. Sepilian, V. P., & Wood, E. (2011, March 8). *Ectopic pregnancy.* Retrieved from http://emedicine.medscape.com/article/258768-overview
3. Puscheck, E. E. (2011, September 7). *Early pregnancy loss.* Retrieved from http://emedicine.medscape.com/article/266317-overview
4. Gibson, P., & Carson, M. P. (2011, March 29). *Hypertension and pregnancy.* Retrieved from http://emedicine.medscape.com/article/261435-overview
5. Ross, M. G. (2010, May 20). *Eclampsia.* Retrieved from http://emedicine.medscape.com/article/253960-overview
6. Marx, J. A., Hockberger, R., & Walls, R. (2010). *Rosen's emergency medicine: Concepts and clinical practice* (7th ed.). St. Louis, MO: Mosby.
7. Roggensack, A., Jeffries, A. L., & Farine, D. (2008). Management of meconium at birth. *SOGC Technical Update, 224,* 353–354.
8. Mason, D. L. (2009). Obstetric emergencies. In P. K. Howard & R. A. Steinmann (Eds.), *Sheehy's emergency nursing: Principles and practice* (6th ed., pp. 619–629). St. Louis, MO: Mosby.
9. Kattwinkle, J. (2006). Textbook of neonatal resuscitation (5th ed.). Elk Grove Village, IL: American Academy of Pediatrics and American Heart Association.

Gynecologic Emergencies

Linda Kelly

Health issues related to women can be quite different from those experienced by men. For example, women have a high incidence of heart disease but with an entirely different set of symptoms. Diseases such as lupus and rheumatoid arthritis occur far more often in women. This chapter focuses on clinical problems unique to women seen in the emergency department (ED).

> A good resource for comprehensive information related to many aspects of caring for women is available at www.womenshealth.gov/health-professionals.

ABNORMAL UTERINE BLEEDING

Abnormal uterine bleeding is one of the most common gynecologic complaints in the ED and one of the most frequent complaints for which women seek care in EDs. Life-threatening bleeding must be quickly ruled out as well as pregnancy-related causes of vaginal bleeding. Medical treatment of patients with vaginal bleeding is influenced by a number of clinical factors, including the patient's age, pregnancy status, severity of bleeding, comorbidities, and current medications. Emergency management focuses on identifying issues that present an immediate threat to the patient's well-being. Dysfunctional uterine bleeding and other non–life-threatening causes are best addressed in the outpatient setting. See Table 47-1 for differential diagnoses related to vaginal bleeding.

Patient Assessment

- Patient history
  - Usual menstrual history, including date of last menstrual period
  - Possible pregnancy
  - Anticoagulant use or clotting disorder
- Current bleeding episode
  - Duration of current bleeding
  - Color of the blood (bright red, dark)
  - Frequency of tampon or pad change over the past 12 to 24 hours
  - Quantity of bleeding (i.e., are the pads saturated?)
  - Presence or absence of clots
- Medical or gynecologic history
- Current contraception use, particularly if intrauterine device used
  - Recent unprotected sexual intercourse
- Obstetric history
  - Recent delivery or abortion
- Associated symptoms
  - Lower abdominal pain
  - Fever or chills
  - Urinary tract symptoms—hemorrhagic cystitis may be the cause of bleeding

Diagnostic Procedures

- Complete blood count (CBC), type and crossmatch
- Bleeding times, coagulation panel, platelet count
- Urine or quantitative serum beta human chorionic gonadotropin (hCG) level in women of childbearing age
  - If pregnancy test is positive, Rh determination
- Urinalysis
- Stool guaiac
- Pelvic or transvaginal ultrasound
- Vaginal examination
  - Should be performed if patient is not pregnant or is less than 20 weeks gestation
- Rule out placenta previa by ultrasound before performing a vaginal examination on a woman more than 20 weeks gestation.
- See Chapter 46, Obstetric Emergencies.

TABLE 47-1	**POTENTIAL CAUSES OF ABNORMAL UTERINE BLEEDING**

- Hormonal dysfunction
- Hemorrhagic cystitis
- Coagulopathies
  - Disseminated intravascular coagulopathy (DIC)
  - Von Willebrand disease
  - Leukemia
  - Thrombocytopenia
- Neoplasms, primarily in postmenopausal women
- Trauma
- Uterine or vaginal foreign body
- Sexual assault
- Uterine or cervical polyps, uterine fibroids, urethral prolapse
- Gynecologic infections
  - Gonorrhea
  - Chlamydia
  - Trichomoniasis
  - Cervicitis
- Complications of pregnancy
  - Ectopic pregnancy
  - Spontaneous abortion
  - Placental abruption
  - Placenta previa
  - Postpartum hemorrhage

Data from Estephan, A., & Sinert, R. H. (2010, February 1). *Dysfunctional uterine bleeding.* Retrieved from http://emedicine.medscape.com/article/795587-overview

TABLE 47-2	**POSSIBLE CAUSES OF PELVIC PAIN**

- Ectopic pregnancy
- Ruptured ovarian cyst
- Endometriosis
- Pelvic inflammatory disease
- Urinary tract infection
- Kidney stones
- Diverticulitis
- Appendicitis
- Ovarian neoplasm
- Mittelschmerz (pain with ovulation)

Data from Kapoor, D., Ghoniem, G. M., & Davila, G. W. (2010, November 9). *Gynecologic pain.* Retrieved from http://emedicine.medscape.com/article/270450-overview

Therapeutic Interventions

- If the patient is hemodynamically unstable, intervene immediately to stabilize airway, breathing, and circulation.
- Administration of blood products, including packed red blood cells, platelets, or fresh frozen plasma, may be indicated if bleeding is copious.
- Uterine curettage may be indicated.
- High-dose estrogen therapy is the treatment of choice for acute vaginal bleeding.

PELVIC PAIN

In addition to vaginal bleeding, pelvic pain is a common chief complaint of women presenting to the ED. Table 47-2 lists possible causes of pelvic pain to be considered in this patient.

Ectopic Pregnancy

Ectopic pregnancy occurs when a fertilized egg becomes implanted at a site other than the endometrium of the uterine cavity; most often the ectopic location is the fallopian tube. Clinical manifestations of ectopic pregnancy typically appear 6 to 8 weeks after the last normal menstrual period but can occur later. See Chapter 46, Obstetric Emergencies, for additional information related to ectopic pregnancy.

Ruptured Ovarian Cyst

Ovarian cysts are more common during childbearing years because of the cyclic changes of the ovary associated with menstruation.[1] They are generally benign and asymptomatic until hemorrhage, rupture, or torsion occurs. A ruptured ovarian cyst may leak serous fluid or can be hemorrhagic and can be confused with an ectopic pregnancy because the signs and symptoms are similar. Appendicitis, diverticulitis, ovarian torsion, and pelvic inflammatory disease also must be considered (see Table 47-2).

Signs and Symptoms

- Severe pelvic or abdominal pain
  - Sudden, sharp, unilateral
  - Rupture and pain may occur during sexual intercourse or following exercise or trauma
- Vaginal bleeding may or may not be present
- Signs of peritoneal irritation
  - Involuntary guarding
  - Rebound tenderness
- Low-grade fever
- If excessive bleeding, signs of hemorrhagic shock

Diagnostic Procedures

- Urine or serum beta hCG to rule out pregnancy
- CBC, possibly type and crossmatch
- Palpable mass on pelvic examination
- Transvaginal ultrasound
- Abdominal computed tomography (CT) to rule out other causes of pelvic pain

Therapeutic Interventions

- Administer supplemental oxygen.
- Initiate intravenous therapy with lactated Ringer solution or normal saline solution.
- Administer analgesics.
- Antibiotics may be considered.
- Prepare the patient for surgical intervention if hemodynamically unstable.

Endometriosis

Endometriosis is a major cause of disability and decreased quality of life in many women and teenage girls.[2] A common cause of pelvic pain, endometriosis occurs when endometrial tissue cells grow outside the uterus, primarily on the pelvic peritoneum, ovaries, and rectovaginal septum. The resulting inflammatory response leads to adhesions, fibrosis, scarring, pain, and infertility.

Signs and Symptoms

- Dysmenorrhea
- Chronic pelvic pain with acute exacerbations
  - Unpredictable, intermittent, or continuous
  - Dull, throbbing, or sharp in nature
  - Exacerbated by physical activity[2]
- Dysuria, hematuria
- Dyspareunia (painful intercourse)

Diagnostic Procedures

Diagnosis of endometriosis is not made in the ED; typical ED studies include pregnancy test, CBC, and urinalysis. Laparoscopic visualization and endometrial biopsy are performed by a gynecologist and used to diagnose endometriosis definitively.

Therapeutic Interventions

- Nonsteroidal antiinflammatory drugs (NSAIDs) to relieve dysmenorrhea
- Oral contraceptives (cyclic or continuous)
- Refer patient for gynecologic follow-up; surgical intervention may be necessary

Gestational Trophoblastic Disease

Gestational trophoblastic disease refers to a group of rare tumors arising from abnormal cells in tissue that would normally become the placenta. These tumors may be benign, as is usually the case with hydatidiform mole, or locally invasive and metastatic, as in the case of a choriocarcinoma.[3] Hydatidiform mole, also called a molar pregnancy, is the most common form of gestational trophoblastic disease.

Choriocarcinomas may originate from a hydatidiform mole or from tissue that remains in the uterus following abortion or normal delivery. These tumors can spread from the uterus to other parts of the body. Fortunately, choriocarcinoma is among the cancers most sensitive to chemotherapy, and even with metastasis the cure rate is 90% to 95%.[4] In the early stages the clinical manifestations of these diseases cannot be distinguished from those of normal pregnancy. Later, vaginal bleeding occurs in most cases.

Signs and Symptoms

- Often diagnosed by routine ultrasound in the first trimester before the onset of signs and symptoms[4]
- Uterine enlargement greater than appropriate for gestational age
- Absent fetal heart tones
- Intermittent or continuous vaginal bleeding
- Hyperemesis gravidarum
- Signs of preeclampsia that may appear at an early gestational age
- Pelvic pressure or pain

Diagnostic Procedures

- High beta hCG levels related to trophoblastic proliferation
- CBC and clotting studies to detect possible anemia or coagulopathy
- Transvaginal ultrasound demonstrates no evidence of a fetus
- Chest radiograph to rule out metastasis to lungs

Therapeutic Interventions

- If bleeding is heavy or the patient is dehydrated from vomiting, monitor vital signs and administer intravenous fluid.
- The patient may require transfusion for anemia or coagulopathy.
- Prepare for uterine evacuation (dilation and curettage or dilation and evacuation).
- Manage symptoms of preeclampsia, particularly hypertension.

GYNECOLOGIC INFECTIONS

Pelvic Inflammatory Disease

Pelvic inflammatory disease (PID) refers to acute infections of the upper genital tract structures involving the fallopian tubes, ovaries, pelvic peritoneum, or some combination of these sites. PID occurs as a result of upward migration of bacteria from the lower reproductive tract. It can be caused by sexually transmitted organisms or by flora indigenous to the lower genital tract. The bacteria most often isolated are *Neisseria gonorrhoeae* (25% to 80% of cases) and *Chlamydia trachomatis*.[5] PID can lead to chronic abdominal pain, ectopic pregnancy, or infertility.

Predisposing factors of PID include:
- Young age
- Multiple sexual partners
- Recent abortion
- Presence of intrauterine device[5]
- Previous diagnosis of PID

Signs and Symptoms

- Lower abdominal pain is the most common
  - Dull, aching, cramping, constant in nature
  - Begins soon after onset of last menstrual period
  - Exacerbated by movement or sexual activity
- Rebound tenderness or involuntary guarding may indicate peritonitis
- Abnormal mucopurulent vaginal discharge
- Temperature greater than 38°C (100.4°F)
- Nausea and vomiting

Diagnostic Procedures

- CBC showing elevated white blood cell count
- Elevated erythrocyte sedimentation rate (ESR) and C-reactive protein (CRP)
- Urinalysis to rule out urinary tract infection
- Pregnancy test
- Pelvic examination
  - Uterine tenderness
  - Adnexal tenderness
  - Cervical motion tenderness
- White blood cells on microscopic examination of vaginal secretions
- Transvaginal ultrasound may show fluid-filled tubes or free pelvic fluid or identify tubo-ovarian abscess[5]

Therapeutic Interventions

- Administer agents for pain management and initiate fluid replacement as appropriate.
- Administer broad-spectrum antibiotics.
- Treat current and recent sexual partners.

- May require hospitalization depending on severity of infection and symptoms.

Toxic Shock Syndrome

Toxic shock syndrome (TSS) refers to a toxin-mediated systemic response usually caused by a toxigenic strain of *Staphylococcus aureus*.[1] TSS was initially associated with the use of hyperabsorbent tampons or contraceptive sponges. When these products were made less absorbent, the incidence of toxic shock syndrome dropped dramatically. Nonmenstrual TSS is now reported in just less than half of the cases.[1] Group A *Streptococcus* infections can also produce TSS, usually secondary to soft tissue infections such as necrotizing fasciitis and burn injury. See Chapter 21, Sepsis, for a more complete discussion of management of the patient with severe sepsis.

Signs and Symptoms

- Sudden onset of fever greater than 38.8°C (101.8°F) and chills
- Hypotension (systolic blood pressure less than 90 mm Hg)
- Nausea and vomiting
- Headache and myalgias
- Diarrhea
- Classic rash
- Confusion
- Multisystem organ failure

Diagnostic Procedures

- CBC
  - Leukocytosis, thrombocytopenia, and anemia
- Chemistry, coagulation panels, and lactate level
  - Elevated creatinine, hypocalcemia, metabolic acidosis
- Urinalysis may reveal hemoglobinuria
- Blood and wound cultures
- Chest radiograph, if signs of respiratory failure

Therapeutic Interventions

- Initiate contact isolation if appropriate.
- Support the patient's airway, breathing, and circulation.
- Administer supplemental oxygen to maintain a PaO_2 greater than 60 mm Hg; endotracheal intubation may be necessary.
- Begin aggressive fluid resuscitation with intravenous crystalloids.
- Identify and remove potential sources of infection.
  - Remove tampon or wound or nasal packing and perform wound debridement.
- Initiate immediate antibiotic administration.

- Anticipate insertion of an arterial line and central venous catheter.
- Consider vasopressors for support of blood pressure.
- Facilitate admission or transfer to a critical care unit.

INFECTIONS OF THE EXTERNAL GENITALIA

When the ecology of the vagina is disturbed (such as by antibiotic use or diabetes), vaginal infections can occur. Some sexually transmitted infections cause vulvovaginitis, as do various chemicals found in bubble baths, soaps, and perfumes. Factors such as poor hygiene and allergens contribute to the proliferation of organisms that thrive in warm, damp, dark environments. Sexual abuse should be considered in children with unusual infections and recurrent episodes of unexplained vulvovaginitis.

Vaginal Infections

Vaginal infections are not an emergency. Nonetheless, because the condition is annoying, patients with such infections frequently present to the ED for treatment. These individuals should be directed to gynecologic offices and clinics where they can receive follow-up care once they have been seen and treated. Table 47-3 compares the symptoms, diagnosis, and management of various vaginal infections.

Bartholin's Cyst Abscess

The Bartholin glands are located on either side of the vaginal opening. Obstruction of the Bartholin duct may result in formation of a cyst; infection of the cyst can result from aerobic and anaerobic vaginal organisms as well as sexually transmitted infections such as *N. gonorrhoeae* or *C. trachomatis*.

Signs and Symptoms

- Painful cystic mass or swelling
- Vulvar swelling and tenderness

Therapeutic Interventions

- Warm compresses
- Sitz baths
- Incision and drainage

TABLE 47-3 COMPARISON OF VAGINAL INFECTIONS

	SYMPTOMS	EXAMINATION FINDINGS	TREATMENT	COMMENTS
Bacterial vaginosis	• 50% are asymptomatic • Milky, white to gray vaginal discharge with fishy odor	• Vaginal pH >4.5 • 20% of epithelial cells are clue cells	• Oral metronidazole (Flagyl) for 7 days • Clindamycin (Cleocin) cream	• Presence of bacterial vaginosis has been shown to be a risk factor for premature labor and perinatal infection • Instruct patient about potential interaction of metronidazole (Flagyl) and warfarin (Coumadin), and that clindamycin (Cleocin) cream may weaken a condom • Advise the patient not to drink alcohol while taking metronidazole (Flagyl) and for 24 hours after completing this medication
Candidiasis	• Vaginal burning and itching • Dyspareunia • Dysuria • "Cheesy" vaginal discharge	• Vulvovaginal erythema and swelling • Normal vaginal pH	• Topical clotrimazole or terconazole • Oral fluconazole (Diflucan)	• *Candida albicans* is the most common causative organism • Risk factors for vulvovaginal candidiasis include recent antibiotic use, uncontrolled diabetes, and HIV infection

Continued

TABLE 47-3 COMPARISON OF VAGINAL INFECTIONS—cont'd

	SYMPTOMS	EXAMINATION FINDINGS	TREATMENT	COMMENTS
Trichomoniasis	• Vaginal itching and burning • Foul-smelling, frothy vaginal discharge • Dyspareunia • Postcoital bleeding	• Vulvovaginal erythema • Positive culture	• Metronidazole (Flagyl)	• Highly transmissible • Associated with other STIs • May increase risk of acquiring HIV[a]
Atrophic vaginitis	• Patient may be asymptomatic • Vaginal irritation • Dyspareunia • Thin, clear or bloody discharge	• Parabasal epithelial cells on microscopic exam of wet prep • Vaginal pH 5 to 7	• Topical (cream, tablet, ring) estrogen	• Due to estrogen deficiency in menopause
Nonspecific vulvovaginitis	• Irritation, itching of genital area • Vaginal discharge with foul odor • Dysuria	• Inflammation of labia majora, labia minora, or perineal area • Cultures to determine chlamydia or gonorrhea as possible causes	• Symptomatic treatment if vaginitis is noninfectious • Antibiotics if microscopic examination identifies causative organism	• Seen in all age groups but greatest frequency is prepuberty • May be associated with poor genital hygiene with an overgrowth of *Escherichia coli*

[a]Owen, M. K., & Clenney, T. L. (2004). Management of vaginitis. *American Family Physician, 70*, 2125–2132.
HIV, Human immunodeficiency virus; *STI*, sexually transmitted infection.

TABLE 47-4 CONTRACEPTIVE EMERGENCIES

TYPE	PROBLEM	THERAPEUTIC INTERVENTION
Unprotected sex or contraceptive failure	Potential pregnancy	Emergency contraception with levonorgestrel (Plan B, Preven), a "morning-after pill," is effective for up to 72 hours after unprotected intercourse. This oral agent prevents ovulation, disrupts fertilization, and inhibits implantation. This medication will not cause an abortion if the embryo is already implanted.
Diaphragm	Unable to remove	Remove with ring forceps.
Intrauterine device (IUD)	Unable to remove	Remove with ring forceps.
	Lost string	Use abdominal radiographs or ultrasound to determine IUD position; may be removed with an IUD hook.
	Partial expulsion	Remove; advise an alternate form of contraception.
	Abdominal cavity migration	Use abdominal radiographs or ultrasound to determine IUD position; may require exploratory laparotomy.
Oral contraceptives	Thrombophlebitis	Encourage bed rest and local heat application; administer anticoagulant therapy.
	Pulmonary embolus	ABCs; administer oxygen, intravenous fluids, analgesia, bronchodilators, and heparin; provide reassurance.
	Stroke	

ABCs, Airway, breathing, and circulation.
Data from Samra-Latif, O. M., & Wood, E. (2011, August 24). *Contraception.* Retrieved from http://emedicine.medscape.com/article/258507-overview

- Insertion of Word catheter to promote drainage
- Culture of drainage to identify causative organism
- Possible antibiotic administration depending on culture results
- If cysts are recurrent or occur in women older than 40 years, carcinoma must be ruled out by biopsy

CONTRACEPTIVE EMERGENCIES

Occasionally, a patient with a contraceptive emergency will present to the ED. Table 47-4 lists some of the more common contraceptive emergencies.

REFERENCES

1. Tibbles, C. D. (2010). Selected gynecologic disorders. In J. Marx (Ed.), *Rosen's emergency medicine: Concepts and clinical practice* (7th ed.). St. Louis, MO: Elsevier.
2. Giudice, L. C. (2010). Endometriosis. *New England Journal of Medicine, 362*, 2389–2398.
3. Soper, J. T. (2006). Gestational trophoblastic disease. *Obstetrics and Gynecolology, 108*, 176–187.
4. Moore, L. E., & Hernandez, E. (2010, January 27). *Hydatidiform mole.* Retrieved from http://emedicine.medscape.com/article/254657-overview
5. Shepherd, S. M. (2011, May 17). *Pelvic inflammatory disease.* Retrieved from http://emedicine.medscape.com/article/256448-overview

Mental Health Emergencies

Anne P. Manton

For many reasons, the emergency department (ED) has become a frequent source of care for patients with mental health concerns. Over the past several decades psychiatric inpatient capacity has decreased. The numbers of mental health clinics and other outpatient services are insufficient to meet the needs of Americans who at any given time have a diagnosable mental illness, which ranges from 20% to 26.2% of the population.[1,2]

Therefore, EDs have become the point of care for millions of people with exacerbations of mental illness in need of immediate treatment. This situation is difficult for emergency health care providers because care of those with mental health emergencies presents unique challenges. With the exception of substance abuse disorders, there are no diagnostic studies or other procedures that can assist in confirming a mental health diagnosis. Knowing the patient's baseline is helpful, but this is frequently not available in the emergency setting.

> The diagnosis of a psychiatric illness is made through observing behavior and listening to the patient.

The decrease in the number of psychiatric inpatient beds and the insufficient outpatient mental health resources compound the issue of mental health care in the ED. As a recent American College of Emergency Physicians (ACEP) survey demonstrated, difficulties with access to psychiatric care has led to excessive boarding of psychiatric patients in the ED.[3,4]

MENTAL HEALTH TRIAGE

The goal of mental health triage is to determine the severity of the presenting problem while protecting the patient, staff, and others. Individuals with mental health emergencies commonly exhibit intense personal distress, suicidal ideation, and self-neglect that jeopardizes their health and safety.

In addition to psychotic conditions, many other mental health emergencies—such as acute anxiety, panic attacks, severe depression, or substance abuse—can cause disordered or dangerous behavior. Evaluation of the patient with a mental health disturbance differs significantly from the typical triage history-taking process. The Emergency Severity Index (ESI) five-level triage categorizations used in most EDs do not fit as well for mental health emergencies as they do for physiologic complaints.[5] Based on the parameters listed in Table 48-1, individuals with mental health emergencies can be assigned a triage category.

MENTAL HEALTH ASSESSMENT

Initial Assessment

As with physiologic complaints, it is critical to identify those psychiatric patients who require immediate attention. Such patients include those with:
- Prehospital involuntary hold
- Suicidal gestures or attempts
- Homicidal gestures or attempts
- Greatly diminished self-care capacity
- Poor impulse control or violence
- Bizarre and unexplained behavior
- Severe self-injurious behavior
- Drug or alcohol use associated with psychiatric symptoms

Secondary Assessment

The second part of mental health assessment is the Mental Status Examination (MSE), which can be thought of as the mental health equivalent of a physical examination for patients with physiologic complaints. The objective of the MSE is to describe the mental state and behaviors of the

TABLE 48-1	**MENTAL HEALTH TRIAGE SCALE***		
TRIAGE CODE	**TRIAGE CATEGORY**	**DESCRIPTION**	**TYPICAL PRESENTATION**
1	Emergent	• Actively suicidal or homicidal • Severe behavioral disturbance	• Violent behavior • Possession of a weapon • Self-injurious behavior • Extreme agitation • Verbally aggressive • Grave disability; greatly diminished self-care capacity • Requires restraint • Poor impulse control; fighting • Drug or alcohol abuse with psychiatric symptoms
2	Urgent	• Possible danger to self or others • Moderate behavioral disturbance	• Agitated; restless • Intrusive behavior • Confusion • Withdrawn; uncommunicative • Suicidal ideation without a plan • Verbal or auditory hallucinations • Delusions • Paranoia • Severe depression or anxiety • Elevated or irritable mood
3	Semi-urgent	Moderate distress	• No agitation or restlessness • Cooperative • Gives a coherent history • Suicidal ideation but is accompanied by a capable friend or family member • No suicidal ideation • Irritable without aggression
4	Nonurgent	No acute distress	• Cooperative • Communicative • Compliant • Known patient with chronic symptoms
5	Nonurgent	No distress	• Medication request or refill

*Note that the Mental Health Triage Scale does not necessarily fall in line with five-scale triage systems currently in use at most emergency departments. Use your best judgment and critical thinking skills to determine the best category for patients presenting to the emergency department with mental health emergencies and follow hospital and departmental policies.
Adapted from Broadbent, M., Jarman, H., & Berk, M. (2002). Improving compliance in mental health triage. *Accident and Emergency Nursing, 10*, 155–162.

patient presenting with psychiatric symptoms. Included in the MSE are both observations by the clinicians (objective data) and information given by the patient (subjective data). Components of the MSE include observation of the following:
- Appearance
  - Appropriateness of dress
  - Grooming and hygiene
  - Posture—slumped, tense, rigid
  - Facial expression—provocative, threatening
- Behavior
  - Psychomotor activity (e.g., restlessness, fidgeting)
  - Eye contact

- Abnormal movements, tremor
- Speech
  - Rate—increased or decreased
  - Rhythm—slurred, monotone
  - Volume—loud, soft
  - Content—few words, talkative, fluent
- Mood
  - Emotional state as reported by the patient
    - Depressed, sad, angry, happy, irritable
- Affect
  - Emotional state observed
    - Type—euthymic (normal), depressed, anxious, elated

- Range—full (normal) versus restricted, flat, or labile
- Congruency—Does it match mood as reported by patient?
- Thought process
  - How are thoughts connected? Do they flow logically?
    - Normal—logical, coherent
    - Abnormal—disorganized, loose connections, incoherent
- Thought content
  - What is the content of thoughts? This may include:
    - Preoccupations (death, suicide, homicide)
    - Illusions—misinterpretation of the environment
    - Ideas of reference—the misinterpretation of outside events having direct personal reference to patient
    - Hallucinations—false sensory perceptions (auditory, visual, tactile, or olfactory)
    - Delusions—fixed, false beliefs firmly held despite contradictory evidence
- Cognition
  - Level of consciousness
  - Attention and concentration
  - Memory—immediate, short and long term
  - Abstract or concrete thinking
  - Intellectual impairment
- Insight
  - Awareness of self and illness
- Judgment
  - Appropriateness of decisions and choices

Patient History

History of Present Illness

- Why is patient seeking help now?
- Events leading to perceived need for treatment
- Suicidal or homicidal ideation or gestures
- Who brought patient to ED?
- Usual source of primary and psychiatric care
- Current medication regimen and date and time of last medication

Psychiatric History

- Psychiatric diagnosis
- Psychiatric hospitalizations
- Suicide attempts
- Medications prescribed
- Conformity with medication regimen

Medical and Surgical History

- Medical diagnoses and treatment
- Allergies
- History of surgical procedures

Family History

- Support system
- Family history of mental illness
- Family history of suicide

Substance Abuse History

- Current substance use: drug of choice, amount and frequency, last use
- Past substance abuse
- Previous detoxification admissions, self-help group participation (Alcoholics Anonymous or Narcotics Anonymous)[6]

GENERAL APPROACH TO THE PATIENT

The primary concerns of emergency care providers are to evaluate the degree of dysfunction of the patient with a mental health emergency, to carry out measures to provide for the patient's safety, and to administer appropriate treatment modalities. Treatment interventions may include therapy and medication administration. The goal of treatment is to ensure patient safety, alleviate acute distress, and help the patient establish a sense of self-control. Once this is achieved, referral can be made for more extensive care.

> The goal of emergency treatment is to ensure patient safety, alleviate acute distress, and help the patient establish a sense of self-control.

When caring for patients with mental health emergencies the following are useful guidelines:
- Attempt to establish a therapeutic alliance and rapport
- Use direct eye contact (within cultural considerations)
- Appear relaxed
- Convey respect
- Let the patient know that there is genuine concern for him or her as a person
- Listen attentively (active listening) but redirect as needed
- Speak clearly and without using jargon
- Encourage patient participation in decision making when possible
- Be honest and genuine
- Expect safe behavior and state this clearly
- Anticipate the emotional component (such as anger, crying, or grief)
- Explain procedures and medications to the patient
- Take the patient seriously
- Validate feelings

- Do not be afraid to admit ignorance
- Include the patient's family and significant other if possible

Do not hesitate to ask for help if you feel physically threatened.

MENTAL HEALTH EMERGENCIES WITHOUT PSYCHOSES

Table 48-2 shows the classification of mental health emergencies used in this chapter.

Anxiety Disorders

Anxiety is a diffuse, unfocused response that alerts an individual to an impending threat, real or imagined. Fear, on the other hand, is a natural psychological and physiologic reaction to an actual or potential threat.[7] Fear is object focused, whereas anxiety involves a faceless, nonspecific threat; no identifiable object can be isolated. Anxiety disorders include panic disorder, obsessive-compulsive disorder, post-traumatic stress disorder, generalized anxiety disorder, and phobias (social phobia, agoraphobia, and specific phobias). Anxiety disorders frequently co-occur with depressive disorders or substance abuse. Approximately 40 million American adults aged 18 years and older, or about 18.1% of people in this age group in a given year, have an anxiety disorder.[2]

TABLE 48-2	CLASSIFICATION OF MENTAL HEALTH EMERGENCIES
MENTAL HEALTH EMERGENCIES WITHOUT PSYCHOSIS	**MENTAL HEALTH EMERGENCIES WITH PSYCHOSIS**
Anxiety disorders	Acute psychotic reactions
• Panic disorder	Schizophrenia
• Generalized anxiety disorder	Paranoia
• Obsessive-compulsive disorder	Bipolar disorder—mania
• Post-traumatic stress disorder	
• Phobias	
Depressive disorders	
• Major depressive disorder	
• Acute grief	
Suicide	

Panic Disorder and Acute Anxiety Attacks

Approximately 6 million adults aged 18 years and older, or about 2.7% of people in this age group, have a panic disorder in a given year.[2] Onset is usually in early adulthood (median age of onset is 24 years).[2] Women are twice as likely to be affected as men.[2]

Panic attacks begin without any warning, commonly during activities that are routine and nonthreatening. The person will experience sudden intense fear, palpitations, chest pain, shortness of breath, and dizziness. These symptoms are accompanied by the feeling that he or she is going to die, go insane, or completely lose control. Panic attacks typically peak within 10 minutes or less and symptoms dissipate within 30 minutes. During the time of the panic attack the individual does not lose contact with reality, but insight and judgment are impaired.

Signs and Symptoms

- Feelings of impending danger, death, or "going crazy"
- Tachycardia, palpitations
- Precordial discomfort, feeling of chest pressure
- Hyperventilation, feeling of breathlessness
- Paresthesias
- Choking sensation, difficulty swallowing (dysphagia)
- Diaphoresis
- Dry mouth
- Urinary frequency
- Tremors
- Hyperactivity
- Attempts to exit location immediately

Therapeutic Interventions. The goal of emergency care for persons experiencing a panic attack or acute anxiety attack is to promote an environment in which the individual can feel safe and supported and achieve an adequate degree of self-control. Nursing interventions to help decrease feelings of extreme anxiety include the following:

- Provide general emotional support.
- Rule out physiologic causes of symptoms.
- Resolve concerns about safety but avoid false reassurance.
- Identify and treat hyperventilation—encourage slow, regular breathing.
- Maintain a calm appearance.
- Encourage the patient to talk.
- Attend to physical symptoms.
- Direct the patient toward reality.
- Consider the use of antianxiety medications.
- Emphasize the importance of mental health treatment on a nonemergency basis.
- Make referrals to mental health providers and agencies.

TABLE 48-3	**SIGNS AND SYMPTOMS OF POST-TRAUMATIC STRESS DISORDER**	
RE-EXPERIENCING SYMPTOMS	**AVOIDANCE SYMPTOMS**	**HYPERAROUSAL SYMPTOMS**
Flashbacks—reliving the trauma over and over Bad dreams or nightmares Frightening thoughts	Staying away from places, events, and objects that are reminders of the experience Feeling emotionally numb Feeling strong guilt, depression, or worry Loss of interest in activities that were previously enjoyed Difficulty remembering the traumatic event	Easily startled Feeling tense or "on edge" Difficulty sleeping Angry outbursts

Obsessive-Compulsive Disorder

Symptoms of obsessive-compulsive disorder (OCD) often begin during childhood or adolescence. According to the National Institute of Mental Health (NIMH), approximately 2.2 million American adults aged 18 years and older, or about 1% of people in this age group, have OCD.[2] One third of adults with OCD developed symptoms as children and research indicates that OCD may have familial tendencies. It affects men and women in roughly equal numbers.[2,8] Diagnostic criteria for OCD generally involve obsessions and compulsions. *Obsessions* are recurrent thoughts, images, and impulses that invade the mind, causing intolerable anxiety. These preoccupations make no sense and may be repulsive or revolve around themes of violence and harm. *Compulsions* are devised to relieve the anxiety and doubt generated by an obsession. The person will be driven to perform specific repetitive, ritualized behaviors calculated to temporarily reduce discomfort. These behaviors can take on a life of their own, imprisoning the individual in a pattern of activities. Common compulsions include the following:
- Hand washing
- Showering or house cleaning
- Excessive ordering and arranging
- Incessant checking and rechecking
- Repetitive counting, touching, and activity rituals
- Excessive slowness in activities such as eating or tooth brushing
- Constant searching for reassurance that the perceived threat has been removed

Persons with OCD are not delusional and are not having hallucinations; they simply cannot control the compulsive responses to their anxiety.[8]

Post-traumatic Stress Disorder

Post-traumatic stress disorder (PTSD) is an anxiety disorder that can develop after exposure to a terrifying event or ordeal in which grave physical harm occurred or was threatened. Traumatic events that may trigger PTSD include violent personal assaults such as rape, mugging, and domestic violence; natural or human-caused disasters; accidents; and military combat.

Patients with PTSD experience emotional, physical, behavioral, and psychological impairment. In PTSD, the "fight or flight" response is changed or damaged. People who have PTSD may feel stressed or frightened when they are no longer in danger.[9]

It is estimated that approximately 7.7 million American adults aged 18 years and older, or about 3.5% of people in this age group, have PTSD in a given year. It can develop at any age, including during childhood.[2] Individuals who have PTSD may be at increased risk for substance abuse, impaired relationships, and suicide.

Signs and Symptoms. Symptoms of PTSD can be categorized as re-experiencing, avoidance, and hyperarousal. Table 48-3 lists these signs and symptoms.

Therapeutic Interventions
- Provide a quiet environment.
- Remain calm and relaxed.
- Assess risk for suicide.
- Assess potential for violence.
- Allow patient to verbalize feelings and concerns.
- Identify the traumatic event if appropriate.
- Assist the patient to identify and use a support system.
- Administer antidepressants and anxiolytics as indicated.
- Help patient identify community resources.
- Facilitate consultations and referral.

Depressive Disorders

Patients with depressive disorders are commonly encountered in emergency care settings. Depressive conditions include major depressive disorder and dysthymic disorder. Depressive disorders have a high prevalence in the general population; major depressive disorder affects approximately 14.8 million American adults, or about 6.7% of the U.S. population aged 18 years and older in a given year.[2] Major depressive disorder is more prevalent in women than in men and is the leading cause of disability in the United States for people aged 15 to 44 years.[2] Dysthymic disorder, which is a chronic, mild depression, affects approximately 3.3 million American adults (1.5% of the population).[2]

Normal sadness, grief, and emotional responses to life's difficulties must be distinguished from a depressive disorder. For the diagnosis of major depressive disorder to be made, depressive symptoms must be present during all or most of the day, every day, for at least 2 weeks.[10] A sad or depressed mood is only one of the indictors of clinical depression.

Major Depressive Disorder

Signs and Symptoms

- Feelings of worthlessness, loneliness, helplessness, sadness
- Decreased interest or pleasure in usual activities
- Feelings of guilt
- Physical fatigue, loss of energy
- Psychomotor retardation or agitation
- Sleep disturbances (insomnia or hypersomnia)
- Difficulty with decision making
- Weight change (gain or loss) of 5% of body weight in 1 month
- Decreased libido
- Irritability (especially children and adolescents)
- Feelings of hopelessness
- Decreased ability to concentrate
- Suicidal ideation, preoccupation with death

Therapeutic Interventions

- Provide for the patient's safety and security.
- Assess risk for suicide.
- Do *not* isolate the patient.
- Decrease excessive environmental stimuli.
- Avoid forced decision making.
- Encourage expression of feelings.
- Explore sources of emotional support.
- Involve family members, with the patient's permission.
- Be genuine and empathetic—not judgmental.
- Refer the patient for psychiatric and medication evaluation and psychotherapy.
- Inform the patient and family of the community resources available.

Acute Grief

Grief is an expected response to a significant loss, such as the loss of a loved one, one's health, a job, or a way of life or a major financial loss. Acute grief reactions are frequently seen in the emergency setting following a patient's death. The grieving process is influenced by many variables, such as the individual's cultural background, personality style, history of losses, coping ability, and other individual factors. Emergency nurses must anticipate psychological and physiologic grief reactions and be prepared to provide physical and emotional support to patients and family members.

Signs and Symptoms

- Shock, disbelief, denial
- Emotional lability with overt tears, moaning, or wailing
- Diminished or slow speech
- Inability to concentrate
- Anger, sadness, guilt
- Increased focus on the lost "person or object"
- Feeling of helplessness
- Anorexia or changes in appetite and weight
- Sleep disturbances (insomnia or hypersomnia)

Therapeutic Interventions

- Accept the individual's response as normal and provide supportive dialogue.
- Encourage expression of feelings, especially sadness and loss.
- Provide privacy in a room with normal lighting but decreased stimuli.
- Stress the importance of proper nutrition and fluid intake, even if appetite is decreased.
- Explore sources of emotional support.
- Encourage the individual to seek out friends, family members, or a bereavement group to discuss feelings of grief.
- Make referrals to counseling or community resources as appropriate.

Suicide

The most recent available statistics related to suicide in the United States report that 33,300 persons killed themselves in 2006.[2,11] This represents an increase from previous years. Suicide is the eleventh ranking cause of death in the United States and the third highest cause of death for the young (under age 24 years).[11] The data show that in the United States one person committed suicide every 15.8 minutes.[11] In addition, it is estimated that there are approximately 832,500 suicide attempts per year that do not have a fatal outcome.[11] Those figures translate to one attempt every 38 seconds. Use of firearms accounted for more than 50% of completed suicides.[11] Additionally, a survey conducted in 2008 found that an estimated 8.3 million adults aged 18 years or older had serious thoughts of suicide in the past year.[12] The highest percentage with serious thoughts and plans of suicide were young adults aged 18 to 25 years.[2,11] It should be noted that suicide affects not only the person who dies, but also his or her entire social structure. Suicide is indeed a major public health problem.[11,13]

Assessment of Suicide Potential

Gender
- Females attempt suicide three times more often than do males.[2]
- Males are four times more likely to succeed at suicide than are women.[2]
- Approximately 70% of all suicide deaths involve Caucasian men.[11]

Age[11]
- The elderly made up 12.5% of the population in 2006 but represented 15.9% of the suicides.
- The young made up 14.2% of the population in 2006 and represented 12.6% of suicides.
- Non-Hispanic Caucasian men over the age of 85 years are the most likely to die of suicide. The rate of 49.8 per 100,000 is greater than in any other age group.

Family History
- There is an increased risk for suicide in families with a history of suicide attempts.
- A family history of mental disorder or substance abuse is a risk factor for suicide.
- History of childhood abuse is a risk factor for suicide.

Seasonal Variations
- The incidence of suicide is highest in spring.[14]

Other Risk Factors for Suicide[14]
- Substance use (or abuse) greatly increases the risk for suicide.
- The risk of lethality is greater if the person has access to a weapon (firearms in the home) or has a well thought-out plan.
- Previous suicide attempts.
- Mental illness is present in most people who die by suicide, especially:
  - Depression (especially feeling hopeless)
  - Bipolar illness
  - Schizophrenia
  - Substance abuse
- Chronic physical illness is a risk factor for suicide.

Signs and Symptoms of Increased Risk
- Feelings of worthlessness, hopelessness, helplessness
- Confusion, impaired insight and judgment
- Restlessness, agitation, irritability
- Indifference, fatigue, insomnia
- Decreased physical activity
- Withdrawal, social isolation

Approach to the Suicidal Patient
The goal of emergency care for suicidal patients is to provide a physically and psychologically protective environment and establish empathetic rapport. All patients presenting with suicidal ideation or a suicide attempt are considered to require emergent care and should be placed in an examination room immediately. One-on-one observations should be instituted and appropriate documentation maintained. Care of the patient who presents after an overdose, hanging, or other type of serious suicide attempt focuses initially on the immediate medical needs of the patient.[13] Once life-threatening issues have been stabilized, the focus of care then becomes the mental health and safety of the patient.

Therapeutic Interventions[15]
- Undress the patient and remove any items from the environment that may pose a danger.
- Encourage the patient to talk about the problem that led to the suicide attempt.
- Evaluate the problem with the patient.
- Assist the patient in looking for alternative solutions.
- Help to manage chronic illness if present.
- Administer medications if appropriate.
- Try to involve family or friends in discussion, with the permission of the patient.
- Prepare the patient for admission to the hospital.
- Obtain psychiatric consultation.
- Ensure that the patient and family have the suicide hotline phone number: 1-800-784-2433.

MENTAL HEALTH EMERGENCIES WITH PSYCHOSES

Acute Psychotic Reactions
Acute psychosis is an emergency condition requiring rapid, accurate assessment and diagnosis. It is important to determine whether the psychosis is of organic or psychiatric etiology. Possible organic causes include dementia, delirium, brain tumor, or substance use or abuse. Individuals with organic causes for the psychosis will require different interventions than persons experiencing an acute schizophrenic episode. An important intervention for acute psychosis regardless of the etiology, however, is ensuring the patient's safety.[16]

Psychosis is a bizarre state of profoundly altered thinking and behavior involving deterioration of thought processes, effective responses, and the individual's ability to maintain connection with reality. Without intervention, deterioration can continue to a point where the patient can no longer communicate with or relate to others.

Signs and Symptoms[17]
- Delusions
- Hallucinations (may involve any of the senses but most frequently auditory)

- Disorganized speech reflecting disordered thinking
- Grossly disordered behavior

Therapeutic Interventions

- Decrease external stimuli.
- Attempt to form a caregiver–patient alliance.
- Undress the patient and remove from the environment any items that may pose a danger.
- Administer antipsychotic medication as indicated.
- Apply restraints only as last resort to protect the patient and others.

Schizophrenia

Schizophrenia is a devastating brain disease that in the acute phase involves a psychotic episode. The word *schizophrenia* means "to split the mind," a phrase that aptly describes the break between reality and psychotic thought processes. Onset of schizophrenia is typically in the young adult years. The prevalence of schizophrenia is estimated to be about 1% of the total population, or close to 3 million people in the United States.[2] Schizophrenia should not be thought of as a single illness but as a disease process that includes different subtypes with varying symptoms. The five subtypes of schizophrenia are:

- Paranoid
- Disorganized
- Catatonic
- Undifferentiated
- Residual

Signs and Symptoms

The signs and symptoms of schizophrenia are commonly thought of in terms of positive and negative symptoms.[18] Table 48-4 lists these symptoms.

Therapeutic Interventions

- Monitor the environment and the patient's behavior for threats to self or others.
- Promote safety of the patient and others; undress the patient and remove from the environment any items that may pose a danger.
- Establish a therapeutic alliance.
- Use simple, concrete expressions and brief sentences.
- Avoid figures of speech that are subject to misinterpretation.
- Project a confident but nonthreatening manner to reassure the patient of the health care providers' ability to control themselves and the environment.
- Listen as the patient talks to gain clues regarding thought distortions.

TABLE 48-4	SIGNS AND SYMPTOMS OF SCHIZOPHRENIA	
POSITIVE SYMPTOMS	**NEGATIVE SYMPTOMS**
Hallucinations—false sensory perceptions that do not exist in reality	Apathy—feelings of indifference
Delusions—fixed false beliefs that have no basis in reality	Alogia—speaking little with minimal content
Thought disorganization—frequently changes topics, irrelevant responses (non sequitur), impaired communication	Flat affect—absence of facial expressions of emotions or mood
Bizarre dress or behavior—disheveled or idiosyncratic dress, regressive or agitated behavior	Anhedonia—feeling no joy or pleasure
Perseveration—persistent adherence to a single idea or topic	Avolition—lack of will, ambition, or drive to accomplish task
Ideas of reference—false belief that external events have special meaning	
Ambivalence—having seemingly contradictory beliefs about the same person or thing	

Adapted from O'Brien, P. G., Kennedy, W. Z., & Ballard, K. A. (2008). *Psychiatric mental health nursing: An introduction to theory and practice.* Boston, MA: Jones & Bartlett.

- If the patient is paranoid, avoid closed doors or blocked doorways to prevent the patient from feeling "cornered."
- Administer antipsychotic medications as indicated.
- Observe for medications' desired and adverse effects.
- Reduce environmental stimuli.
- Explain all actions.

Paranoia

Paranoia is a symptom of schizophrenia and several other psychiatric conditions. A paranoid person demonstrates a loss of reality through a delusional thought system, generally persecutory or grandiose and with a coherent theme. The persecutory delusions may generate feelings of suspicion, fear, anxiety, anger, hostility, or violence. Grandiose delusions may lead the patient to engage in high-risk behaviors.

Signs and Symptoms

- Pervasive mistrust and suspiciousness
- Guarded, hypervigilant
- Projective delusions (blames others for difficulties)
- Feelings of uniqueness or grandiosity
- Difficulty with relationships
- Illogical thought processes
- Obsessive thinking
- Restlessness, agitation
- Combative or assaultive behavior

Therapeutic Interventions

- Promote patient safety and the safety of others; undress the patient and remove from the environment any items that may pose a danger.
- Avoid psychological threats or challenges.
- Use simple, concrete expressions.
- Set limits on the patient's behavior.
- Explain actions in advance.
- Remain calm and authoritative.
- Sit or stand at the same level as the patient to avoid a power discrepancy.
- Minimize environmental stimuli.
- Encourage the patient to verbalize concerns (distorted or illogical thinking).
- Do not validate false beliefs but do not try to convince the patient that delusions are erroneous.

Bipolar Disorder—Mania

Bipolar disorder affects approximately 5.7 million American adults, or about 2.6% of the U.S. population aged 18 years or older in a given year.[2] Bipolar disorders are manifested by episodes of depression and episodes of mania or hypomania.

Bipolar I disorder is characterized by at least one episode of acute mania, usually accompanied by at least one severe depressive period. The manifestations of the illness tend to follow a characteristic pattern for each individual, with certain persons tending more toward mania and others tending toward depression.

Bipolar II disorder is characterized by at least one major depressive episode but never a full manic episode; rather, there is the experience of a hypomanic episode. Manic and hypomanic episodes are similar in symptoms but differ in severity and duration. While hypomanic episodes are noted to be a significant change from the patient's usual functioning, they are not severe enough to require hospitalization. In bipolar I mixed disorder, patients exhibit signs of mania and depression simultaneously.

For many, bipolar disorder is a lifelong chronic illness. More than half of all individuals with these disorders will have some functional disability that persists throughout their lives. According to NIMH's National Comorbidity Survey Replication (NCSR), bipolar disorder was the most seriously disabling mental disorder.[19] As a rule, the more episodes a person has, the more likely he or she is to experience future episodes.

> Studies have shown that up to 50% of people with bipolar disorder will have a suicide attempt at some point in their lives; 20% of people with the disorder will complete suicide.[20]

Traditionally, medications for management of bipolar disorder have been lithium (Lithobid) or antiepileptic drugs such as divalproex (Depakote), lamotrigine (Lamictal), or carbamazepine (Tegretol). Recently a number of the atypical antipsychotic medications have been approved for the treatment of bipolar disorder. When a patient with bipolar disorder is in the emergency setting, medication levels should be measured to determine whether the drug is in the therapeutic range.

Signs and Symptoms of Mania

- Elation or increased mental excitement that is unstable
- Irritability, irrational anger
- Pressured speech (rapid, difficult to interrupt)
- Racing thoughts, flight of ideas
- Increased motor activity (restless, increased energy)
- Decreased need for sleep
- Grandiosity
- Disinhibition
- Impulsivity
- Impaired insight and judgment
- High-risk behaviors
- Sexual acting out or preoccupation with sex
- Preoccupation with ideas—may evolve into delusional thinking

Therapeutic Interventions

- Institute safety mechanisms for the patient and staff.
- Guard the patient, caregivers, and others against physical harm.
- Decrease environmental stimuli.
- Assume an authoritative, nonthreatening manner.
- Provide a safe room to allow for pacing or other motor activity.
- Do not encourage patient to talk; ask succinct questions.
- Medicate as indicated.

- Mechanical restraints as a last resort to ensure safety of the patient and staff.

THE VIOLENT PATIENT

The management of acutely agitated, aggressive individuals in the ED is a major issue. Initial management should focus on attempts to calm the patient through empathetic yet firm verbal means and by establishing a collaborative relationship with the patient. It is important to appear calm, unthreatened, and in control and to be concerned about personal safety.[16]

Impulsivity and aggression are not limited to any specific psychiatric disorder or even to the presence of a disorder. There are numerous mechanisms that can lead to agitation and aggression, increasing the risk of violence, including the following[21]:

- Mania, PTSD, anxiety and panic, dementia, delirium, psychosis, personality disorders, and substance intoxication or withdrawal.
- Medical conditions—including metabolic imbalances, infections, trauma, brain tumors, and neurologic or endocrine dysfunction—can serve as causes of aggression and violence.
- Societal influences such as poverty, discrimination, exposure to violence, and physical abuse can all play contributory roles in the origin of violence.

> Threats of violence, from whatever cause, should always be taken seriously.

Patient Factors That Increase Risk for Violent Behavior

Psychological

- Anxiety or fear for personal safety
- Feelings of being overwhelmed or unable to cope
- History of physical or sexual abuse

Organic

- Alcohol or drug intoxication
- Medication side effects
- Inadequate symptom control (e.g., pain)
- Delirium

Psychiatric

- Delusional beliefs of persecution
- "Command" hallucinations to hurt others (auditory hallucinations)

- Depression and acute suicidal attempt
- Mania

Therapeutic Interventions[21]

- Threats of violence must always be taken seriously.
- Obtain unobstructed access to the patient. Clear away movable furniture and objects that can be used as potential weapons.
- Confiscate any real or potentially harmful objects.
- Ask bystanders to leave quietly.
- Do not hurry the patient. Most violent or psychotic patients can be "talked down" if given time.
- If possible, engage the patient in conversation; attempt to establish a therapeutic alliance.
- Speak in simple, direct sentences.
- Allow verbalization of complaints. That may be all that is needed.
- Speak calmly. Many people experiencing psychosis are frightened and feel out of control. Reassure the patient to help him or her regain self-control.
- Be clear, nonthreatening, and honest.
- Avoid confrontation.
- Stand sideways to the patient. This is less threatening and provides a smaller target.
- Keep hands visible so it will be obvious to the patient that you are not concealing a weapon.
- Caregivers should position themselves in the treatment room so they are between the patient and the door. The patient should never be in a position to block access to the room's exit.
- Do *not* try to cope with a violent patient alone. Obtain help as quickly as possible.

MENTAL HEALTH EMERGENCIES DUE TO A MEDICAL OR NEUROLOGIC DISORDER

When a patient comes to the ED with what appears to be a psychiatric disorder, it is important to identify any possible medical or organic causes. A thorough medical and neurologic evaluation, including laboratory and radiographic procedures, often is indicated. In addition, an MSE is indicated.

- Unless the patient has a known history of psychiatric illness consistent with the presenting symptoms, an organic cause should always be strongly considered.
- A key assessment finding in patients with organic disorders is that the behavioral symptoms are completely out of character for the individual or are fluctuating.
- According to Petit,[6] patients with an alteration in behavior, emotion, or cognition or with psychotic symptoms

should always be assessed for underlying medical conditions or medication interactions before ascribing the symptoms or findings to a primary psychiatric disorder. Assessing medical conditions should be standard practice for all patients presenting to the ED with behavioral or mental health symptoms.[4]

- Medical conditions capable of inducing behavioral or mental status changes or psychosis include the following:
  - Cerebral tumors
  - Head injuries
  - Epilepsy
  - Migraine headache
  - Acquired immune deficiency syndrome (AIDS)
  - Other infections (especially in the elderly)
  - Hypothyroidism or hyperthyroidism
  - Hypoglycemia or hyperglycemia
  - Hepatic or renal disease

Dementia and delirium are two neurologic conditions frequently encountered in the ED that can mimic psychosis. For additional information about dementia and delirium, refer to Chapter 53, Geriatric Considerations in Emergency Nursing.

DRUG-RELATED MENTAL HEALTH EMERGENCIES

The function of emergency personnel in an acute, drug-induced crisis involves rapid intervention, critical observation, and supportive therapeutic communication. Clinical findings are as diverse as the substances to which a patient may have been exposed. It should be noted that substance abuse is a comorbidity of many mental illnesses, especially bipolar disorder.[12,19]

Questions to Ask

The emergency nurse should ask the following questions of or about a patient who is experiencing a drug-induced psychiatric crisis:

- To what type of substance was the patient exposed?
- When and how much?
- What has happened since the drug was taken (symptoms, interventions)?
- Was there only one substance involved?
- Has the patient also consumed alcohol?
- What is the patient's history of drug use?
- Is this part of a chronic pattern of abuse or an isolated incident?
- How did the exposure occur (i.e., orally, parenterally, inhalation, or absorption)?
- Where was the substance obtained (i.e., over the counter, prescription, street drug)?

Signs and Symptoms

- Central nervous system: depression, tremors, confusion, decreased level of consciousness, agitation, seizures, coma
- Respiratory system: tachypnea, hyperpnea, hyperventilation, hypoventilation, apnea
- Autonomic nervous system: increased or decreased temperature, pulse, blood pressure
- Pupil size: increased or decreased
- Behavioral and psychiatric: mood distortion, altered thought patterns, hallucinations, delusions, agitation, aggression
- Gastrointestinal: anorexia, nausea, vomiting, diarrhea, bleeding, hepatic failure
- For additional information regarding specific drug- and toxin-related emergencies, see Chapter 30, Toxicologic Emergencies.

ADVERSE REACTIONS TO PSYCHIATRIC DRUGS

Dystonic Reactions

Occasionally the drug of choice for treatment of a mental heath condition produces more stress than relief for the patient. An example of this is the severe extrapyramidal symptoms (EPS) of some major psychotropic medications. These symptoms are also referred to as dystonic symptoms. Most antipsychotic medications can produce these symptoms but they are more commonly experienced with first-generation antipsychotics, such as haloperidol (Haldol), than with the newer class of antipsychotic medications referred to as atypical antipsychotics, such as olanzapine (Zyprexa) or quetiapine (Seroquel).

Signs and Symptoms[22]

- Dystonia (disordered muscle tone), including:
  - Oculogyric crisis (deviation of the eyes in all directions)
  - Blepharospasm (spasm of the eyelid muscles)
  - Buccolingual crisis (spasm of the face, jaw, and pharynx muscles)
  - Opisthotonos (spasm of the paravertebral muscles, forcing the trunk and neck into hyperextension)
  - Torticollis (spasm of the neck muscles with twisting of the neck to one side)
  - Tortipelvic crisis (forced spasm of the trunk and pelvic muscles causing bizarre body postures)
  - Akathisia (the urge to move about constantly, inability to sit still)
- It should be noted that mental status and vital signs are usually unaffected.

- When a patient arrives at the ED with any of these signs and symptoms, it is important to ask about a medication history.
  - Extrapyramidal side effects are commonly mistaken for hypocalcemia, tetany, or seizures.
  - Dystonic reactions are more likely to occur during the initial phase of psychotropic drug therapy (within 1 hour to 5 days).
  - The appearance of EPS can be anxiety provoking and may be enough to cause patients to refuse all future prescribed medications. Emergency personnel can help these individuals understand that antipsychotic drug therapy requires patience and persistence to achieve a satisfactory response.

> Akathisia is often misdiagnosed as psychotic agitation; treating the patient with a neuroleptic medication such as haloperidol only makes the condition worse.

Therapeutic Interventions

- Inform the patient that the symptoms are reversible and will resolve with medication (or spontaneously).
- Administer diphenhydramine (Benadryl) or an antiparkinson drug such as benztropine mesylate (Cogentin) or trihexyphenidyl (Artane).
- Propranolol (Inderal) is used to treat akathisia.
- Provide a quiet room with decreased stimuli while the patient waits for antagonist drug to take effect.
- Monitor the patient until symptoms have subsided.

Neuroleptic Malignant Syndrome

Neuroleptic malignant syndrome (NMS) is a rapidly developing, life-threatening syndrome of profound muscle stiffness, hyperthermia, and tremor produced by the use of an antipsychotic agent. This condition requires immediate medical management. NMS onset can occur within days or months of initiating neuroleptic therapy. Within a space of a few hours, a person can become completely immobile, unable to swallow, to speak, or to move.[19]

Signs and Symptoms[23]

- Hyperthermia
- Mental status changes (often the first symptom)
- Severe muscle rigidity (lead pipe rigidity)
- Autonomic instability (tachycardia, respiratory distress, hypoxia, labile blood pressure)
- Diaphoresis

- Leukocytosis
- Elevated creatinine kinase (CK) levels (may indicate rhabdomyolysis)
- Renal failure

Therapeutic Interventions

- Stop administering the antipsychotic medication.
- Initiate life support measures as indicated—stabilize blood pressure, normalize body temperature, correct hypoxia.
- Reduce muscular rigidity by administering bromocriptine (Parlodel) or dantrolene (Dantrium).
- Arrange for inpatient admission.

Serotonin Syndrome

Serotonin syndrome is another potentially fatal drug reaction that resembles NMS in presentation but does not involve a neuroleptic (antipsychotic) agent. It occurs when high levels of serotonin accumulate. It can be the result of polypharmacy or an issue with drug metabolism. One known contributor is the herbal supplement St. John's wort; when combined with a prescribed selective serotonin reuptake inhibitor (SSRI) antidepressant, this amounts to "double dosing." St. John's wort also has the potential to induce mania. Patients should be asked about their use of herbal supplements. Since many of the symptoms of serotonin syndrome are similar to NMS, it is important to determine the patient's medication regimen to assist with determining the correct diagnosis.[19]

Signs and Symptoms

- Agitation or restlessness
- Confusion
- Tachycardia
- Diaphoresis
- Diarrhea
- Headache
- Shivering
- Piloerection (goose bumps)
- Hyperthermia
- Seizures
- Cardiac dysrhythmias
- Loss of consciousness

Therapeutic Interventions

- Discontinue all SSRIs and other medications and contact the prescriber.
- Initiate life support measures as indicated.
- Hydration to prevent rhabdomyolysis.
- If recent ingestion or overdose, consider gastrointestinal decontamination with activated charcoal.

Sudden Cardiac Death

The use of psychiatric medications has been linked to sudden cardiac death.[24] Most frequently implicated are antipsychotic medications, especially atypical or second-generation antipsychotics. Sudden cardiac death associated with the use of antipsychotic medications is a concern especially in older people with dementia and dementia-related psychosis. Atypical antipsychotics carry a black box warning label; however, typical (first-generation) antipsychotics also carry risk of sudden cardiac death. In older adults the use of antipsychotic medications should be restricted to treatment of psychosis or mania.

It is known that a prolonged QTc interval is a risk factor for sudden cardiac death, and antipsychotic medications lengthen the QT interval. The cardiac danger is dose dependent and increases in the presence of previous cardiac conditions. Prior to the initiation of antipsychotic medications, the patient should be thoroughly evaluated for potential risk factors.

Pretreatment evaluation should include the following:
- Medical history, especially for heart disease (including conduction delays) or metabolic abnormalities
- Current medications—increased caution with medications that extend the length of the cardiac cycle (procainamide, amiodarone, amitriptyline)
- Baseline electrocardiogram (ECG) and periodic ECGs if antipsychotic therapy is continuing
- Physical examination with emphasis on cardiac and neurologic evaluation
- Vital signs
- Fasting blood glucose
- Lipid panel
- Basic metabolic panel
- Renal and liver function

PEDIATRIC MENTAL HEALTH EMERGENCIES

In the United States about one in five children has a mental disorder.[25] Of these, approximately 5% to 9% of children aged 9 to 17 years are affected by a serious mental disturbance that causes severe functional impairment.[25] The most common mental disorders among children are anxiety disorders, mood disorders, and disruptive disorders.[25] Despite the prevalence of mental disorders, approximately 79% of children aged 6 to 17 years with mental disorders do not receive mental health care.[25]

Suicidal ideation, feeling out of control, aggression, and drug-related antisocial behavior are also common presenting problems for children with behavioral emergencies. The young psychiatric patient presents additional challenges for emergency nurses because of the following:
- The impulsiveness associated with the patient's age.
- Involvement of other systems (e.g., family, school, courts, social services).
- The limited availability of inpatient care beds for children and adolescents.

Therapeutic Interventions

- The emergency nurse must identify the child's legal guardian before initiating treatment or determining disposition.
- Whether the child has been brought to the ED because of aggressive behavior or not, always ask about a history of violence.
- The emergency nurse must attempt to form a therapeutic alliance with the child but the child must know that aggressive behavior will not be tolerated; setting limits is essential.
- If the child is unable to cooperate, steps must be taken to ensure safety for the child and others. Medication may be appropriate.
- The child's usual medication regimen should be followed if possible.
- Seclusion or restraint should be an intervention of last resort, as it ultimately may cause additional psychological trauma.
- It is important to provide support for the parents or caregivers, who also may become very emotional.

MENTAL HEALTH PATIENT DISPOSITION

Perhaps the single most important question in the management of patients with mental health emergencies is: "Does this patient require hospitalization?" An important factor to consider is the presence or absence of a solid support system. Does the patient have competent family members or friends who are willing to observe and supervise the individual? Patients who cannot be discharged safely must be placed on a psychiatric hold, usually by a psychiatrist. Mental health holds typically are limited to 72 hours in most states. Involuntary hold criteria differ somewhat from state to state but most states require mandatory hospitalization if the patient meets the following criteria:
- A serious, imminent risk to health and safety exists because the patient is completely unable to provide self-care.
- The patient is at risk for suicide.
- The patient is a physical threat to others.

Even when psychiatric patients have been "admitted" they frequently remain in the ED as boarders for many hours or for days. This presents many challenges for both patients and staff. In 2008 the American College of Emergency Physicians (ACEP) issued a press release based on the results of a survey that found that "[p]eople with psychiatric illnesses, including children, who are admitted to the hospital from the emergency department can wait 24 hours or longer for an inpatient bed principally because of a lack of psychiatric beds."[3,4]

Some strategies that EDs have implemented to help meet the needs of both the patients and the department include the following[23,26]:

- Having a dedicated "psychiatric hold" area—may be locked or simply a geographic area of the department.
- Including a psychiatric nurse in ED staffing.
- Developing protocols and care plans for the care of psychiatric boarders so that their physical needs (e.g., hygiene, nutrition, medication, communication, safety) as well as their psychiatric needs are met.
- Employing case managers to become involved in the care of psychiatric patients seen the ED.
- Maintaining a supply of materials, such as art supplies, board games and playing cards, books, magazines, and writing paper, that psychiatric patients can use while in the ED.
- Staff education in de-escalation techniques.
- Staff education about the care of psychiatric patients to increase the level of compassion and respect for these patients.[27]

The Emergency Nurses Association position statement related to the care of psychiatric patients states that patients with psychiatric and addictive disorders "deserve the same timely and compassionate care that all patients receive … [they] should be treated with respect, dignity, care and compassion in a non-judgmental manner."[28]

REFERENCES

1. Doheny, K. (2010, November 18). Mental illness affects 1 in 5 Americans. *WebMD Health News*. Retrieved from http://www.webmd.com/mental-health/news/20101118/mental-illness-affects-1-in-5-americans

2. National Institute of Mental Health. (2008, June). The numbers count: Mental disorders in America. Retrieved from https://www.apps.nimh.nih.gov/health/publications/the-numbers-count-mental-disorders-in-america.shtml

3. American College of Emergency Physicians. (2010, June 28). *Psychiatric patients, including children, routinely boarded in emergency departments*. Retrieved from http://www.acep.org/content.aspx?id=39170

4. American College of Emergency Physicians. (2008). *ACEP psychiatric and substance abuse survey 2008*. Retrieved from http://www.acep.org/uploadedFiles/ACEP/Advocacy/federal_issues/PsychiatricBoardingSummary.pdf

5. Gilboy, N., Tanabe, P., Travers, D. A., Rosenau, A. M., & Eitel, D. R. (2005). *Emergency severity index, version 4: Implementation handbook*. Rockville, MD: Agency for Healthcare Research and Quality.

6. Petit, J. R. (2004). *Handbook of emergency psychiatry*. Philadelphia, PA: Lippincott Williams & Wilkins.

7. Davison, G. C., Neale, J. M., & Kring, A. M. (2004). Anxiety disorders. In *Abnormal psychology, with cases* (9th ed., pp. 133–171). Hoboken, NJ: John Wiley & Sons.

8. National Institute of Mental Health. (n.d.). *Obsessive-compulsive disorder*. Retrieved from http://www.nimh.nih.gov/health/topics/obsessive-compulsive-disorder-ocd/index.shtml

9. National Institute of Mental Health. (n.d.). *Post-traumatic stress disorder*. Retrieved from http://www.nimh.nih.gov/health/topics/post-traumatic-stress-disorder-ptsd/index.shtml

10. Zieve, D., & Merrill, D. B. (2011, March 15). *Major depression*. Retrieved from http://www.nlm.nih.gov/medlineplus/ency/article/000945.htm

11. McIntosh, J. L. (2009). *U.S.A. suicide 2006: Official final data*. Washington, D.C.: American Association of Suicidology.

12. Substance Abuse and Mental Health Services Administration. (2009, September 17). *Suicidal thoughts and behaviors among adults*. Retrieved from http://www.oas.samhsa.gov/2k9/165/Suicide.htm

13. Perhats, C., & Valdez, A. M. (2008). Suicide prevention in the emergency department. *Journal of Emergency Nursing, 34*, 251–253.

14. Soreff, S. (2011, January 11). *Suicide introduction and definitions*. Retrieved from http://emedicine.medscape.com/article/288598-overview

15. Ramadan, M. (2007). Managing psychiatric emergencies. *The Internet Journal of Emergency Medicine, 4*(1). Retrieved from http://www.ispub.com/ostia/index.php?xmlFilePath=journals/ijem/vol4n1/psycho.xml

16. Hendrick, J. (2004, April 1). A REMINDER for assessing psychosis. *Current Psychiatry, 3*(4). Retrieved from http://www.currentpsychiatry.com

17. O'Brien, P. G., Kennedy, W. Z., & Ballard, K. A. (2008). *Psychiatric mental health nursing: An introduction to theory and practice*. Boston, MA: Jones & Bartlett.

18. National Institute of Mental Health. (n.d.). *Questions and answers about the national comorbidity survey replication (NCSR) study*. Retrieved from http://www.nimh.nih.gov/health/topics/statistics/ncsr-study/questions-and-answers-about-the-national-comorbidity-survey-replication-ncsr-study.shtml

19. Kimmel, R. (2010, February). Serotonin syndrome or NMS? Clues to diagnosis. *Current Psychiatry, 9*(2). Retrieved from http://www.currentpsychiatry.com

20. Granello, D. H., & Granello, P. F. (2007). Suicide: An essential guide for helping professionals and educators. Boston, MA: Pearson, Allyn & Bacon.

21. Citrome, L. L. (2011, June 28). *Aggression*. Retrieved from http://emedicine.medscape.com/article/288689-overview

22. Nochimson, G. (2010, December 7). *Toxicity, medication-induced dystonic reactions*. Retrieved from http://emedicine.medscape.com/article/814632-overview

23. Walker-Cillo, G., Jones, C., & McCoy, E. (2008). Psychiatric nurse: A role in overcrowding. *Journal of Emergency Nursing, 34*, 455–457.

24. Ray, W. A., Chung, C. P., Murray, K. T., Hall, K., & Stein, C. M. (2009). Atypical antipsychotic drugs and the risk of sudden cardiac death. *New England Journal of Medicine, 360*, 225–235.

25. Bazelon Center for Mental Health Law. (n.d.). *Facts on children's mental health.* Retrieved http://www.bazelon.org/LinkClick.aspx?fileticket=Nc7DS9D8EQE%3D&tabid=378

26. Bender, D., Pande, N., & Ludwig, M. (2008, October 29). *A literature review: psychiatric boarding.* Retrieved from http://aspe.hhs.gov/daltcp/reports/2008/PsyBdLR.pdf

27. Manton, A. (2010). Psychiatric patients in the emergency department: The dilemma of extended lengths of stay. *ENA Connection, 34*(3), 22.

28. Emergency Nurses Association. (2010, July). *Medical evaluation of psychiatric patients* [position statement]. Retrieved from http://www.ena.org/SiteCollectionDocuments/Position%20Statements/MEDICAL%20EVALUATION%20OF%20PSYCHIATRIC%20PATIENTS.pdf

Abuse and Neglect

Shelley Cohen

An attentive emergency nurse undresses the one year old for examination of symptoms related to a runny nose and cough. During her assessment, she identifies round marks about the size of a dime that look like burns. Her assessment and documentation may have saved the life of this child who was not only being burned with cigarettes, but also was not consistently fed. The child is now 11 years old, thriving in his adoptive home, because of the assessment and intervention of an emergency nurse. This child was just one of the estimated 872,000 children in the United States that are identified as victims of abuse and neglect.[1]

Although child maltreatment has always existed, Western culture has recognized it as a problem only since the 1962 landmark article "The Battered Child Syndrome."[2] What surprises many emergency health care workers is that most of these patients are victims of neglect rather than abuse. An estimated 3.5 million American children received an investigation or assessment by Child Protective Services in 2007.[3] Of these, 22.5% were validated as maltreatment, 59% were categorized as neglect, 10.8% as physical abuse, 7.6% as sexual abuse, and 4.2% as emotional abuse.[3] Data from 2007 also revealed that approximately 1760 children died because of abuse or neglect.[3] More than 75% of the children who were killed were younger than 4 years of age.[4]

Child Maltreatment Facts[3]

Of an estimated 872,000 child victims:
- 75.4% were "first-time" victims
- 31.9% of victims were less than 4 years of age
- 59% were neglected
- 10.8% were physically abused
- 7.6% were sexually abused
- 4.2% were psychologically maltreated

2007 Child Maltreatment and Neglect Fatality Statistics[5]
- 34.1% of fatalities were related to neglect
- 35.2% of fatalities were related to multiple maltreatment types
- 26.4% of fatalities were related to physical abuse
- 42.2% of fatalities occurred in children younger than 1 year of age

---

CHILD MALTREATMENT

Child maltreatment is defined as any harm that occurs to a child as a result of physical, emotional, or sexual abuse or neglect. Maltreatment can take many forms, and minors are regularly the victims of more than one type of abuse.

Types of Maltreatment

Neglect

Neglect involves failure (intentional or unintentional) to provide basic needs such as food, shelter, clothing, schooling, and medical care. Figure 49-1 depicts failure to thrive as a consequence of neglect. Neglect commonly is subcategorized as follows:

- Medical: This type of neglect consists of failure to provide medical care, including immunizations, necessary surgical procedures, and emergency interventions. Cases of alleged medical neglect because of a family's philosophical or religious beliefs may require resolution in court.
- Physical: This type of neglect exists when caregivers either fail to protect the child from harm or do not provide for basic needs.
- Emotional: The caregiver fails to maintain a nurturing environment that will meet the emotional and

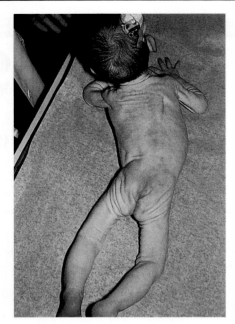

Fig. 49-1   Failure to thrive as a result of neglect. (From Newberry, L. [2010]. *Sheehy's emergency nursing: Principles and practice* [6th ed.]. St. Louis, MO: Mosby.)

TABLE 49-1	EMOTIONAL ABUSE
ABUSIVE ACTION	**CHILD'S RESPONSE**
Verbal abuse	Withdrawal
Verbal threats	Eating disorders
Constant criticism	Head banging
Unreasonable and outrageous expectations	Rocking
	Learning difficulties
Use of child to manipulate other adults	Enuresis
	Suicidal behavior
Extreme behaviors (anger, passivity)	Self-destructive or risk-taking behaviors
Lack of affection toward child	
Use of the child as a bargaining tool between parents	

developmental needs of the minor. This type of neglect is difficult to recognize and define.

- Educational: Poor school attendance or failure to provide necessary specialized education constitutes educational neglect.
- Mental health: Caregivers may fail to obtain necessary care for a child with emotional or behavioral problems.

Physical Abuse

Physical abuse, or intentional trauma, is defined as injury intentionally inflicted on a child. This includes trauma that results from discipline, punishment, torture, maiming, or the use of unreasonable force.

Sexual Abuse

According to the American Academy of Pediatrics, sexual abuse "occurs when a child is engaged in sexual activities that he or she cannot comprehend, for which he or she is developmentally unprepared and cannot give consent, and/or that violate the law or social taboos of society."[6] Abusive behaviors may be violent, coercive, or even nontouching (e.g., pornographic photography).

Emotional Abuse

Unlike emotional neglect, in which the child's needs are simply not met, emotional abuse is deliberate. In reality, it may be difficult to draw a distinction between the two. Table 49-1 lists emotionally abusive strategies used by abusers and common responses to abuse. Table 49-2 describes factors that contribute to child maltreatment.

Duty to Report

The duty of health care providers to report actual or suspected child maltreatment exists in all 50 states. Local law enforcement or child welfare agencies must be notified of any suspicion of abuse or neglect. Persons who disclose suspected maltreatment in good faith are immune from prosecution. Refer to Chapter 1, Legal Issues for Emergency Nurses, for a more detailed discussion of the responsibilities and ramifications associated with duty to report. Be sure to document to whom this information was transmitted and the date and time the information was relayed. Importantly, the reporter is under no obligation to prove the allegation but only to describe it. Abuse laws vary from state to state; become familiar with regulations in your practice area. Reporting procedures also vary by institution. Know how to access facility-specific protocols.

In general, the following information should be included in a maltreatment report:
- The child's name (and any other names the child may be using)
- The child's address and telephone number
- The child's date of birth
- Where the child is now living (if this is different from the stated address)
- The names of the child's parents or other caregivers
- The reasons for your suspicions
- The alleged cause of injury or the nature of the neglect

TABLE 49-2 FACTORS THAT CONTRIBUTE TO CHILD MALTREATMENT

SOCIOLOGICAL	CAREGIVER	SITUATIONAL	CHILD
Dangerous living environment	Unemployment	Alcohol or drug abuse by caregiver	Child of multiple birth
Inadequate housing	Perception of child as "different"	Inadequate support system	Chronically ill
Poverty	Attention-seeking behavior	Intimate partner abuse in the home	Developmental delays
Social isolation	Belief in corporal punishment	Many small children in the home	Feeding difficulties
	Female (62% of the time)[a]	Parental discord	Mental deficits
	History of abuse as a child		Physically disabled
	Inability to be nurturing		Prenatal drug addiction
	Lack of self-control		Preterm delivery
	Low self-esteem		Psychosocial disabilities
	Physical or psychological illness		
	Single parent		
	Unmet emotional needs		
	Unrealistic expectations of child		

[a]The National Center for Victims of Crime. (n.d.). *Child maltreatment.* Retrieved from http://www.ncvc.org/ncvc/main.aspx?dbName=DocumentViewer& DocumentID=38709

- The circumstances surrounding the incident
- Where the alleged incident occurred
- A description of the child, including any injuries or other signs of maltreatment
- The extent of abuse or neglect
- The name or any description of the suspect
- The suspect's address and telephone number
- The name, work address, and work telephone number of the person making the report

Signs and Symptoms of Child Maltreatment

The primary goals of therapeutic intervention in the emergency department are to identify and address the immediate needs and safety of the child, prevent further harm, facilitate investigation of potential abuse, and assist the child and family to deal with the crisis. A thorough assessment of behavioral and physical signs and symptoms and a well thought-out interview are important initial steps in providing protection for the child.

Behavioral Signs

Behavioral signs of child maltreatment include the following:
- The caregiver delays seeking treatment for illness or injury in the child
- The caretaker is also a child
- Evidence of caregiver ignorance or carelessness exists
- Descriptions of events are confusing, conflicting, ever-changing, or improbable
- The caregiver focuses on the child's behavior instead of the child's injury or presenting illness

- The caregiver denies knowledge of how the injury occurred
- A change in caregivers has occurred recently
- The caregiver emphasizes unimportant details or minor problems not directly related to the present situation
- The caregiver focuses on self-absorbed concerns rather than on the needs of the child
- The caregiver bypassed a closer emergency department to seek treatment
- Tension or outright hostility exists between caregivers
- Caregivers exhibit tension, hostility, or aggressiveness toward emergency department staff members
- The caregiver is uncooperative and demanding
- The child has a history of multiple emergency department visits
- Caregivers describe the child as clumsy or accident prone
- The child exhibits low self-esteem
- The child displays attention-seeking behavior
- The caregiver lacks any sense of guilt, remorse, or culpability for the incident (rather than the caregiver stating, "If only I had …")
- The child appears fearful of adults or is unusually unafraid
- The child is fearful of the caregiver
- The caregiver displays anger toward the child regarding the injury or illness
- Answers to questions are vague
- The caregiver refuses to leave a verbal child alone with health care providers

- The child's age (chronological or developmental) does not correlate with the reported history of injury

Physical Manifestations

The list of physical manifestations suggestive of abuse or neglect is extensive. Table 49-3 describes many possible assessment findings. Figures 49-2 to 49-4 provide examples of retinal hemorrhage, cigarette burns, and pattern bruises related to abuse.

The Interview

When dealing with the patient with suspected child maltreatment, the manner in which the initial emergency department interview is handled will set the tone for the rest of the evaluation process. The emergency nurse cannot obtain the entire story in the triage area. Avoid excessive questioning at this time. Perpetrators who detect suspicion may flee with the child or become violent. The triage nurse should fully document whatever the caregiver states to facilitate comparison of stories once a more thorough assessment and history have been obtained.

Move suspected maltreatment patients to a treatment room as quickly as possible. The emergency nurse will find it much easier to calm and contain the victim and potential perpetrator in a treatment room. With children who have the capacity to understand and verbalize their feelings, attempt to ask safety questions in the absence of those accompanying the child. Options to accomplish this include walking the child to the bathroom for a specimen, referring the adult to the cafeteria, or distracting the adult with a hallway discussion.

Methods of interviewing the child vary depending on the patient's developmental age. If possible, interview multiple caregivers separately and away from the child to check the consistency of the stories.

The following are tips for patient and family interviews in a potential child maltreatment situation.

- Listen closely and watch interactions between child and caregivers
- Evaluate the child's state of cleanliness, nutrition, and dress
- Pay particular attention to patients with a history of multiple emergency department visits
- Be nonjudgmental and nonaccusatory; cooperation is more likely if discussions are held in a nonthreatening manner
- Speak in easy-to-understand language
- Ask open-ended questions at first
- Attempt to determine an event timeline
- Establish whether similar situations have occurred in the past
- Initially avoid questions that deal with the alleged assault

- Inquire about other children in the family
- Carefully document objective assessment findings and any statements made by the patient or caregivers.

The Examination

Undressing the child completely for the examination is important to identify potential undisclosed injuries. Be sure to provide privacy and protect the child's modesty. Explain each part of the examination as it is being done. Physical assessment, diagnostic testing, and therapeutic interventions depend on the chief complaint, the child's general condition, and the type of abuse suspected. Consider each of the following components, as appropriate:

- Primary and secondary assessments
- Be aware of cultural remedies and health care practices that can mimic abuse; see Table 49-4 for an explanation of some of these practices
- Radiographic procedures for patients with suspicious injuries (especially preverbal or nonverbal children)
- Laboratory procedures: complete blood count, glucose, serum chemistries, toxicology screens, urinalysis, and pregnancy testing
- Visual acuity, eye examination
- Neurologic examination
- Growth and development level (compared with normative charts)

Conditions That Mimic Child Maltreatment
Blood dyscrasias and coagulation disorders
Cultural and ethnic practices that produce physical marks
Complementary and alternative therapies that delay appropriate care or cause actual harm
Sudden infant death syndrome
Failure to thrive
Congenital dermal melanocytosis (Mongolian spots)
Reye's syndrome

If any potential evidence is collected during the examination, strictly follow the institutional guidelines for evidence preservation and custody. Do not allow the chain of custody to be broken.

Documentation

Documentation is an essential part of the medical-legal process in any case of suspected child maltreatment. Documentation by health care professionals is viewed as objective third-party evidence in legal proceedings. As such, documentation needs to be complete, accurate, and legible and should also follow institutional guidelines.

Tips for clinicians to facilitate successful prosecution include the following:

TABLE 49-3   **POSSIBLE MANIFESTATIONS OF PHYSICAL ABUSE AND NEGLECT**

AREA OR INJURY	MANIFESTATIONS
Fractures	Ribs, scapulae, distal clavicle
	Fingers and femur in nonmobile children
	Fractures in various stages of healing
	Any fracture in a child <3 years of age
Head	Traumatic alopecia
	Uneven hair growth (various lengths in different spots)
	Subgaleal hematomas
	Head injuries
	Subdural hematomas
	Skull fractures
	Unexplained unconsciousness
	Unexplained cardiopulmonary arrest
Ear, eye, nose	Displaced nasal cartilages
	Bleeding from nasal septum
	Retinal hemorrhages
	Detached retina
	Hyphema
	Periorbital ecchymosis
	Ruptured tympanic membrane
	Postauricular hematoma (Battle sign)
Throat	Fractured mandible
	Lacerated frenulum
	Loose or missing teeth not appropriate for age
	Petechiae around the head or neck (from choking)
Burns	Burns on lips and tongue
	Burns on rectum or perineum
	Cigarette burns
	Chemical burns
	Electrical burns
	Lines of demarcation, limited injury to protected area, and uniform burn depth
	Burns in the shape of an object (iron, heating grate, stove coils)
	Splash burns of nonuniform depth involving various body parts
Bruising	In various stages of healing
Ecchymosis	In the shape of identifiable objects (hand print, extension cord, belt buckle)
Lacerations	Human bite marks
Genitalia and perineal	Genital or perineal trauma
	Discharge: vaginal or rectal (possible sexually transmitted infection)
	Bleeding
	Pain
	Urinary tract infection symptoms
Behavioral	Post-traumatic stress disorder
	Attention deficit hyperactivity disorder
	Secondary enuresis or fecal soiling in toilet-trained child (encopresis)
	Nightmares
	Inappropriate sexual behavior
Poisoning	Ingestion of alcohol or other drugs
	"Morning-after" poisoning (ingestion of drinks left over from a party the night before)
	Intentional poisoning by a parent, caregiver, or other adult

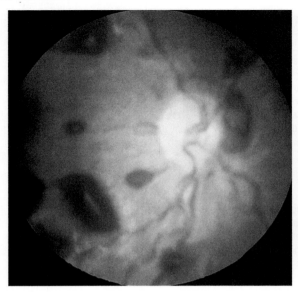

Fig. 49-2 Retinal hemorrhages caused by abusive head trauma. (From Zitelli, G. J., & Davis, H. W. [1997]. *Atlas of pediatric physical diagnosis* [3rd ed.]. St. Louis, MO: Mosby. Courtesy of Stephen Ludwig, Children's Hospital of Philadelphia.)

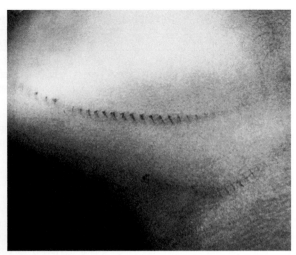

Fig. 49-4 Child was struck with a chain, leaving a clear imprint of the links. (From Zitelli, G. J., & Davis, H. W. [1997]. *Atlas of pediatric physical diagnosis* [3rd ed.]. St. Louis, MO: Mosby.)

- If computer documentation is not used, write legibly.
- Place quotation marks around statements made by the victim or caregiver. Identify who is being quoted with words such as "Father states, 'I walked into the room…'"
- Ensure that law enforcement personnel obtain photographs pertinent to the child's presentation. The skill and knowledge of victim photography is essential to ensure that the photos are acceptable to the court. Some emergency departments are fortunate to have a Sexual Assault Nurse Examiner (SANE) who has been trained in appropriate photography collection and documentation. Follow institutional policy and procedures for photographic evidence collection.
- Draw injuries on body maps to indicate their locations, size, and potential age.
- Use medical terms when charting. Avoid legal terms such as *alleged perpetrator* or *assailant.*
- Objectively describe emotional and mental states, behaviors, and physical problems.
- Record dates and times accurately.
- Provide detailed descriptions of injuries.
- Document only facts.

Prevention of Child Maltreatment

It is vital that health care professionals recognize and report instances of abuse and neglect to prevent future morbidity and mortality. Maltreatment that results in the death of a child is almost always preceded by prior instances of abuse.

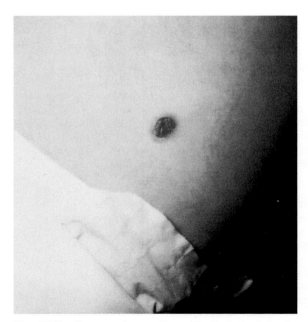

Fig. 49-3 Cigarette burns. (From Zitelli, G. J., & Davis, H. W. [1997]. *Atlas of pediatric physical diagnosis* [3rd ed.]. St. Louis, MO: Mosby.)

TABLE 49-4 CULTURAL PRACTICES AND ALTERNATIVE THERAPIES THAT MAY PRODUCE PHYSICAL MARKS

	PROCEDURE	PURPOSE	PHYSICAL MARK
Cupping	Heated glass cups applied to skin (generally the back) to create a localized vacuum	Increase blood flow to draw toxins out of the body	Circular discolorations similar to a bruise
Coining	Skin is lubricated and a coin is firmly rubbed along the skin	A dermabrasive therapy to relieve nausea, vomiting, chills, fever, aches, and pains	Linear pattern of blood under the skin
Moxibustion	Bundle of burning herb (mugwort) used to heat the skin at acupuncture points	Radiant heat restores balance and flow of vital energy	Reddened, burned, blistered, or scarred area of skin

Early identification of at-risk children and appropriate referral is essential. Many educational programs and informational materials are available that address parenting techniques, anger management, and child abuse prevention. Emergency departments can post information where it will be visible and easily obtainable in waiting rooms and treatment areas.

MUNCHAUSEN SYNDROME BY PROXY

Munchausen syndrome by proxy (MSP) is a psychiatric disorder occasionally seen in caregivers. This form of child maltreatment is often missed (or even unintentionally abetted) by health care providers. In MSP, an adult caregiver (frequently the mother) fabricates a child's illness or actually creates symptoms through a variety of mechanisms. Health care personnel, particularly nurses, also have been perpetrators of MSP. These individuals can operate in any setting in which the victim is vulnerable. After first causing or faking an illness, the clinician or perpetrator can then glory in the attention received from "saving" the child or the "kindness" bestowed on grieving parents.[7]

The traditional and most accepted explanation for MSP is the secondary gain (attention) received by the perpetrator. Attention is garnered from medical professionals, family members, and friends who laud the caregiver's care, devotion, and selflessness. MSP is a serious disorder that ends in the death of up to 10% of child victims.[8] Several rationales for MSP have been posited in the medical literature. The perpetrator may have the following characteristics:

- Believes that an ill child will bring about an improved relationship with the spouse (many of these children have distant, uninvolved fathers)
- Had an emotionally deprived childhood and was physically abused herself or himself

- Uses the child's illness as a means of escaping the responsibilities and realities of life
- Gains gratification and a sense of importance in the presence of medical professionals[9]
- Insists on being included in health care decision making, further reinforcing attention and support

The caregiver may also display any of the following signs and symptoms:

- Is extremely attentive and refuses to leave the child alone; he or she may initially appear to be the "perfect" caregiver
- Demands an extensive workup and will not accept a minor diagnosis
- Is unusually calm and does not appear worried about the child's condition
- Is knowledgeable about health care, uses medical terminology, and frequently has a health care background
- Appears to enjoy the hospital environment, engaging in gossip with staff members and involving herself or himself in the details of other patients' problems; is inordinately concerned about the personal and professional lives of the staff members
- Spends more time with the staff than with the child; works to form close relationships with the staff but appears to have few other friends or support persons
- Is either highly supportive of medical personnel or angry and devaluing, demanding more treatments and procedures
- Is emotionally distant from the spouse
- Comes from a dysfunctional family setting
- May report a history of dramatic, negative events in his or her life
- Brings the child to the emergency department frequently
- Is not concerned about subjecting the child to painful diagnostic tests or treatments

- Requires much adulation and may even seek public acknowledgement
- Treats the child as if the child has a disability when no true disability is present
- Is overly attached to the child

The child, on the other hand, may exhibit some of the following signs:

- One or more medical problem unresponsive to therapy
- A medical course that is puzzling and unexplainable
- Symptoms that manifest only in the presence of the caregiver; seizures witnessed only by the caregiver and unresponsive to anticonvulsants
- Multiple "allergies"
- A general appearance that does not correspond with laboratory results
- A sibling with similar illness or unexplained death[9]

Physical findings vary widely and tend to be incongruent, inappropriate, and inconsistent with known pathophysiology. Symptomatology associated with MSP is often bizarre and multisystem; the imagination of the perpetrator is the only limiting factor. Table 49-5 lists several common symptoms with possible causes.

Forensic Munchausen syndrome by proxy[10] is a situation in which, as a part of a divorce proceeding and custody battle, one parent falsely claims that the child has been sexually abused by the other. The child is then forced to undergo physical examination and intensive interviewing as a result of these accusations.

Making the diagnosis of MSP is always a challenge. This disorder can often be overlooked, but some argue that the label is applied too quickly whenever a caregiver is anxious or overly concerned, provides an inaccurate history, has unusual coping mechanisms, or knows more about a disease than the health care professionals. Needless to say, detection of this unusual condition and obtaining treatment for the caregiver are necessary to prevent further abuse, and even death, of the child victim.

ELDER AND DEPENDENT ADULT ABUSE

Abuse of elderly and dependent adults is considered together because the issues involved for each group are similar. Adults who are elderly or otherwise dependent have limited ability to report maltreatment or have compelling reasons not to report it. Sadly, 90% of abusers are family members; two thirds are the victim's adult child or spouse.[11] Frequently, even if the dependent individual can describe the situation and identify the abuser, there is no arrest, prosecution, or conviction because the disabled victim is unable to testify effectively on his or her own behalf.

TABLE 49-5	PHYSICAL FINDINGS IN PATIENTS WITH MUNCHAUSEN SYNDROME BY PROXY
SYMPTOMS	**POSSIBLE CAUSES**
Bleeding	Warfarin (Coumadin) poisoning
	Laxative abuse
	Use of colored substances
Poisoning	Phenothiazines
	Hydrocarbons
	Iron
	Salts
Central nervous system depression	Insulin
	Sedatives and sleeping aids
	Barbiturates
	Aspirin
	Diphenhydramine (Benadryl) or other antihistamines
	Tricyclic antidepressants
	Acetaminophen
	Hydrocarbons
	Diphenoxylate hydrochloride and atropine sulfate (Lomotil)
	Suffocation
Diarrhea or vomiting	Syrup of ipecac
	Laxatives
	Salt administration
	Lying (symptoms do not actually exist)
Rashes	Drug poisoning
	Scratching
	Caustics (oven cleaners)
	Skin painting
Seizures	Intoxication
	Suffocation
	Poisoning
	Carotid sinus pressure
	Lying (symptoms do not actually exist)
Infection	Needlesticks
	Intravenous line contamination
	Bladder catheterization
Apnea	Suffocation
	Poisoning
	Lying (symptoms do not actually exist)
Fever	Injection of contaminates into the blood through intravenous line
	Falsifying temperatures in chart

The National Center on Elder Abuse (NCEA) has described seven categories of elder abuse[12]:

- Physical abuse
- Emotional or psychological abuse
- Financial abuse
- Neglect
- Sexual abuse
- Self-neglect
- Abandonment

In 2004 Adult Protective Services (APS) across the country received 565,747 reports of elder and vulnerable adult abuse. Of those investigated, 191,908 were substantiated. This 34% occurrence is broken down into the following categories[13]:

- Self-neglect: 37.2%
- Caregiver neglect: 20.4%
- Emotional or psychological abuse: 14.8%
- Financial exploitation: 14.7%
- Physical abuse: 10.7%
- Sexual abuse: 1%

Financial Exploitation

Financial exploitation of an elder or dependent adult is difficult to determine. This practice can involve stealing money or other possessions. The older individual also may be coerced into signing a contract, changing a will, assigning durable power of attorney, and transferring assets to family members or caregivers. Financial abuse of elders is part of the marketing scheme of corporations that prey on those who simply do not understand things such as computer technology or complicated payment plans. Table 49-6 lists some red flags for financial exploitation of elders.

Signs and Symptoms

In many ways, abuse of elders and dependent adults is similar to that of children. Table 49-7 outlines risk factors for elder and dependent adult abuse. Manifestations of these abuses vary greatly and may include any of the following physical findings:

- Soft tissue trauma: bruises, welts, lacerations
- Sprains, dislocations, fractures
- Burns
- Untreated injuries and medical problems
- Sexually transmitted infections, genital infections
- Vaginal or rectal bleeding
- Stained or bloody underwear
- Dehydration, malnutrition, decubitus ulcers
- Overdose or underdose of medications
- Changes in mentation or personality
- Withdrawal, decreased communication

TABLE 49-6	FINANCIAL EXPLOITATION RED FLAGS

- Patient is unaware of their financial situation and they do have the capacity to understand
- Discrepancy between financial resources and their lifestyle
- Prescriptions not being filled while they have the financial resources
- Sudden bank account changes
- Additional unexplained names on an elder's bank signature card
- Disappearance of funds or valuable possessions
- Provision of substandard care despite adequate finances
- Sudden transfer of assets or changes in a will
- An elder's report of financial exploitation

Data from Purcell, B. (n.d.). *Financial exploitation of seniors.* Retrieved from http://www.elder-abuse-information.com/abuse/abuse_financial.htm

TABLE 49-7	RISK FACTORS FOR ELDER AND DEPENDENT ADULT ABUSE

- Shared living arrangement
- Psychopathology of abuser (alcoholism, drug abuse)
- Caregiver stress and burnout
- Extensive care needs of persons with dementia, major physical deficits, or developmental limitations
- Transmission of abuse from one generation to another
- Caregiver inexperience
- Financial distress
- Lack of caregiver support system or social isolation
- The sudden and unpredictable nature of the needs of elder and dependent adults
- Poor physical living conditions

- Social isolation
- Lack of personal hygiene
- Signs of unsafe or unclean living conditions (lice, fleas, soiled clothing)

Identifying and reporting abuse of elderly and dependent adults is just as important as recognizing and intervening in cases of child abuse. Individuals who rely on others for their well-being deserve optimal care. Emergency nurses must be aware of state reporting laws and individual policies and practices regarding elder and dependent adult abuse.

Long-Term Care Issues

With more than 17,000 licensed nursing homes and more than 45,000 residential-type care facilities, a large vulnerable population remains at risk. Many are dependent on others for their activities of daily living and survival. Mental health challenges, diseases such as Alzheimer's, and communication disabilities prevent many of these adults from seeking help or speaking out. Dr. Catherine Hawes, a professor of health policy and management at Texas A&M University, reported to the U.S. Senate in 2003[14] on the prevalence of abuse and neglect in the long-term setting. Dr. Hawes' testimony is a firm reminder of the lack of reliable data in this area. She reports that data from various studies reveal the following[13]:

- Of 80 residents in 23 Georgia nursing homes, 44% reported that they had been abused and 48% reported that they had been treated roughly.
- More than one third of the 577 nursing home staff members from 31 facilities reported witnessing at least one incidence of physical abuse.
- 81% of staff interviewed reported observing verbal or psychological abuse.

In an effort to improve nursing home quality of care, several studies were undertaken. Among these, a common thread was noted of inadequate staffing being a major cause of abuse and neglect.[14]

Accurate and current statistics are difficult to ascertain, as there is no consistent definition for elder abuse and the incidence of abuse is thought to be grossly underreported.[13] It is known that nearly one third of nursing homes or other long-term facilities have been cited for violations and that 10% of these were cited for actual physical abuse. Underreporting occurs in 20% of instances, partly because of the cognitive impairment of many residents.[15] In 2008 2.1 million emergency department visits were made by residents of long-term care settings.[16] These patients look to the emergency nurse for care. Using critical thinking and assessment skills can raise suspicion for maltreatment. Assess, intervene, and report concerns for elder adult abuse and neglect.

REFERENCES

1. Schneider, D. (2011, April 19). *President's FY 2008 budget appropriations for the Administration for Children and Families* [testimony]. Retrieved from http://www.hhs.gov/asl/testify/2007/03/t20070308n.html

2. Kempe, C. H., Silverman, F. N., Steele, B. F., Droegemueller, W., & Silver, H. K. (1962). The battered child syndrome. *Journal of the American Medical Association, 181,* 17–24.

3. Administration for Children and Families. (2009). *Child maltreatment 2007.* Retrieved from http://www.acf.hhs.gov/programs/cb/pubs/cm07/index.htm

4. The National Center for Victims of Crime. (n.d.). *Child maltreatment.* Retrieved from http://www.ncvc.org/ncvc/main aspx?dbName=DocumentViewer&DocumentID=38709.

5. Child Welfare Information Gateway. (2010). *Child abuse and neglect fatalities: Statistics and interventions.* Retrieved from http://www.childwelfare.gov/pubs/factsheets/fatality.cfm

6. Kellogg, N., & Committee on Child Abuse and Neglect. (2005). Clinical report: The evaluation of sexual abuse in children. *Pediatrics, 116*(2), 506–512.

7. Brown, P., & Tierney, C. (2009). Munchausen syndrome by proxy. *Pediatrics in Review, 30,* 414–415.

8. The Cleveland Clinic. (n.d.). *Munchausen syndrome by proxy.* Retrieved from http://my.clevelandclinic.org/disorders/factitious_disorders/hic_munchausen_syndrome_by_proxy.aspx

9. Abdulhamid, I., & Siegel, P. T. (2011, August 13). *Pediatric Munchausen syndrome by proxy.* Retrieved from http://emedicine.medscape.com/article/917525-overview

10. Naegele, T., & Clark, A. (2001). Forensic Munchausen syndrome by proxy allegations: An emerging subspecies of child sexual abuse. *The Forensic Examiner, 10*(3–4), 21–23.

11. Teaster, P. B., Dugar, T. A., Mendiondo, M. S., Abner, E. L., & Cecil, K. A. (2006). *The 2004 survey of state adult protective services: Abuse of adults 60 years of age and older.* Retrieved from http://www.ncea.aoa.gov/NCEARoot/Main_Site/pdf/2-14-06%20FINAL%2060+REPORT.pdf

12. Sellas, M. I., & Krouse, L. H. (2011, June 8). *Elder abuse.* Retrieved from http://emedicine.medscape.com/article/805727-overview.

13. Wood, E. (2006). *The availability and utility of interdisciplinary data on elder abuse.* Retrieved from http://ncea.aoa.gov/ncearoot/Main_Site/pdf/publication/WhitePaper060404.pdf

14. Hawes, C. (2003). Elder abuse in residential long-term care setting: What is known and what information is needed? In R. J. Bonnie & R. B. Wallace (Eds.), *Elder mistreatment: Abuse, neglect, and exploitation in an aging America* (pp. 446–500). Washington, D.C.: The National Academies Press.

15. Fashbaugh, J. (n.d.). *Nursing home abuse statistics.* Retrieved from http://ezinearticles.com/?Nursing-Home-Abuse-Statistics&id=2064764

16. Pitts, S. W., Niska, R. W., Xu, J., & Burt, C. W. (2008, August 6). *National Hospital Ambulatory Medical Care Survey: 2006 emergency department summary.* Retrieved from http://www.cdc.gov/nchs/data/nhsr/nhsr007.pdf

Intimate Partner Violence

Shelley Cohen

Intimate partner violence (IPV), also known as domestic violence, is defined as a pattern of assaultive and coercive behavior by an individual against a current or former intimate partner. Intimate partners may be heterosexual or homosexual. Eighty-five percent of the time, IPV involves a woman being abused by a male partner.[1] However, violence against men by women and violence against a partner in a same-sex relationship also occur. IPV may also extend to dating violence.

Intimate partner violence is a global health problem. It is estimated that, one in every five women worldwide has been abused physically by a current or former partner.[2] Numerous studies report that American women experience a similar incidence of physical or sexual abuse.[3]

- Women account for 85% of the victims of IPV; men account for approximately 15%.[4]
- Women are much more likely than men to be killed by an intimate partner. IPV accounts for 33.5% of murders of women, but less than 4% of murders of men.[5]
- For many complex reasons, including embarrassment and fear, IPV is underreported. Underreporting is especially prevalent in same-sex relationships and among abused men.

The emergency nurse must understand that IPV can be found in all economic, racial, religious, educational, and age groups. Victims have no specific personality type, occupation, or sexual orientation profile. Factors that place women at increased risk for IPV include the following[6]:

- Young age (16 to 25 years)
- Low socioeconomic status
- Recent separation from a partner
- Young children (<12 years of age) in the home
- Homelessness

In the United States, African-Americans experience IPV at rates higher than those of other racial groups.[1] Nearly one third of black American women experience IPV in their lifetimes compared with one quarter of white American women.[7] Most victims are not identified unless a health care provider directly and sensitively asks about the possibility of IPV.

TYPES OF INTIMATE PARTNER VIOLENCE

Intimate partner violence takes many forms, including physical abuse, emotional abuse, psychological abuse, and sexual abuse and economic control. Although it is possible to experience only a single type of abuse, those in IPV situations commonly report multiple categories of abuse over time, particularly if the relationship remains unchanged. Table 50-1 summarizes common manifestations of IPV.

Teen Dating Violence

According to the Centers for Disease Control and Prevention (CDC), dating violence is a type of IPV. The underpinnings of this power and control relationship are similar to those that occur with adults.[8] Research by the Liz Claiborne Corporation[9] showed the following astonishing IPV facts:

- One in five teens who have been in a serious relationship have been hit, slapped, or pushed by their partner.
- One in three girls expressed concern for physical harm from their partner.
- One in four teens in a serious relationship have experienced a situation in which their partner (both boys and girls) tried to keep them from spending time with friends or family.
- One in four girls in a relationship reported sexual activity as a result of pressure.

A 2006 CDC survey confirms that both males and females may be victims of physical dating violence.[10] Of the 14,956 students surveyed, prevalence was 8.9% for males and 8.8% for females.[10] Teenagers at risk for dating violence include those whose partner is depressed and known to have aggressive behaviors.

TABLE 50-1	MANIFESTATIONS OF INTIMATE PARTNER VIOLENCE
Physical	Repetitive; increases in frequency and severity over time
	Pushing, shoving, slapping, kicking, choking, restraining
	Leaving victim in a dangerous situation
	Delaying or refusing care or help when sick or injured
Emotional	May occur independent of physical abuse or as a part of it
	Perpetrator uses shame, guilt, helplessness, and loss of self-worth as means to control the victim
	Physical and social isolation from family and friends
	Threats of physical harm
	Extreme jealousy
	Economic deprivation
	Acts of intimidation, humiliation, and degradation
Sexual	Completed or attempted sexual acts against the victim's will
	Any form of nonconsensual physical contact
Economic	Excluding victim from access to family income
	Requiring victim to ask for money or an allowance
	Appropriating victim's assets
	Preventing victim from getting or keeping a job

Warning Signs for Perpetrator of Dating Violence[8]
- Poor social skills
- Inability to manage anger and conflict
- Belief that this violent behavior is acceptable
- Witnesses violence in his or her own home
- Use of alcohol
- Behavior problems in other areas

Same-Sex Intimate Partner Abuse

In 2008 Brown[11] reported on same-sex IPV, which led to changes in how IPV is assessed in the emergency care setting. Studies have found the following[11]:
- IPV is the third largest problem facing gay men.
- IPV occurs at similar and possibly higher frequency in the gay, lesbian, bisexual, and transgender community.

Although many elements of IPV are similar for same-sex relationships as for heterosexual relationships, some key differences exist including the following[12]:
- Same-sex victims have more difficulty finding support because of their sexual orientation.
- Making use of resources and services for help may involve the victim revealing his or her sexual orientation to others who may not have been aware of it.
- The silence about domestic violence in this community further isolates the victim.
- The risk of losing children to another party is higher for lesbian and gay couples.

Facts Related to Same-Sex Intimate Partner Violence[12]
- Incidence of domestic violence is 25% to 33%.
- Many shelters and safe houses for battered women deny services to same-sex victims.
- Only seven states define domestic violence to include same-sex victims.
- Perpetrators use the threat of "outing" their partner to family and friends as a means of control and power.
- One in eight rape victims is male.
- Eighty-one percent of male victims had their protection order violated.

IDENTIFYING INTIMATE PARTNER VIOLENCE

Victims of IPV present to emergency departments (EDs) with a multitude of complaints ranging from multiple trauma to milder physical and mental health symptoms. Chronic medical and psychological conditions, minor and serious injuries, depression, suicidal behavior, sexually transmitted infections, substance abuse, and even death are only a few of the health consequences of IPV. In addition to physical injuries, a number of stress-related conditions have been linked to IPV, such as chronic neck and back pain, recurrent headaches, chronic pelvic pain, indigestion, diarrhea, constipation, gastritis, and spastic colon. Overall, victims of IPV have more surgeries, medical visits, and hospitalizations than persons without a history of abuse.[13]

Signs and Symptoms Suggestive of Abuse

The following signs and symptoms potentially suggest IPV as the cause:
- The patient describes the alleged "accident" in a hesitant, embarrassed, or evasive manner, or avoids eye contact.
- The extent or type of injury is inconsistent with the explanation offered by the patient.
- The victim has a history of traumatic injuries or frequent ED visits.
- The patient denies physical abuse but has unexplained bruises; areas of erythema or bruises in the shape of a hand or other object; lacerations, burns, scars, fractures,

or multiple injuries in various stages; mandibular fractures; or a perforated tympanic membrane.
- The patient expresses a fear of returning home or concern for the safety of his or her children.
- Injuries are in areas hidden by clothing or hair (e.g., head, chest, breasts, abdomen, genitals). Unintentional trauma generally involves injuries to the extremities, whereas IPV often involves truncal, head, and neck injuries.
- The partner (or suspected abuser) accompanies the patient, insists on staying close to the patient, and tries to answer all questions directed to the patient.
- The patient admits to past or present physical or emotional abuse as a victim or as a child witness.
- The woman is pregnant. Homicide is the leading cause of death for pregnant women, and intimate partners are the most common perpetrators.[14]
- The victim shows evidence of sexual assault.
- The patient is the caregiver of an abused child.
- A substantial delay occurred between the time of injury and presentation for treatment. The patient may have been prevented from seeking medical attention sooner or may have had to wait for the batterer to leave.
- The patient has psychosomatic complaints such as panic attacks, anxiety, a choking sensation, or depression.
- A complaint of chronic pain (especially back or pelvic pain), with no substantiating physical evidence, often signifies fear of impending or actual physical abuse.

Assessment of Victims

The Emergency Nurses Association recommends the development of routine protocols and procedures for the assessment and identification of IPV.[15] Intervention goals for victims include the following:
- Treat presenting complaints of injuries
- Offer emotional support
- Help victims establish a safety plan and identify available options
- Give victims information regarding legal protection, including assault documentation
- Provide information about available support services and community resources

Identification of IPV victims requires sensitivity, understanding, and a high index of suspicion. The psychological effects of battering are complex and can be difficult to understand. Victims are made to feel worthless. Abusers repeatedly tell their victims that no one cares and that more violence will follow if the abuse is revealed. For these reasons, it can be extremely difficult for victims to take the first step toward revealing abuse. However, breaking through the barrier of silence and denial will begin the process of physical and psychological healing. Many

TABLE 50-2	**SCREENING QUESTIONS FOR ADULT PATIENTS**

- Is anyone in your home being hurt, hit, threatened, frightened, or neglected?
- Do you feel safe in your current relationship?
- Do you ever feel afraid at home? Are you afraid for your children?
- Sometimes patients tell me that they have been hurt by someone close to them. Could this be happening to you?
- You seem frightened of your partner. Has he (she) ever hurt you?
- Have there been times during your relationship when you have had physical fights?
- Do your verbal fights ever include physical contact?
- Have you been hit, punched, kicked, or otherwise hurt by someone within the past year? If so, by whom?
- You mentioned that your partner uses alcohol (drugs). How does he (she) act when drinking (on drugs)?
- Does your partner consistently control your actions or put you down?
- Sometimes when others are overprotective and as jealous as you describe, they react strongly and use physical force. Is this happening in your situation?

victims will acknowledge abuse openly if questioned in a nonjudgmental manner in a safe environment. When not asked directly, abused patients are generally hesitant to bring up the subject.

Screening with explicit but nonthreatening questions increases disclosure rates. Nonetheless, victims may require several visits and screenings before they feel comfortable revealing abuse. Table 50-2 lists some screening questions that can be asked of adult patients.

Therapeutic Interventions

- Find a quiet, safe, private environment to assess the patient and screen for violence.
- Interview the patient privately, not in the presence of family members or other accompanying individuals.
- Universally screen all teenage and adult patients for IPV regardless of the presenting complaint.
- Have the patient undress completely so that any hidden injuries will be exposed.
- Take a careful history. Begin a IPV screen with a statement such as the following:
  - "Domestic violence has come to be recognized as an important, often overlooked health issue in our society. So many people are affected directly or indirectly. Sometimes we are even afraid to say anything. We care about our patients and want to help

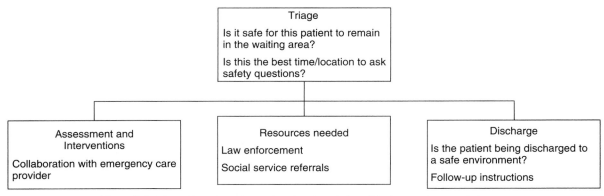

Fig. 50-1 Considerations for caring for the victim of intimate partner violence.

everyone in need. We screen every patient who comes to the emergency department for abuse because it is so common, so I would like to ask you a few questions."

- "Does your current partner or a partner from a previous relationship make you feel unsafe now?"
- "Are you here today because of an illness or injury related to violence from a partner or ex-partner?"
- "Has your partner ever controlled your actions? Threatened you? Hit, shoved, punched, kicked, or otherwise physically hurt you? Forced you to have unwanted sexual contact?"
- Following these questions, ask patients if they want additional information on IPV or would like to discuss their situation with someone.
- Examples of other direct, nonthreatening questions are the following:
  - Do you feel safe to go home today when we discharge you?
  - You seem frightened of your partner. Has he (she) ever hurt you?
  - Sometimes patients tell me someone close to them has hurt them. Could this be happening to you?
  - Your partner seems overly concerned and anxious. Is he (she) responsible for your injuries?
  - I notice you have a number of bruises. Did someone hit you?
- Assessment of the patient's safety is important in terms of reducing the danger faced by the patient after discharge.
  - Determine whether the patient has a safe place to go and the necessary resources (e.g., medications).
  - Ask if the patient needs help locating a shelter.

- Offer to find a social worker or medical advocate to talk with the patient.
- Let the patient know that IPV is against the law and that a police report can be made and a temporary restraining order can be obtained.
- Explain to the patient the physical and emotional sequelae of chronic battering for both the patient and his or her children.
- Stress the importance of follow-up for medical, legal, and social support.
- Emphasize that the cycle of violence *can* be broken and that help is available.

Figure 50-1 summarizes considerations for caring for the victim of IPV.

ADVOCACY AND SUPPORT SERVICES

Advocates for victims of IPV have specialized training in abuse issues and are dedicated to providing victim assistance. Their role is to be available to help and support the patient whenever needed, from the initial ED visit through the critical days or months ahead.

- The advocate offers a victim the opportunity to explore various available options, such as crisis intervention, a safe home network, and legal representation.
- The advocate works with the victim to support his or her choices, regardless of whether the advocate agrees with the decision. Many times a victim will choose to return to an unsafe and potentially violent environment. For a variety of complex reasons (low self-esteem, guilt, fear, loneliness, lack of support systems, insufficient funds) victims are frequently unprepared to separate from violent partners. The advocate's role is to provide unconditional support so that victims feel they are no longer alone.

- With the patient's permission, notify a local advocacy service to initiate contact and support while the patient is still in the ED (if possible).
- Provide the patient with the telephone number of the abuse hotline in the area. Various social services can be contacted to help the patient identify programs and options available.

LEGAL OBLIGATIONS

The emergency nurse must be familiar with IPV reporting laws in the state or location in which he or she is employed. Expectations vary between jurisdictions:

- Is it mandatory to report nonfatal but life-threatening injuries (gunshot wounds or strangulations)?
- Is there an obligation to report non–life-threatening injuries?
- Does your facility have policies and procedures in place regarding IPV reporting?

Every state in the United States has some form of legislation that offers protection to IPV victims. Be aware of state laws and services for abuse victims in the area.

Documentation

Accurate and concise documentation of suspected IPV is essential from medical and legal perspectives. The medical records can provide evidence of injury, escalating violence, or patterns of abuse. These records can be subpoenaed for subsequent criminal hearings. The patient's injuries should be documented clearly in the medical record by licensed health care professionals. The following are things to consider for documentation:

- Record the size, pattern, description, and location of all injuries.
- Use a body injury map for documentation, especially when numerous wounds are present.
- Be as specific as possible. For example, "multiple contusions and lacerations" will not convey a clear picture to a judge or jury but "three oval contusions and one 5-cm laceration at the base of the anterior neck" will back up allegations of attempted strangulation.
- Record other evidence of abuse, such as torn clothing and broken jewelry.
- Document the patient's demeanor and behavior objectively.
- If the patient states that the injury was caused by abuse, record the information verbatim and write "Patient states" before the quotation. For example, record: "Patient states she was 'hit in the face by my husband's fist.'"

Example of a triage note: *Crying—sits with knees drawn up to chest, makes no eye contact, trembling. Patient states, "I can't believe he did this to me."*

Example of a discharge note: *Left ambulatory with sister. Patient states, "I feel very safe with her and in her apartment."*

Documentation Tips

- Use actual quotes by the patient.
- Only document what is seen, heard, smelled, or touched.
- Use descriptive terms to paint a picture of the victim.
- Document where the patient is going after discharge.
- Document with whom the patient left if he or she did not leave alone.
- Document all resources provided to the patient.

Photographs should be taken with the permission of the victim as a means of supplementing (not replacing) the written documentation in the medical record. Follow institutional guidelines regarding photography of injuries; the following are some general guidelines:

- Whenever possible, use the law enforcement's expertise for photography related to injuries.
- The patient does not need to sign for permission for photographs taken by law enforcement personnel; the nurse is responsible for documenting the fact that they were taken and by whom.
- If the ED staff is responsible for obtaining photographs, patient permission is required. If the victim is a minor, permission from his or her legal guardian is needed.
- Additional information regarding written and photographic documentation of injuries can be found in Chapter 6, Forensics.

Often the process of follow-up photography is omitted from discharge instructions. If law enforcement was used for photography, arrangements should be made as to when the victim should report to law enforcement for additional photography. Wounds and bruises may appear differently 24 to 48 hours later and some bruises, not evident at the time of the emergency department visit, may reveal themselves later on.

MAKING AN IMPACT

Emergency nurses affect patients and their lives in many ways. The victim of IPV needs an emergency nurse by his or her side, not only to act as an advocate but to ensure appropriate assessment, intervention, and discharge planning. This patient population can be helped both proactively and during their presentation post-violence. Figure 50-2 illustrates other ways to positively affect care for the victim of IPV.

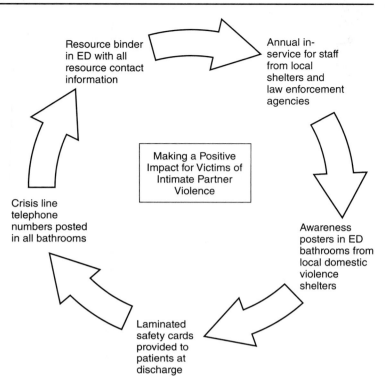

Fig. 50-2 Making a positive impact for victims of intimate partner violence.

REFERENCES

1. Bureau of Justice Statistics. (2011, February 23). *Intimate partner violence in the U.S.* Retrieved from http://bjs.ojp.usdoj.gov/content/intimate/victims.cfm
2. World Health Organization. (2005). *Addressing violence against women and achieving the Millennium Developmental Goals.* Geneva, Switzerland: Author. Retrieved from http://whqlibdoc.who.int/hq/2005/WHO_FCH_GWH_05.1.pdf
3. American Bar Association Commission on Domestic Violence. (n.d.). *Survey of recent statistics.* Retrieved from http://new.abanet.org/domesticviolence/Pages/Statistics.aspx
4. Domestic Violence Resource Center. (n.d.). *Domestic violence statistics.* Retrieved from www.dvrc-or.org/domestic/violence/resources/C61/
5. Violence Policy Center. (2008). *When men murder women: An analysis of 2006 homicide data.* Washington, DC: Author. Retrieved from http://vpc.org/studies/wmmw2008.pdf
6. Dryden-Edwards, R. (n.d.). *Domestic violence.* Retrieved from http://www.emedicinehealth.com/domestic_violence/article_em.htm
7. Institute on Domestic Violence in the African American Community. (n.d.). *Fact sheet: Intimate partner violence (IPV) in the African American community.* Retrieved from http://www.idvaac.org/media/publications/FactSheet.IDVAAC_AAPCFV-Community%20Insights.pdf
8. Centers for Disease Control. (2010). *Understanding teen dating violence.* Retrieved from http://www.cdc.gov/violenceprevention/pdf/TeenDatingViolence_2010-a.pdf
9. Dating abuse statistics. (n.d.). Retrieved from http://www.loveisrespect.org/is-this-abuse/dating-violence-statistics
10. Centers for Disease Control and Prevention. (2006). Physical dating violence among high school students—United States, 2003. *Morbidity and Mortality Weekly Report, 55*(19), 532–535.
11. Brown, C. (2008). Gender role implications on same-sex intimate partner abuse. *Journal of Family Violence, 23*(6), 457–462.
12. University of Wisconsin–Stout. (n.d.). *Same gender violence statistics.* Retrieved from http://www.uwstout.edu/cvpp/same_gender_stats.cfm
13. Bonomi, A. E., Thompson, R. S., Anderson, M., Reid, R. J., Carrell, D., Dimer, J. A., & Rivara, F. P. (2006). Intimate partner violence and women's physical, mental, and social functioning. *American Journal of Preventive Medicine, 30*(6), 458–466.
14. Campbell, J. C., Glass, N., Sharps, P. W., Laughon, K., & Bloom, T. (2007). Intimate partner homicide: Review and implications of research and policy. *Trauma, Violence, and Abuse, 8*(3), 246–269.
15. Emergency Nurses Association. (2006). *Intimate partner and family violence, maltreatment, and neglect* [position statement]. Retrieved from http://www.ena.org/SiteCollectionDocuments/Position%20Statements/Violence_-_Intimate_Partner_and_Family_-_ENA_PS.pdf

Sexual Assault

Barbara Weintraub

The U.S. Department of Justice defines rape as "[f]orced sexual intercourse including both psychological coercion as well as physical force. Forced sexual intercourse means penetration by the offender(s). This definition includes attempted rapes, male as well as female victims, and both heterosexual and homosexual rape. Attempted rape includes verbal threats of rape."[1] While each state has its own definition of rape, all states include in their definition the element of force and lack of consent. Although the terms "rape" and "sexual assault" are frequently used interchangeably, the Rape, Abuse, and Incest National Network (RAINN)[2] refines this definition, classifying sexual assault as unwanted sexual contact that stops short of rape or attempted rape. Most state statutes currently define rape as "nonconsensual oral, anal, or vaginal penetration of the victim by body parts or objects using force, threats of bodily harm, or by taking advantage of a victim who is incapacitated or otherwise incapable of giving consent."[3]

Although the total number of sexual assaults has dropped nearly 60% in the United States in the past decade[2], the incidence is still staggering. It is estimated that one in six American women will have been the victim of an attempted or completed rape some time in her life and that someone is sexually assaulted in America every 2 minutes.[2] In 2010, there were 188,380 incidents of rape or sexual assault.[4] A 2006 study noted that 22% of women report having been forced to do "something sexual" in their lifetimes.[5] According to the 2000 National Violence Against Women Survey,[6] a very conservative estimate of the number of female rape victims treated by emergency department (ED) personnel in the 12 months preceding the survey was almost 129,000.

GENERAL APPROACH

Given these statistics, it is nearly inevitable that an emergency nurse will be responsible for the care of a sexual assault survivor at some time during his or her career. The emergency nurse is a key member of the treatment team and is instrumental in coordinating the multiple activities necessary to ensure that the simultaneous goals of compassionate emergency care and forensic evidence collection are met.[7] The Emergency Nurses Association (ENA) advocates that these at-risk victims "receive appropriate and sensitive care that addresses their medical, emotional, and legal needs."[7] It is important to recognize that sexual assault is a crime of violence, not of sexual gratification[8] and, as such, can cause concomitant physical injuries as well as long-lasting detrimental effects on the survivor's psychological well-being and future interpersonal relationships. Because the ED is the first point of contact for many of these survivors, emergency nurses play a key role in their care, not only as that of health care provider but as that of evidence collector as well.[9] As such, it is imperative that the emergency nurse approach the patient as well as the examination from an integrated, holistic psychological-social-legal perspective.

The Sexual Assault Nurse Examiner

Because of the intensely personal needs and legal implications inherent in the care of the sexual assault survivor, many EDs have adopted the Sexual Assault Nurse Examiner (SANE) model of care. SANE programs grew out of a need recognized by health professionals who care for sexual assault victims. These professionals recognized that the services provided in the ED to sexual assault victims were not at the same standard of care as for other populations of emergency department patients.[10] The first SANE programs were established in Memphis, Tennessee, in 1976 and they have grown in number from 3 in the 1970s to more than 600 as of June 6, 2010.[11] In addition, 17 schools offer forensic nurse degree programs at this time.

The benefit of SANE services was evidenced in a retrospective analysis of sexual assault victims presenting to a pediatric ED in a study by Bechtel, Ryan, and Gallagher.[12] They found that patients whose care was directed by a SANE as compared to those whose care was not were more likely to have a full genitourinary examination documented. They were also more likely to have had appropriate testing for sexually transmitted infections, to have received pregnancy prophylaxis treatment, and to have been referred to a rape crisis center.[12] Research has shown that additional benefits of a SANE program include the following:

- More victims make a police report and follow through with prosecution.
- Survivors experience a shortened treatment time in the ED.
- The emergency nurse and physician have more time to care for other patients.
- Survivors report that they feel a higher level of satisfaction and a decreased level of feeling victimized during the ED examination.
- A better chain of evidence is maintained and conviction rates are as good, if not better, than with non-SANE care.[10]

Triage

In addition to any physical pain from injuries incurred during the assault, patients presenting for treatment following sexual assault are in extreme emotional pain. Using a five-tier triage system that the ENA and American College of Emergency Physicians (ACEP) jointly recommend,[13] these patients should be assigned a triage category of 2 on a scale of 1 to 5 (with 1 meaning resuscitation). These patients warrant a level 2 categorization because of the time-sensitive nature of their required treatment as well as the severity of their psychological pain.[14] Following identification of the chief complaint, these patients should bypass the remainder of the triage process and be taken to a private treatment room if at all possible. This provides them with the maximum amount of privacy and assists in the preservation of forensic materials. In EDs with access to SANE services, the SANE should be notified at this time.

> Each sexual assault survivor is not only a crime victim but a crime scene as well.

Primary Assessment

Aside from patients who present with obvious immediate threats to life, assessment should proceed in the usual manner, with an initial assessment of airway, breathing, and circulation. Sexual assault patients may sustain a wide array of physical injuries, dependent on the number of attackers, whether foreign objects were employed, and the overall violence of the incident. The Centers for Disease Control and Prevention (CDC)[15] found that among sexual violence victims aged 18 years and older, 31.5% of women and 16.1% of men reported a physical injury as a result of a rape. While life-threatening injuries should be attended to immediately, care of other non–life-threatening injuries should wait until evidence collection has been completed, to maintain the integrity of any evidence collected.[10]

HISTORY

Following the initial assessment for life threats, a more detailed history and physical examination pertinent to the assault itself should take place. The history should include "an accurate and detailed description of the incident, which will guide forensic evidence collection."[16] In addition to a standard patient history, an obstetric and gynecologic (OB/GYN) history as well as additional elements specific to the assault should be attained. Elements to obtain are outlined next.[8]

Obstetric and Gynecologic History

- Gravida para status; for maximum information this ideally is recorded in the format of gravida (total pregnancies)/para (pregnancies carried to 20 weeks gestation), or $G_\#P_{TPAL}$.[17] See Chapter 46, Obstetric Emergencies, for more information.
- Last menstrual period
- Current method of birth control
- Time of last consensual intercourse

Assault History

- Date, time, and place of the assault
- Events surrounding or leading up to the assault
- Description of the assailant and number of assailants
- Information regarding all acts perpetrated by the attacker
  - Verbal and physical threats
  - Use of weapons and restraints
  - Sites of penetration
  - Sites of ejaculation if known
  - Whether a condom was used
- Injuries associated with the assault
- Post-assault activities by victim (e.g., bathing, wound care, douching, eating, drinking, and clothing changes)

PHYSICAL ASSESSMENT

Care of the sexual assault survivor differs from care of other patients in that the responsibility to maintain the integrity of forensic evidence is equal to or greater than the responsibility for timely and accurate patient assessment and treatment. This remains true regardless of the survivor's current desire to report the attack or make a police report. While the decision to make a police report can occur at any time, the ability to collect intact evidence cannot. For this reason, once immediate life threats have been ruled out, evidence collection should be completed prior to the full patient assessment and treatment of other injuries. Even the collection of routine vital signs can disrupt potential evidence and, as such, should be delayed until the forensic evidence is collected if the patient is stable.

Basic Principles of Sexual Assault Evidence Collection

Because of the intensely personal and highly traumatic nature of sexual assault, many survivors delay seeking treatment. While patients may present at any time following an assault, in general a sexual assault evidence collection kit should be completed only when the attack has occurred within the previous 96 hours. If the assault took place more than 96 hours prior to the patient presenting for treatment, an evidence collection kit is generally not used, as the presence of any trace evidence is unlikely at that point. This time limit may change in the future, as it is dependent on the current sensitivity of forensic testing. Deoxyribonucleic acid (DNA) from suspects has been found in epithelial cells in the vaginal vault of patients for as long as 3 weeks post-assault and on the clothing for years.[18]

Absence of kit use, however, does not negate the value of careful assessment and documentation. Documenting findings obtained during the sexual assault examination (e.g., contusions, lacerations), photographing injuries and bite mark impressions, and recording patient statements about the assault gather evidence that can be of legal value.

In conducting a sexual assault examination, it is necessary to keep in mind some baseline concepts. It is critical that the examination be conducted in a compassionate and objective manner that meets the needs of the sexual assault survivor while at the same time being carried out in an organized and systematic manner so as not to compromise potential forensic evidence. Conducting an examination in this manner means allowing choices, even the declining of any or all evidence collection; proceeding at a pace determined by the survivor; and taking breaks as needed by the survivor.

It is also important to keep in mind that for each patient there is only one opportunity for evidence collection. Therefore when in doubt, collect. In most states, standardized examination kits have been developed or purchased for evidence collection. Generally included in these kits is information regarding specimen collection, instructions for maintaining the chain of custody, and a list of documentation requirements. Standardized sexual assault evidence collection kits are packaged according to Food and Drug Administration regulations; instructions must be followed and all evidence collected should be placed and sealed in the containers provided in the approved kit to maintain its viability as evidence.

Some basic principles include the following:[18]

- Whenever possible, unbutton or unzip any clothing for removal.
- If the patient is able, have her or him undress while standing on a sheet so that trace evidence will fall on the sheet. The sheet is then preserved.
- If clothes must be cut, do not slice through stains, holes, tears, or buttonholes.
- Air-dry all physical evidence of the crime collected from the victim. Heat degrades biological samples. Fold clothing without shaking. Take care not to cross-contaminate the surfaces. Place individual items in paper collection containers that are sealed and labeled as described below.
- When moisture is needed to collect biological samples, slightly moisten (versus saturate) the tip of a cotton swab with sterile water. Moisture dilutes biological samples thereby reducing the chance of detecting scant amounts of DNA. Separate items as they are collected so that there is no transfer of trace evidence between objects. Dry the samples and place them in a separate, labeled envelope obtained from the sexual assault kit.
- For the vaginal examination, lubricate the speculum with tap water only, as other lubricants may affect test results and decrease sperm motility. A vaginal speculum is never used in prepubertal children without general anesthesia.
- Collect biological samples before any activity or procedure (catheter insertion, voiding, eating, smoking, drinking) that could result in the destruction of evidence. Dry the sample and place it in a separate, labeled envelope obtained from the evidence collection kit.
- Never place moist evidence in plastic or glass containers. Heat and moisture promote growth of mold and other organisms that destroy evidence. Collect and store specimens using paper or glass only, never plastic. Plastic does not breathe, and mold will grow.[19]
- After drying, place each cotton-tipped applicator (bulb end first) into a separate, labeled envelope obtained from

the evidence collection kit. Ensure that all envelopes are sealed properly.[19]
- Properly seal all envelopes; do not lick or your DNA will be on the envelope.
- If the specimen was once living (e.g., blood or other body fluids), refrigerate it after collection.[19]
- Do not touch objects that may contain fingerprints (i.e., knife, gun, bullet, cartridge case). Package the evidence to preserve the prints.[19]
- Sterile collection is not essential but it is important to change gloves between sites to avoid cross-contamination.[19]

Penile Specimen Collection[19]

In the event of an assault involving a male victim's penis, collect biological evidence from the penile area following these steps:
- Inspect the external structures of the penis for injury or disease using colposcopy if possible.
- With a cotton-tipped applicator, thoroughly swab the penile shaft and glans area.
- If the assault included oral contact with the penis, swab along the penile shaft hairline and scrotal sack for saliva.
- Prepare a slide smear as directed by the forensic laboratory.
- Dry all penile swabs and slides and place them in separate, labeled envelopes provided in the kit.
- Properly seal all envelopes; do not lick or your DNA will be on the envelope.

Labeling Specimens

Initial all specimens and label them with the following information:
- The hospital name, patient name, and patient identification number
- The date and time of collection
- A description of the specimen and its collection site
- The name and signature of the person collecting the evidence

Individually place any objects (e.g., knife, bullets, or clothing) removed from the patient in a paper evidence bag, sealed and labeled.

Alternate Light Source Screening

- When available, a Wood's lamp or another alternate light source (i.e., infrared, ultraviolet) is used in a darkened room to screen the body and clothing for biological stains and injury.
  - Take swabs or scrapings from any sites identified.
- Use an alternate light source to assist in identifying findings.

- Be observant for redness, abrasions, bruises, swelling, lacerations, fractures, bites, burns, and other forms of physical trauma.
- Note areas of tenderness and induration.
- On dark-skinned individuals, it may be difficult to identify these areas and they may need to be sought out carefully.

Documentation

While documentation standards regarding sexual assault examinations vary from state to state, there are consistencies. According to the U.S. Department of Justice, "[g]ood documentation, whether or not the patient initially wants to report to law enforcement, can provide the basis for prosecution or other legal action at a later time."[16] While most institutions have developed their own sexual assault forms for medical record documentation, sample forms are available to assist institutions wishing to devise their own. One such site is the Sexual Assault Forensic Examiner Technical Assistance website, administered by the International Association of Forensic Nurses.[20]

> Documentation of the assault should always be written in the patient's own words and placed in quotation marks.

The medical record also serves as a legal document and, as such, must reflect that a sexual assault examination was conducted, the extent of the examination, as well as physical findings, diagnostic procedures performed, treatment provided, patient education, and recommended follow-up care.[19] Careful objective and legible documentation is essential, as the medical record may be the only tool the emergency nurse has to recall a case should he or she be called to court. Documentation should not include any subjective opinions or conclusions as to whether a crime has occurred. Terms to avoid include the following:[19]
- "In no acute distress"
- "No evidence of rape"
- "Rule out rape"
- "Alleges" or "claims"

Assessment and accurate injury documentation is a critical feature in the care of sexual assault patients. Injuries not in the genital area are generally easier to visualize. Although they are usually minor in nature, they can have immeasurable forensic value and, as such, should be accurately and objectively documented. Forensic photography and body diagrams can support injury documentation; however, they should be considered only as tools to augment the medical record and not take the place of complete, competent documentation. Documentation of injuries should include the following:

- Site of the injury, clearly stated in appropriate anatomic terms, specifying right or left if applicable.
- Type of injury (e.g., contusion, burn, stab, bite).
- Size of injury, both length and width. Use the same unit of measurement throughout the document.
- Shape of the injury. If a specific shape is recognized, it should be documented (e.g., circular, curvilinear, triangular). Injuries can have a shape and pattern of the causative objective. This is called a patterned injury and should be documented as such.
- Color of the injury. The color of bruises has been shown to have poor correlation to age of injury and should not be used to estimate the age of the injury.[19]

Record all physical findings on body diagram forms:
- Observable or palpable tissue injuries
- Physiologic changes
- Foreign materials such as grass, sand, and stains
- Dried or moist secretions or positive fluorescence

Using colposcopy during the external genital examination can enhance visualization of microscopic trauma and can assist in providing photographic documentation. In some jurisdictions, toluidine blue dye may be used to detect trauma, either with or without the use of colposcopy. Use of toluidine blue dye is contraindicated in the prepubertal patient secondary to pain and burning.[18]

Forensic Photography

When injuries are found on examination, photography may enhance the written description and body diagrams. This is important for both genital and nongenital injuries because:
- The physical evidence may be short-lived and, if not visually recorded, may be lost.
- The appearance of injuries can change significantly with time.
- Photographs create a permanent record of the acute injury and reduce subjectivity and observer interpretation.
- Photographs serve as an aid to memory when a case goes to court years later.
- Photographs permit the court and jurors to see the evidence "as it was."

Key points related to forensic photography include the following:
- Patients must give specific consent for photography; exceptions occur in cases where "implied consent" applies and in situations where a court order has been issued.
- Note in the medical record that photographs were taken, how many were taken, and by whom they were taken.
- Follow institutional policy and procedures regarding forensic photography.

Chain of Custody

Chain of custody is a legal term referring to "the order of places where, and the persons with whom, physical evidence was located from the time it was collected to its submission at trial."[21] To maintain the chain of custody, an evidence collection kit and the specimens it contains must be accounted for from the moment collection begins until the moment it is introduced in court as evidence.[19] Accurately maintaining and accounting for the chain of custody is essential for the evidence to be admissible in a court of law. Each item of evidence must be properly labeled to include the following:
- The initials of every person who handled it
- The date it was collected
- A description of the evidence
- The source of the specimen
- The name of the examiner who collected the evidence
- The name of the patient

Evidence not included in the kit (e.g., clothing, photographs) must be individually packaged in paper, sealed, and labeled with a description of the item. Never leave the patient alone with the evidence. Do not allow family members or support persons (e.g., advocates) to handle or transport evidence after it has been collected. The examiner is responsible for maintaining the chain of custody during the examination. Chain of custody is essential to be able to swear to the integrity of the evidence in court.[19] Evidence must remain with the person who collected it until the police take custody of it. Both the collector and the receiving officer verify with their signatures that the chain of custody was maintained.

DIAGNOSTIC PROCEDURES

While the diagnostic procedures ordered for any patient must be appropriate for that patient, there are baseline diagnostic procedures routinely required in the care of sexual assault survivors. When a survivor presents to the ED a short time after the assault, results of these tests are looking for baseline conditions rather than conditions incurred as a result of the assault. Table 51-1 lists the recommendations for diagnostic procedures related to potential infectious complications of sexual assault.

Routine toxicology testing for patients is not recommended for sexual assault victims unless there is suspicion of a drug-facilitated sexual assault (DFSA). In this situation, permission must be obtained from the victim. Indicators of possible DFSA include the following:
- Unexplained drowsiness, fatigue, light-headedness, dizziness, hypotension, or impaired motor skills

TABLE 51-1 ROUTINELY RECOMMENDED DIAGNOSTIC PROCEDURES

POSSIBLE COMPLICATION	RECOMMENDATION	JUSTIFICATION	TEST TO PERFORM
Pregnancy	With their consent, perform pregnancy test on all women with reproductive capability, except when the patient is clearly pregnant.[a]	Treatment options for pregnancy prophylaxis and HIV treatment may be altered if patient is pregnant.	Serum or urine pregnancy test
Sexually transmitted infection	The CDC[b] recommends that the decision to obtain baseline tests for detection of STIs be made on an individual rather than a routine basis	The baseline testing of survivors for STIs is controversial. Although all 50 states have laws strictly limiting the evidentiary use of a survivor's sexual history, including evidence of previous STIs, there are occasional, exceptional situations where these diagnoses may later be accessed and brought to light during courtroom proceedings in an effort to undermine the credibility of the survivor's testimony. Thus many experts advise against baseline testing. Survivors may be significantly concerned about contracting an STI from the assailant; testing for previous presence of an STI may alleviate this particular concern.[c]	Culture or FDA-cleared NAAT for *Neisseria gonorrhoeae* and *Chlamydia trachomatis* from any sites of penetration or attempted penetration. NAAT offers the advantage of increased sensitivity in detection of *C. trachomatis.*[b] Wet mount and culture of a vaginal swab for *Trichomonas vaginalis.* If vaginal discharge, malodor, or itching is evident, test wet mount for evidence of bacterial vaginosis and candidiasis.[b] Serum sample for evaluation of syphilis[b]
Hepatitis B	Perform in the previously immunized patient Not indicated in the nonimmunized patient	Confirms adequate antibody formation in the previously immunized patient. If hepatitis B surface antibody is present, no vaccination is necessary.	Hepatitis B surface antibody
HIV	Baseline HIV testing is not generally considered a routine exam component.[d] However, each situation is different; assess the risk for HIV infection in the assailant on an individual basis. Evaluate assault characteristics that could raise the risk for HIV transmission. Regardless of the results of this assessment, some survivors may wish to be tested and treated.[a]	When the survivor presents within 72 hours of the assault and wishes to start antiretroviral therapy, establish a baseline HIV status.[d]	HIV antibody test at original assessment and again at 6 weeks, 3 months, and 6 months. Baseline CBC and serum chemistry if considering initiation of antiretroviral therapy. Do not delay initiation of PEP pending results.

[a]Bechtel, K., Ryan, E., & Gallagher, D. (2008). Impact of sexual assault nurse examiners on the evaluation of sexual assault in a pediatric emergency department. *Pediatric Emergency Care, 24*(7), 442–447.

[b]Centers for Disease Control and Prevention. (2006). Sexually transmitted diseases treatment guidelines. *Morbidity and Mortality Weekly Report, 55*(RR-11), 1–94.

[c]U.S. Department of Justice Office of Violence Against Women. (2004). *A national protocol for sexual assault medical forensic examinations: Adults/adolescents.* Washington, DC: Author.

[d]American College of Emergency Physicians. (2008). *Evaluation and management of the sexually assaulted or sexually abused patient.* Dallas, TX: Author.

CBC, Complete blood count; *CDC,* Centers for Disease Control and Prevention; *FDA,* Food and Drug Administration; *HIV,* human immunodeficiency virus; *NAAT,* nucleic acid amplification test; *PEP,* post-exposure prophylaxis; *STI,* sexually transmitted infection.

- Complaints of amnesia, lapse of time surrounding events
- Patient or accompanying person states a suspicion that the patient may have been drugged
- Patient found with clothes on differently or not at all
- Patient may note a "salty" taste in a drink, which may indicate presence of gamma-hydroxybutyric acid.

Routine testing is not recommended, as it can reveal drugs that the patient took voluntarily and this may be discoverable by defense. If toxicology testing is done, consider the following:

- Urine collection must be done within 96 hours of ingestion of the suspected drug.
    - The victim's first urine is critical to obtain if at all possible.
    - Do not use the clean-catch method of urine collection and collect as much urine as possible, up to 100 mL.[12]
- The drugs used in DFSA are eliminated quickly from the body. Obtain a blood sample if drugs have been ingested within 24 hours before the examination.
- If the patient vomits, the emesis can be sent for toxicology testing.

THERAPEUTIC INTERVENTIONS

To assist in the standardization of patient treatment and adherence to current CDC guidelines, some facilities have developed a standardized order sheet for the care of sexual assault patients.[22] See Figure 51-1 for an example of such a form.

Pregnancy Prophylaxis

- Five percent of women who are raped become pregnant.[23]
- Emergency contraceptives are 57% to 89% effective when used within 72 hours postcoitus.[5] Optimally, the treatment should be initiated within 12 hours after the assault.[10]
- Acceptable treatment options may vary according to a patient's age and social, cultural, and religious background. A careful, nonbiased dialogue must be conducted so as not to sway the patient's decision.
- Counsel female patients about options for prophylaxis against pregnancy resulting from sexual assault (also known as emergency contraception or "morning-after" pill) and the importance of timely action. Ensure that female patients are properly informed of the effectiveness rates, risks, and benefits associated with the provision of emergency contraception to prevent pregnancy resulting from sexual assault.

- Provide female patients with appropriate information to make an informed choice regarding emergency contraception and ensure that such services are provided upon request to the patient without delay, unless medically contraindicated.

Sexually Transmitted Infections

- Trichomoniasis, bacterial vaginosis, gonorrhea, and chlamydial infection are the most frequently diagnosed infections among women who have been sexually assaulted.[5]
- Presumptive treatment is aimed at treatment of these pathogens. Either of two regimens is recommended[23]:
    - Regimen 1
        - Ceftriaxone (Rocephin) 250 mg intramuscularly in a single dose **PLUS**
        Metronidazole (Flagyl) 2 g orally in a single dose **PLUS**
        Azithromycin (Zithromax) 1 g orally in a single dose
        OR
    - Regimen 2
        - Doxycycline (Vibramycin) 100 mg orally twice a day for 7 days

> The likelihood of developing any sexually transmitted infection as result of sexual assault is 26.3%.[24]

Hepatitis B

- In the previously unvaccinated patient, administer a hepatitis B vaccination. Follow-up vaccine doses should then be administered at 1 to 2 months and 4 to 6 months after the first dose.
- Administration of hepatitis B immune globulin (HBIG) is not recommended.[24]

Human Immunodeficiency Virus

The danger of exposure to human immunodeficiency virus (HIV) is real and very frightening. The examiner should recommend HIV post-exposure prophylaxis (PEP) to patients reporting sexual assault when significant exposure may have occurred. Significant exposure is defined as direct contact of the vagina, anus, or mouth with the semen or blood of the perpetrator, with or without physical injury, tissue damage, or presence of blood at the site of the assault. Offer PEP as soon as possible following exposure, ideally within 1 hour and not more than 36 hours after exposure.[23]

- If PEP is being considered, consult with a specialist in HIV treatment. If the survivor is at risk for HIV transmission and chooses to start PEP, the following should be adhered to:

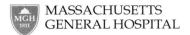

MASSACHUSETTS
GENERAL HOSPITAL

ADULT SEXUAL ASSAULT ORDER SHEET

ALLERGIES: DATE:

TIME	MEDICATION ORDERED	MD SIGNATURE	MEDICATION ADMINISTRATION RECORD	COMMENTS
	STD PROHPHYLAXIS: **Gonorrhea:** • Ceftriaxone 250 mg IM × 1		Time / Initial / Dose / Site	
	OR if allergic to PCN or cephalosporins and no pharyngeal contact • Spectinomycin 2 gm IM × 1		Time / Initial / Dose / Site	
	OR if allergic to PCN or cephalosporins and with pharyngeal contact • Azithromycin 2 gm po × 1		Time / Initial / Dose / Site	
	Chlamydia: • Azithromycin 1 gm po × 1 (unless already given 2 gm Azithromycin for gonorrhea)		Time / Initial / Dose / Site	
	OR if allergic to macrolide antibiotics • Doxycycline 100 mg po BID × 7 days		Time / Initial / Dose / Site	
	Trichomoniasis: • Flagyl 2 g po × 1		Time / Initial / Dose / Site	
	Hepatitis B: (see comments) • Recombivax 10 mcg/1ml IM for age ≥ 20 • For age < 20: age specific dosing		Time / Initial / Dose / Site	Recombivax not needed for patients with known immunity - either had the vaccine or had the disease.
	PREGNANCY PROHYLAXIS: (see comments) • PLAN B (levonorgestrel) 0.75 mg 1 tab now and 1 tab 12 hours later if Hcg is negative.		Time / Initial / Dose / Site	Plan B may be given up to 120 hours after assault.
	OTHER: • Tetanus Toxoid 0.5 ml IM × 1 PRN		Time / Initial / Dose / Site	
	• Antiemetic (when giving Azithromycin, Plan B or Flagyl) (specify): _____		Time / Initial / Dose / Site	
	HIV PROPHYLAXIS: (see comments) • HIV PEP med: _____		Time / Initial / Dose / Site	MD should page ID needle stick beeper (36222) for recommendation. Patient must call 617-726-3906 to schedule follow up visit with ID
	• HIV PEP med: _____		Time / Initial / Dose / Site	within 2-3 days of ED visit. MD will dispense adequate supply of PEP medication until ID visit.

TIME	REQURIED LABS	MD SIGNATURE	RN	COMMENTS
	PREGNANCY TEST: • Urine HCG (HCG serum only when kiosk closed)			
	HEPATITIS SCREEN: • Hepatitis B surface antigen & antibody • Hepatitis C antibody			**NO HOSPITAL TOXICOLOGY SCREEN** (unless medically necessary)
	If starting HIV PEP: (see comments) • CBC with diff, Lytes, Cal, Phos, Mg, LFTS.			**NO HIV TESTING IN THE ED**
INIT.	NURSE'S SIGNATURE.	INIT.	NURSE'S SIGNATURE.	INIT. NURSE'S SIGNATURE.

White - Medical Record Copy   Yellow - Department Copy   84291 (1/04)

Fig. 51-1 Sample adult sexual assault order form. (From Finkel, M., Mian, P., McIntyre, J., Sellas-Ferer, M. I., McGee, B., & Balch, N. (2005). An original, standardized, emergency department sexual assault medication order sheet. *Journal of Emergency Nursing, 31,* 271.)

- Discuss antiretroviral prophylaxis, including toxicity and lack of proven benefit.
- Provide enough medication for the next 3 to 7 days following the initial assessment.
- Facilitate reevaluation of the survivor by an infectious disease physician on the third through seventh day to assess tolerance of the medication.
- Assistance with PEP decisions can be obtained by calling the National Clinician's Post-Exposure Prophylaxis Hotline (PEPline): 1-888-448-4911.

EMOTIONAL SUPPORT FOR SEXUAL ASSAULT VICTIMS

Care of the victim of sexual assault must address the emotional aspects of this traumatic event. Patients' responses to assault vary greatly; some victims have an expressive reaction: crying, shaking, and exhibiting restless, tense, and anxious behavior. Others may appear to be "in control" of their emotions, speaking in a detached or rational manner.

Rape trauma syndrome consists of three characteristic phases: acute, outward adjustment, and long-term reorganization. How successfully the victim progresses through these phases depends in part on the support of friends and family and on professional follow-up. Prepare the patient for possible reactions and symptoms of the acute phase:

- Shock, disbelief
- Guilt and shame
- Fear
- Anxiety, depression
- Flashbacks and nightmares
- Physical symptoms such as stomach pains, loss of appetite, headache, sleep disturbances

Provide the victim with resources to deal with this common syndrome. Refer students to their school or university counseling center. Most cities or towns have a nearby crisis or rape center where counseling services are offered free of charge.

It may be helpful to give the victim the telephone number of the National Sexual Assault Hotline (1-800-656-HOPE). The call is automatically routed to the nearest assault or crisis center and conversations are anonymous and confidential.

FOLLOW-UP

After the initial post-assault examination, follow-up examinations provide an opportunity to:

- Detect new infections acquired during or after the assault.
- Complete hepatitis B immunization, if indicated.
- Complete counseling and treatment for other sexually transmitted infections.
- Monitor side effects of and adherence to PEP medication, if prescribed.

Examination for sexually transmitted infections should be repeated within 1 to 2 weeks of the assault. Because infectious agents acquired through assault may not have produced sufficient concentrations of organisms to result in positive test results at the initial examination, testing should be repeated during the follow-up visit unless prophylactic treatment was provided. If treatment was provided, testing should be conducted only if the survivor reports having symptoms. If treatment was not provided, follow-up examination should be conducted within 1 week to ensure that results of positive tests can be discussed promptly with the survivor and that treatment is provided. Serologic tests for syphilis and HIV infection should be repeated at 6 weeks, 3 months, and 6 months after the assault if initial test results were negative and infection in the assailant could not be ruled out. Educate the patient on the importance of this follow-up and provide the patient with information on where to obtain these follow-up services.

REFERENCES

1. U.S. Department of Justice Office of Violence Against Women. (2004). *A national protocol for sexual assault medical forensic examinations: Adults/adolescents.* Washington, DC: Author.
2. Rape, Abuse, & Incest National Network. (n.d.). *Statistics.* Retrieved from http://www.rainn.org/statistics
3. U.S. Department of Justice. (2011, September 19). *Key facts at a glance.* Retrieved from http://bjs.ojp.usdoj.gov/content/glance/rape.cfm
4. Truman, J. L. (2011, September). *National Crime Victimization Survey: Criminal victimization, 2010.* Retrieved from http://www.bjs.gov/content/pub/pdf/cv10.pdf
5. Tjaden, P., & Thonnes, N. (2006). *Extent, nature, and consequences of rape victimization: Findings from the National Violence Against Women Survey.* Washington, DC: U.S. Department of Justice.
6. Tjaden, P., & Thoennes, N. (2000). *Full report of the prevalence, incidence and consequences of violence against women: Findings from the National Violence Against Women Survey.* Washington, DC: U.S. Department of Justice.
7. Emergency Nurses Association. (2010). *Care of sexual assault and rape victims in the emergency department* [position statement]. Retrieved from http://www.ena.org/SiteCollection Documents/Position%20Statements/SexualAssaultRape Victims.pdf
8. Ernoehazy, W. Jr., & Murphy-Lavoie, H. (2009, December 3). *Sexual assault.* Retrieved from http://emedicine.medscape.com/article/806120-overview

9. Polak, T., & Lindner, H. (2006). Nursing documentation standards and practice in cases of sexual assault. *The Oregon Nurse*, *71*(1), 2.

10. New York State Department of Health. (2004, November). *State of New York protocol for the acute care of the adult patient reporting sexual assault: DNA evidence collection*. Retrieved from http://www.health.state.ny.us/professionals/protocols_and_guidelines/sexual_assault/docs/adult_protocol.pdf

11. Straight, J. D., & Heaton, P. C. (2007). Emergency department care for victims of sexual offense. *American Journal of Health-System Pharmacy*, *64*(17), 1845–1850.

12. Bechtel, K., Ryan, E., & Gallagher, D. (2008). Impact of Sexual Assault Nurse Examiners on the Evaluation of Sexual Assault in a Pediatric Emergency Department. *Pediatric Emergency Care*, *24*(7), 442–447.

13. Emergency Nurses Association. (2010, July). *Standardized ED triage scale and acuity categorization: Joint ENA/ACEP statement*. Retrieved from http://www.ena.org/SiteCollection Documents/Position%20Statements/STANDARDIZEDED TRIAGESCALEANDACUITYCATEGORIZATION.pdf

14. Gilboy, N., Tanabe, P., Travers, D. A., Rosenau, A. M., & Eitel, D. R. (2005). *Emergency Severity Index: Implementation handbook, version 4*, Rockville, MD: AHRQ Publication No. 05-0046-2: Agency for Healthcare Research and Quality.

15. Centers for Disease Control and Prevention. (2008). *Sexual violence: Facts at a glance Spring 2008*. Retrieved from http://www.cdc.gov/violenceprevention/pdf/SV-DataSheet-a.pdf

16. U.S. Department of Justice. (2008, July). *Sexual assault resource service*. Retrieved from http://www.sane-sart.com/staticpages/index.php?page=20031023141144274

17. Beebe, K. R. (2005). The perplexing parity puzzle. *AWHONN Lifelines*, 9, 396.

18. American College of Emergency Physicians. (2008). *Evaluation and management of the sexually assaulted or sexually abused patient*. Dallas, TX: Author.

19. Plichta, S. B., Clements, P. T., & Houseman, C. (2007). Why SANEs matter: Models of care for sexual violence victims in the emergency department. *Journal of Forensic Nursing*, *3*(1), 15–23.

20. Ledray, L. (1999). *Sexual assault nurse examiner (SANE) development and operation guide*. Washington, DC: U.S. Department of Justice, Office for Victims of Crimes.

21. International Association of Forensic Nurses. (n.d.). *Welcome to the SAFEta forms library*. Retrieved from http://www.safeta.org/displaycommon.cfm?an=1&subarticlenbr=69

22. Wild, S. E. (2010). *Webster's new world law dictionary*, Hoboken, NJ: Wiley Publishing, Inc.

23. Centers for Disease Control and Prevention. (2010). Sexually transmitted diseases treatment guidelines, 2010. *Morbidity and Mortality Weekly Report*, *59*(RR-12), 1–110.

24. Finkel, M., Mian, P., McIntyre, J., Sellas-Ferer, M. I., McGee, B., & Balch, N. (2005). An original, standardized, emergency department sexual assault medication order sheet. *Journal of Emergency Nusring*, *31*(3), 271–275.

Pediatric Considerations in Emergency Nursing

Colleen Andreoni

Pediatric patients present a unique challenge to the emergency nurse because of the physiologic and anatomic differences and the vast growth and developmental characteristics specific to this population. Table 52-1 provides information about physical and psychosocial characteristics of the growing child along with guidelines for nursing assessment.[1] In addition, keep in mind that family plays an important role in a child's health care experience.

PEDIATRIC TRIAGE (PRIORITIZATION OF CARE)

There are four components in pediatric triage (or prioritization of care): the pediatric assessment triangle (PAT), focused assessment (objective information), focused pediatric history (subjective information), and assignment of an acuity rating decision.

Pediatric Assessment Triangle

The PAT is a simple observational tool for performing a rapid, visual, across-the-room assessment of children presenting to the emergency department (ED) regardless of presenting complaint.[2] The PAT consists of the following three components:

- Appearance: Muscle tone, consolability, spontaneous movements, speech or cry, distress level
- Breathing: Respiratory distress, abnormal airway sounds
- Circulation: Skin color, such as pale, mottled, cyanotic, or flushed

Allow the caregiver to remain with the patient, as appropriate. Look for additional assessment cues that will prioritize care for each pediatric patient, such as:

- Patient's developmental stage: Is this current behavior in line with his or her typical behavior?
- Significant developmental delays

- Illnesses and injuries common to different developmental ages
- Risk factors for maltreatment
- Compensatory mechanisms of pediatric patients that may mask serious illness or injury
- Risk level for rapid deterioration

The rationale for additional history may include the following:

- Caregiver concerns and perceptions: crying and "fussiness" are vague symptoms
- Rashes that may be a concern for potentially contagious diseases
- Delay in definitive care and nonuse of emergency medical services because of the portability of children
- Use of cultural and home treatments prior to arrival at the ED
- Lack of primary care provider or lack of preventive care (immunization status)

Focused Assessment and History

Following the rapid visual across-the-room assessment, the next step in triage is the focused assessment, which includes the primary and secondary assessments. Refer to Chapter 44, Pediatric Trauma, for more information. Systematically obtain a history, which can be done by using the pneumonic CIAMPEDS (Table 52-2).

Vital Signs

For pediatric patients, obtain a full set of vital signs, including weight in kilograms; obtain a measured weight whenever possible. If circumstances do not permit a measured weight using a scale or length-base resuscitation tape, the weight may be estimated using the following formula: Weight in kilograms = $(3 \times Age) +7$.[3] The nurse should be

Text continued on page 552.

TABLE 52-1 PEDIATRIC GROWTH AND DEVELOPMENT

AGE GROUP	PHYSICAL CHARACTERISTICS	MOTOR SKILLS	PSYCHOSOCIAL CHARACTERISTICS	COMMUNICATION	PAIN AND REFLEXES	ASSESSMENT GUIDELINES
Infant (birth to 1 yr)	Period of the most rapid growth. Weight doubles by 6 mo; triples by 12 mo. Head circumference is 1–2 cm larger than the chest. The posterior fontanel closes by 2–3 mo. Can distinguish odors, including mother's scent. Visual acuity is 20/400 at birth but nears adult acuity levels by 8 mo. The neonatal bladder capacity is ≤15 mL	3 mo: lifts head while prone. 5 mo: turns from abdomen to back. 7 mo: turns from back to abdomen; transfers objects from one hand to the other. 9 mo: sits unsupported. 12 mo: walks with one hand; crawls quickly; sits from a standing position; uses pincer grasp; eats with fingers	Trust versus mistrust. 6 mo: fears separation and strangers. Coping skills: sucking, crying, cooing, babbling, thrashing	Cries in response to needs. Is most interactive during the quiet-alert stage. 12 mo: uses a three-word vocabulary, one-word sentences. Touch is important. Responds to rocking, holding, patting	Experiences pain. Withdraws from pain. Reflexes present at birth: Babinski's reflex: Fans toes up and outward (disappears at 9 mo). Moro (startle): Sudden extension of the arms with return to midline when startled (disappears at 4 mo). Rooting reflex: Turns head toward the stimulated side when the face is stroked	Allow a caregiver to hold the pediatric patient or maintain eye contact (when possible). Allow the infant to keep a security object. Approach gently and quietly. Use distraction techniques. Obtain a rectal temperature at the end of the examination
Toddler (1 to 3 yr)	Growth slows. Average weight gain is ≤5 lb/yr. Brain is 90% of adult size by 2 yr. The anterior fontanel closes by 18–24 mo	12 mo: learning to walk. 15 mo: able to walk alone, begins climbing, has a wide-based gait. 24 mo: can dress self with simple clothing; can kick a ball without losing balance. 2.5 yr: can build a tower of six blocks; draws stick figures	Autonomy versus shame and doubt. Expresses independence as "no!" Possessive of toys and parents. Temper tantrums are common. Transitional objects may help decrease separation anxiety. Spends most of the time playing. Focuses on potty training. Very curious. Fears: separation, loss of control, pain, altered rituals	2 yr: can almost communicate verbally. Attention span is ~2 min at 2 yr. Literally believes what is heard. Uses short, concrete terms when describing or explaining	No formal concept of pain, may react as intensely to painless procedures as to painful ones. Reacts with resistance, aggression, and regression. Is rarely able to fake pain. Gives unreliable answers when questioned about pain	Approach gradually; establish a relationship. Allow the toddler to remain with the caregiver as much as possible. Allow the patient to handle equipment before use. Use play to interact with the patient. Keep skin exposures minimal. Praise the patient for cooperating and when the assessment is finished

(3 to 5 yr)	Limbs grow more than the trunk	undresses self Coordination and muscle strength increase rapidly Jumps rope, skips, plays catch Learns to ride a bike Uses scissors, prints name, can tie shoes	Greater independence Imitates parents and other adults Age of discovery Trial and error leads to learning Magical thinking May see injury or illness as a punishment Fears: mutilation, loss of control, death, dark, ghosts Coping skills: denial, somatization, regression, displacement, projection, fantasy	cause and effect >2100 word vocabulary Uses five-word complete sentences Counts to 10; knows the days of the week, name, and address May benefit if given the chance to ask questions Attention span: ~10 min at 3 yr; ~30 min at 5 yr	punishment Does not understand that painful procedures are necessary to get better All pain is perceived as "bad pain" Reacts to pain with aggression and often "I hate you"	close to caregivers Allow the patient to handle equipment before use Allow the patient to undress self; respect the child's modesty Expose skin only as necessary for assessment Use play and games to elicit cooperation
School age (6 to 12 yr)	Gains ~5.5 lb/yr Lymph tissue grows until 9 yr Frontal sinuses develop at 7 yr Puberty may begin in late school age Increased myelinization improves fine motor skills	Musculoskeletal growth allows greater coordination and strength Involved in active play, sports, and games Performs activities requiring balance and strength Beginning team sports Improved hand-eye coordination Learning new skills	Industry versus inferiority Takes pride in accomplishments Interacts best with same-sex, same-age friends Becoming competitive in games Remains dependent on parents for love and security Beginning to take responsibility Fears: separation from friends, loss of control, physical disability	Attention span >30 min Learns to write in cursive Begins to think logically Understands past, present, and future Growing vocabulary allows description of feelings and thoughts May be unable to verbalize the need for parental support	Reactions to pain are often guided by past experiences Able to talk about pain in simple, descriptive terms May exaggerate pain because of fears of more pain or death	Help foster self-esteem by frequent and sincere praise Opinions of health care are often guided by past experiences Allow privacy and time to compose oneself Explain the purpose of the assessment, relating it to the patient's illness or injury Diagrams and teaching aids are helpful Give older school-age patients the choice of having caregivers remain during the assessment

Continued

TABLE 52-1	PEDIATRIC GROWTH AND DEVELOPMENT—cont'd					
AGE GROUP	**PHYSICAL CHARACTERISTICS**	**MOTOR SKILLS**	**PSYCHOSOCIAL CHARACTERISTICS**	**COMMUNICATION**	**PAIN AND REFLEXES**	**ASSESSMENT GUIDELINES**
Adolescent (12 to 21 yr)	Final growth spurt Experiences puberty Sweat gland function increases; acne is common Increased muscle mass Weight problems and eating disorders often develop at this age	Greater coordination of gross and fine motor skills	Identity versus role confusion Transition from child to adult Peers are important and provide a sense of belonging Moody Developing own values Very private Seeks independence Family dissent is common Involved in risk-taking behaviors Developing sexual orientation Thinking of vocational goals, college Fears: changes in physical appearance or functioning, dependency, loss of control	Memory fully developed Able to project to the future Can see the consequences of actions Uses language to convey ideas, beliefs, values Language includes slang	Accurately locates and describes pain May be hyperresponsive to pain Associates pain with possible changes in appearance or function Usually has good self-control during painful procedures	Give the patient the choice of having caregivers remain during the assessment Explain the purpose of the examination and all equipment Allow the patient to undress in private Provide feedback, especially normals, during the assessment

Data from Andreoni, C., & Klinkhammer, B. (2000). *Quick reference for pediatric emergency nursing.* Philadelphia, PA: Saunders.
lb, Pound; *min,* minute; *mo,* month; *yr,* year.

TABLE 52-2 CIAMPEDS MNEMONIC

	DEFINITION	DESCRIPTION
C	Chief complaint	Reason for the pediatric patient's ED visit and duration of complaint (e.g., fever for past two days).
I	Immunizations	Evaluation of the pediatric patient's current immunization status.
		The completion of all scheduled immunizations for the patient's age should be evaluated.
		If the pediatric patient has not received immunizations because of religious or cultural beliefs, document this information.
I	Isolation	Evaluation of the pediatric patient's exposure to communicable diseases (e.g., meningitis, chickenpox, shingles, whooping cough, and tuberculosis)
		A pediatric patient with active disease or who is potentially infectious must be placed in respiratory isolation on arrival to the ED.
		Other exposures that may be evaluated include exposure to meningitis and scabies.
A	Allergies	Evaluation of the pediatric patient's previous allergic or hypersensitivity reactions.
		Document reactions to medications, food, products (e.g., latex), and environmental allergens. The type of reaction must be documented.
M	Medications	Evaluation of the pediatrics patient's current medication regimen, such as prescription medications, over-the-counter medications, and herbal and dietary supplement, including: • Dose administered • Time of last dose • Duration of use
P	Past medical history	A review of the pediatric patient's health status, including prior illnesses, injuries, hospitalizations, surgical procedures, and chronic physical and psychiatric illnesses. Use of alcohol, tobacco, drugs, or other substances of abuse should be evaluated as appropriate. The medical history of the neonate should include the prenatal and birth history: • Maternal complications during pregnancy or delivery • Infant's gestational age and birth weight • Number of days infant remained in the hospital after birth • The medical history of the menarche of the female patient should include date and description of her last menstrual period The medical history for sexually active patients should include the following: • Type of birth control used • Barrier protection • Prior treatment for sexually transmitted infections • Gravida (pregnancies) and para (pregnancies carried to the 20th week of gestation)
P	Caregiver's impression of the pediatric patient's condition	Evaluation of the caregiver's concerns and observations of the patient's condition. These factors are especially significant when evaluating the special needs pediatric patient. Consider cultural differences that may affect the caregiver's impressions.
E	Events surrounding the illness or injury	Evaluation of the onset of the illness or circumstances and mechanism of injury. Time and date injury occurred: • M: Mechanism of injury, including the use of protective devices (seat belts and helmets) • I: Injuries suspected • V: Vital signs in the prehospital environment • T: Treatment by prehospital providers Description of circumstance leading to injury. Witnessed or unwitnessed. Illness • Length of illness, including date and day of onset and sequence of symptoms • Treatment provided before the ED visit

Continued

TABLE 52-2 CIAMPEDS MNEMONIC—cont'd

	DEFINITION	DESCRIPTION
D	Diet	Assessment of the pediatric patient's recent oral intake and changes in eating patterns related to the illness or injury.
		Time of last meal and last fluid intake.
		Changes in patterns or fluid intake.
		Usual diet: Breast milk, type of formula, solid foods, diet for age and developmental level, and cultural differences.
		Special diet or diet restrictions.
D	Diapers	Assessment of the patient's urine and stool output:
		• Frequency of urination during the past 24 hours and changes in frequency
		• Time of last void
		• Changes in odor or color of urine
		• Last bowel movement and color and consistency of stool
		• Change in the frequency of bowel movements
S	Symptoms associated with the illness or injury	Identification of symptoms and progression of symptoms since the onset of the illness or injury event.

Reprinted from Emergency Nurses Association. (in press). *Emergency nursing pediatric course* (4th ed.). Des Plaines, IL: Author.
ED, Emergency department.

TABLE 52-3 NORMAL RESPIRATORY AND HEART RATES BY AGE GROUP

AGE GROUP	NORMAL RESPIRATORY RATE, BREATHS PER MINUTE	NORMAL HEART RATE, BEATS PER MINUTE
Infant (1 to 12 months)	30–60	100–160
Toddler (1 to 3 years)	24–40	90–150
Preschooler (3 to 5 years)	22–34	80–140
School-aged child (5 to 11 years)	18–30	70–120
Adolescent (11 to 18 years)	12–16	60–100

Reprinted from Emergency Nurses Association. (in press). *Emergency nursing pediatric course* (4th ed.). Des Plaines, IL: Author.

aware of the normal vital signs for a pediatric patient and recognize when vital signs deviate from normal. Normal heart and respiratory rates are described in Table 52-3.

Temperature

- Obtain temperature via an appropriate route considering the pediatric patient's age and condition.
- Avoid rectal temperatures in immunocompromised patients.

- Fever can be associated with abnormal activity, respiratory patterns, or dermal warning signs, such as rashes, cyanosis, or mottling.
- Temperature variations that may indicate a serious condition include the following:
  - Rectal temperature greater than 38.5°C (101.3°F) in infants younger than 1 month of age[4]
  - Rectal temperature greater than 40°C (104°F) in infants aged 3 months to 2 years, with no localized sign of infection
  - Rectal temperature less than 34.2°C (93.2°F)[4]

Blood Pressure

Determine the minimum normal systolic blood pressure for pediatric patients using the following formula: Systolic blood pressure = 70 + (Age in years × 2).

A blood pressure change in children is considered a late change and not always reliable. Blood pressure should be determined by serial measurements, not a single reading.

Acuity Rating Decision

The final step in the prioritization of care process is the triage nurse's interpretation of the pediatric patient's assessment, resulting in an acuity rating decision. The determination of the acuity rating decision provides conclusion for the urgency and order for care. Follow your institution's guidelines for which acuity rating system to use.

MEDICATION ADMINISTRATION AND INTRAVENOUS THERAPY

Because virtually all pediatric medications are dosed according to the pediatric patient's weight, obtain an accurate measurement as part of the focused assessment. If this is not possible, use a length-based resuscitation tape to calculate estimated body mass or use the formula described above. Pediatric patients present unique risk factors that can contribute to medication errors; therefore reducing or managing these risk factors is important. The age and developmental stage of the pediatric patient are essential to consider whenever administering medications. Not only will age influence drug absorption, distribution, and excretion, but the patient's age will often determine the best route for administration and appropriate developmental approaches.[5]

Oral Medications

Children who cannot or will not swallow pills present a nursing challenge. Tips for successful oral medication administration include the following:

- Ask the caregiver how the patient usually takes oral medication.[5]
- Mix or dilute medications in a minimal amount of fluid, applesauce, or chocolate syrup to encourage the patient to ingest the entire dose. When mixing medication with food or liquids use as little diluent as possible.[5]
  - For infants, consider administration of liquid medication through a nipple followed by 5 mL of water. Avoid mixing medication with formula or breast milk because it may lead the infant to refuse formula later.[5]
- Demonstrate to caregiver how to use a syringe to administer medications in the young pediatric patient's buccal cavity.
  - Place the syringe between the gum and cheek. Administer no more than 0.5 mL at a time.[5]
- Administer oral medication while the pediatric patient's head is raised or while the patient is in a sitting position to prevent asphyxiation.[5]
- Consult the pharmacist before opening capsules for administration.[5]
  - Do not crush enteric-coated tablets or caplets.[5]
  - Do not open sustained-release capsules.[5]

Intramuscular Medications

When determining an injection site, consider the pediatric patient's age, weight, and muscle mass, along with the medication volume and viscosity. Table 52-4 provides information regarding intramuscular injections in children.

TABLE 52-4 PEDIATRIC INTRAMUSCULAR INJECTION SITES

SITE	RECOMMENDED AGE
Vastus lateralis	Infant
	Can be used at any age and is the preferred site in children younger than 3 years
	Considerations
	Large muscle mass, free of important nerves and blood vessels
	Acceptable injection volumes: Infants, 0.5–1 mL; older children, up to 2 mL
	Use a 22- to 25-gauge needle (length, ⅝ to 1 inch)

SITE	RECOMMENDED AGE
Ventrogluteal	Child
	Consider for children older than 3 years
	Considerations
	Large muscle mass, free of important nerves and blood vessels
	Easily accessible site
	Injection volume up to 2 mL
	Use a 20- to 25-gauge needle (length, 1 to 1.5 inch)

SITE	RECOMMENDED AGE
Deltoid	Infant
	Considerations
	Small muscle mass, easily accessible, with a rapid absorption rate
	Danger of radial nerve injury in young children
	Injection volumes of 0.5–1 mL
	Use a 22- to 25-gauge needle (length, ½ to 1 inch)

Data from Bindler, R., & Howry, L. (2005). *Pediatric drug guide*. Upper Saddle River, NJ: Pearson Education.

Subcutaneous Injections

- Sites considered include the upper lateral arm, the anterior thigh, and the anterior abdominal wall.[5]
- Limit the injection volume to 0.5 to 1 mL, depending on the age of the patient and the site of the injection.[5]
- Insert needle at a 45- to 60-degree angle in a thin pediatric patient with little subcutaneous tissue or at a 90-degree angle in the patient with generous amounts of subcutaneous fat.[5]

Veins on the dorsum of the hand or foot are the preferred sites for infants and children, while the scalp vein is ideal for infants for over-the-needle intravenous catheter insertion (24 gauge or larger).

Intravenous Therapy

Establishing and maintaining vascular access in the young pediatric patient is one of the most difficult and stressful emergency nursing tasks. Tips for successful intravenous (IV) therapy include the following[6]:

- Provide emotional support to patients and their care-givers; this procedure is anxiety-provoking for both. Give caregivers permission to stay with the patient or leave the room during the procedure.
- Infants tend to have deep veins that are well covered with subcutaneous tissue. In these patients, scalp veins are an excellent alternative to extremity sites.
- In the presence of volume depletion, younger pediatric patients may have no visible peripheral veins, even after a tourniquet has been applied.
- Quickly consider an intraosseous site if the patient is critically ill or injured and requires emergent vascular access. Intraosseous lines offer many benefits and few drawbacks. Refer to Chapter 10, Intravenous Therapy, for more information.
- When selecting a site, try to avoid the antecubital fossa, veins over joints, or the dominant hand.
- Use a warm pack (consider use of a commercially available heel warmer) to dilate potential veins.
- Immobilize the pediatric patient's extremity before veni-puncture if possible. A padded pediatric armboard works well.
- Insert the IV device into the skin at an angle, generally 10 degrees, although this may vary. Flush the catheter with a small amount of saline to ensure patency.
- Inserting the IV device with a bevel down can minimize the risk of puncturing the distal wall.
- Once venous access is obtained, be sure to secure the device well according to hospital guidelines.
- Always use extension tubing and an infusion pump with pediatric IV infusions.
- Volume loss is treated by administering isotonic crystallized fluid boluses (lactated Ringer solution or normal saline). The amount of the bolus is usually cal-culated at a rate of 20 mL/kg and may be repeated based on the patient's response.
- After any volume losses have been replaced, run the patient's IV at maintenance rate. This rate is calcu-lated based on the patient's age and weight. Table 52-5 provides pediatric maintenance formulas.

TABLE 52-5 MAINTENANCE INTRAVENOUS FLUID RATES IN CHILDREN

WEIGHT	AMOUNT PER HOUR (ML)
1–10 kg	100 mL/kg/24 hr
10–20 kg	1000 mL plus 50 mL/kg for each additional kilogram over 10 (up to 20 kg), given over 24 hr
≥21 kg	1500 mL plus 20 mL/kg for each additional kilogram over 21, given over 24 hr

Data from National Institutes of Health. (2008, June 23). *Intravenous fluid management*. Retrieved from http://www.cc.nih.gov/ccc/pedweb/pedsstaff/ivf.html

When starting an intravenous line, the characteristic "pop" may not be felt in small children. The blood flashback seen with a suc-cessful venipuncture may be minimal.

Nasal Administration

Nasal administration of medication may be used to treat respiratory conditions or induce anesthesia. Nasal medica-tions are best administered in infants and toddlers with the patient's head slightly hyperextended on a caregiver's lap. For older children, position the patient with pillows under his or her shoulders to create the hyperextension. Administer drops slowly to prevent choking.

Dermal Administration

- Wear gloves.
- Apply a thin layer of medication and spread in the direction of hair growth.
- If applying an anesthetic cream, apply an occlusive dressing and have a caregiver hold the dressing in place and distract the patient for 30 to 60 minutes.

PEDIATRIC CARDIOPULMONARY ARREST

The pediatric patient in respiratory failure or shock is at high risk for further decompensation and subsequent car-diopulmonary arrest. Advanced life support interventions must be implemented emergently. Begin with basic life support (BLS) maneuvers by immediately opening the airway, assisting ventilations, and initiating cardiac com-pressions as needed. Refer to current American Heart Asso-ciation Basic Life Support and Pediatric Advanced Life Support (PALS) guidelines for pediatric resuscitation.[7] Be sure to facilitate family presence at the bedside and to arrange for transfer to a higher level of care, such as admission to a pediatric intensive care unit (PICU) or to another facility. Start this process early.

Apparent Life-Threatening Events

An apparent life-threatening event (ALTE) is defined as an episode that is frightening to the observer because of a change in the infant's breathing.[8] Previously this condition was referred to as a "near-miss" sudden infant death syndrome (SIDS). ALTEs are characterized by a combination of the following:

- Apnea: central (no respiratory effort) or obstructive
- Color change: cyanosis or pallor
- Marked change in muscle tone (limp)
- Choking or gagging

Parents may fear that the child has died. Reversal or recovery of the condition occurs after the child is stimulated or resuscitated. A detailed and precise description of the event is of paramount importance; the emergency nurse should identify and address any underlying causes such as:

- Events immediately preceding the ALTE (e.g., recent illness, immunizations, daily activities)
- Usual sleep conditions (e.g., position, bedding, bed sharing)
- Precise time when ALTE occurred and association with time of last feeding or presence of fever
- Place where ALTE occurred (e.g., caregiver's arms, crib, bed, car)
- State of infant when found (e.g., awake or asleep; position of sleep, face covered or uncovered)
- If awake, activities during ALTE (e.g., feeding, bathing, crying)
- Reason that led to discovery of the infant (e.g., abnormal cry)
- Caretakers who discovered or witnessed ALTE

Etiology

- Sepsis
- Seizures
- Upper airway abnormalities
- Gastroesophageal reflux disease
- Hypoglycemia
- Poisoning
- Metabolic disorders
- Allergic reaction
- SIDS: 5% to 6% of children with SIDS have a history of an ALTE[9]

Diagnostic Procedures

- Complete blood count (CBC) with differential
- Platelet count
- Arterial blood gases (ABGs)
- Serum chemistry panel
- Chest radiograph
- 12-lead electrocardiogram
- Toxicologic studies

Therapeutic Interventions

Begin continuous cardiorespiratory monitoring and initiate BLS and PALS measures as indicated. Most infants with ALTE should be hospitalized for more evaluation and observation. If home monitoring is started, it is typically terminated following a 6-week period free of recurrent events or when the infant is at least 6 months old. Caregiver education is essential, as is providing a safe disposition on discharge.

Sudden Infant Death Syndrome

SIDS is the sudden death of a child (generally <12 months old) that remains unexplained after postmortem examination, investigation of the death scene, and review of the patient's case history. SIDS is a diagnosis of exclusion. The peak SIDS incidence is between 2 and 4 months of age.[10]

Etiology

The cause of SIDS is unknown, but several different factors may cause infant death. SIDS incidents occur most often between the ages of 0 and 6 months, with Native Americans and African Americans having the highest incidence.[10] It occurs most often in the winter months, with January having the peak incidence.[11] SIDS affects boys more often than girls.[10] Almost all SIDS deaths occur without any warning or symptoms and usually when the infant is thought to be asleep.[11]

The following have been linked to an increased risk of SIDS:

- Exposure to cigarette smoke while in the womb or following birth
- Babies who sleep on their stomachs
- Late or no prenatal care
- Teen mothers
- Multiple-birth babies
- Babies who have soft bedding in their cribs
- Babies who sleep in the same bed as their parents

Therapeutic Interventions

Pacifiers at naptime and bedtime can reduce the risk of SIDS.[12] It is thought that the pacifier may keep the airway open more and also that the infant does not fall into a deep sleep. Other preventative measures include the following:

- Teach the parents infant cardiopulmonary resuscitation.
- Implement BLS and PALS resuscitation guidelines.

Because of the poor prognosis, prehospital protocols may allow the pronouncement of death at the scene without initiation of futile resuscitation efforts.

Most therapeutic interventions are directed toward the grieving family. These include the following:

- Permit the family to say goodbye before discontinuing resuscitation.
- Allow family members to hold the deceased infant (as permitted by municipal rules related to handling of the body by family members); do not rush them.
- Provide mementos such as a lock of hair, footprints, or handprints (these also can be obtained from the funeral home).
- Consult with the antepartum and postpartum nursing staff as they may have a protocol for infant loss that may be helpful in the loss of an infant in the ED.
- Explain to the family that it is unlikely they did anything to cause the infant's death and that there was nothing they could have done to prevent it.
- Describe what will happen next: autopsy, then release to the funeral home.
- Encourage follow-up grief counseling and support groups.
- Many SIDS websites are available as resources for distraught families and staff members.

Despite a 50% decline in the number of SIDS deaths since 1992, thought to be because of the "Back to Sleep" initiative, SIDS remains the leading cause of postneonatal infant death in the United States.[12]

GENERAL PEDIATRIC EMERGENCIES

Pediatric Fever

Fever is the most common single complaint in pediatric patients and accounts for as many as 20% to 25% of pediatric visits to the ED.[13] Fever is defined in a neonate as 38°C (100.4°F).[14] Hyperthermia has a variety of causes, most commonly infection, but it also can result from poisoning, dehydration, heat exposure, metabolic disorders, or collagen-vascular diseases. The presence of fever on presentation, or fever reported at home, may influence triage and treatment decisions in pediatric patients who are at increased risk for sepsis or other serious illness (e.g., neonate, immunocompromised).

Signs and Symptoms

- Rapid pulse
- Flushed skin
- Tachypnea
- Agitation
- Diaphoresis

Therapeutic Interventions

- Administer fluids (oral, subcutaneous, or IV) based on the pediatric patient's need.
- Dress the patient in a minimal amount of lightweight clothing.
- Administer antipyretic medications as indicated[14]:
  - Acetaminophen 15 mg/kg initially
  - Ibuprofen 10 mg/kg (avoid ibuprofen in the infant less than 6 months and the child who has been vomiting)
  - Do not administer aspirin to a child under 12 years of age.
- Give the patient a tepid bath or shower.
- Identify and treat the cause of the elevated temperature.
- A fever of unknown cause in an infant under 3 months of age requires a septic workup that includes blood cultures and urine culture (urine must be obtained via urinary catheterization). A lumbar puncture is also performed in most febrile infants less than 2 to 3 months of age without an identified source of fever.

RESPIRATORY EMERGENCIES

Airway Obstruction

A common cause of respiratory distress in pediatric patients is airway obstruction. If the patient is in distress but still moving some air, attempt to identify the cause of the obstruction. Consider airway obstruction in any sudden onset of airway distress. Perform a rapid assessment, checking for the following:

- Level of consciousness: alert, irritable, lethargic
- Skin signs: color, temperature, moistness
- Signs of hypoxia: circumoral or general cyanosis, rapid respiratory rate
- Upper airway obstruction: stridor, object in the mouth, oropharyngeal edema
- Nasal plugging (infants)
- Use of accessory muscles of respiration: retractions, abdominal muscle use, nasal flaring
- Unusual breath odors: ketones, chemicals, ethanol
- Decreased air movement
- Abnormal lung sounds: wheezes, stridor, crackles, absent
- Vital signs (be sure to include temperature and pain assessment)
- Evidence of dehydration: poor skin turgor, dry mucosa, lack of tears, sunken fontanel
- Signs of trauma: chest, neck, face, head

Nasopharyngeal Obstruction

Obstruction may be caused by the following:
- Foreign body: beads, beans, food, small toy parts
- Impacted nasal secretions (especially in young infants)
- Edema: trauma, infection, swollen adenoids

Signs and Symptoms
- Nasal obstruction: young infants are obligate nose breathers until 6 months of age. Obstruction can be life-threatening.
- Respiratory distress
- Cyanosis

Therapeutic Interventions
- Administer high-flow oxygen by any means the patient will tolerate.
- Assist with foreign body removal and nasal suctioning.
- Use airway adjuncts as indicated, based on level of consciousness and level of distress (an oral airway or an endotracheal tube).

Oropharyngeal Obstruction

Obstruction may be caused by the following:
- Facial trauma
- Swelling of the tongue (anaphylaxis)
- Burns
- Foreign body or aspiration

Signs and Symptoms
- Noisy respirations: gargling, snoring, stridor
- Little or no air movement or respiratory distress
- Tripod positioning: leaning forward with neck and chin extended
- Insistence on a sitting position
- Cyanosis
- Difficulty speaking or hoarseness
- Dysphagia, drooling

Therapeutic Interventions
- Administer moist, high-flow oxygen by any means the patient will tolerate.
- Keep the patient and caregiver calm.
- If the patient is moving air, encourage him or her to cough but do not attempt to remove the foreign body and do not force the patient to change position.
- If there is no air movement in a patient with a known foreign body obstruction, perform the following maneuvers:
  - Infant: Hold the patient prone, with head lower than the trunk; administer five back blows followed by up to five chest thrusts (stop if the object is dislodged).
  - Child: Administer a series of up to five subdiaphragmatic abdominal thrusts (Heimlich maneuver).

- Attempt to ventilate the patient.
- Repeat the steps above until the foreign body is expelled or prepare to assist with an invasive method of removal (i.e., direct laryngoscopy) or cricothyrotomy.

Upper Airway Disorders

Upper airway conditions are associated with varying degrees of obstruction and are characterized by hoarseness and inspiratory stridor. The disorders involved include acute epiglottitis, acute laryngotracheobronchitis (LTB), acute spasmodic laryngitis, and acute tracheitis. Of these, bacterial epiglottitis is the most life-threatening, but acute viral LTB is the most common cause of stridor in children.

Epiglottitis[15]

Epiglottitis is defined as an acute inflammation of the epiglottis. This condition occasionally is seen in connection with upper airway burns and direct trauma but most frequently it is the result of a rapidly progressive, potentially lethal bacterial infection of the epiglottis and surrounding structures. *Haemophilus influenzae* type B was previously considered the usual causative organism. Today, no single organism is considered the usual cause of epiglottitis.

> The number of cases of epiglottitis has declined sharply since 1988 when childhood *Haemophilus influenzae* type B vaccination became routine in developed countries. In fact, the incidence of epiglottitis is now greater among adults than children.[15]

Signs and Symptoms[16]
- Typically seen in unimmunized children of 2 to 5 years of age
- Abrupt onset of symptoms
- Temperature higher than 39.5°C (103.1°F)
- Sore throat, muffled voice ("hot potato" voice)
- Inspiratory stridor, respiratory difficulty
- Neck extended and chin extended ("turtle sign" or "sniffing position")
- Anxious appearance, agitation
- Absent cough
- Pallor, tachycardia

> The three D's of epiglottitis are drooling, dysphagia, and distress.

Diagnostic Procedures
- Diagnosis generally is based on history and examination.
- Lateral soft tissue neck radiographs will demonstrate massive epiglottal swelling, giving it a "thumb" shape. Exercise caution when obtaining radiographs in patients

highly suspicious for epiglottitis. Unnecessary agitation may worsen the airway obstruction.

- An accurate history and physical examination may be adequate for diagnosis.

Therapeutic Interventions

- Administer high-flow humidified oxygen by any means the patient will tolerate. Nebulized racemic epinephrine may be given until the airway is definitively controlled.
- Patients may require emergent endotracheal intubation. Coordinate care between anesthesia, otolaryngology, and pediatric intensivists whenever possible. The preferred location for definitive airway management is an operating suite, with a highly experienced clinician to perform the intubation.
- Institute continuous cardiorespiratory monitoring.
- Keep the patient as calm as possible; crying stimulates laryngospasm and airway obstruction.
- Do not attempt to look in the patient's mouth; doing so could possibly aggravate spasm and progress to complete airway obstruction.
- Delay invasive diagnostic tests and procedures (e.g., IV access) until the airway is secure.
- Ensure that the equipment for emergent endotracheal intubation and cricothyrotomy is available at the patient's bedside.
- Administer antibiotics as soon as the airway is secured.
- Corticosteroids may reduce swelling in the first 24 hours.
- Prepare for PICU admission.

Acute Laryngotracheobronchitis[15]

Acute LTB, commonly referred to as "croup," is the most frequent cause of upper airway obstruction in children. Acute LTB is a viral infection of the trachea and larynx (which may extend to the bronchi) that causes edema and inflammation of the laryngotracheal mucosa. Transmission occurs through direct contact with respiratory secretions. The incidence of infection is highest in the fall and winter months, and severity ranges from mild (stage I) to severe (stage IV). Various tools for scoring the severity of croup have been developed; however, their use remains controversial.[15]

Signs and Symptoms

- Patient age: usually 6 months to 3 years of age, with peak incidence at 2 years of age[15]
- Signs of an upper respiratory tract infection
- Several-day history of increasing nocturnal respiratory distress
- Overall appearance of being active and well
- Low-grade fever
- Loud "barking" cough
- Hoarse voice, inspiratory stridor

- Tachypnea, sternal retractions
- Tachycardia

Diagnostic Procedures

- Diagnosis is based on history and examination.
- Subglottic narrowing ("steeple sign") may be present on anterior-posterior neck radiographs, although it is absent in up to 50% of patients with LTB.[15]

Therapeutic Interventions

- Administer cool, high-flow humidified oxygen by any means the patient will tolerate. Recent research has not validated the efficacy of this treatment for moderate to severe LTB; however, it continues to be used in many facilities.
- Nebulized racemic epinephrine can be given until the airway is definitively controlled. Effects of treatment are seen within 30 minutes and last for 2 hours. Symptoms can return when the effects of epinephrine wear off. Patients treated with epinephrine should be observed for at least 3 to 4 hours in the ED before discharge.[16]
- Institute continuous cardiorespiratory monitoring.
- Systemic steroids are the mainstay of treatment. Corticosteroids reduce airway swelling and thus the severity and duration of mild to severe LTB episodes.[14] They may be administered nasally, orally, or parenterally. Oral and parenteral administration have similar results.[14] The ease of oral administration is often preferred in the ED. Dexamethasone (0.6 mg/kg) as a one-time dose has been proven effective in many cases of moderate to severe croup.[17]

Bronchiolitis[18]

Bronchiolitis is a term representing a set of symptoms related a viral infection of the lower respiratory tract responsible for inflammation of the smaller airways. It is particularly prevalent in children under 4 years of age, especially infants. This condition is most pervasive in the winter months and in early spring. Patients at highest risk are those who were less than 34 weeks gestational age at birth, had a low birth weight, were exposed to tobacco smoke, and have compromised cardiac, pulmonary, neurologic, or immune systems.

Etiology

- Respiratory syncytial viruses (RSV) are the most common infective organisms in bronchiolitis.
- Other pathogens include adenoviruses, parainfluenza, rhinovirus, and influenza. (Human metapneumovirus is the most common cause of non-RSV bronchiolitis in infants.)
- Most often seen in the winter and early spring.
- Infants who are premature or ones who have cardiac or pulmonary disease are at greatest risk.

Signs and Symptoms
- History of mild respiratory infection, rhinorrhea
- Worsening of symptoms noted first 3 to 5 days, with gradual improvement afterward
- Respiratory difficulty: prolonged expiratory phase, dyspnea
- Diminished breath sounds, wheezing, crackles
- Frequent coughing
- Rhinorrhea
- Pharyngitis
- Intercostal and subcostal retractions, nasal flaring
- Poor feeding
- Apneic spells

Diagnostic Procedures
- Chest radiographs show hyperinflation, interstitial infiltrates, or atelectasis
- CBC with differential
- Nasal swab or nasal washing for respiratory syncytial virus antigens
- Rapid immunofluorescent antibody testing
- Enzyme-linked immunoabsorbent assay
- Viral cultures (may take several days to get results)

Racemic epinephrine is the agent of choice for aerosolized bronchodilator therapy.

Therapeutic Interventions
- Place the patient on contact and droplet isolation.[19]
- Obtain a nasal swab specimen.
- Institute continuous cardiac, respiratory, and oxygen saturation monitoring.
- Management is directed toward symptom and supportive care.
- Administer humidified oxygen to keep saturation greater than 95%.
- Administer aerosolized bronchodilator therapy (patient response to this intervention varies).
- Corticosteroid administration has not been proven to be beneficial.
- Palivizumab is indicated for high-risk infants or young children with chronic lung disease, a history of prematurity, or a history of congenital heart disease.[20]
- For patients with severe tachypnea, provide IV rehydration.
- Endotracheal intubation and positive pressure ventilation may be required for patients in severe distress.
- Antiviral therapy with ribavirin may be an option for patients refractory to conventional therapy.

Disposition
- Indications for admission include persistent desaturation below 95%, tachypnea, and age under 6 months.

- Upon discharge to home, follow-up with the patient's pediatric primary care provider is recommended in 1 to 2 days.

Pertussis

Commonly referred to as whooping cough, pertussis is a highly contagious, acute bacterial infection caused by *Bordetella pertussis* with an incubation period of 7 to 10 days.

Signs and Symptoms
- Paroxysmal spasms of coughing with thick mucous in the tracheobronchial tree
- Long inspiratory effort with high-pitched whoop
- Cyanosis (which may occur during a paroxysm of coughing)
- Vomiting and fatigue after each episode
- Ill and distressed appearance when coughing
- Appears normal when not coughing

Therapeutic Interventions
- Initiate droplet precautions
- Provide supportive care
- Administer medications as ordered. Erythromycin is the antibiotic of choice and may be given to all close contacts.[20]
- Counsel caregivers about the need to obtain a booster or begin immunizations for others in the home, especially when a newborn is present.

Pneumonia

Pneumonia is an inflammation of the lung parenchyma caused by a variety of infectious agents, including viruses, bacteria, and mycoplasma. Table 52-6 gives characteristics of various pneumonia types.

Therapeutic Interventions
- Perform serial respiratory assessments.
- Place the patient in a position of comfort.
- Hydrate as necessary with oral and IV fluids.
- Administer humidified oxygen to maintain saturation greater than 95%.
- Administer antibiotics.
- Give antipyretics as needed.
- Treat bronchospasm with bronchodilators.

Disposition
- Most pediatric patients with pneumonia can be treated and released from the ED.
- Consider admission for patients who meet the following criteria:
  - Apneic, cyanotic, or greatly fatigued
  - At high risk for complications
  - Has a concomitant pleural effusion
  - Requires supplemental oxygen

TABLE 52-6   **TYPES OF PNEUMONIA WITH CHARACTERISTIC FEATURES**

	VIRAL	BACTERIAL	MYCOPLASMAL
Causative agent	Respiratory syncytial virus, parainfluenza, influenza, adenovirus, rhinovirus	*Streptococcus pneumoniae, Staphylococcus aureus, Haemophilus influenza*	*Mycoplasma pneumoniae*
Age	All ages, most common in children <5 years	All ages	Most common in children <5 years
Onset	Gradual	Rapid	Gradual
Fever	Moderate	High, often with chills	Low
Cough	Dry	Productive	Dry, hacking, especially at night
Breath sounds	Few crackles, few wheezes	Decreased, crackles, rhonchi	Fine crackles, rare wheezes
Other signs or symptoms	Severity varies; myalgias	Pleuritic pain, anorexia	Headache, pharyngitis, malaise, anorexia
	Chest radiograph: diffuse or patchy infiltrates	Chest radiograph: diffuse or patchy infiltrates	Chest radiograph: may show areas of consolidation
	White blood cells normal	White blood cells increased, often with increased bands	White blood cells normal
Specific emergency department treatment	Supportive care	Supportive care	Supportive care
	Susceptible to a secondary infection	Antibiotics	Antibiotics

Data from Andreoni, C., & Klinkhammer, B. (2000). *Quick reference for pediatric emergency nursing.* Philadelphia, PA: Saunders and Centers for Disease Control and Prevention. (2011, November 7). *Pneumonia.* Retrieved from http://www.cdc.gov/features/Pneumonia/

The three pathologic components of asthma are bronchospasm, inflammation, and mucous plugging.

Asthma

Asthma is a recurrent reactive airway disease associated with reversible obstruction. The airways of asthmatic patients are hyperresponsive to a variety of triggers that stimulate the release of inflammatory mediators. Hypoxia and hypercarbia result from a mismatch between ventilation and perfusion produced by these conditions. Children at high risk for life-threatening exacerbations include those with a history of the following:

- Prior endotracheal intubation or PICU admission for asthma
- Two or more asthma hospitalizations in the past year
- Three or more visits to the ED for asthma within the last 12 months
- A visit to the ED or inpatient admission for asthma within the past month
- Daily oral corticosteroid use

Etiology and Triggers

- Allergens
- Environmental irritants
- Cold air
- Respiratory infections
- Exercise

Signs and Symptoms

The following signs and symptoms depend greatly on the severity of the exacerbation:

- Shortness of breath, cough, dyspnea, tachypnea
- Use of accessory muscles, retractions
- Nasal flaring, grunting
- Chest discomfort
- Diminished breath sounds
- Prolonged expiration
- Expiratory wheezes (also may have inspiratory wheezing)
- No expiratory sounds (silent chest) if air movement is minimal
- Tachycardia
- Exercise intolerance
- Hypocapnia initially; hypercapnia develops as the patient decompensates

---

Routine chest radiographs are *not* indicated for asthma.

Diagnostic Procedures

- Oxygen saturation (pulse oximetry)
- Serial peak expiratory flow rate measurements (before and after each intervention)
- Obtain chest radiographs only for patients with the following:

- The first episode of wheezing
- Suspected pneumonia, pneumothorax, or other respiratory disorder
- Unilateral wheezing (to rule out foreign body)
- Severe exacerbations unresponsive to treatment.
- ABGs (for severe exacerbations only)

Therapeutic Interventions

- Institute continuous cardiac, respiratory, and oxygen saturation monitoring.
- Administer supplemental oxygen to maintain saturation above 95%.
- Administer an inhaled beta$_2$-agonist (albuterol or levalbuterol).
    - These drugs relax smooth airway muscles and have a 5-minute onset of action.
- Inhaled beta$_2$-agonists can be given using the following:
    - A metered dose inhaler with spacer. Observe for correct technique. Administer every 20 minutes as needed.
    - A nebulizer. Administer continuously or every 20 minutes as needed.
    - Initiate vascular access for severe exacerbations.
- Bronchodilators treat only the bronchospastic component of asthma.
- Anti-inflammatory agents address the inflammatory component and have been shown to reduce the rate of relapse.
- Administer corticosteroids as soon as possible for moderate to severe exacerbations.
- Administer anticholinergics (e.g., ipratropium bromide). These medications decrease vagal stimulation of the airways. Ipratropium bromide can be administered by metered dose inhaler with a spacer or by nebulizer. The drug may be mixed with albuterol.
- Consider administration of epinephrine, terbutaline, ketamine, or heliox (although the effectiveness of most of these agents is not well supported in the literature) for severe, refractory exacerbations.
- Consider administration of magnesium sulfate, as it inhibits calcium channel smooth muscle contraction and reduces acetylcholine release.
- Consider noninvasive positive pressure ventilation (e.g., biphasic positive airway pressure) or endotracheal intubation and mechanical ventilation for severe exacerbations.
- Initiate antibiotic therapy if indicated, but most exacerbations are associated with viral, not bacterial, infections.
- Do not allow asthmatics to become hypoxic, hypercarbic, or acidotic. Once patients have reached this state,

intubation is associated with a high incidence of mortality. Permissive hypercarbia in pediatric patients is acceptable if the patient maintains normal mental status; intubation in the pediatric asthma population is not done as early as in the adult asthma population.[21]

> Oral steroid preparations are just as effective as parenteral (intravenous or intramuscular) steroid administration. All routes have an onset of action of about 6 hours, so initiation of therapy should not be delayed.

Disposition

- Prepare to admit any pediatric patient who remains symptomatic, hypoxic, or fatigued. Consider PICU admission.
- Discharge those with improved peak expiratory flow rates and minimal symptoms.
- Encourage follow-up with the patient's pediatric primary care provider in 2 days.
- Provide patient education and discharge instructions.
- Observe, coach, and correct patient's peak expiratory flow rate measurement technique and metered dose inhaler technique.
- Emphasize the importance of routine peak expiratory flow rate monitoring and having an individualized action plan.
- Discuss the appropriate use of corticosteroids (oral and inhaled) and beta$_2$-agonists (long-acting and short-acting).
- Emphasize early signs of exacerbation and red flags.
- Teach trigger avoidance strategies.

NEUROLOGIC EMERGENCIES

The Unconscious Pediatric Patient

Evaluation of the pediatric patient with a severely altered level of consciousness must be rapid, systematic, and thorough. Determining the cause is crucial but immediate priority is given to supporting airway, breathing, and circulation. Refer to Chapter 44, Pediatric Trauma, for the pediatric patient with unconsciousness related to injury.

Possible Etiologies

Central Nervous System
- Trauma
- Infection
- Seizures

Cardiovascular
- Heart failure
- Congenital heart disease
- Infection

Respiratory

- Acute respiratory failure, obstruction, or hypoxia
- Trauma
- Allergy
- Infection

Shock

- Septic
- Hypovolemic
- Neurogenic
- Cardiogenic
- Anaphylactic

Gastrointestinal

- Vomiting and diarrhea (dehydration)

Metabolic

- Ketoacidosis
- Hypoglycemia
- Toxic exposure
- Reye's syndrome
- Renal or hepatic failure

Endocrine

- Addisonian crisis
- Diabetes mellitus

Signs and Symptoms

- Poor muscle tone
- Decreased level of responsiveness
- Loss of bladder or bowel control (in a toilet-trained child)
- Lack of awareness of the surroundings; poor interaction with environment
- Pallor, mottling, cyanosis
- Delayed capillary refill
- Tachypnea, apnea
- Bradycardia, tachycardia
- Hypothermia, hyperthermia

Diagnostic Procedures

- CBC with differential
- Chemistry panel
- Bedside glucose level
- Ammonia level
- Toxicology screen, ethanol level
- ABGs
- Lumbar puncture
- Computed tomography (CT) scan of the brain
- Chest radiograph

Therapeutic Interventions

- Initiate cardiorespiratory monitoring.
- Obtain intravascular access.
- Monitor oxygen saturation, administer oxygen as necessary, and consider endotracheal intubation.

- Determine serum glucose. Treat hypoglycemia with dextrose.
- Measure temperature.
- Perform neurologic assessments, including serial pediatric Glasgow Coma Scale scoring (Table 52-7).
- Obtain a history and description of events from the family, caregivers, or prehospital personnel.
- Insert a gastric tube and decompress the stomach.
- Place an indwelling urinary catheter
- Maintain normothermia; warm or cool as needed.
- Definitive treatment depends on the cause of unconsciousness.

Febrile Seizures

The most common cause of seizures in young children is fever. Febrile seizures usually occur between the ages of 6 months and 3 years, with a peak incidence at 18 months.[22] These seizures are associated with a febrile illness, most often viral. However, other seizure causes must be excluded before a definitive diagnosis is made. Seizure causes include hypoglycemia, hypoxia, central nervous system infections, toxins, epilepsy, metabolic disorders, developmental defects, and head trauma. In addition, seizures in the pediatric population are frequently idiopathic. Refer to Chapter 25, Neurologic Emergencies, for further information on seizure disorders.

> "Febrile seizures" is not a seizure disorder, although 30% to 40% of children who experience a febrile seizure will have another.[22]

Signs and Symptoms

- History of a preceding illness with a rapidly elevating fever
- Self-limited, generalized, tonic-clonic motor activity
- Duration less than 15 minutes, usually followed by a postictal period
- Normal level of consciousness that returns after the postictal period

> A febrile seizure usually occurs within 24 hours of the onset of fever.[22]

Diagnostic Procedures

- Serum glucose level.
- Consider a chemistry panel, CBC with differential, and blood cultures.
- Lumbar puncture is indicated if the seizure cause is unclear, the patient is highly symptomatic, or a central nervous system infection is suspected.
- Send cerebrospinal fluid (CSF) to laboratory for cell count, Gram stain, culture, protein, and glucose.

TABLE 52-7	**PEDIATRIC GLASGOW COMA SCALE**		
Eye Opening	**0–1 Year** **4:** Spontaneously **3:** To verbal command **2:** To pain **1:** No response	**≥1 Year** **4:** Spontaneously **3:** To verbal command **2:** To pain **1:** No response	
Best Motor Response	**0–1 Year** **5:** Localizes pain **4:** Flexion–withdrawal **3:** Flexion–abnormal (decorticate rigidity) **2:** Extension (decerebrate rigidity) **1:** No response	**≥1 Year** **6:** Obeys **5:** Localizes pain **4:** Flexion–withdrawal **3:** Flexion–abnormal (decorticate rigidity) **2:** Extension (decerebrate rigidity) **1:** No response	
Best Verbal Response	**0–2 Years** **5:** Cries appropriately, smiles, and coos **4:** Cries **3:** Inappropriate crying or screaming **2:** Grunts **1:** No response	**2–5 Years** **5:** Appropriate words and phrases **4:** Inappropriate words **3:** Cries or screams **2:** Grunts **1:** No response	**>5 Years** **5:** Oriented and converses **4:** Disoriented and converses **3:** Inappropriate words **2:** Incomprehensible sounds **1:** No response

Note: Score is the sum of the individual scores from eye opening, best motor response, and best verbal response, using age-specific criteria.
A score of 13 to 15 indicates mild neurologic dysfunction; 9 to 12 indicates moderate neurologic dysfunction; and 8 or less indicates severe neurologic dysfunction.
Data from Barkin, R. M., & Rosen, P. (2003). *Emergency pediatrics: A guide to ambulatory care* (6th ed.). St. Louis, MO: Mosby.

Therapeutic Interventions

Generally, patients with a febrile seizure will recover by the time they arrive at the ED. The presence of continued seizures or a prolonged postictal period strongly suggests a nonfebrile cause. Treatment is largely symptomatic and is focused on airway, breathing, circulation, and seizure control.

Interventions include the following:
- Protect seizing or postictal patients from injury.
- When possible, place the child in a lateral decubitus position.
- Suction secretions as needed to maintain airway patency. A nasopharyngeal airway can be inserted even in patients with a clenched jaw.
- Administer 100% oxygen by mask or blow-by during the seizure and postictal period to maintain saturation.
- Assist ventilations as indicated.
- If the seizure is prolonged, initiate vascular access for anticonvulsant infusion. Consider an intraosseous site.
- Anticonvulsants can be administered by intramuscular and rectal routes, but absorption is slow and unreliable.

- Prepare for endotracheal intubation if there is a delayed return of spontaneous respirations. Rapid sequence intubation is necessary if the patient is still seizing. (See Chapter 15, Procedural Sedation, for more information.)
- Correct hypoglycemia.

Disposition

- Consider admission for children less than 1 year of age.[23]
- Parental reassurance and education is essential upon discharge from the ED.
- Discharge patients that are stable after febrile seizure that do not have a serious infectious cause.
- Admit patients who remain symptomatic and those with a first-time seizure of questionable cause.
- Administer antipyretics and antibiotics as directed.
- Encourage follow-up with the patient's pediatric primary care provider in 2 to 5 days.
- Instruct caregivers in ways to manage seizures at home.

Meningitis

Meningitis is an acute inflammation of the meninges from a viral or bacterial infection. Infection can progress rapidly and may invade the cerebral ventricles. Continued inflammation leads to increases in intracranial pressure. Infection can progress rapidly and may invade the ventricles. The clinical presentation of meningitis varies with the age of the child and the severity of the illness. Viral meningitis is generally much less severe than bacterial.[24] Neurologic sequelae are common in those who survive bacterial meningitis. The most common bacterial organisms are *H. influenzae*, *Streptococcus pneumoniae*, and *Neisseria meningitidis*. Table 52-8 highlights signs and symptoms of bacterial meningitis by age group.[1]

Like epiglottitis, the declining incidence of viral meningitis has been attributed to the introduction of routine *H. influenzae* type B immunization. Symptoms tend to be similar to those of bacterial meningitis but are considerably milder. Common findings include fever, stiff neck, and headache. Symptom severity dictates the extent of diagnostic studies and therapeutic interventions.

Diagnostic Procedures

- CBC with differential
- Chemistry panel
- Bedside glucose level
- Urinalysis and urine culture
- ABGs
- Coagulation profile
- Blood cultures
- Lumbar puncture: send CSF for cultures, Gram stain, protein, glucose, and cell count
- CT scan of the brain
- Chest radiograph

Therapeutic Interventions

- Initiate respiratory isolation.
- Maintain airway, breathing, and circulation.
- Administer supplemental oxygen.
- Obtain vascular access and administer the following:
  - Fluid boluses (20 mL/kg) for hypotension and poor perfusion
  - Antibiotics
  - Antipyretics
  - Analgesics
- Administration of dexamethasone for suspected *H. influenzae* meningitis has not been proven to be a beneficial adjunct in improving outcomes.[25]
- Perform ongoing neurologic assessments and document Pediatric Glasgow Coma Scale score.

TABLE 52-8	SIGNS AND SYMPTOMS OF BACTERIAL MENINGITIS

Neonate
- Symptoms are often vague, nonspecific, or absent
- Fever or hypothermia
- Irregular respiratory patterns, apnea
- Altered level of consciousness: lethargy, irritability
- Bulging or tense fontanel
- Weak cry
- Meningeal signs possibly absent
- Opisthotonus (head, neck, and spine are arched backward)
- Poor muscle tone
- Seizures
- Petechia or purpura
- Poor feeding
- Weak suck
- Vomiting, diarrhea

Infant to Toddler
- Altered level of consciousness: lethargy, irritability
- Fever
- Bulging fontanel
- High-pitched cry
- Meningeal signs may be absent in child less than 2 years of age
- Petechia or purpura
- Poor feeding
- Vomiting
- Ataxia

Preschooler to Adolescent
- Altered level of consciousness: confusion, lethargy, irritability
- Fever
- Headache
- Photophobia
- Meningeal signs:
  - Positive Brudzinski sign (passive flexion of head produces flexion of the hips)
  - Positive Kernig sign (pain with flexion of the hip and extension of the knee)
- Seizures
- Purpura
- Myalgias
- Anorexia, nausea, vomiting, diarrhea

Data from Andreoni, C., & Klinkhammer, B. (2000). *Quick reference for pediatric emergency nursing*. Philadelphia, PA: Saunders; and Kim, K. S. (2010). Acute bacterial meningitis in infants and children. *Lancet Infectious Diseases, 10*(1), 32–42.

- Consider placing a gastric tube and indwelling urinary catheter.
- Institute seizure precautions.
- Assist with lumbar puncture after CT scan.
  - Arrange the older pediatric patient or young infant in a sitting or side-lying position. Place younger pediatric patients in a lateral decubitus position to provide maximal control.
  - Avoid airway compromise during the procedure; continuously monitor heart rate and oxygen saturation.
  - Number CSF specimens as they are drawn and send the tubes for testing in the following order:
    1. Culture and Gram stain
    2. Protein and glucose
    3. Cell count
    4. Miscellaneous tests as ordered

> Do *not* hold antibiotics if the lumbar puncture or blood cultures are delayed in the patient with suspected meningitis.

Disposition

- Facilitate PICU admission for the patient with an abnormal cardiorespiratory or neurologic status.
- Stable patients with viral meningitis may be discharged.
- Provide caretakers with information regarding the disease course, symptomatic treatments, and comfort measures.

Meningococcemia

Meningococcemia is a systemic bacterial infection caused by *N. meningitidis.* Sepsis occurs with or without concomitant meningitis. Meningococcemia is a rapidly progressive disease capable of producing death from shock and coagulopathies within hours of symptom onset.

Signs and Symptoms

- Fever (or hypothermia in the neonate and young infant)
- Chills
- Rash: petechia, purpura
- Headache, irritability, altered level of consciousness, coma
- Hypotension
- Diffuse bleeding

Diagnostic Procedures

- Lumbar puncture: send CSF for cultures, Gram stain, protein, glucose, and cell count
- CBC with differential

- Chemistry panel
- Glucose
- Erythrocyte sedimentation rate
- Urinalysis, urine culture
- Coagulation profile and disseminated intravascular coagulation screen

Therapeutic Interventions

- Immediate recognition and intervention.
- Implement droplet isolation precautions.
- Institute continuous cardiorespiratory monitoring.
- Provide supplemental high-flow oxygen.
- Obtain vascular access and give isotonic crystalloid boluses (20 mL/kg) for hypotension and poor perfusion.
- Rapidly initiate antibiotic administration.

Disposition

- Facilitate PICU admission.
- Consider antibiotic prophylaxis for family, friends, and staff members with potential droplet exposure.

Ventriculoperitoneal Shunt Emergencies

Children with hydrocephalus often are brought to the ED with a problem related to their ventriculoperitoneal (VP) shunt. These catheters are placed surgically to redirect CSF from the ventricles to the peritoneal cavity in patients with inadequate ventricular drainage. The two most common problems are shunt malfunction and shunt infection. Malfunction involves catheter obstruction, disconnection, or distal tip migration.

Signs and Symptoms

Ventriculoperitoneal Shunt Malfunction in Infants
- Vomiting
- Increased head circumference, separation of the cranial sutures
- Bulging or tense fontanels
- Irritability, lethargy

Ventriculoperitoneal Shunt Malfunction in Older Children
- Altered level of consciousness
- Vomiting
- Headache
- Ataxia
- Seizures

Signs and Symptoms of Ventriculoperitoneal Shunt Infection
- Nausea
- Headache
- Fever
- Malaise, altered level of consciousness
- Signs and symptoms consistent with meningitis

TABLE 52-9   DEHYDRATION SEVERITY

SIGNS AND SYMPTOMS	MILD (<5% LOSS)	MODERATE (5% TO 10% LOSS)	SEVERE (10% TO 15% LOSS)
Mucous membranes	Somewhat dry	Dry	Very dry
Skin turgor	Normal	Poor	Very poor
Anterior fontanel	Normal	Sunken	Sunken
Eye appearance	Normal	Sunken	Sunken
Heart rate	Normal	Increased moderately	Increased greatly
Respiratory rate	Normal	Increased	Increased
Blood pressure	Normal	Minimally decreased	Decreased
Skin	Pale, warm	Very pale to mottled, cool	Mottled to cyanotic, cool
Capillary refill	Normal	Minimally delayed	Delayed
Urine output	Normal	Decreased	Decreased to none
Mental status	Normal	Normal to lethargic	Lethargic to unresponsive

Diagnostic Procedures

- Radiographic: views of the lateral neck, chest, and abdomen (shunt series)
- CT scan of the head
- Other tests may be performed in patients with a possible coexisting infection.

> Ventriculoperitoneal shunt infections most commonly occur 1 to 2 months after catheter insertion.

Disposition

Patients with VP shunt malfunction frequently require PICU admission and surgical shunt revision. Children with shunt-related infections are treated aggressively with antibiotic therapy in a PICU.

GASTROINTESTINAL EMERGENCIES

Vomiting and Diarrhea

A variety of conditions may cause vomiting and diarrhea in children, the most common of which is self-limiting viral gastroenteritis. Intractable vomiting occurs with increased intracranial pressure, Reye's syndrome, gastroesophageal reflux, pyloric stenosis, toxicities, or bowel obstruction.

Diarrhea is defined as three or more liquid stools in a day. Viruses, bacteria, parasites, toxins, gastrointestinal bleeding, medications, malabsorption syndromes, certain diets, and bowel disorders can produce diarrhea. Regardless of the cause, diarrhea generally stops within a week. Serious episodes are characterized by voluminous stools, bloody diarrhea, and coexisting vomiting. Decompensation can progress rapidly. Although most cases of vomiting and diarrhea are mild and self-limiting, gastroenteritis is the leading cause of childhood mortality in developing nations.

Etiology

- Infectious causes are viral, bacterial, or parasitic.
- Transmission is by the oral-fecal route or person to person.
- The incidence of viral gastroenteritis is highest during the winter months.
- Bacterial gastroenteritis is more common in the summer.
- Noninfectious causes are toxins, gastrointestinal bleeding, malabsorption syndromes, certain diets, bowel disorders, cathartic abuse, and medications (e.g., antibiotics).

Signs and Symptoms

- Abdominal pain, often cramping
- Fever
- Dehydration (Table 52-9)
- Dry mucous membranes
- Limited tearing
- Decreased urine output
- Sunken anterior fontanel
- Sunken-appearing eyes
- Weight loss
- Thirst
- Poor skin turgor
- Listlessness
- Prolonged capillary refill
- Hypovolemic shock

Diagnostic Procedures

- The scope and extent of diagnostic testing in the child with vomiting and diarrhea depends on the duration and severity of symptoms and their probable cause.
- Testing includes the following:
  - CBC with differential
  - Chemistry panel

TABLE 52-10 ORAL REHYDRATION THERAPY (ORT) FOR MILD TO MODERATE DEHYDRATION

Using Oral Rehydration Solution (ORS)[a]

Option 1	100 mL/kg of ORS over 4 hours		
Option 2	ORS in the amount of two times the estimated stool volume over 6 to 12 hours		
Option 3	10 mL/kg of ORS for each diarrheal stool		
Maintenance fluid therapy: after adequate rehydration			
Administer orally: ORS, breast milk, soy-based formula, or half-strength milk			
Weight	1 to 10 kg	10 to 20 kg	Next 21 kg
Amount	4 mL/kg/hour	4 + 2 mL/kg/hour	4 + 2 + 1 mL/kg/hour
Diarrheal stool replacement	5 to 10 mL/kg for each liquid stool	5 to 10 mL/kg for each liquid stool	5 to 10 mL/kg for each liquid stool

Adapted from King, C., Glass, R., Bresee, J., & Duggan, C.; Centers for Disease Control and Prevention. (2003). Managing acute gastroenteritis among children: Oral maintenance, and nutritional therapy. *MMWR Recommendations and Reports, 52*(RR-16), 1–16.
[a]Larson, C. (2000). Safety and efficacy of oral rehydration therapy for the treatment of diarrhea and gastroenteritis in pediatrics. *Pediatric Nursing, 26*(2), 177–179; King, C., Glass, R., Bresee, J., & Duggan, C.; Centers for Disease Control and Prevention. (2003). Managing acute gastroenteritis among children: Oral maintenance, and nutritional therapy. *MMWR Recommendations and Reports, 52*(RR-16), 1–16; Centers for Disease Control and Prevention. (2008, September 14). *Guidelines for the management of acute diarrhea.* Retrieved from http://emergency.cdc.gov/disasters/hurricanes/pdf/dguidelines.pdf

- Urinalysis
- Stool for culture, ova, parasites, *Escherichia coli*, and *Clostridium difficile*

In children with vomiting and diarrhea, avoid sugary drinks and salty soups. Encourage continuation of breastfeeding in infants.

Therapeutic Interventions

- Administer ondansetron intravenously or by oral dissolving tablet as indicated for vomiting.
- Institute oral rehydration in patients capable of drinking. Administer oral rehydration solution (Pedialyte, Rehydralyte, Infalyte, Ricelyte) every hour or after each diarrheal stool (Table 52-10).[26] Give the total volume in small amounts (sips of 1 to 2 tsp) to facilitate absorption and discourage vomiting.
- Consider hypodermoclysis, or subcutaneous rehydration. Adding hyaluronidase enhances fluid absorption.
- In the presence of moderate or severe dehydration (greater than 10%), establish vascular access.
- Administer an isotonic crystalloid fluid bolus (20 mL/kg); reassess and give another bolus as needed. Several boluses may be required.
- Following rehydration, reduce IV fluid administration to maintenance levels (see Table 52-5).
- Closely monitor intake and output.

Vomiting in small amounts does not contraindicate administering oral rehydration therapy (ORT). Encourage the caregivers to give the ORT slowly (e.g., 1 tablespoon every 5 minutes).

Disposition

- Patients with mild to moderate dehydration who have been successfully rehydrated in the ED may be discharged home with responsible caregivers. Ensure they have clear understanding of oral replacement therapy to be continued at home and when to bring the patient back to the ED (signs and symptoms indicating a need for aggressive rehydration).
- Follow-up with the patient's primary care provider is necessary in 1 to 2 days.
- Severe dehydration often requires admission to the pediatric unit and continued IV infusions.

Pyloric Stenosis

Infants with pyloric stenosis have a history of projectile vomiting after feeding. Congenital hypertrophy of the pyloric muscles leads to obstruction at the pyloric sphincter. This results in forceful vomiting in which gastric contents can be ejected to a distance of up to 4 feet. The force of vomiting intensifies as the extent of obstruction increases. The cause of pyloric stenosis remains controversial.

Signs and Symptoms[27]

- Age of the infant usually 2 to 5 weeks
- Projectile vomiting after feedings (70% to 94%)
- Continued hungry behavior
- No indications of pain
- Poor weight gain
- Few stools
- Visible peristaltic waves on the abdomen, left to right

- Palpable abdominal mass above the umbilicus, in the right upper quadrant (about the size of an olive)
- Signs of dehydration (31% to 69%)

Diagnostic Procedures[27]

- Diagnosis usually based on history and examination
- Abdominal ultrasound is study of choice; demonstrates an elongated, thickened pylorus
- Barium swallow (after surgical consultation)
- CBC with differential
- Chemistry panel (also to assess for metabolic alkalosis [31% to 69%])
- Urinalysis

Therapeutic Interventions

- Initiate IV fluid replacement. Patients may require potassium replacement as well.
- Monitor intake and output.
- Insert a gastric tube to decompress the stomach.

Disposition

- Prepare for admission and surgical repair.

Appendicitis

Appendicitis is the most common cause of abdominal pain and abdominal surgery in children. It is rare in patients less than 2 years old. Symptoms can be difficult to interpret and diagnosis is complicated in the very young child. See Chapter 28, Abdominal Pain and Emergencies, for more information.

Signs and Symptoms[28]

- Pain typically originates in the periumbilical area and then localizes in the right lower quadrant (McBurney's point) within 24 to 48 hours of onset (70% to 94%).
- The patient's preferred position is supine with the legs flexed.
- Positive iliopsoas (or psoas) test: The psoas test is said to be positive if, when lying on the left side, hyperextension of the right hip produces pain (6% to 30%).
- Loss of appetite: If anorexia is not present, appendicitis is unlikely (70% to 94%).
- Nausea and vomiting may occur (31% to 69%).
- Constipation.
- Right lower quadrant guarding and pain with movement are present (31% to 69%).
- Peritoneal signs will be present if the appendix has ruptured.

Diagnostic Procedures[28]

- CBC with differential
- C-reactive protein
- Chemistry panel

- Urinalysis
- Abdominal ultrasound
- Abdominal CT scan with contrast has a sensitivity and specificity of 94% to 100%
- Chest radiograph (to rule out lower lobe pneumonia as the cause of abdominal pain)

Therapeutic Interventions

- Maintain nothing by mouth (NPO) status.
- Establish vascular access.
- Administer the following:
  - Analgesics
  - Antipyretics
  - Antibiotics (begin before transferring the child to the operating room)

Disposition

- Prepare the patient for surgery and admission.

Intussusception

Intussusception is the telescoping of one segment of the bowel into another. This disorder is most common in children between 3 months and 5 years of age. The typical location is the ileocecal valve. Intussusception may follow a viral infection, especially in younger children.

Signs and Symptoms[28]

- Sudden, acute, crampy, episodic abdominal pain occurs (94% to 100%).
- Flexed knees (70% to 94%).
- The patient may be pain-free between episodes.
- Vomiting occurs after the onset of pain (70% to 94%).
- Patient passes "currant jelly" stool with bloody mucus (6% to 30%).
- Abdominal distension is present (31% to 69%).
- A sausage-shaped mass is palpable in the right upper quadrant (31% to 69%).
- Early examination may appear normal.
- Later signs include fever, tachycardia, lethargy, and dehydration.

Diagnostic Procedures[28]

- Abdominal radiographs
- CBC with differential
- Chemistry panel
- Barium enema can both diagnose and reduce an intussusception. Air enema is replacing barium enema, as it is considered safer and more efficacious in reduction.
- CT scan of the abdomen may be obtained.

Therapeutic Interventions

- Maintain NPO status.
- Establish vascular access.

Disposition

- Admit for surgery if the barium or air enema failed to reduce the intussusception or if it reoccurs.

Volvulus

Malrotation of the bowel is a congenital anomaly involving abnormal bowel rotation and mesenteric attachment. This twisting (volvulus) of the small intestine can result in strangulation of the superior mesenteric artery and bowel infarction. Volvulus most commonly occurs in the first month of life but can appear later in childhood.

Signs and Symptoms[28]

- Bilious vomiting.
- Signs of abdominal pain. The pain can be severe and constant if the volvulus is complete and ischemic (95% to 100%).
- Abdominal distension.
- Bloody stools.
- Hematemesis.
- Visible peristaltic waves.
- Peritoneal signs if the bowel is perforated.

Diagnostic Procedures

- CBC with differential
- Chemistry panel
- Urinalysis
- Upper gastrointestinal series if the patient is stable
- CT scan of the abdomen may be obtained

Therapeutic Interventions

- Establish vascular access.
- Give analgesics as needed.
- Administer IV antibiotics before transferring the child to the operating room.
- Insert a gastric tube to decompress the stomach.

Disposition

- Prepare the patient for surgery and admission.

REFERENCES

1. Andreoni, C., & Klinkhammer, B. (2000). *Quick reference for pediatric emergency nursing*. Philadelphia, PA: Saunders.
2. Dieckman, R. A., Brownstein, D., & Gausche-Hill, M. (2010). The pediatric assessment triangle: A novel approach for the rapid evaluation of children. *Pediatric Emergency Care, 26*(4), 312–315.
3. Luscombe, M. D., Owens, B. D., & Burke, D. (2011). Weight estimation in paediatrics: A comparison of the APLS formula and the formula "weight = 3(age) + 7." *Emergency Medicine Journal, 28*(7), 590–593.
4. Emergency Nurses Association. (2009). *Core curriculum for pediatric emergency nursing* (2nd ed.). Des Plaines, IL: Author.
5. Emergency Nurses Association. (in press). *Emergency nursing pediatric course* (4th ed.). Des Plaines, IL: Author.
6. Frey, A. (1997). Tips for pediatric IV insertion. *Nursing, 97*(9), 32.
7. American Heart Association. (n.d.). *Pediatric advanced life support course*. Retrieved from http://www.americanheart.org/presenter.jhtml?identifier=3012001
8. National Sudden and Unexpected Infant/Child Death & Pregnancy Loss Resource Center. (2010, March). *Apparent life-threatening events and sudden infant death syndrome: A selected annotated bibliography*. Retrieved from http://www.sidscenter.org/TopicalBib/ALTE.html
9. Meštrović, J. (2008). Insight into pathophysiology of sudden infant death syndrome. *Signa Vitae, 3*(Suppl 1), S41–S43.
10. Mayo Clinic. (2011, June 11). *Sudden infant death syndrome (SIDS)*. Retrieved from http://www.mayoclinic.com/health/sudden-infant-death-syndrome/DS00145
11. American SIDS Institute. (n.d.). *Home page*. Retrieved from http://www.sids.org/
12. Esposito, L., Hegyi, T., & Ostfeld, B. (2007). Educating parents about the risk factors of sudden infant death syndrome. *Journal of Perinatal and Neonatal Nursing, 21*(2), 158–164.
13. Graneto, J. W. (2010, May 20). *Pediatric fever*. Retrieved from http://emedicine.medscape.com/article/801598-overview
14. Fleisher, G. R., & Ludwig S. (2010). *Textbook of pediatric emergency medicine* (6th ed.). Philadelphia, PA: Lippincott Williams & Wilkins.
15. Sobol, S. E., & Zapata, S. (2008). Epiglottitis and croup. *Otolaryngologic Clinics of North America, 41*(3), 551–566.
16. Muñiz, A., Molodow, R. E., & Defendi, G. L. (2011, September 15). *Croup*. Retrieved from http://emedicine.medscape.com/article/962972-overview
17. Neuman, M. I. (2006). Neck pain/Masses. In M. A. Davis, V. W. Chiang, & S. Manzi (Eds.), *Signs and symptoms in pediatrics: Urgent and emergent care*. St. Louis, MO: Elsevier.
18. Willis, K. (2007). Bronchiolitis: Advanced practice focus in the emergency department. *Journal of Emergency Nursing, 33*(4), 346–351.
19. Harris, J., Huskins, W. C., Langley, J., & Siegel, J. (2007). Health care epidemiology perspective on the October 2006 recommendations of the Subcommittee on Diagnosis and Management of Bronchiolitis. *Pediatrics, 120*(4), 890–892.
20. American Academy of Pediatrics. (2006). Diagnosis and management of bronchiolitis. *Pediatrics, 118*, 1774–1793.
21. García Martínez, J. M. (1999). Round table: Severe asthma in pediatrics: Treatment of acute crises. *Allergologia et Immunopathologia, 27*(2), 53–62.
22. Leung, A., & Robson, W. (2007). Febrile seizures. *Journal of Pediatric Health Care, 21*(4), 250–255.
23. Armon, K., Stephenson, T., MacFaul, R., Hemingway, P., Werneke, U., & Smith, S. (2003). An evidence and consensus based guideline for the management of a child after a seizure. *Emergency Medicine Journal, 20*(1), 13–20.

24. Centers for Disease Control. (2011, March 11). *Meningitis questions and answers.* Retrieved from http://www.cdc.gov/meningitis/about/faq.html

25. van de Beek, D., Farrar, J. J., de Gans, J., Mai, N. T., Molyneux, E. M., Peltola, H., ... Zwinderman, A. H. (2010). Adjunctive dexamethasone in bacterial meningitis: A meta-analysis of individual patient data. *Lancet Neurology, 9*(3), 254–263.

26. Larson, C. (2000). Safety and efficacy of oral rehydration therapy for the treatment of diarrhea and gastroenteritis in pediatrics. *Pediatric Nursing, 26*(2), 177–179.

27. Waltzman, M. L. (2006). Vomiting. In M. A. Davis, V. W. Chiang, & S. Manzi (Eds.), *Signs and symptoms in pediatrics,* St. Louis, MO: Elsevier.

28. Peña, B. M. G. (2006). Abdominal pain. In M. A. Davis, V. W. Chiang, & S. Manzi (Eds.), *Signs and symptoms in pediatrics,* St. Louis, MO: Elsevier.

Geriatric Considerations in Emergency Nursing

Karen L. Rice and Maria Albright

Older adults, particularly those 75 years and older, use emergency department (ED) services more than any other group. However, many times this vulnerable patient group is treated using guidelines that were tested in the general adult population and this may lead to poor clinical outcomes. The ED is the greatest source of hospital admissions in older adults; according to the National Center for Health Statistics, about 15% of all visits to the ED result in hospital admission.[1] Most hospital admissions via the ED result from an inadequate transition linked to either a prior hospitalization or a visit to the ED.[1] This chapter provides content to increase awareness about the vulnerability of older adults presenting to the ED and guidelines to improve clinical outcomes.

AGE-RELATED CHANGES AFFECTING VULNERABILITY

Older patients discharged home from the ED are at significant risk for adverse outcomes such as functional decline, return to the ED, hospitalization, and death.[1,2] Age-related physiologic changes affect all organ systems (Fig. 53-1), which potentially has important implications in clinical management of patients in the ED.

Knowledge of these physiologic changes is important in caring for this vulnerable population in the ED[3] (Table 53-1).

Age-related changes in pharmacokinetics that predispose older adults to adverse drug events are described in Table 53-2.[3]

Creatinine Clearance

The Cockcroft-Gault formula is used to measure creatinine clearance in older adults with stable kidney function.

$$\text{Creatinine clearance (mL/min)} = \frac{(140 - \text{age in years}) \times \text{body weight in kg}}{72 \times \text{serum creatinine}}$$
(in females, multiply the result by 0.85)

Normal range of creatinine clearance is 97 to 137 mL/min in men and 88 to 128 mL/min in women.

CROSS-CULTURAL ISSUES IN THE ELDERLY

Emergency departments generally provide care to a variety of culturally diverse groups that represent the community they serve. However, the urgency of rapid assessment and intervention associated with emergency services may prevent individualization of care from a cross-cultural perspective. Irrespective of the elderly patient's ethnic background, verify individual preferences and beliefs. Remember the following tips:

- Elderly persons within every ethnic group can differ greatly.
- Individual preferences may differ from those of persons of shared cultural heritage.
- Differences between ethnic groups differ widely regarding:

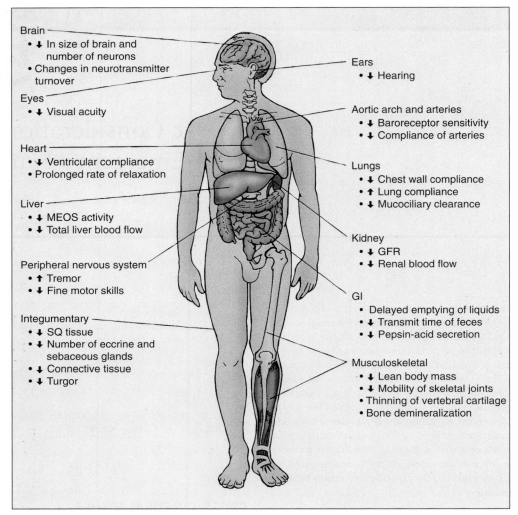

Brain
- ↓ In size of brain and number of neurons
- Changes in neurotransmitter turnover

Eyes
- ↓ Visual acuity

Heart
- ↓ Ventricular compliance
- Prolonged rate of relaxation

Liver
- ↓ MEOS activity
- ↓ Total liver blood flow

Peripheral nervous system
- ↑ Tremor
- ↓ Fine motor skills

Integumentary
- ↓ SQ tissue
- ↓ Number of eccrine and sebaceous glands
- ↓ Connective tissue
- ↓ Turgor

Ears
- ↓ Hearing

Aortic arch and arteries
- ↓ Baroreceptor sensitivity
- ↓ Compliance of arteries

Lungs
- ↓ Chest wall compliance
- ↑ Lung compliance
- ↓ Mucociliary clearance

Kidney
- ↓ GFR
- ↓ Renal blood flow

GI
- Delayed emptying of liquids
- ↓ Transmit time of feces
- ↓ Pepsin-acid secretion

Musculoskeletal
- ↓ Lean body mass
- ↓ Mobility of skeletal joints
- Thinning of vertebral cartilage
- Bone demineralization

Fig. 53-1 Summary of the physiologic changes that occur in all systems and that the critical care nurse must consider in caring for the elderly patient in the critical care unit. *GFR,* glomerular filtration rate; *GI,* gastrointestinal; *MEOS,* microsomal enzyme oxidative system; *SQ,* subcutaneous. From Urden, L. D., Stacy, K. M., & Lough, M. E. (Eds.). [2010]. *Critical care nursing: Diagnosis and management* [6th ed.]. St. Louis, MO: Elsevier.

- Involvement of family and friends in decision making
- Disclosing medical information about condition and prognosis
- End-of-life decision making and preferences about care

Table 53-3 describes cross-cultural issues for 15 ethnic groups[4]; however, never make assumptions about a patient based on a cultural or ethnic label.

QUALITY INDICATORS FOR OLDER ADULT EMERGENCY CARE

In 2009 the Society for Academic Emergency Medicine and the American College of Emergency Physicians identified three conditions as having quality gaps in the care that older adults receive in the ED.[5] These conditions include cognitive impairment, pain management, and transitional care.

TABLE 53-1   AGE-RELATED PHYSIOLOGIC CHANGES

AGE-RELATED CHANGES	CLINICAL CONSIDERATIONS	NURSING INTERVENTIONS
Cardiovascular system • ↓ Inotropic and chronotropic myocardial response to catecholamine stimulation • ↓ Baroreceptor sensitivity • ↓ Blood vessel compliance	• Stress- and exercise-induced increases in cardiac output rely on diastolic filling • Increased tendency for orthostatic hypotension with position change, particularly if on antihypertensive medications • ↑ Peripheral vascular resistance and BP	• Closely monitor vital signs (be alert for tachyarrhythmias), oxygen saturation, and cognitive function when administering vasoactive drugs and in patients presenting with heart failure • Evaluate each patient's response to BP reductions, as some may not tolerate a "normal" BP
Respiratory system • ↓ PaO_2 level	• ↓ Ventilatory response to hypoxia and hypercapnia • ↑ Sensitivity to opioids and benzodiazepines	• Monitor oxygen saturation, including exhaled CO_2 if available, when administering opioids and benzodiazepines • "Start low and go slow" when administering high-risk drugs, especially in patients with cardiovascular, pulmonary, and cognitive disorders
Renal system • ↑ Glomerular filtration rate • ↓ Ability to concentrate and conserve H_2O • ↓ Ability to excrete salt and H_2O loads, urea, NH_3, and drugs	• ↑ Sensitivity to drugs cleared by kidneys (i.e., antibiotics, contrast agents) • ↑ Risk for dehydration and hypernatremia • ↑ Risk for fluid overload and drug reactions	• Certain antibiotics administered in the ED may require renal dosing. Estimate creatinine clearance as a measurement of renal function rather than serum creatinine (normal value does not mean normal renal function because age-related loss of muscle mass affects serum creatinine) • Monitor oxygen saturation, cardiac rhythm, vital signs, and cognition for mental status changes in patients being treated for dehydration or fluid overload • Fluid resuscitation should be slower than for younger patients
Liver • ↓ Total hepatic blood flow	• ↑ Adverse drug interactions	• Observe for any changes in vital signs, cardiac rhythm, and cognitive function following administration of medications
Neurologic system • ↑ Cranial dead space • Changes in neurotransmitter function	• Symptoms associated with hemorrhage take a long time to manifest • Delayed or impaired processing of sensory and motor information	• Be aware that normal mental status–neurologic examinations do not confirm the absence of serious injury • Quiet the environment and limit distractions while completing mental status–neurologic examinations
Musculoskeletal • ↓ Lean body mass • Thinning of intervertebral cartilage with compression of the spinal column • ↓ Joint mobility	• ↑ Risk for deconditioning and functional decline with acute and chronic illness • ↑ Risk for fractures	• Encourage independence with assistance as needed while in the ED rather than "doing it for them" • Educate patient and families about importance of home safety and preventing functional decline associated with acute illness and injury

BP, Blood pressure; *CO_2*, carbon dioxide; *ED*, emergency department; *H_2O*, water; *NH_3*, ammonia; *PaO_2*, partial pressure of oxygen in arterial blood.

TABLE 53-2 AGE-RELATED PHARMACOKINETIC CHANGES

PHARMACOKINETIC PARAMETER	Age-related change	OTHER FACTORS EXERTING EFFECT
Absorption—impacts uptake of the drug into tissue	↓ Absorptive surface of small intestine ↓ Splanchnic blood flow ↑ Gastric acid pH ↓ GI motility	• Achlorhydria (primary disorder or resulting from prolonged histamine [H_2] blockers or proton-pump inhibitors) • Administering multiple medications together • Tube feedings
Distribution—tissue into which the free form of the drug is distributed	↓ Lean body mass and total H_2O ↑ Total body fat ↓ Serum albumin ↑ α_1-acid glycoprotein	• Heart failure • Ascites
Metabolism—chemical change that renders the drug active or inactive	↓ Liver mass and blood flow ↓ Microsomal drug-metabolizing enzyme system that affect CYP 450 enzymes	• Tobacco abuse • Alcohol and caffeine • Drugs that inhibit or induce CYP 450 enzyme activity
Excretion—removal of drug by elimination	↓ Renal blood flow and glomerular filtration rate (GFR) ↓ Distal renal tubular secretory function	• Acute and chronic renal disease
Pharmacodynamics—physiologic response to a drug	↓ Predictability in drug response at usual or lower concentrations of many drugs	• Drug-drug interactions • Drug-disease interactions

CYP 450, cytochrome P450; *GI*, Gastrointestinal; *H_2O*, water.
Adapted from Rice, K. L., & Winterbottom, F. (2010). Gerontological alterations and management. In L. D. Urden, K. Stacy, & M. E. Lough (Eds.), *Critical care nursing* (6th ed.). St. Louis, MO, Mosby.

Table 53-4 describes quality indicators associated with cognitive impairment, pain management, and transitional care.

Cognitive Impairment

- Older adults frequently present to the ED with mental status changes.
- Approximately 25% of older patients in the ED have some type of cognitive impairment.[6]
  - About 10% present with delirium.[6]
  - About 20% present with some type of dementia or chronic memory impairment.[6]

Pain Management[5]

- Pain is a common chief complaint in the ED, with approximately 75% reporting moderate or severe pain.
- Unrelieved acute pain is associated with poor clinical outcomes, including functional decline and an increased risk for developing delirium.
  - Advanced age is the strongest independent predictor that a patient will not receive any analgesia in the ED.
  - Thirty-three percent of patients presenting with hip or long-bone fracture do not receive analgesia in the ED and only 57% receive opioids.

Transitional Care from the Nursing Home[5]

- More than 2.7 million nursing home residents visit an ED each year. Therefore it is critical that communication channels are open between the ED and nursing home to optimize clinical outcomes.
- Nursing home residents are frequently transported to and from the ED without essential information.
  - Nursing home residents are frequently sent to the ED without adequate documentation, including the reason for the visit to the ED.
  - Many nursing home residents are returned from the ED without any written information.

PRIMARY ASSESSMENT OF THE GERIATRIC PATIENT

Although older adults seek emergency care for a variety of complaints, they frequently present with acute pain, psychiatric disorders, urosepsis, and dehydration. This section will describe tips for assessing each of these conditions, including therapeutic interventions, and diagnostic considerations that focus on the unique needs of older adults.

Text continued on page 580.

TABLE 53-3	A GUIDE TO CROSS-CULTURAL HEALTH CARE FOR OLDER ADULTS				
ETHNIC GROUP	**PREFERRED CULTURAL TERM**	**RESPECTFUL NONVERBAL COMMUNICATION**	**TRADITION AND HEALTH BELIEFS**	**DECISION-MAKING**	**END-OF-LIFE CARE**
African-Americans	African-American or Black	• Maintain eye contact • Close proximity during dialogue	• Diverse health beliefs	• Family usually involved • May include non-blood kin or clergy	• Aggressive therapies usually preferred • May resist DNR orders because of religious beliefs or mistrust of health care system
American Indians and Alaskan Natives	American Indian Alaska Native Note: Be aware of tribal affiliation Avoid "Native American"	• Avoid attitude of physical domination • Delay personal touching	• Seeks balance with self, nature, family, community • Disease is the result of invading object or loss of personal spirit • Rituals, herbal remedies and statements of intent form basis of treatments • Dementia is not viewed as a disease but rather a "change"	• Close or distant relatives or kinsmen may be involved	• Avoid life expectancy predictions • Desires to stay with family and maintain hopeful, positive attitude
Arab-Americans	Arab-American Note: Immigrants from Afghanistan and Turkey are not included	• Handshake appropriate for men, but not for many Muslim women • Women may avoid smiling/eye contact • Use conservative demeanor	• Most are Muslim, but many are Christian • Cleanliness and prayer important • Blood transfusions accepted • Mental illness is feared (evil) • Preventive medicine viewed with suspicion • Typically refuse gynecological examinaton by male	• Males make decisions • Bad news often held back from patient	• Medical care balanced with acceptance of God's will • Traditions about washing and wrapping of dead body

Continued

TABLE 53-3   A GUIDE TO CROSS-CULTURAL HEALTH CARE FOR OLDER ADULTS—cont'd

ETHNIC GROUP	PREFERRED CULTURAL TERM	RESPECTFUL NONVERBAL COMMUNICATION	TRADITION AND HEALTH BELIEFS	DECISION-MAKING	END-OF-LIFE CARE
Asian Indian Americans	Asian Indian (even if born in U.S.)	• Physician is expected to take control and uncertainty is perceived as incompetence • Expects to be questioned for health information rather than to volunteer it	• May follow western health practices • May believe in karma, reincarnation, illness as payment for sins • Seek permission before removing religious clothing, amulets, etc.	• Family and friends may be involved • Emphasis is on interconnectedness vs. patient autonomy	• Voicing thoughts about death is feared as self-fulfilling • Prefer to die at home • End-of-life care is an unfamiliar concept
Cambodian Americans	Cambodian American	• Greet with palms together and slight bow • Avoid steady eye contact • Avoid touching head, location of person's spirit	• Buddhist outlook • Disease is caused by spirits, spells, imbalance • Herbal remedies, dermal coining, pinching, special foods • Expect to receive medications from western physicians	• Elders usually live with family and family acts as decision maker • Family may shield patient from bad news	• Home death preferred • Heroic interventions considered "bad death"
Chinese Americans	Chinese, Chinese American, or Asian Avoid "Oriental"	• Politeness • Smiling and/or nodding may conceal patient's lack of understanding	• Disease caused by yin/yang • Traditional remedies usually accepted • Mental illness caused by spirits • Fearful of blood draws and surgery	• Decisions made by family • Older male takes primary role • Patient is usually not told of cancer diagnosis	• Diverse beliefs • Speaking of death may be perceived as "bad luck" • May prefer to die in hospital rather than at home
Filipino Americans	Philipino or Philipino American	• Genuine smile, eye contact, handshake • Avoid prolonged eye contact • Head nodding means respect rather than understanding by patient	• Traditional view of illness includes imbalance, divine retribution, spirits, witches • Traditional and western medicine generally accepted	• Extended family may be involved • May protect the patient from bad news	• Usually Roman Catholic beliefs • May be resistant to organ donation and autopsy • Hospice and DNR infrequently used

Cultural group	Communication	Health beliefs	Decision making	End-of-life care
Haitian Americans	• Firm handshake • Avoid African American	• Most are Roman Catholic but also voodoo/spirit beliefs • Folk remedies • Mental illness/dementia carry social stigma	• Extended family usually involved • Physician is expected to make decisions	• Prefer to die at home • DNR may be an acceptable option if explained adequately
Hispanic Americans	• Refer to country of origin, such as Cuban, Puerto Rican, or use Hispanic, Latino, Chicano, Mexican-American • Patient may avoid eye contact with authority figure • Smiling and nodding may conceal understanding • Avoid overly firm handshake or continuous eye contact	• Some believe in spirits impacting health • Western beliefs frequently accepted	• Patriarchal family structure with oldest male making decisions • Religion and prayer usually considered in making decisions	• Aggressive treatment usually preferred • Palliative care accepted • Fear of losing all care if DNR given • Organ donation usually avoided • Amenable to DNR as death approaches
Japanese Americans	• Restrained, avoid open confrontation	• Yin/yang responsible for health/illness • Complementary medicine, such as acupuncture, massage, accepted	• Oldest male is decision maker • May hide bad news from patient • Discussion about death is usually avoided	
Korean Americans	• Respect sense of space • Handshake may be accepted with a simultaneous bow • Avoid extended eye contact	• "Han bang" or "Han yak" (similar to yin/yang) • Acupuncture, herbs, cupping used • Believe causes of illness due to failures in rituals, ancestral anger and spirits	• Family unit involved with oldest son making decisions • Bad news often withheld from patient	• Belief that discussion of death with patient hastens it • Less aggressive treatment options usually preferred
Pakistani Americans	• Approach respectfully with door left open • Only males shake hands • Restrict unnecessary touching	• Health depends on avoiding sins, rituals, spirits • Traditional and western health systems accepted together • Cleanliness and prayers important to well-being	• Acceptance of Allah's decisions • Elders often defer decisions to children • Bad news, such as cancer, often withheld from patient	• End-of-life planning threatening • Prefer to die at home with family/friends • Withholding food is forbidden

Continued

TABLE 53-3 A GUIDE TO CROSS-CULTURAL HEALTH CARE FOR OLDER ADULTS—cont'd

ETHNIC GROUP	PREFERRED CULTURAL TERM	RESPECTFUL NONVERBAL COMMUNICATION	TRADITION AND HEALTH BELIEFS	DECISION-MAKING	END-OF-LIFE CARE
Portuguese Americans	Portuguese American or Portuguese	• Direct eye contact, handshake	• Expect prescriptions • Mental illness is a stigma • May use spirits, amulets, cards, laying on of hands by healers	• Prefer physician to guide decisions • Family plays important role with deferment to children • Bad news often withheld because of fear of self-fulfillment	• May favor resuscitation in fear of neglect • May agree with DNR if perceived as "God's will"
Russian-Speaking Americans	Avoid "Russian" as many that still speak Russian were the victim of Russian persecution. Use terms such as Ukrainian, Armenian, or other term reflecting the area of Russian from where they immigrated	• Use of first name alone is considered impolite • Eye contact with genuine smile	• Prefer western medical system • May use massage, herbal remedies, chicken broth • Expect aggressive treatment with hospitalization vs. home care when ill • Depression and anxiety are considered stigma	• Physician is the decision maker • Asking for patient/family input suggests physician inadequacy	• Planning for end-of-life care is taboo • DNR orders and palliative treatment rare
Vietnamese Americans	Vietnamese American or Vietnamese	• Reserved demeanor with slight bow • Use both hands when giving an object • Keep arms crossed or hands folded in front • Avoid direct eye contact, shaking hands and loud voice	• Diseases are due to religious and spiritual causes • Balance sought with yin/yang, hot/cold • Cupping and coining are traditional remedies	• Family may make decisions • Younger relatives frequently assume control	• Aversion to dying in hospital • End-of-life support may be considered an insult to ancestors or contributor to death • Belief that a difficult death is karmic justice

Data from American Geriatrics Society. (2001). *Doorway thoughts: Cross-cultural health care for older adults.* Sudbury, MA: Jones & Bartlett.
DNR, Do Not Resuscitate.

TABLE 53-4   **QUALITY INDICATORS FOR OLDER ADULT EMERGENCY CARE**

CONDITION	QUALITY INDICATORS	RATIONALES
Cognitive impairment (includes acute mental status changes and memory impairment)	1. Include level of alertness and orientation in baseline cognitive assessment. 2. Assessment of patients with acute mental status changes: Focus on documenting the presence or absence of delirium-related symptoms (Table 53-6 and Table 53-7). 3. For patients with an acute mental status change who are discharged home: Document the name of the support person who is responsible for the plan of care and medical follow-up. 4. Determine whether cognitive impairment has been previously diagnosed by a health care provider, screen for dementia (see Table 53-7) if appropriate, or refer for follow-up.	1. Cognitive impairment is common in patients in the ED and screening for impairment is feasible. 2. An acute mental status change is a key feature of delirium. Although delirium is potentially life-limiting, it is frequently missed. 3. Delirious patients discharged home are at an increased risk for death in the months following discharge[a] without appropriate management. 4. Chronic mental status changes frequently play a role in why the patient presents to the ED (i.e., nonadherence to medical regimen, traumatic injury). However, many patients who present with a baseline cognitive impairment have no prior history of abnormal mental status changes.
Pain management	1. Formal assessment of acute pain within 1 hour of arrival at ED. 2. Pain assessment every 1 to 2 hours as appropriate but within 6 hours if still in ED. 3. Pain reassessment prior to discharge home. 4. Initiate pain treatment for moderate to severe pain (numeric pain score of 4 or higher) or document why treatment was not initiated. 5. Provide instructions about a bowel regimen to all patients discharged from the ED who receive a prescription for opioids or document why a bowel regimen was not provided.	1, 2, and 3. Appropriate assessment of pain fosters effective treatment. 4. Consider opioids (other than meperidine and propoxyphene) when nonopioid analgesia is ineffective. 5. Constipation is a side effect of opioid analgesia.
Transitional care	1. Critical information from nursing homes transferring patients to the ED includes: • Reason for transfer • Resuscitation (code) status • Medication allergies • Medication list • Contact information for nursing home • Primary care and on-call physician • Resident's legal health care representative, family member 2. When patients are discharged back to the nursing home, critical information the ED should communicate includes: • Diagnosis • Test results and pending results • Recommendations regarding medication regimen • Any follow-up required by primary care	1. Individualized information is essential to make treatment decisions. 2. Communication between providers is critical to ensure continuity of care.

ED, Emergency department.

[a]van Zyl, L. Y., & Davidson, P. R. (2003). Delirium in hospital. An underreported event at discharge. *Canadian Journal of Psychiatry, 48,* 555–560.

Pain

The International Association for the Study of Pain defines pain as "an unpleasant sensory and emotional experience associated with actual or potential tissue damage."[7] Acute pain has rapid onset with limited duration usually related to apparent pathology. Chronic pain persists for long periods of time and may not be related to disease process. Among older community dwellers, more than 50% report living with pain while at least 85% of nursing home residents experience some form of pain.[8] The high prevalence of chronic and acute pain in older adults necessitates adequate pain assessment in the ED. Pain management is considered a quality indicator in managing older adults in the ED (Table 53-4).

Pain Assessment

Important points to be aware of in performing a comprehensive pain assessment in older adults include the following:

- Pain is not part of the aging process.
- Involve family members in all aspects of assessment and planning.
- Assessment may be challenging because of multiple concurrent disease processes.
- Patient report is the most reliable evidence.
  - Adapt for sensory and cognitive impairment by using simple questions and observe nonverbal cues such as grimacing, restlessness, guarded movement, and rubbing a particular area.
- Pain is frequently associated with depression, sleep disturbance, withdrawal, and impaired mobility—these disorders may indicate pain rather than a report of pain.
- Gait disturbances, malnutrition, falls, and slow rehabilitation are exacerbated by pain.
- Reassess regularly and document findings (see Table 53-4).

History and Physical

- Refer to the pain assessment guide in Chapter 11, Care of the Patient with Pain.
- Ask the patient to pick a word that best describes his or her pain.[8] A verbal descriptor is preferred in older adults.[9]
- Determine if this is new onset or chronic pain.
- Screen for depression, anxiety, or mental status if needed.
- Obtain analgesic history: over-the-counter (OTC), natural or complementary remedies, prescription.
- Determine the effectiveness of nonpharmacologic treatment.

Rapid General Assessment

- Assess for changes in level of consciousness.
- Assess for vital sign changes that may or may not be present in older adults.
  - Increases in heart rate, respirations, and blood pressure may be associated with mild to moderate pain.
  - Decreased blood pressure, pallor, bradycardia, dizziness, nausea, and vomiting may be associated with severe pain.
- Assess factors that aggravate or alleviate the pain.

Diagnostic Procedures

In many instances a history and physical examination is all that is required to assess pain in older adults. However, the following diagnostic procedures may be indicated:

- Laboratory studies (i.e., urinalysis for flank pain; serum cardiac enzymes, troponin for chest pain)
- Radiographs (i.e., abdominal, chest for musculoskeletal pain)
- Computed tomography (CT) or magnetic resonance imaging (MRI)

Therapeutic Interventions

Nonpharmacologic interventions provide a benefit in minimizing the need for or dosage of pharmacologic agents in effectively managing pain in older adults. Examples include:

- Heat or cold application
- Distraction (TV, music, guided imagery)
- Repositioning for comfort
- Relaxation techniques

Guidelines for pharmacologic interventions for pain in older adults include the following[10]:

- Oral agents are always the preferred route.
  - Avoid intramuscular administration because of decrease in muscle and fatty tissue.
- Begin with nonopioids such as acetaminophen or nonsteroidal anti-inflammatory drugs (NSAIDs). Always start with low doses and increase dosage slowly, evaluating effects.
- Progress to stronger agents as needed. Avoid agents that are considered potentially inappropriate for older adults.
- See Table 53-5 for pharmacologic recommendations.
- Epidural and intrathecal techniques may be administered safely in older adults by anesthesia personnel as smaller doses of opioids are given using these methods. However, these drugs likely should not be

TABLE 53-5	**GUIDELINES FOR MANAGEMENT OF PERSISTENT PAIN IN OLDER ADULTS**		
INDICATION	**TYPE**	**MEDICATION AND PRECAUTIONS**	**DOSE**
Mild pain	Nonopioids	Acetaminophen: first-line therapy	325–500 mg po every 4–6 hours
		Contraindicated in liver failure	not to exceed 4g/24 hours
		Ibuprofen*	200 mg po 3 times/day
		Naproxen*	220 mg po every 12 hours
		Celecoxib (Celebrex)*	100 mg po daily
		Nabumetone (Relafen)*	1 g po daily
		Monitor for GI side effects	
Mild to moderate pain	Opioids	Oxymorphone	5 mg po every 6 hours
		Extended release	0.5 mg intravenously every 4–6 hours
		Significant interactions with food and alcohol toxicity	5 mg po every 12 hours
		Hydrocodone	2.5–5 mg po every 4–6 hours
		Oxycodone (Oxycontin)	2.5–5 mg po every 4–6
Moderate to severe pain		Morphine	2.5–10 mg po every 4 hours
			1–2 mg intravenously every 4–6 hours
		Morphine (sustained release)	15 mg po every 8–24 hours
		Limited use in patients with renal insufficiency	
		Significant interactions with food and alcohol	
		Transdermal	12–25 mcg/hour patch every 72 hours
		Fentanyl (Duragesic)	
		18–24 hours to peak	
		Hydromorphone	1–2 mg po every 3–4 hours
			0.5–1 mg intravenously every 3–4 hours

*Use with caution in heart disease, heart failure, gastropathy, and chronic kidney disease.
GI, Gastrointestinal; *po,* by mouth.

used older adults being discharged home because of the risk for sedation and respiratory depression in the first 24 hours.

- Regional neural blocks are being administered by anesthesia personnel for hip fracture with increased frequency in the ED because of evidence that supports significantly less use of opioids to manage pain effectively and a reduction in the incidence of delirium. A major limitation has been having trained personnel available to complete the neural blocks in the ED.
- Effective pain management is usually associated with a scheduled administration of pain medication around the clock before pain incidents occur versus "as needed" dosing.
- Monitor older adults frequently for signs of sedation, respiratory depression, confusion, and hallucinations.

> Although analgesics can contribute to the development of delirium, pain itself can also cause delirium.

Psychiatric Disorders

Although patients frequently present to the ED with a primary complaint related to a medical disorder, many have underlying psychiatric problems that significantly contribute to the presenting problem yet go undiagnosed. Delirium is either missed or misinterpreted as dementia or depression more than 30% of the time and is associated with significant increases in mortality and morbidity.[11] In addition, older adults may present with a psychosis that is related to a preexisting psychiatric disorder.

- Delirium is an acute, potentially reversible disturbance in consciousness, attention, cognition, and perception that is caused by a general medical condition, a substance, or a combination of factors. Patients at highest risk for delirium are those with a prior history of delirium or a diagnosis of dementia.[11]
- Dementia is a chronic neurocognitive disorder in which a significant loss of intellectual abilities, such as memory impairment, interferes with social and occupational functioning.[12]

TABLE 53-6 THE DIFFERENCES BETWEEN DELIRIUM, DEMENTIA, AND DEPRESSION

FEATURE	DELIRIUM	DEMENTIA	DEPRESSION
Onset	Acute and abrupt	Slow and insidious	Recent and situational
Duration	Hours to days	Months to years	Chronic
Attention	Impaired (hallmark symptom)	Usually normal	Generally normal
Consciousness	Fluctuating and reduced	Clear	Clear
Speech	Disorganized	Ordered, anomic and aphasic	May be slow
Alertness	↑ or ↓, varied	Labile	Flat
Orientation	Usually impaired, fluctuates between normal and abnormal	Often impaired	Usually normal

TABLE 53-7 SCREENING FOR DELIRIUM, DEMENTIA, AND DEPRESSION IN THE EMERGENCY DEPARTMENT

	DELIRIUM	DEMENTIA	DEPRESSION
Screening strategies	Confusion Assessment Method[a] 1. Acute mental status change that fluctuates 2. Inattention 3. Disorganized thinking 4. Altered level of consciousness	Two-Step Mini-Cog[b] 1. Use three-word recall to test the patient's memory; state three words (apple, penny, table) and have the patient repeat them back. Inform the patient he or she is to remember the words. 2. Draw a circle to represent a clock. Instruct the patient to insert all numbers in the clock; then tell him or her to place the hands of the clock at a specific time (e.g., 11:45).	Patient Health Questionnaire 2 (PHQ-2)[c] Over the past month: 1. Have you often had little interest or pleasure in doing things? 2. Have you often been bothered by feeling down, depressed, or hopeless? Assess for suicide risk (see Chapter 48, Mental Health Emergencies).
Interpreting screening results	In the absence of a preexisting psychiatric disorder responsible for these symptoms, the presence of 1 and 2 and either 3 or 4 is suggestive of delirium.	In the absence of acute mental status change, chronic cognitive impairment is suspected if the patient is unable to recall words and if the clock is abnormal; referral for diagnostic workup is indicated.	"Yes" to either of these questions is suggestive of depression. Follow-up is indicated using a structured self-assessment scale (e.g., Geriatric Depression Scale).

[a]Waszynski, C. (2001). Confusion Assessment Method (CAM). *Try this: Best practices in nursing care to older adults*, (13), 1–2.
[b]Doerflinger, D.M.C. (2007). How to try this: The mini-cog. *American Journal of Nursing 107*(1), 62–71.
[c]Kroenke, K., Spitzer, R.L., & Williams, J.B. (2003). The Patient Health Questionnaire-2: Validation of a two-item depression screener. *Medical Care*, (41), 1284–1294.

- Depression is a mood disorder in which feelings of sadness, discouragement, and lack of self-worth get in the way of everyday life and have been present for at least 2 weeks.[12]
- Psychosis is a condition of the mind in which there is a loss of reality as evidenced by abnormal thinking, hallucinations, or delusions.[12] Although patients with delirium, dementia, and depression may be psychotic, other psychiatric disorders (i.e., schizophrenia, bipolar disorder) may be responsible.

Table 53-6, Table 53-7, and Table 53-8 provide information on the difference between delirium, dementia, and

TABLE 53-8 USING THE MNEMONIC DELIRIUM TO IDENTIFY CAUSES OF DELIRIUM

D	Drugs	• Opioids, steroids, benzodiazepines, antipsychotics, H_1 and H_2 blockers, anticonvulsants, anti-Parkinson, anticholinergics, quinolone and macrolide antibiotics, cardiac glycosides, beta-blockers, ACE inhibitors, calcium channel blockers, salicylates
	Drug toxicity	• Lithium, salicylates, anticonvulsants
	Drug withdrawal	• Withdrawal from alcohol, benzodiazepines, and opioids
E	Endocrine	• Diabetes, thyroid, parathyroid, adrenal dysfunction
	Epilepsy	• New and chronic seizures
L	Lung disease	• Hypoxia, pneumonia, COPD, sleep apnea
I	Infection	• Encephalitis, meningitis, syphilis, HIV, sepsis
	Injury	• Concussion, subdural, extradural hemorrhage, burns, surgery
	Intracranial lesions	• Tumor, increased intracranial pressure
R	Renal	• Acute and chronic renal failure
I	Intestinal	• Cancer, obstruction, ileus
U	Unstable circulation	• Arrhythmias, myocardial infarction, hypertensive encephalopathy, hypoperfusion, stroke, blood loss, shock
M	Metabolic	• Electrolyte disturbances (sodium, calcium, magnesium, phosphorus)

ACE, Angiotensin-converting enzyme; *COPD*, chronic obstructive pulmonary disease; *HIV*, human immunodeficiency virus.

depression; different screening strategies for each of these disorders; and use the mnemonic DELIRIUM to identify potential causes of delirium.

Patient Behaviors That Are Clues for Dementia
- Appears disoriented
- "Poor historian"
- Defers to family member for answers to questions
- Repeats information
- Difficulty finding the correct words or makes inappropriate responses
- Difficulty following conversation

Family Questionnaire to Detect Dementia
The following questions provide information as to the degree cognitive dysfunction may be affecting the patient's functional level of independence.

Ask family or significant to answer whether or not the patient frequently does any of the following*:
1. Repeating or asking the same thing over and over?
2. Forgetting appointments, family occasions, holiday?
3. Writing checks, paying bills, balancing the checkbook?
4. Shopping independently for clothing or groceries?
5. Taking medications according to instructions?
6. Getting lost while walking or driving in familiar places?
7. Making decisions that arise in everyday living?

*From Mezy, M., & Maslow, K. (2007). *Try this: Recognition of dementia in hospitalized older adults*. Retrieved from http://consultgerirn.org/uploads/File/trythis/try_this_d5.pdf

Therapeutic Interventions

Therapeutic interventions associated with caring for older adult patients manifesting a psychiatric disorder focus on facilitating the following:
- A therapeutic environment that ensures a quiet and nonthreatening climate
- An environment that is safe to both the patient and family and the staff
- Pharmacologic management only when behavioral interventions fail to promote patient and staff safety (see Table 53-9 for pharmacologic recommendations)

Behavioral Interventions for Psychiatric Disorders in the Older Adult
- Quiet environment
- Limit traffic in and out of examination room
- Encourage familiar person to stay at bedside
- May use music or television if it reduces anxiety
- Frequent checks or constant visualization when required to keep patient safe

Urosepsis

Urosepsis is a systemic blood infection that develops when a urinary tract infection (UTI) pathogen enters the bloodstream and disseminates through the body. It is the most severe form of a UTI; therefore management is different than with an uncomplicated UTI. In the elderly, this

TABLE 53-9 PHARMACOLOGIC MANAGEMENT OF DELIRIUM AND AGITATION IN OLDER ADULTS

DRUG CLASS/DRUG AND DOSE	INDICATION	PRECAUTIONS
Traditional antipsychotic: Haloperidol (Haldol) • 0.5–1 mg twice daily with additional dose every 4 hours as needed (peak effect in 4 to 6 hours) OR • 0.5–1 mg IM or IV, can repeat in 30–60 minutes (peak effect 20 to 40 minutes)	• Agitation not responsive to behavioral interventions • Goal is to elicit calming effect not sedation	• IV initially has more pronounced effect but a very short half life compared to IM dosing • Increased risk for extrapyramidal symptoms if dose > 3 mg/day • Avoid in patients with withdrawal syndrome, hepatic insufficiency, history of neuroleptic malignant syndrome • Be alert for prolonged QT interval on ECG
Atypical antipsychotics: • Risperidone (Risperdal) 0.5 mg twice daily • Olanzapine (Zyprexa) 2.5–5 mg once daily • Quetiapine (Seroquel) 25 mg twice daily Benzodiazepine • Lorazepam (Ativan) 0.5–1 mg IV titrating for calming effect vs. sedation or orally with additional doses every 4 hours as needed	• Small uncontrolled studies suggest a benefit of calming patients with delirium • Second-line agent • Reserve for use in patients with withdrawal syndrome, those with Parkinson's disease, and those with neuroleptic malignant syndrome • Goal is to elicit calming effect not sedation	• Associated with increased mortality rate among older patients with dementia • Extrapyramidal effects less prevalent than with haloperidol • Be alert for prolonged QT interval on ECG • Paradoxical excitation, respiratory depression, oversedation • Clinical trials support the potential for prolongation or worsening of delirium-related symptoms

ECG, Electrocardiogram; *IM,* intramuscular; *IV,* intravenous.
Data from Inouye, S. K. (2006). Delirium in older persons. *New England Journal of Medicine, 354*(11), 1157–1165.

condition gives rise to morbidity and mortality rates up to 40%, warranting prompt attention.[13]

In older adults, decreased alertness or confusion may be the first and only sign associated with a UTI. UTIs are more common in women and in patients with indwelling catheters, particularly those residing in long-term care facilities. However, as men age, UTI incidence rises and approaches that of women (20% to 50%) as a result of prostate enlargement, prostatism, and debilitation as well as instrumentation in the urinary tract.[14]

Signs and Symptoms

- Decreased alertness (often first sign)
- Dysuria and frequency of urination
- Symptomatic bacteremia: fever, chills, hypotension (only one third present with fever, chills, hypotension)[14,15]

Diagnostic Procedures

- Urinalysis: positive for red blood cell, white blood cell, and a bacterial count >100,000/mL.
- Urine culture: *Escherichia coli, Proteus, Enterobacter,* and *Klebsiella* are common.
- Obtain two sets of blood culture before antibiotics are given.
- Ultrasound may be indicated to define kidney size and evaluate prostate gland.
- CT and MRI may be indicated to identify suspected abscesses and necrosis.

Therapeutic Interventions

- Start antibiotics in the ED and continue for 10 to 21 days.
- Administer intravenous fluids to establish fluid and electrolyte balance.

- Maintain urine output at 0.5 mL/kg per hour.
- Maintain systolic blood pressure greater than 90 mm Hg and mean arterial pressure greater than 65 mm Hg with intravenous fluids or vasopressors.
- If condition deteriorates, it should be treated as septic shock (see Chapter 20, Shock).

Dehydration

Dehydration is defined as the loss of body water content resulting from pathologic fluid losses, diminished water intake, or both. Older adults are at increased risk for dehydration because of diminished thirst perception and physical, cognitive, and other age-related impairments.[8] When older adults are stressed by physical or emotional conditions, the risk for dehydration escalates. Some factors that predispose older patients to dehydration are age greater than 85 years, polypharmacy, stroke, dementia, renal disease, surgery, trauma, residing at a long-term care facility, and previous history of dehydration.[12]

Signs and Symptoms

- Dry mucous membranes
- Tongue furrows present
- Decreased saliva
- Sunken eyes
- Elevated heart rate compared to baseline
- Orthostatic hypotension
- Decreased urine output (<30 mL per hour)

> Skin turgor is *not* a valid assessment finding in older adults because of age-related loss in skin elasticity.[16]

Diagnostic Procedures

- Urine sodium often less than 10 mEq/L
- Serum sodium greater than 150 mEg/L
- Blood urea nitrogen–creatinine ratio often greater than 20
- Serum osmolality greater than 300 mmoL/kg

Therapeutic Interventions

- Administer 5% dextrose in 0.45% normal saline with potassium intravenously as needed; assess for fluid overload.
- If hemodynamically unstable, give 0.9% saline 500 mL bolus and 200 m per hour until systolic blood pressure is greater than 100 mm Hg, then switch to 5% dextrose in 0.45% normal saline with potassium.[8,12] Monitor closely for fluid overload. Monitor patient intake and output, weights, and laboratory values. Older adults are at increased risk for fluid overload with rapid

intravenous infusion, especially those with a history of heart failure or diastolic dysfunction.

SECONDARY ASSESSMENT OF THE GERIATRIC PATIENT

Although the primary complaint of older adults presenting to the ED is usually related to an acute medical illness, trauma-related injury, or psychiatric disorder, special attention is warranted in observing and screening for potential problems that frequently are underdetected in this vulnerable population. A brief overview of problems and tips for secondary assessment are provided in addressing adverse drug reactions and polypharmacy, fall risk, abuse and neglect, and immunizations.

Adverse Medication Reactions and Polypharmacy

Adverse medication reactions occur when medications interact with one another or with something that is ingested.

- The most common adverse medication reactions prompting an ED visit in older adults are related to warfarin (Coumadin) and insulin.[15]
- More than 400,000 OTC medications are available in the United States and older adults are the largest group of users.[15,17] Since age-related changes contribute to a significant increase in risk for both renal and liver toxicity, OTC agents for pain management pose a particular risk to older adults. For examples, see Table 53-10.

The Beers complete list of potentially inappropriate medications for older adults can be found at http://www.dcri.duke.edu/ccge/curtis/beers.html. Avoid these medications in this high-risk population. Although many

TABLE 53-10	OVER-THE-COUNTER DRUGS ASSOCIATED WITH TOXICITY AND ADVERSE EFFECTS
DRUG	**ADVERSE EFFECT**
Aspirin and aspirin-containing analgesics	• Bleeding • Gastritis, gastric ulcers • Tinnitus
Nonsteroidal anti-inflammatory drugs (NSAIDs) (ibuprofen, ketoprofen, naproxen)	• Gastritis, gastric ulcers • Gastrointestinal bleeding • Renal failure
Acetaminophen	• Liver toxicity

TABLE 53-11 POTENTIALLY INAPPROPRIATE MEDICATIONS COMMONLY ADMINISTERED IN THE EMERGENCY DEPARTMENT

DRUG CLASSIFICATION	POTENTIALLY INAPPROPRIATE MEDICATION	BETTER ALTERNATIVE
Antiemetic Analgesia for mild to moderate pain	• Promethazine (Phenergan) • Propoxyphene (Darvon, Darvocet)	• Ondansetron (Zofran) • Acetaminophen (Tylenol) • Ibuprofen (Motrin, Advil) • Oxycodone immediate release (Percolone) or with acetaminophen (Percocet) • Hydrocodone with acetaminophen (Vicodin, Lortab)
Analgesia for severe pain	• Meperidine (Demerol)	• Morphine • Hydromorphone
Antihistamine	• Diphenhydramine (Benadryl)	• Loratadine • Fexofenadine
Benzodiazepine	• Diazepam (Valium)	• Lorazepam (Ativan) (for benzodiazepine or alcohol withdrawal) • Haloperidol (Haldol) (0.5 to 2 mg po or IM) • Note: Peak effect for parenteral dosing is 20–40 minutes; therefore can repeat IM dose every 1 hour
Muscle relaxant	• Cyclobenzaprine (Flexeril)	• Complementary therapy (e.g., moist heat, massage)

IM, Intramuscular; *po*, by mouth.

medications on this list are not commonly used in the ED, six have been identified as frequently administered in the ED and 7% of patients are discharged from the ED with new prescriptions for potentially inappropriate medications.[15,17–19] Table 53-11 describes potentially inappropriate medications frequently used in the ED and suggestions for better alternatives.

Polypharmacy is the use of more medication than is clinically indicated or warranted. The more medications a patient takes, the higher the risk for an interaction with another medication within the treatment regimen. The incidence of drug interactions increases from 6% in patients taking two medications a day to around 50% in patients taking five medications.[20] Most older adults seeking treatment in the ED are taking a significant number of medications. Therefore, exercise caution in discontinuing, adjusting dosage, or adding medications to their regimen. The following is important information to remember when older adults are treated in the ED:

• Use the visit as an opportunity to discontinue potentially inappropriate medications that may be responsible for the patient's primary complaint.
• Select medications to avoid because of their side effect profile rather than their approved indication.
• Educate the patient and family about the importance of adhering to the new regimen because of the risk for withdrawal symptoms associated with both discontinuing or reducing the dose of certain medications (opioids, benzodiazepines, alcohol, antidepressants, antipsychotics).
• Educate the patient and family about consulting with a pharmacist before adding OTC medications to the medication regimen.

Fall Risk

Falls are a leading predictor of mortality and morbidity among older adults. They are the leading cause of injurious death, the eighth leading cause of injury, and the most common cause of hospital admissions for this vulnerable age group.[21,22] Among this group, 1.8 million visits to the ED occur in the United States each year for falls.[19] One third of older adults living in the community and 50% to 75% of nursing home residents fall each year.[22] Although a fall may not be the immediate reason the patient is in the ED, a fall risk screening should be completed to help prevent further injuries both in the ED and after discharge.

Assessment for Fall-Related Risk Factors

• Age greater than 75 years
• Cognition—acute and chronic mental status changes (i.e., confusion, dementia, delirium)
• History of falling
• Gait instability

- Medications—polypharmacy
- Elimination—incontinence, diarrhea
- Sensory impairment—glasses, hearing aids
- Assistive devices—walkers, canes
- Environmental barriers—unfamiliar environment, unsafe home environment
- Footwear—should have nonskid or rubber soles, increased risk with slippers or flip-flops
- Substance use—alcohol, opioids, benzodiazepines, antipsychotics

Preventing Falls in the Emergency Department[23]

- Identify patients at risk for falls upon admission to the ED, communicate this to all staff members, and institute preventive measures when appropriate.
- Be aware of environmental risk factors (wet, shiny, or uneven floors).
- Frequently or constantly monitor of patients with cognitive dysfunction.
- Identify and correct any of the following:
  - Equipment that is faulty (i.e., bedrails, rolling intravenous poles)
  - Areas with poor lighting or glare
  - Bathrooms without bars
  - Patients with inappropriate footwear
- Use brakes on beds and wheelchairs.
- If patient is at risk upon discharge:
  - Educate patient and family about fall prevention (instruction, brochure, web-based resources).
  - Provide referrals as needed (social worker, case manager, community-based programs).

Elder Abuse and Neglect

Abuse and neglect are serious problems for older people and often go undetected. As many as 1.2 million older adults are affected in the United States annually.[24] In 90% of cases the abuser is a family member such as an adult child or spouse. Only 1 in 10 cases is reported, and there is significant underreporting by clinical professionals.[24] Cognitive impairment and shared living arrangements are the biggest contributor to elder abuse.

Risk Factors for Inadequate Care or Abuse by Caregivers[12]

- Cognitive impairment in patient, caregiver, or both
- Financial or psychological dependency of caregiver
- Family conflict
- Family history of abusive behavior (alcohol or drug abuse, mental illness)
- Financial instability

- Isolation of patient or caregiver
- Depression
- Malnutrition
- Inadequate living arrangements to support needs
- Stressful life events (death of significant other or close friends, loss of employment)

General Screening[24]

The following is a list of circumstances that may provide a clue that the patient is a victim of abuse or neglect.
- Seeking care long after the injury occurred
- Wounds or fractures that have healed without appropriate medical treatment
- Numerous visits to the ED
- Poor hygiene
- Unexplained bruises or bruises in various stages of healing
- Cigarette or rope burns
- Explanations that do not match injury
- Patient is anxious, fearful, and nervous

When abuse or neglect is suspected, always interview the patient without family or caregiver present. See Chapter 49, Abuse and Neglect.

Helpful Questions to Ask the Patient When Assessing for Abuse and Neglect[24]

- Is there anyone you can call that can come take care of you?
- Has anyone at home ever hurt or hit you?
- Has anyone ever taken your things?
- Are you receiving enough care at home?
- Has anyone ever threatened you or made fun of you?

Be aware that in some cultures sharing a home is common practice and questioning the patient alone is not accepted (see Table 53-3 for a list of cross-cultural issues in health care).

Interventions in Addressing Abuse and Neglect

- The nurse is legally responsible to report suspected or actual abuse.
- Patient safety is your first concern.
- Identify and prioritize the patient's needs.
- Make appropriate referrals.

Immunizations

Administration of vaccines plays an important role in both primary and secondary prevention of diseases in geriatric patients. Table 53-12 describes recommendations,

TABLE 53-12　A GUIDE TO COMMON IMMUNIZATIONS FOR OLDER ADULTS

VACCINE	RECOMMENDATION	INDICATIONS	PRECAUTIONS	DOSING AND ADMINISTRATION	SIDE EFFECTS	TALKING POINTS WITH PATIENT
Pneumococcal polysaccharide vaccine (PPSV)	Single dose is usually sufficient for a lifetime if administered ≥65 years of age	• All persons ≥65 years • A second dose if previously vaccinated before age 65 years and ≥5 years has elapsed • One-time second dose after 5 years in patients with chronic renal failure, nephritic syndrome, sickle cell disease, splenectomy, and immunocompromising conditions	• Do not administer if prior reaction to vaccine or components • Use caution in cases of moderate or severe acute illness • Pneumococcal conjugate vaccine (PCV) not approved for use in older adults	• 0.5 mL either IM or SQ • Can be given concurrently with other vaccines at different sites	• Soreness or redness at the injection site lasting 1–2 days	• PPSV is 60% to 70% effective against pneumococcal disease but not other types of pneumonia • Medicare covers the cost of the vaccine and administration
Influenza (flu)	Single dose annually for each influenza-specific type of vaccine	• All persons ≥65 years • Any person with a high-risk condition (COPD, CV disease [except hypertension], chronic hepatitis, renal disease, immunosuppression, metabolic disorders, neurologic or neuromuscular disorders) • All nursing home and chronic care facility residents • All household contacts of high-risk adults	• Do not administer if prior reaction to vaccine or components • Do not give live vaccine to persons ≥50 years • Do not give to patients with a history of Guillain-Barré syndrome within 6 weeks of any previous dose	• 0.5 mL IM using a needle length ≥1 inch • Administer just prior to annual flu season	• Soreness/redness at the injection site lasting 1–2 days • Hoarseness, sore or red eyes, cough, itchiness, fever aches	• Vaccination is effective in preventing 47% of deaths and 27% of hospitalizations related to flu in community dwellers

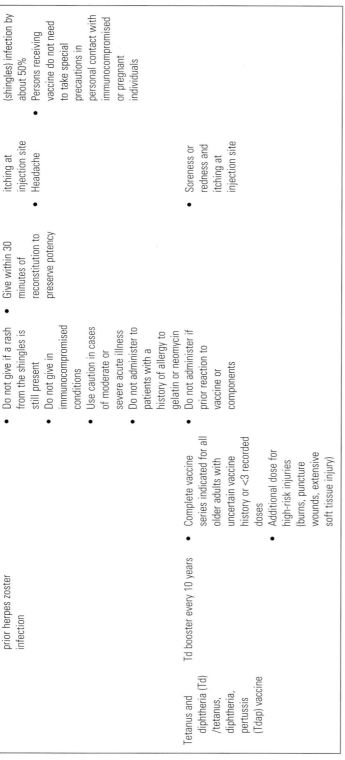

Vaccine	Schedule	Indications/Contraindications	Administration	Side Effects	Patient Education
Herpes zoster (shingles)	Single lifetime dose regardless of history of prior herpes zoster infection	• All persons ≥60 years	• Not indicated as treatment of shingles • Do not give if a rash from the shingles is still present • Do not give in immunocompromised conditions • Use caution in cases of moderate or severe acute illness • Do not administer to patients with a history of allergy to gelatin or neomycin • Do not administer if prior reaction to vaccine or components	• 0.65 mL SQ in upper arm • Give within 30 minutes of reconstitution to preserve potency	• Soreness or redness and itching at injection site • Headache	• Vaccine reduces the risk for herpes zoster (shingles) infection by about 50% • Persons receiving vaccine do not need to take special precautions in personal contact with immunocompromised or pregnant individuals
Tetanus and diphtheria (Td)/tetanus, diphtheria, pertussis (Tdap) vaccine	Td booster every 10 years	• Complete vaccine series indicated for all older adults with uncertain vaccine history or <3 recorded doses • Additional dose for high-risk injuries (burns, puncture wounds, extensive soft tissue injury)		• Soreness or redness and itching at injection site	

Adapted from Immunization Action Coalition. (2011, April). *Summary of recommendations for adult immunization*. Retrieved from http://www.immunize.org/catg.d/p2011.pdf

COPD, Chronic obstructive pulmonary disease; *CV*, cardiovascular; *IM*, intramuscular; *SQ*, subcutaneous.

TABLE 53-13 **WEB-BASED RESOURCES**	
RESOURCE	**WEBSITE**
Evidence-based geriatric clinical nursing website sponsored by the Hartford Institute for Geriatric Nursing; provides multiple resources.	http://consultgerirn.org
General Assessment	http://consultgerirn.org/resources
Try This series that includes assessment tools and videos demonstrating the use of these instruments.	
Try This topics of particular interest to emergency nurses include:	
• Mental status assessment: The Mini-Cog	
• Confusion Assessment Method to detect delirium	
• Geriatric Depression Scale	
• Assessing pain in older adults	
• Assessment of elder mistreatment	
• Beers criteria for potentially inappropriate medications	
Pain management in older adults	http://consultgerirn.org/topics/pain/want_to_know_more
American Academy of Pain Medicine	http://www.painmed.org/
American Pain Society	http://www.ampainsoc.org/pub/cp_guidelines.htm
American Academy of Pain Management	http://www.aapainmanage.org/
Geriatric Pain	http://www.GeriatricPain.org

indications, precautions, dosing and administration guidelines, side effects, and talking points for the pneumococcal, influenza, herpes zoster, and tetanus and diphtheria vaccines.

Emergency nurses face many challenges on a daily basis in addressing the unique needs of a vulnerable older adult population. Emergency nurses are strategically positioned to champion post-discharge quality clinical outcomes in this high-risk population. However, it is imperative that nurses develop an accurate understanding and appreciation of age-related changes and are knowledgeable about the problems for which older adults frequently seek care in the ED. Additional resources related to the care of geriatric patients can be found in Table 53-13.

REFERENCES

1. Snow, V., Beck, D., Budnitz, T., Miller, D. C., Potter, J., Wears, R. L., ... Williams, M. V.; American College of Physicians; Society of General Internal Medicine; Society of Hospital Medicine; American Geriatrics Society; American College of Emergency Physicians; Society of Academic Emergency Medicine. (2009). Transitions of care consensus policy statement American College of Physicians–Society of General Internal Medicine–Society of Hospital Medicine–American Geriatrics Society–American College of Emergency Physicians–Society of Academic Emergency Medicine. *Journal of General Internal Medicine, 24*(8), 971–976.

2. Hastings, S. N., & Heflin, M. T. (2005). A systematic review of interventions to improve outcomes for elders discharged from the emergency department. *Academic Emergency Medicine, 12*(10), 978–986.

3. Rice, K. L., & Winterbottom, F. (2010). Gerontological alterations and management. In L. D. Urden, K. Stacy, & M. E. Lough (Eds.), *Critical Care Nursing* (6th ed.). St. Louis, MO: Mosby.

4. American Geriatrics Society. (2001). *Doorway thoughts: Cross-cultural health care for older adults.* Sudbury, MA: Jones & Bartlett.

5. Terrell, K. M., Hustey, F. M., Hwang, U., Gerson, L. W., Wenger, N. S., & Miller, D. K.; Society for Academic Emergency Medicine (SAEM) Geriatric Task Force. (2009). Quality indicators for geriatric emergency care. *Academic Emergency Medicine, 16*(5), 441–449.

6. Wilber, S. T. (2006). Altered mental status in older emergency department patients. *Emergency Medicine Clinics of North America, 24*, 299–316.

7. Classification of chronic pain syndromes and definitions of pain terms. Prepared by the International Association for the Study of Pain, Subcommittee on Taxonomy. (1986). *Pain, 3*(Suppl), S1–S226

8. Capezuti, E., Zwicker, D., Mezey, M., Fulmer, T., & Gray-Miceli, D. (Eds.). (2007). *Evidence-based geriatric nursing protocols for best practice.* New York, NY: Springer.

9. Springhouse. (2002). *Handbook of geriatric nursing care.* Springhouse, PA: Author.

10. American Geriatrics Society Panel on the Pharmacological Management of Persistent Pain in Older Persons. (2009). Pharmacological management of persistent pain in older persons. *Journal of the American Geriatrics Society, 57*(8), 1331–1346.

11. Inouye, S. K. (2006). Delirium in older persons. *New England Journal of Medicine, 354*(11), 1157–1165.

12. Reuben, D. B., Herr, K. A., Pacala, J. T., Pollock, B. G., Potter, J. F., & Semla, T. P. (2009). *Geriatrics at your fingertips* (11th ed.). New York, NY: American Geriatrics Society.

13. Kalra, O. P., & Raizade, A. (2009). Approach to patient with urosepsis. *Journal of Global Infectious Disease, 1*(1), 57–63.

14. Brusch, J. L., Cunha, B. A., Howes, D. S., Pillow, M. T., Salomone, J. A. III, & Sinert, R. H. (2011, July 7). *Urinary tract infection in males.* Retrieved from http://emedicine. medscape.com/article/231574-overview

15. Budnitz, D. S., Shehab, N., Kegler, S. R., & Richards, C. L. (2007). Medication use leading to emergency department visits for adverse drug events in older adults. *Annals of Internal Medicine, 147*(11), 755–765.

16. Vivanti, A., Harvey, K., Ash, S., & Battistutta, D. (2008). Clinical assessment of dehydration in older people admitted to hospital: What are the strongest indicators? *Archives of Gerontology and Geriatrics, 47*(3), 340–355.

17. Nixdorff, N., Hustey, F. M., Brady, A. K., Vaji, K., Leonard, M., & Messinger-Rapport, B. J. (2008). Potentially inappropriate medications and adverse drug effects in elders in the ED. *American Journal of Emergency Medicine, 26*(6), 697–700.

18. Hustey, F. M. (2008). Beers criteria and the ED: An adequate standard for inappropriate prescribing? *American Journal of Emergency Medicine, 26*(6), 695–696.

19. Hustey, F. M., Wallis, N., & Miller, J. (2007). Inappropriate prescribing in an older ED population. *American Journal of Emergency Medicine, 25*(7), 804–807.

20. Wooten, J. M., & Galavis, J. (2005). Polypharmacy: Keeping the elderly safe. *Modern Medicine.* Retrieved from http://www. modernmedicine.com/modernmedicine/article/articledetail. jsp?id=172920

21. American Physical Therapy Association. (2007, November). *Impact of falls among older adults.* Retrieved from http:// phoenix.gov/fallprevention/issuesbrief.pdf

22. Centers for Disease Control and Prevention. (2010, December 8). *Falls among older adults: An overview.* Retrieved from http://www.cdc.gov/HomeandRecreationalSafety/Falls/ adultfalls.html

23. Terrell, K., Weaver, C., Giles, B., & Ross, M. (2009). Emergency room patient falls and resulting injuries. *Journal of Emergency Nursing, 35*(2), 89–92.

24. Fulmer, T. (2005). Elder abuse and neglect assessment. *Dermatological Nursing, 16*(5), 473.

Considerations for the Patient with Morbid Obesity

Valerie Aarne Grossman

In 2005 the World Health Organization indicated that 1.5 billion people over the age of 15 were overweight (body mass index [BMI] >24) and at least 400 million were obese (BMI >29).[1] By 2015 an estimated 2.3 billion adults will be overweight, and more than 700 million will be obese.[1] In 2008 the rate of obesity among adults averaged 32%[2] and was up to 18% for children aged 6 to 19 years.[3] While obesity-related mortality rates have many variables, most studies show similar findings: The death rate increases in relation to the degree of obesity and the related comorbidities. On average, an overweight person lives 3 years less and an obese person lives 7 years less than a person of average weight. For those obese persons who also smoke, life expectancy is 14 years less than for a person of average weight.[4]

Obesity in health care is a challenge from every perspective. Treating this population with the same degree of dignity used with any special needs patient is essential in building a trusting rapport with the patient and his or her family. Understanding the physiologic differences and comorbidities is essential to optimal care for the obese patient.

If you are uncertain as to how to best adapt care to the obese patient, consider asking the following:
- "How do you do this at home?"
- "How would you like us to help you?"

ASSESSING AND TREATING THE SPECIAL NEEDS OF THE PATIENT WITH MORBID OBESITY

Airway Management

Because of redundant upper airway soft tissue, increased body mass, and increased airway resistance, managing the airway can be difficult in patients with morbid obesity. The following sections offer suggestions for ways to manage the airway and discuss potential difficulties the health care provider may encounter.

Bag-Mask

- Higher pressures are required to effectively ventilate the obese patient, and it can be difficult to maintain a good seal with the mask. Two people may be needed to ensure proper positioning and seal of the mask.
- Unless contraindicated, it is best to use an oropharyngeal or nasopharyngeal airway when bag-mask ventilation is required.

Endotracheal Intubation

- Administer the highest possible concentration of oxygen via the best available means prior to intubation.
- The "ramped position" (reverse Trendelenburg) is more effective for optimal glottis visualization than the traditional "sniff" position.[5]
- Rapid sequence intubation carries a higher risk of aspiration pneumonia in the obese patient.

- When possible, attempt to visualize the vocal cords while the patient is awake to determine if rapid sequence intubation is safe.
- Consider awake intubation for patients who are poor candidates for rapid sequence intubation.
- Nasotracheal intubation is not typically recommended in this population.
- Cricothyrotomy can be extremely difficult in the morbidly obese patient, as traditional landmarks are masked by excess soft tissue and conventional tubes may be too short.

Ventilation

- The heavy noncompliant chest wall of a patient with morbid obesity makes ventilation difficult.
- Static pulmonary compliance is decreased.
- Keeping the head of the bed elevated will facilitate ventilation and decrease the risk of aspiration. For acute management, place the patient in the reverse Trendelenburg position (if possible) to reduce abdominal pressure on the diaphragm and improve chest wall and diaphragm excursion.
- Target oxygen levels may be difficult to reach because of an increase in oxygen consumption.
- Oxygen desaturation occurs quickly in the obese patient because of decreased functional reserve capacity.

Medication Administration

Obesity alters the pharmacokinetics and pharmacodynamics of many medications. Because of fat stores, obese patients have a larger volume of distribution for lipophilic drugs; however, they have a decrease in lean body mass and tissue water compared to patients of normal weight. Consider the following when administering medications to obese patients:

- Dosage of medications used for rapid sequence intubation should be based on lean body mass. Insufficient sedation may occur if ideal body mass is used, and excessive sedation may occur if total body weight is used for dosage calculations.
- Care should be taken with thiopental and benzodiazepines, as they have prolonged effects in the obese patient because of their lipophilicity.
- Subtherapeutic or toxic responses to medication are common.
- Dosing medications can be difficult; some examples of proper dosing are:
  - Ideal body mass calculations for digoxin (Lanoxin), beta-blockers, penicillins, cephalosporins, histamine blockers, corticosteroids, and vecuronium (Norcuron).

- Total body weight calculations for succinylcholine, atracurium (Tracrium), unfractionated heparin, and fentanyl (Sublimaze).
- Longer intramuscular needles may be required.
- The ventrogluteal site should be used.

Body Mass Index (BMI)

BMI is a simple index of weight-for-height that is commonly used in classifying overweight and obese individuals. It is defined as the weight in kilograms divided by the square of the height in meters (kg/m^2). To determine BMI using pounds and inches, the following formula is used: [Weight (pounds) / Height (inches)^2] × 703. Normal BMI is considered to be 18.9 to 24.5.

Dosing Weight

Dosing weight = Ideal body mass + 0.4 × [Total body weight − Ideal body mass]

Vascular Access

- Central line placement can be difficult because of obscured anatomic landmarks. The distance from the skin to the vessel is longer in the obese patient than most prepackaged central line kits are designed for, and the angle of approach may be too steep to allow cannulation once the vessel is reached.
- The use of ultrasound when placing an internal jugular central venous catheter will facilitate successful completion of the procedure.
- Peripherally inserted central catheters (PICC) work well in this population, as they are fairly easy to place accurately.
- Avoid the groin for central line access, as many obese patients have intertrigo and this greatly increases the infection risk.

Imaging Studies

- A 2007 study by Massachusetts General Hospital reported that patients who weighed more than 450 pounds experienced repeated delays in diagnosis and treatment because of an inability to obtain standard, modern radiographic studies.[6]
- Most radiology tables are designed for patients who weigh less than 300 pounds. Some hospitals have tables with weight limits up to 680 pounds, yet patients may still be too large to fit into the opening of the computed tomography or magnetic resonance imaging (MRI) scanners.
- The utility of ultrasound is limited because of reduced transmission of sound waves through the extensive subcutaneous and intraperitoneal adipose tissue.

- More than one film cartridge may be required to obtain a complete image with some diagnostic radiographic procedures.
- Intravenous radioisotopes are weight based, with a maximum allowable safe dose; obese patients may require longer exposures to complete the study while the radioisotope circulates.
- Additional preparations—including longer catheters, sedation, and airway management necessitating additional staff—may need to be considered prior to a procedure.[7]

Equipment Requiring Bariatric Consideration

The following equipment should be properly sized for the morbidly obese patient:

- Blood pressure cuff
- Scale
- Bed; stretcher; wheelchair; recliner; examination table; dental or ear, nose, and throat (ENT) chair; walker; and cane
  - Rooms and doorways must accommodate larger beds and wheelchairs
- Clothing: gown, nonslip socks, wristbands, and incontinence briefs
  - Compression sleeves, antiembolism stockings
- Toilets (floor mounted versus wall mounted), commodes, and bed pans
  - Floor-mounted toilets are safer for patients who weigh more than 250 pounds (as they do not fall off the wall)
- Ceiling-mounted lifts, lateral transfer systems, and the use of lift teams
- Longer catheters, surgical supplies, and procedural equipment, including longer needles for lumber punctures (5.5 inches)

Few home scales will accurately weigh a patient over 250 pounds. Obese patients can gain or lose a great deal of weight and not realize it since the time they were last accurately weighed. Do not rely on their stated weight, especially for drug dosing.

Use a blood pressure cuff instead of a tourniquet for phlebotomy or intravenous catheter placement.

STAFF SAFETY

In one study, patients with a BMI of 35 made up only 10% of the patient population but were associated with 30% of staff injuries related to patient handling.[8] Emergency departments should consider establishing the following practices to reduce the incidence of staff injury:

- Develop bariatric policies and procedures for safety of staff and patient handling.
- Mobilize proper equipment prior to initiating patient care.
- Wait for proper number of staff before trying to assist a bariatric patient.
  - Use of "Lift teams" or "transfer teams"[9]
- Communicate a "game plan" before initiating patient care.[10]

Under ideal conditions the maximum limit for manual patient handling is 35 pounds. The leg of a 250-pound patient weighs about 39 pounds. Multiple caregivers may be needed for some tasks, such as positioning for urinary catheter insertion.[8]

The limit for manually pushing or pulling loads is 20% of the caregiver's weight.[8]

DISEASE RISK IN THE OBESE POPULATION

Endocrine System

Prediabetes

In 2010, 79 million Americans over the age of 20 years were classified as having "prediabetes,"[11] and obesity increases this risk. The condition is defined by elevated blood glucose levels not high enough to be diagnosed as diabetes.[11]

- Fasting blood glucose level of 100 to 125 mg/dL
- Two-hour post–oral glucose tolerance test of 140 to 200 mg/dL

Metabolic Syndrome

Metabolic syndrome results from a combination of obesity and genetics. This condition progresses to type 2 diabetes if left untreated. It is identified by a cluster of symptoms, including the following:

- Proinflammatory state
- Truncal obesity: higher BMI, but more so central adiposity, increases the risk of ischemic (not hemorrhagic) stroke in adults. The direct correlation is not entirely clear.
- Atherogenic dyslipidemia
- Elevated blood pressure
- Insulin resistance
- Glucose intolerance
- Prothrombotic state

Type 2 Diabetes

Eighty percent of type 2 diabetes can be attributed to obesity.[12] This results, in part, from the fact that cells in the muscles, liver, and fat do not use insulin properly to process glucose into energy. Eventually the pancreas is unable to make enough insulin to meet the body's needs.

- Laboratory values:
  - Symptomatic patients (polyuria, fatigue, weight loss, etc.) may have a random serum glucose greater than 200 mg/dL.
  - Asymptomatic patients with a random serum glucose greater than 140 mg/dL suggests diabetes.
  - Hemoglobin A1c greater than 6.5% is indicative of diabetes.

Cardiovascular System

Heart Disease

Weight is a major risk factor for heart disease in younger patients. Other possible links between increased risk of heart disease and obesity include the following:

- The distribution of body fat is an important determinant of risk, as those patients with central or truncal obesity have a higher risk of heart disease.
- The greater the BMI, the higher the incidence of fatty streaks and raised atherosclerotic lesions in the right and left anterior descending coronary arteries.[13]
- The higher a patient's BMI, the higher the myocardial triglyceride content as seen on MRI.[14] This directly contributes to the structural (left ventricular hypertrophy) and functional (hyperdynamic circulation) cardiac changes seen in the obese patient.
- Obesity has a strong effect on lipoprotein metabolism. As weight increases, there are higher levels of triglycerides and low-density lipoprotein cholesterol and a lower level of high-density lipoprotein cholesterol.
- Heart failure occurs more often in the obese patient because of the following:
  - Increase in cardiac workload
  - Diastolic dysfunction occurs and can then be followed by systolic dysfunction resulting from excessive wall stress
- Eccentric hypertrophy occurs more in the obese patient. There is more likely to be an increased chamber radius and wall thickness leading to both volume and pressure overload.

Hypertension

An estimated 75% of all hypertension cases can be attributed directly to obesity, although the precise mechanism is not fully understood.[15] There is increasing belief that obesity stresses the sympathetic nervous system, which then stresses the renal system, in turn raising the blood pressure.

- Highest rates are in those with upper body and abdominal obesity, perhaps because of the higher correlation with truncal obesity and insulin resistance, impaired glucose tolerance, and hyperinsulinemia.
  - Hyperinsulinemia may then lead to higher blood pressure by increasing sympathetic activity, renal sodium reabsorption, or vascular tone.
- Dyslipidemia.

Cardiac Dysrhythmias

Obese patients may show the following difference on their electrocardiogram (ECG) tracings[16]:

- The P, QRS, and T wave axes are more leftward
- Prolonged QT interval
- Multiple ECG criteria for left ventricular hypertrophy and left atrial abnormality and T wave flattening in the inferior and lateral leads are more common
- Atrial fibrillation or flutter
  - Patients with a BMI greater than 30 are more likely to have atrial fibrillation or flutter
  - The greater the weight, the higher the association for sustained atrial fibrillation or flutter rather than transient episodes

Venous Thrombosis

- Risk of deep vein thrombosis and pulmonary embolus increases by 2% to 3%.[16]
- Central or truncal obesity more indicative than BMI of deep vein thrombosis and pulmonary embolism risk.
- Plasma fibrinogen concentrations and other prothrombotic factors increase or elevate and platelet function is altered, particularly in women.

Pulmonary System

Sleep Apnea

Obese persons have a higher incidence of sleep apnea. Sleep apnea increases, inflames, and stiffens vessel walls, which in turn increases the risk of hypertension, arrhythmias, coronary heart disease, heart failure, and stroke. Other considerations in obese patients with sleep apnea include the following:

- The use of alcohol increases apnea frequency in the obese person and worsens nocturnal oxyhemoglobin desaturation.
- Benzodiazepines, opiates, and barbiturates should be used with care in this group of patients, as they may worsen ventilatory responsiveness, upper airway patency, or arousal mechanisms.

- Patients who are being admitted to the hospital should be advised to bring their continuous positive airway pressure (CPAP) mask with them.

Hypoventilation Syndrome[16]

Hypoventilation syndrome occurs because of extreme obesity and alveolar hypoventilation while the patient is awake. The patient fails to generate adequate tidal volume to sufficiently eliminate carbon dioxide, preventing a diurnal elevation in the $PaCO_2$. About 90% of these patients also have sleep apnea. Other signs of hypoventilation syndrome include the following:
- Increased abdominal pressure on the diaphragm, which leads to a decreased residual lung volume
- Decreased lung compliance
- Increased chest wall impedance
- Ventilation-perfusion abnormalities
- Reduced strength and stamina of respiratory muscles
- Depressed ventilatory drive

Asthma

- The lungs tend to underexpand and the size of the breath is smaller, making it more likely that the airways of an obese person will structurally narrow.
- Chronic low-grade systemic inflammation affects the smooth muscle in the airways, causing them to narrow excessively.
- Obesity affects key asthma-related hormones:
  - Leptin is a pro-inflammatory hormone and morbidly obese and asthmatic patients tend to have a higher than normal level of this hormone.
  - Adiponectin is an antiinflammatory hormone and levels tend to be lower in morbidly obese patients.

Gastrointestinal System
Cholelithiasis

- As BMI increases, so does the incidence of symptomatic cholelithiasis.
- Approximately 20 mg of additional cholesterol is synthesized daily for every extra kilogram of body weight. Excess cholesterol is excreted in the bile.
- High biliary concentrations of cholesterol relative to bile acids and phospholipids increase the likelihood of gallstone production.
- Sudden weight loss may also put a person at risk for gallstones, because of the flux of cholesterol through the biliary system.

Fatty Liver Disease

- When triglyceride synthesis exceeds clearance, there will be an abnormal accumulation of triglyceride fat cells in the liver.

- In the beginning, the liver cells fill with fat that does not displace the cell's nucleus. If this process continues, fatty cysts will develop into irreversible liver lesions.

Gastroesophageal Reflux Disease

- Gastroesophageal reflux disease (GERD) is common in the obese patient because of the large volume of gastric fluid, the increased abdominal pressure, and the increased gastroesophageal gradient.
- GERD is more common in patients with a hiatal hernia, and hiatal hernia is more common in obese persons.
- Vagal nerve function abnormalities associated with obesity may cause a higher output of bile and pancreatic enzymes, which makes the refluxed stomach acids more toxic to the esophagus lining.

Musculoskeletal System
Gout

Obesity is associated with the increased production of uric acid and its decreased elimination from the body and, therefore, with an increased incidence of gout.

Osteoarthritis

There is a correlation between an increasing BMI and risk of osteoarthritis. The stress of obesity alters the cartilage and bone metabolism in all joints, including hands, back, hips, knees, and ankles. The severity of osteoarthritis in the lower extremities is influenced by additional factors, including alignment of extremities and how the burden of carrying the excess weight traumatizes those joints.

Infections

There is a decreased immune response and a deactivation of macrophages (scavenger cells) to destroy bacteria and foreign organisms in the obese population, resulting in a higher risk for infection. Obese diabetic patients are at high risk for malignant (or necrotizing) otitis externa. Patients present with severe ear pain, otorrhea, and no fever, yet this infection is a rapidly progressing, invasive disease that becomes lethal by attacking cranial nerves, meninges, and the mastoid.

Cancer Risks

Certain forms of cancer occur more frequently in those who are overweight, and mortality rate increases by 20% to 40% in those persons diagnosed with cancer.[17] Tables 54-1 and 54-2 highlight cancers that have increased incidence and higher death rates in obese persons.

TABLE 54-1	CANCERS WITH INCREASED INCIDENCE AMONG OBESE PERSONS

Occurrence rates are approximately 5% higher among obese patients than among ideal body mass patients for the following cancers:

- Esophagus
- Stomach
- Colon
- Pancreas
- Breast
- Endometrium and/or ovarian
- Kidney
- Prostate
- Gallbladder
- Thyroid
- Non-Hodgkin lymphoma
- Multiple myeloma
- Leukemia

Data from Adams, K. F., Schatzkin, A., Harris, T. B., Kipnis, V., Mouw, T., Ballard-Barbash, R., ... Leitzmann, M. (2006). Overweight, obesity, and mortality in a large prospective cohort of persons 50 to 71 years old. *New England Journal of Medicine, 355*(8), 763–778.

TABLE 54-2	CANCERS WITH HIGHER DEATH RATES AMONG OBESE PERSONS

Death rates are higher among obese men and women than among ideal body mass patients for the following cancers:

- Esophagus
- Colon or rectal
- Liver
- Gallbladder
- Pancreas
- Kidney
- Non-Hodgkin lymphoma
- Multiple myeloma
- Stomach (men)
- Prostate (men)
- Breast (women)
- Uterus, cervix, and ovary (women)

Data from Adams, K. F., Schatzkin, A., Harris, T. B., Kipnis, V., Mouw, T., Ballard-Barbash, R., ... Leitzmann, M. (2006). Overweight, obesity, and mortality in a large prospective cohort of persons 50 to 71 years old. *New England Journal of Medicine, 355*(8), 763–778.

PEDIATRIC CONSIDERATIONS

It is estimated that nearly 20% of patients under the age of 18 years are over their ideal weight. A 2010 Australian study found that 21.8% of two hospitals' emergency department patients aged 2 to 15 years were overweight or obese.[18]

Until recently, BMI was not considered a reliable equation when identifying ideal weight in pediatric patients. The Centers for Disease Control and Prevention and the American Academy of Pediatrics recommend that BMI be calculated for all patients aged 2 years and older. BMI should be used as a screening tool and as a comparison to age, sex, and percentile charts. Overall, childhood obesity increases the prevalence of "adult diseases" in pediatric patients.

DISEASE RISK IN THE OBESE PEDIATRIC POPULATION

Pediatric Endocrine System

- Impaired glucose tolerance is common in pediatric patients who are over their ideal body mass. Insulin resistance is commonly associated with impaired glucose tolerance in this age group. If left to its own progression, these pediatric patients will develop diabetes.
- Metabolic syndrome risk factors for pediatric patients are similar as for adults, but puberty may alter this diagnosis for a patient (may "grow out of it" or make it worse).
- Diabetes mellitus type 2: Typically thought of as an "adult" disease, an increased incidence is now being seen in pediatric patients. It can be asymptomatic for extended periods of time, but early diagnosis and treatment is essential to slow its effects.

Pediatric Cardiovascular System

Hypertension

- Up to 50% of obese children may have hypertension. This is frequently a missed or masked diagnosis.[19]
- Hypertension predisposes the pediatric patient to cardiovascular morbidity, coronary heart disease, stroke mortality, and renal injury from glomerular hyperperfusion and hyperfiltration.[20]

Dyslipidemia

- Commonly occurs in obese children, especially those with central fat distribution.
- Dyslipidemia predisposes an obese child to insulin resistance and cardiovascular diseases.

Coronary Artery Disease

- Atherosclerosis occurs earlier in adult years among obese pediatric patients.[21]
- Comorbidities of pediatric obesity that increase the risk of coronary artery disease include the following:
  - Hypertension
  - Dyslipidemia
  - Insulin resistance syndrome
  - Nutrition deficiencies
  - Sedentary lifestyle
  - Tobacco smoke exposure
- Other cardiovascular changes seen in obese children include the following:
  - Endothelial dysfunction
  - Carotid intimal thickening
  - Early aortic and coronary arterial fatty streaks and fibrous plaque development
  - Decreased arterial distensibility
  - Increased left atrial diameter

Pediatric Gastrointestinal System

Nonalcoholic Fatty Liver Disease

- Nonalcoholic fatty liver disease (NAFLD) is the most common liver disease in children and is seen in up to 38% of obese children.[22]
- The pathogenesis of NAFLD is not clearly understood but may be related to metabolic syndrome, insulin resistance, dyslipidemia, obesity, and hypertension.[23]
- Most children with NAFLD will be asymptomatic. If symptoms occur, they may include right upper quadrant or nonspecific abdominal pain, hepatomegaly, and fatigue.
- The only established treatment for NAFLD in the obese pediatric patient is weight loss.

Cholelithiasis

- Obesity is the most common cause of gallstones in children.

Pediatric Musculoskeletal System

Obese pediatric patients have an increased risk for the following:
- Slipped capital femoral epiphysis
  - Characterized by displacement of the capital femoral epiphysis from the femoral neck through the epiphyseal ("growth") plate
  - Presents with nonradiating, dull, aching pain in the hip, groin, thigh, or knee with no history of trauma

- Tibia vara (Blount disease)
  - Seen more commonly in obese pediatric patients
  - Characterized by progressive bowed legs and tibial torsion
  - Occurs from stunted growth of the medial proximal tibial growth plate because of excessive abnormal weight bearing
- Fractures
  - Obese pediatric patients have a higher incidence of extremity fractures related to trauma[24]
- Malformation
  - Genu valgum ("knock knees"): condition worsens over time
  - Lower extremity malalignment
  - Obese adolescents can have accelerated linear growth and bone age

Pediatric Neurological System

- Pseudotumor cerebri (idiopathic intracranial hypertension) prevalence is higher in obese pediatric patients. Presentation may include headache, hypertension, obesity, and papilledema.

Additional Resources for Safe Patient Handling and Movement[8]
- VA Sunshine Healthcare Network: http://www.visn8.va.gov/patientsafetycenter/safePtHandling/default.asp
- Centers for Disease Control and Prevention: http://www.cdc.gov/niosh/docs/2009-127
- American Nurses Association: http://www.nursingworld.org/MainMenuCategories/ANAPoliticalPower/State/StateLegislativeAgenda/SPHM/Enacted-Legistation.aspx

---

REFERENCES

1. World Health Organization. (2011, March). *Obesity and overweight.* Retrieved from http://www.who.int/mediacentre/factsheets/fs311/en/index.html
2. Flegal, K. M., Carroll, M. D., Ogden, C. L., & Curtin, L. R. (2010). Prevalence and trends in obesity among U.S. adults, 1999–2008. *Journal of the American Medical Association, 303*(3), 235–241.
3. Ogden, C. L., Carroll, M. D., Curtin, L. R., Lamb, M. M., & Flegal, K. M. (2010). Prevalence of high body mass index in U.S. children and adolescents, 2007–2008. *Journal of the American Medical Association, 303*(3), 242–249.
4. Peeters, A., Barendregt, J., Willekens, F., Mackenbach, J., Mamun, A., & Bonneux, L. (2003). Obesity in adulthood and its consequences for life expectancy: A life-table analysis. *Annals of Internal Medicine, 138*(1), 24–32.
5. Rao, S. L., Kunselman, A. R., Schuler, H. G., & DesHarnais, S. (2008). Laryngoscopy and tracheal intubation in the

head-elevated position in obese patients: A randomized, controlled, equivalence trial. *Anesthesia and Analgesia, 107*(6), 1912–1918.

6. Uppot, R. N., Sahani, D. V., Hahn, P. F., Gervais, D., & Mueller, P. R. (2007). Impact of obesity on medical imaging and image-guided intervention. *American Journal of Roentgenology, 188*(2), 433–440.

7. Grossman, V. (2009). Imaging tips for the large patients. *RN Magazine, 72*(4), 26–29.

8. Menzel, N. N., & Nelson, A. L. (2010). Strengthening your evidence base: Focus on safe patient handling. *American Nurse Today, 5*(7), 38–40.

9. Brown, D. X. (2003). Nurses and preventable back injuries. *American Journal of Critical Care, 12*(5), 400–401.

10. Gallagher-Camden, S., Shaver, J., & Cole, K. (2007). Promoting the patient's dignity and preventing caregiver injury while caring for a morbidly obese woman with skin tears and a pressure ulcer. *Bariatric Nursing and Surgical Patient Care, 2*(1), 77–82

11. Centers for Disease Control and Prevention. (2011). *National diabetes fact sheet: National estimates and general information on diabetes and prediabetes in the United States, 2011*. Atlanta, GA: Author. Retrieved from http://www.cdc.gov/diabetes/pubs/pdf/ndfs_2011.pdf

12. Bray, G. (2011, February 16). *Health hazards associated with obesity in adults*. Retrieved from http://www.uptodate.com/contents/health-hazards-associated-with-obesity-in-adults?source=search_result&selectedTitle=1%7E150

13. McGill, H. C., McMahon, C. A., Herderick, E. E., Zieske, A. W., Malcolm, G. T., Tracy, R. E., & Strong, J. P. (2002). Obesity accelerates the progression of coronary atherosclerosis in young men. *Circulation, 105*(23), 2712–2718.

14. McGavock, J. M., Victor, R. G., Unger, R. H., & Szczepaniak, L. S. (2006). Adiposity of the heart, revisited. *Annals of Internal Medicine, 144*(7), 517–524.

15. Davy, K. P., & Hall, J. E. (2004). Obesity and hypertension: Two epidemics or one? *American Journal of Physiology, 286*(5), R803–R813.

16. Poirier, P., Giles, T. D., Bray, G. A., Hong, Y., Stern, J. S., Pi-Sunyer, X., & Eckel, R. (2006). Obesity and cardiovascular disease. *Arteriosclerosis, Thrombosis, and Vascular Biology, 26*, 968–976.

17. Adams, K. F., Schatzkin, A., Harris, T. B., Kipnis, V., Mouw, T., Ballard-Barbash, R., … Leitzmann, M. (2006). Overweight, obesity, and mortality in a large prospective cohort of persons 50 to 71 years old. *New England Journal of Medicine, 355*(8), 763–778.

18. Considine, J., Craike, M., Waddell, D., Stergiou, H. E., & Hauser, S. (2010). Role of emergency departments in screening for obese and overweight children. *Australasian Emergency Nursing Journal, 13*(4), 105–110.

19. Maggio, A., Aggoun, Y., Marchand, L., Martin, X., Herrmann, F., Beghetti, M., & Farpour-Lambert, N. (2008). Associations among obesity, blood pressure, and left ventricular mass. *Journal of Pediatrics, 152*(4), 489–493.

20. Stabouli, S., & Kotsis, V. (2009). Hypertension and target organ damage in obese children. *Pediatric Health, 3*(1), 3–6.

21. Raghuveer, G. (2010). Lifetime cardiovascular risk of childhood obesity. *American Journal of Clinical Nutrition, 91*(5), 1514–1519.

22. Schwimmer, J., Deutsch, R., Kahen, T., Lavine, J., Stanley, C., & Behling, C. (2006). Prevalence of fatty liver in children and adolescents. *Pediatrics, 118*(4), 1388–1393.

23. Feldstein, A., Charatcharoenwitthaya, P., Treeprasertsuk, S., Benson, J., Enders, F., & Angulo, P. (2009). The natural history of non-alcoholic fatty liver disease in children: A follow-up study for up to 20 years. *Gut, 58*(11), 1538–1544.

24. Rana, A., Michalsky, M., Teich, S., Groner, J., Caniano, D., & Schuster, D. (2009). Childhood obesity: A risk factor for injuries observed at a level-1 trauma center. *Journal of Pediatric Surgery, 44*(8), 1601–1605.

INDEX

Page numbers followed by *b, t,* and *f* indicate boxes, tables, and figures, respectively.